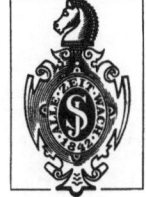

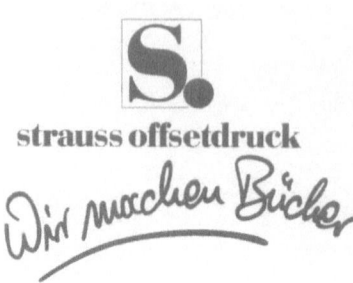

strauss offsetdruck

Wir machen Bücher

Springer-Verlag
z. Hd. Hr. Jöst
Tiergartenstraße 17

69121 Heidelberg

LIEFERSCHEIN   30..05.1995

Anbei erhalten Sie:

das Musterbuch zu dem Titel:

„ASSISTED",Circulation (UNGER)   # 242/95

Strauss Offsetdruck GmbH · Robert-Bosch-Str. 6-8 · 69509 Mörlenbach · Postadresse: Postfach 1108 · 69503 Mörlenbach · Telefon 0 62 09 - 7141-0 · Fax 18 98
Geschäftsführende Gesellschafter: Manfred Strauss, Uwe Scheuermann · HRB 834 Fürth/Odw.
Voba Weinheim 60 22 00 00 (BLZ 67 09 23 00) · Bez. Sparkasse Heppenheim 8047467 (BLZ 509 51 469) · Postscheck Karlsruhe 0235693-754 (BLZ 660 100 75)

Assisted Circulation 3

Edited by Felix Unger

With 343 Figures and 80 Tables

Springer-Verlag Berlin Heidelberg New York
London Paris Tokyo HongKong

Univ. Prof. Dr. med. univ. FELIX UNGER
Herzchirurgie Salzburg
Landeskrankenanstalten, Müllner Hauptstr. 48
A-5020 Salzburg, Austria

ISBN-13:978-3-642-74406-8   e-ISBN-13:978-3-642-74404-4
DOI: 10.1007/978-3-642-74404-4

Library of Congress Catalog Card Number 86-640518.

© Springer-Verlag Berlin Heidelberg 1989
Softcover reprint of the hardcover 1st edition   1989

2127/3130-543210 – Printed on acid-free paper

Preface

It is certainly a great pleasure to edit the third volume of *Assisted Circulation*. In the past 5 years there has been dramatic change in the status of assisted circulation and in our understanding of it. There have now been 513 clinical implantations of pneumatically driven blood pumps, in addition to unknown, uncountable and unregistered implantations of nonpulsatile blood pumps. In view of the clinical experience now accumulated, it is now time to reevaluate and to judge the progress made on the basis of results reported in 1979 and 1984.

A great deal of help is necessary in editing a book, and I want to thank especially St. John's Hospital for their generous support and my co-workers and associates R. Schistek, J. Hager, and P. Ghosh. Special thanks are due to my secretary C. Stutz, who had the burden of reading and typing my manuscripts. I also thank the Kurt Polzer Foundation for their support; Prof. Dr. Kurt Polzer was the nestor of Austrian cardiac research.

Hearty thanks go as well to Dr. J. Wieczorek, Mary Schäfer and Rick Mills, who did the copy editing, and to the Springer staff, who gave this third volume an attractive format and ensured its accuracy as usual.

This volume focuses strongly on clinical experience with cardiac assistance. We hope that the discussion of it here, along with those in the other two volumes will trigger research and clinical investigation of new concepts. I trust that the fourth volume will introduce these new concepts and report improved results in clinical applications.

Salzburg, February 1989   FELIX UNGER

Contents

Part III. Bridging to Transplantation

Part IV. Total Artificial Heart

Part V. Heart Transplantation

List of Authors

ACKER, M. A., Dr., Harrison Department of Surgical Research, Department of Surgery, University of Pennsylvania, Philadelphia, PA 19104, USA

ANDERSEN, J. S., Dr., Harrison Department of Surgical Research, Department of Surgery, University of Pennsylvania, Philadelphia, PA 19104, USA

ANDERSON, W. A., Dr., Harrison Department of Surgical Research, Department of Surgery, University of Pennsylvania, Philadelphia, PA 19104, USA

ATSUMI, K., Prof. Dr., Institute of Medical Electronics, Faculty of Medicine, University of Tokyo, 7-3-1 Hongo, Bunkyo-Ku, Tokyo 113, Japan

AUPETIT, B., Dr., Department of Biochemistry, Hôpital La Pitié, 83 Bd. de l'Hôpital, 75013 Paris, France

AURIOL, A., Dr., Department of Pathology, Hôpital La Pitié, 83 Bd. de l'Hôpital, 75013 Paris, France

BANNER, N. R., Dr., Harefield Hospital, Middlesex UB9 6JH, United Kingdom

BECERRA, E., Dr., University of Cape Town, Medical School, Observatory 7925, Cape Town, Republic of South Africa

BERLOCO, P., Dr., II. Patologia Chirurgica e Propedeutica Clinica, Università di Roma „La Sapienza", Policlinico Umberto I, 00161 Roma, Italy

BERNHARD, W. F., Prof. Dr., Harvard Medical School, Department of Surgery, Children's Hospital, Medical Center, 300 Longwood Ave., Boston, MA 02115, USA

BJÖRK, V. O., Prof. Dr., Department of Thoracic and Cardiac Surgery, Karolinska University of Stockholm, 10401 Stockholm, Sweden

BOEHM, D. H., Dr., University of Cape Town, Medical School, Observatory 7925, Cape Town, Republic of South Africa

BORS, V., Dr., Department of Cardiovascular Surgery, Hôpital La Pitié, 83 Bd. de l'Hôpital, 75013 Paris, France

BOURGEOIS, I., Dr., Université Paris VI, Hôpital Broussais, Département de Chirurgie, Cardio-Vasculaire et Laboratoire d'Etude des Prothèses Cardiaques, 96 Rue Didot, 75014 Paris, France

BRAMM, G., Dr., Fraunhofer-Institut für zerstörungsfreie Prüfverfahren, Hauptabteilung Medizintechnik, Ensheimer Str. 48, 6670 St. Ingbert

BRANDSTAETTER, F., Prof. Dr., Institut für Physik, Universität Innsbruck, 6020 Innsbruck, Austria

BREGMAN, D., Prof. Dr., Department of Surgery, St. Joseph's Hospital and Medical Center, 703 Main Street, Paterson, NJ 07503, USA

BRIDGES, C. R., Dr., Harrison Department of Surgical Research, Department of Surgery, University of Pennsylvania, Philadelphia, PA 19104, USA

CABROL, A., Dr., Department of Anesthesiology, Hôpital La Pitié, 83 Bd. de l'Hôpital, 75013 Paris, France

CABROL, C., Prof. Dr., Service of Thoracic and Cardiovascular Surgery, Hôpital La Pitié, 83 Bd. de l'Hôpital, 75013 Paris, France

CACHERA, J. P., Department of Cardiac Surgery, C.H.U. Henri Mondor, 94000 Creteil, France

CAMPBELL, C. D., Dr., Michael Reese Hospital and Medical Center, Cardiac Surgery, Lake Shore Drive at 31st Street, Chicago, IL 60616, USA

CARPENTIER, A., Prof. Dr., Université Paris VI, Hôpital Broussais, Département de Chirurgie Cardio-Vasculaire et Laboratoire d'Etude des Prothèses Cardiaques, 96 Rue Didot, 75014 Paris, France

CASTAIGNE, A., Prof. Dr., Department of Cardiology, C.H.U. Henri Mondor, 94000 Creteil, France

CEDERWALL, G., Dr., Thoratec Laboratories, 2023 8th Street, Berkeley, CA 94710, USA

CHACHQUES, J. C., Dr., Université Paris VI, Hôpital Broussais, Département de Chirurgie Cardio-Vasculaire d'Etude des Prothèses Cardiaques, 96 Rue Didot, 75014 Paris, France

CHIN, A., Dr., Harrison Department of Surgical Research, Department of Surgery, University of Pennsylvania, Philadelphia, PA 19104, USA

CONNOLLY, M., Dr., Department of Thoracic Surgery, Maimonides Medical Center, 4802 10th Avenue, Brooklyn, NY 11219, USA

COOLEY, D. A., Prof. Dr., Texas Heart Institute of St. Luke's Episcopal and Texas Childrens' Hospital, Houston, TX 77025, USA

COOPER, D. K. C., Prof. Dr., Department of Cardiac Surgery, Baptist Medical Center, Oklahoma City, OK 73126, USA

COPELAND, J. G., Dr., Department of Surgery, Section of Cardiovascular and Thoracic Surgery, University of Arizona, Tucson, AZ 85724, USA

CORTESINI, R., Prof. Dr., Cattedra di Chirurgia esperimentale, University of Rome, Policlinico Umberto I, 00161 Rome, Italy

CUNNINGHAM, J. N., Jr., Dr., Department of Surgery, New York University Medical Center, New York, NY 10016, USA

DELEUZE, P., Dr., Department of Cardiac Surgery, C.H.U. Henri Mondor, 94000 Creteil, France

DE PAULIS, R., Dr., Cattedra di Cardiochirurgia, C. so Polonia 14, 10126 Torino, Italy

DIETZE, O., Dr., Chirurgie I, Universität Innsbruck, 6020 Innsbruck, Austria

DI MEO, F., JR., Dr., Harrison Department of Surgical Research, Department of Surgery, University of Pennsylvania, Philadelphia, PA 19104, USA

DUBOIS RANDE, J. L., Dr., Department of Cardiology, C.H.U. Henri Mondor, 94000 Creteil, France

EMOTO, H., Dr., Department for Artificial Organs, Cleveland Clinic, 9500 Euclid Avenue, Cleveland, OH 44106, USA

FASOL, R., Dr., Chirurgie II, Universität Wien, Spitalgasse 23, 1090 Wien, Austria

FITZGERALD, M., Dr., Harefield Hospital, Middlesex UB9 6JH, United Kingdom

FRAZIER, O. H., Prof. Dr., Cardiac Transplant Service, Texas Heart Institute, Houston, TX 17025, USA

FUJIMOTO, L. K., Dr., Department for Artificial Organs, Cleveland Clinic, 9500 Euclid Avenue, Cleveland, OH 44106, USA

FUJITA, T., Dr., Institute of Medical Electronics, Faculty of Medicine, University of Tokyo, 7-3-1 Hongo, Bunkyo-Ku, Tokyo 113, Japan

FUKUNAGA, S., Dr., First Department of Surgery, Hiroshima University School of Medicine, 1-2-3 Kasumi, Minami-Ku, Hiroshima 734, Japan

GANDJBAKHCH, I., Dr., Service of Thoracic and Cardiovascular Surgery, Hôpital La Pitié, 83 Bd. de l'Hôpital, 75013 Paris, France

GHOSH, P. K., Dr., Herzchirurgie Salzburg, Landeskrankenanstalten, Müllner Hauptstraße 48, 5020 Salzburg, Austria

GOLDING, L. A. R., Prof. Dr., Department of Cardiothoracic Surgery and Artificial Organs, Cleveland Clinic Foundation, Cleveland, OH 44106, USA

GRANDJEAN, P. A., Dr., Université Paris IV, Hôpital Broussais, Départment de Chirurgie Cardio-Vasculaire et Laboratoire d'Etude des Prothèse Cardiaques, 96 Rue Didot, 75014 Paris, France

GRIFFITH, B. P., Prof. Dr., Department of Surgery, University of Pittsburgh, Pittsburgh, PA 15261, USA

HAGER, J., Dr., Chirurgie I, Universität Innsbruck, 6020 Innsbruck, Austria

HAMANAKA, Y., Dr., Research Institute for Artificial Hearts, Hiroshima University, 1-2-3 Kasumi, Minami-Ku, Hiroshima 734, Japan

HAMMOND, R. L., Dr., Harrison Department of Surgical Research, Department of Surgery, University of Pennsylvania, Philadelphia, PA 19104, USA

HILLION, M. L., Dr., Department of Cardiac Surgery, C.H.U. Henri Mondor, 94000 Creteil, France

HINES, H. H., Jr., Prof. Dr., University of Chicago, Medical Center, Chicago, IL 60616, USA

HIRANO, A., Dr., Department of Medical Electronics, Research Institute of Applied Electricity, Hokkaido University, Sapporo 060, Japan

HORIUCHI, T., Dr., Institute of Medical Electronics, Faculty of Medicine, University of Tokyo, 7-3-1 Hongo, Bunkyo-Ku, Tokyo 113, Japan

HUMAN, P. A., Dr., University of Cape Town, Medical School, Observatory 7925, Cape Town, Republic of South Africa

ICENOGLE, T., Dr., Department of Surgery, Section of Cardiovascular and Thoracic Surgery, University of Arizona, Tucson, AZ 85724, USA

ISHIHARA, H., Dr., Research Institute for Artificial Hearts, Hiroshima University, 1-2-3 Kasumi, Minami-Ku, Hiroshima 734, Japan

JAMIESON, S. W., Prof. Dr., Division of Cardiovascular and Thoracic Surgery and Minnesota Heart and Lung Institute, 425 East River Road, Minneapolis, MN 55455, USA

KANTER, K. R., Dr., Department of Surgery, St. Louis University Medical Center, St. Louis, Mo 63104, USA

KANTROWITZ, A., Prof. Dr., Division of Cardiovascular Surgery, Sinai Hospital of Detroit, Suite 309, 14800 W. McNichols Rd., Detroit, MI 48235, USA

KHAGHANI, A., Dr., Harefield Hospital, Middlesex UB9 6JH, United Kingdom

KHALAFALLA, A. S., Dr., International Bio-Technology Dialogue, P.O. Box 6107, Minneapolis, MN 55406, USA

KOLFF, J., Dr., Cardiac Surgical Department, Temple University Hospital, 3401 N. Broad Street, Philadelphia, PA 19140, USA

KOLFF, W. J., Prof. Dr., Division of Artificial Organs and Institute for Biomedical Engineering, University of Utah, Medical Center, Salt Lake City, UT 84112, USA

KOLLER, I., Dr., Herzchirurgie Salzburg, Landeskrankenanstalten, Müllner Hauptstr. 48, 5020 Salzburg, Austria

LANDIS, D. L., Prof. Dr., Division of Artificial Organs, Department of Surgery, College of Medicine, Pennsylvania State University, Hershey, PA 17033, USA

LAWSON, J. H., Dr., Thoratec Laboratories, 2023 8th Street, Berkeley, CA 94710, USA

LEGER, P., Dr., Department of Anesthesiology, Hôpital La Pitié, 83 Bd. de l'Hôpital, 75013 Paris, France

LELLOUCHE, D., Dr., Department of Cardiology, C.H.U. Henri Mondor, 94000 Creteil, France

LEVASSEUR, J. P., Dr., Department of Anesthesiology, Hôpital La Pitié, 83 Bd. de l'Hôpital, 75013 Paris, France

LIMA QUINTANA, O., Dr., Hospital Italiano, Gascon 450, 1181 Buenos Aires, Argentina

LIOTTA, D., Dr., Hospital Italiano, Gascon 450, 1181 Buenos Aires, Argentina

LOISANCE, D., Prof. Dr., Université Paris XII, Faculté de Médicine, Centre de Recherches Chirurgicales, C.H.U. Henri Mondor, 8, Rue du Général Sarrail, 94010 Créteil Cedex, France

LOOP, F. D., Dr., Department of Cardiothoracic Surgery and Artificial Organs, Cleveland Clinic Foundation, Cleveland, OH 44106, USA

MAGOVERN, J. A., Division of Artificial Organs, Department of Surgery, College of Medicine, Pennsylvania State University, Hershey, PA 17033, USA

MALEK, A. M., Dr., International Bio-Technical Dialogue, P.O. Box 6107, Minneapolis, MN 55406, USA

MATSUURA, Y., Dr., Research Institute for Artificial Hearts, Hiroshima University, 1-2-3 Kasumi, Minami-Ku, Hiroshima 734, Japan

McBride, L. R., Dr., Department of Surgery, St. Louis University Medical Center, St. Louis, MO 63104, USA

Mestiri, T., Dr., Department of Cardio-Vascular Surgery, Hôpital La Pitié, 83 Bd. de l'Hôpital, 75013 Paris, France

Mikami, T., Dr., Department of Biomedical Systems Engineering, Graduate School of Engineering, Hokkaido University, Sapporo 060, Japan

Miller, L. W., Dr., Department of Surgery, St. Louis University Medical Center, St. Louis, MO 63104, USA

Mitamura, Y., Dr., Department of Medical Electronics, Research Institute of Applied Electricity, Hokkaido University, Sapporo 060, Japan

Mitchell, A. G., Dr., Harefield Hospital, Middlesex UB9 6JH, United Kingdom

Morea, M., Dr., Cattedra di Cardiochirurgia, C. so Polonia 14, 10126 Turin, Italy

Moulopoulos, S. D., Prof. Dr., Department of Clinical Therapeutics, University of Athens, School of Medicine, Vas. Sofias, K. Lourou Str., Athens, Greece

Navia, J. A., Dr., Hospital Italiano, Gascon 450, 1181 Buenos Aires, Argentina

Nitta, S., Dr., Institute of Medical Electronics, Faculty of Medicine, University of Tokyo, 7-3-1 Hongo, Bunkyo-Ku, Tokyo 113, Japan

Nosé, Y., Prof. Dr., Department for Artificial Organs, Cleveland Clinic, 9500 Euclid Avenue, Cleveland, OH 44106, USA

Novitzky, D., Dr., Department of Cardiac Surgery, Baptist Medical Center, Oklahoma City, OK 73126, USA

Odell, J. A., Dr., University of Cape Town, Medical School, Observatory 7925, Cape Town, Republic of South Africa

Okamoto, E., Dr., Department of Medical Electronics, Research Institute of Applied Electricity, Hokkaido University, Sapporo 060, Japan

Olsen, D. B., Prof. Dr., Division of Artificial Organs, University of Utah, Building 5188, Salt Lake City, UT 84112, USA

Oppell, U. von, Dr., University of Cape Town, Medical School, Observatory 7925, Cape Town, Republic of South Africa

Pae, W. E., Jr., Dr., M.S. Hershey Medical Center, Penn State University, Division of Cardiothoracic Surgery, P.O. Box 850, 500 University Drive, Hershey, PA 17033, USA

Pavie, A., Dr., Service of Thoracic and Cardiovascular Surgery, Hôpital La Pitié, 83 Bd. de l'Hôpital, 75013 Paris, France

Pennington, D. G., Dr., Department of Surgery, St. Louis University Medical Center, St. Louis, Mo 63104, USA

Pierce, W. S., Prof. Dr., Department of Surgery, Division of Cardiovascular and Thoracic Surgery, State University of Pennsylvania, Hershey, PA 17033, USA

Qian, K. X., Dr., Shanghai Second Medical Science University, Shanghai, People's Republic of China

Radley-Smith, R., Dr., Harefield Hospital, Middlesex UB9 6JH, United Kingdom

Reedy, J. E., Dr., Department od Surgery, St. Louis University Medical Center, St. Louis, MO 63104, USA

Reichart, B., Prof. Dr., University of Cape Town, Medical School, Observatory 7925, Cape Town, Republic of South Africa

Reichenspurner, H., Dr., University of Cape Town, Medical School, Observatory 7925, Cape Town, Republic of South Africa

Replogle, R. L., Prof. Dr., Division of Cardiac Surgery, Michael Reese Hospital and Medical Center, Chicago, IL 60616, USA

Riebman, J. B., Dr., Division of Artificial Organs and Institute for Biomedical Enginneering, University of Utah Medical Center, Salt Lake City, UT 84112, USA

Río Del, P., Dr., Hospital Italiano, Gascon 450, 1181 Buenos Aires, Argentina

Rose, A., Dr., Departments of Cardiothoracic Surgery and Pathology, University of Cape Town, Medical Center, Observatory 7925, Cape Town, Republic of South Afrika

Rose, D. M., Dr., Division of Cardiovascular Surgery, St. Vincent's Medical Center, 2800 Main Street, Bridgeport, CT 06606, USA

ROSENBERG, G., Dr., Division of Artificial Organs, Department of Surgery, College of Medicine, Pennsylvania State University, Hershey, PA 17033, USA

SATO, N., Dr., Institute of Medical Electronics, Faculty of Medicine, University of Tokyo, 7-3-1 Hongo, Bunkyo-Ku, Tokyo 113, Japan

SCHIMA, H., Dr., Chirurgie II, Universität Wien, Spitalgasse 23, 1090 Wien, Austria

SCHISTEK, R., Dr., Herzchirurgie Salzburg, Landeskrankenanstalten, Müllner Hauptstr. 48, 5020 Salzburg, Austria

SCHOEN, F. J., Dr., Harvard Medical School, Department of Surgery, Children's Hospital Medical Center, 300 Longwood Avenue, Boston, MA 02115, USA

SEMB, B. K. H., Prof. Dr., Karolinska Sjukhuset, Thoracic and Cardiovascular Surgical Clinic, 10401 Stockholm, Sweden

SEZAI, Y., Dr., Institute of Medical Electronics, Faculty of Medicine, University of Tokyo, 7-3-1 Hongo, Bunkyo-Ku, Tokyo 113, Japan

SHUMAKOV, V. I., Dr., Institute of Transplantology and Artificial Organs, USSR Ministry of Health, Moscow, USSR

SIMONNEAU, F., Dr., Department of Anesthesiology, Hôpital La Pitié, 83 Bd. de l'Hôpital, 75013 Paris, France

SNYDER, A. J., Dr., Division of Artificial Organs, Department of Surgery, College of Medicine, Pennsylvania State University, Hershey, PA 17033, USA

SOLIS, E., Dr., Department of Cardio-Vascular Surgery, Hôpital La Pitié, 83 Bd. de l'Hôpital, 75013 Paris, France

SPENCER, F. C., Prof. Dr., Department of Surgery, New York University Medical Center, New York, NY 10016, USA

STEPHENSON, L. W., Dr., Harrison Department of Surgical Research, Department of Surgery, University of Pennsylvania, Philadelphia, PA 19104, USA

STEWART, R. W., Dr., Department of Cardiothoracic Surgery and Artificial Organs, Cleveland Clinic Foundation, Cleveland, OH 44106, USA

SUEDA, T., Dr., Research Institute for Artificial Hearts, Hiroshima University, 1-2-3 Kasumi, Minami-Ku, Hiroshima 734, Japan

SWARTZ, M. T., Dr., Department of Surgery, St. Louis University Medical Center, St. Louis, MO 63104, USA

SZEFNER, J., Dr., Department of Cardio-Vascular Surgery, Hôpital La Pitié, 83 Bd. de l'Hôpital, 75013 Paris, France

TARRAL, A., Dr., Department of Cardiology, C.H.U. Henri Mondor, 94000 Creteil, France

TAUB, J., Dr., Department of Surgery, St. Louis University Medical Center, St. Louis, MO 63104, USA

THOMA, H., Prof. Dr., Chirurgie II, Universität Wien, Spitalgasse 23, 1090 Wien, Austria

TOLITANO, D. J., Dr., Cardiovascular Surgery, Michael Reese Hospital and Medical Center, Chicago, IL 60616, USA

TRUBEL, W., Dr., Chirurgie II, Universität Wien, Spitalgasse 23, 1090 Wien, Austria

TUNA, I. C., Dr., Department of Surgery, University of Minnesota Hospital, Minneapolis, MN 55455, USA

UNGER, F., Prof. Dr., Herzchirurgie Salzburg, Landeskrankenanstalten, Müllner Hauptstr. 48, 5020 Salzburg, Austria

VAISSIER, E., Dr., Department of Anesthesiology, Hôpital La Pitié, 83 Bd. de l'Hôpital, 75013 Paris, France

VAŠKŮ, J., Prof. Dr., Department of Surgical Research, University of Brno, Brno, CSSR

WATSON, J. T., Dr., National Heart, Lung and Blood Institute, National Institutes of Health, Bethesda, MD 20014, USA

WEBER, K. T., Prof. Dr., Cardiovascular Institute, Michael Reese Hospital and Medical Center, Chicago, IL 60616, USA

WEISS, W., Dr., Division of Artificial Organs, Department of Surgery, College of Medicine, The Milton S. Hershey Medical Center, Pennsylvania State University, Hershey, PA 17033, USA

WOLNER, E., Prof. Dr., Chirurgie II, Universität Wien, Spitalgasse 23, 1090 Wien, Austria

WURZEL, P., Dr., Cardiac Surgical Department, Temple University Hospital, 3401 N. Broad Street, Philadelphia, PA 19140, USA

YACOUB, M. H., Prof. Dr., Harefield Hospital, Middlesex UB9 6JH, United Kingdom

ZILLA, P., Dr., Department of Cardio-Thoracic Surgery, Groote-Schuur-Hospital, University of Cape Town, Cape Town, Republic of South Africa

ZIMIN, N. K., Dr., Institute of Transplantology and Artificial Organs, USSR Ministry of Health, Moscow, USSR

1. The Present Status of Assisted Circulation. Introduction

F. UNGER

It is now 10 years ago that the book *Assisted Circulation* and 4 years ago that the book *Assisted Circulation 2* were issued by Springer-Verlag. The progress in replacing the heart which was made during those years is tremendous, as was evidenced by the content of the two books. The first volume reported on clinical experience with intra-aortic balloon pumping and on several clinical trials with ventricular assist devices. Most of the chapters dealt with animal experiments and considerations for clinical application, and most concluded with hope of a new clinical reality. The cardiac assist devices most frequently employed were pulsatile and were driven pneumatically.

By the second volume, the picture had changed. With intra-aortic balloon pumping having become clinical routine, interest was now focused on the first clinical results with ventricular assist devices. For the first time, the permanent use of a total artificial heart was regarded as a real possibility. The transition from experiment to clinical application had been made, and the experimental results were confirmed by the clinical results. There was also new interest in the nonpulsatile blood pump for cardiac assistance and even as a functional heart replacement.

The picture has now changed again entirely. This new volume covers the latest results with total artificial hearts, and the clinical reality attests to the fact that the artificial heart can be considered as a bridge to transplantation, a concept introduced in 1969 by Cooley; it was discussed in the first two volumes and has now been tried in 127 clinical cases.

Parallel to the efforts made in mechanical replacement of the heart, the concomitant therapy improved remarkably, so that heart transplantation programs have now been established in 188 centers throughout the world. Thanks to cyclosporin and improved techniques, heart transplantation can be considered a routine method for definitive indications.

Newly addressed in this volume are the muscle-powered assist devices and a technique to endothelialize the surfaces with cultured blood cells. The field of biomaterials has produced nothing new in this area of research: the blood pumps are still constructed of the same well-known biomaterials and have the same valves those used 4 or 10 years ago. Most available artificial heart chambers are pneumatically driven, which is sufficient for temporary use. For long-term use mechanical pumps are under construction, and the ultimate goal is to make the devices completely implantable.

Besides reviewing the continuing cardiac assist and replacement program, it is quite interesting to note the number of experimental groups looking for new

Assisted Circulation 3
F. Unger (Ed.)
© Springer-Verlag Berlin Heidelberg 1989

concepts. Indeed, it is very difficult to establish research programs for permanent heart substitutes. Such research requires immense financial support.

The success of such programs depends on a great amount of tenacity, but this same dedication was also required 10 or 20 years ago. The number of groups interested in clinical applications of the artificial heart is constantly increasing, as is the number of transplantation centers. The two concepts of cardiac assistance and replacement are complementary. A barrier to the discussion is the bureaucratic evaluations and exemptions made regarding cardiac assist devices, which have resulted in the uncontrolled use of commercially available nonpulsatile blood pumps. The number of clinical applications made is not available as there is no register; only a few results have come to the surface, like the tip on an iceberg. The industry was at first interested only in intra-aortic balloon pumps. Now there are seven companies on the market offering various types of cardiac devices.

To repair or to replace a heart is a dream which has been realized over the past 30 years with excellent and reliable results. The field of cardiac surgery has grown enormously, especially with "interventional cardiology" as aggressive therapy for acute myocardial infarction. This is reflected by the increasing number of open-heart cases worldwide. To help calculate the present need and demand let us consider the roughly 1 billion people living in Japan, the United States, Europe, The Soviet Union up to the Urals, and Latin America (Table 1). The prevalence of coronary heart disease is estimated at 30 000 cases per million people. This implies that there are 30 million people in this area with a silent lesion of the coronary artery system.

The incidence of acute myocardial infarction per year is 5000 cases per million population, whereby 2000 people per million die of cardiac failure and 8000 per million have a cardiac pump failure which might be treatable. Five hundred patients per million are possible candidates for various devices from the IABP to the TAH. This would imply a total pool in this geographic area of approximately 0.56 million people. Of further interest are the rates of operations per year: 1000 patients per million undergo surgical intervention (Table 2).

Table 1. Estimated world population as of 1986 according to geographic area (total: 4.9 billion)

	Population (in millions)
Europe	496
USSR	279
USA and Canada	264
Latin America	212
Africa	276
Asia	2876
– China	1060
– India	759
– Japan	121
Oceania	25

Table 2. Prevalence of coronary heart disease and rates of operation per year (in millions per billion population)

Prevalence of CHD	30	
Incidence:		
Myocardial infarction	5	
of these, deaths	2	
Angina	8	
Incidence of cardiac OP:	1	(10000 are possible candidates for various assist devices)
CABG	0.7	
Valve failure	0.1	
Congenital heart disease	0.1	
Cardiac transplant	0.01	

The figures in Table 2 are valid only if 1000 patients per million population are operated on; this standard was met in the USA in 1985 and is targeted in Europe. In 1984 the mean worldwide average was 234 per million population, but this is increasing constantly.

The incidence of cardiac failure after open-hart surgery has dropped from 10% in 1975 to maximally 1% now. The most feasible approach is prolonged extracorporeal circulation (ECC) in combination with all types of catecholamines to achieve a wean off. If this is not effective, IABP and then consecutive ventricular assistance by means of such devices as pneumatically driven pumps or non-pulsatile blood pumps are indicated. A total artificial heart is feasible only when there is literally no hope of a recovery and all requirements for a consecutive transplantation can be met.

The clinical indications for cardiac assistance are shown in Fig. 1. Possibilities are counterpulsation by means of intra-aortic balloon pumping with or without extracorporeal oxygenation, cardiac assist devices driven pneumatically with pulsatile flow or driven electrically with nonpulsatile flow, cardiac replacement by means of a total artificial heart, and a cardiac transplant. It is clear that the presently, available mechanical devices are limited to temporary use. To construct and to design permanent devices new concepts are necessary and are under develop-

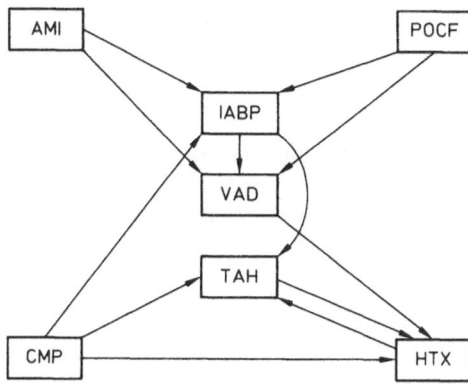

Fig. 1. Management of cardiac failure in *AMI*, Acute myocardial infarction; *POCF*, postoperative cardiac failure; *CF*, cardiac failure; *CMP*, cardiomyopathy; *IABP*, intra-aortic balloon pump; *VAD*, ventricular assist device; *TAH*, total artificial heart; *HTX*, heart transplantation

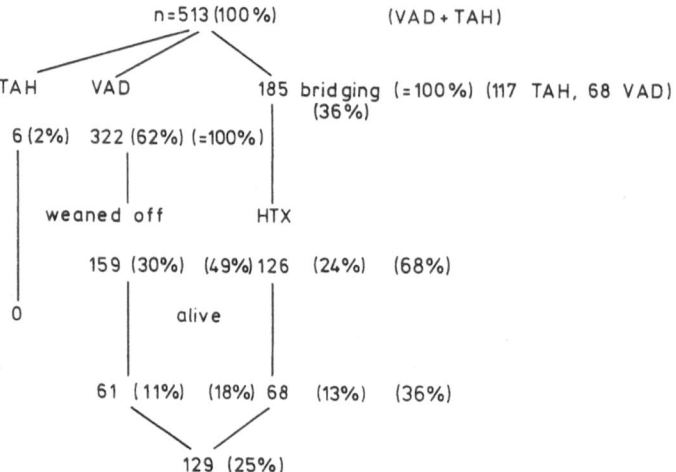

Fig. 2. Pneumatically driven cardiac assist devices in clinical use 1962–1988. *TAH*, Total artificial hearts; *VAD*, left-, right-, and biventricular assist devices

ment. Beside new design requirements, the biomaterials are very limiting, as are the valves.

To date, 513 patients in the world have received pneumatically driven cardiac assist devices (Fig. 2). Of these, 117 were total artificial hearts (TAH) and 396 were ventricular assist devices (VAD). A consecutive transplantation was planned for 185 patients and performed in 126, of whom 68 survived. Ventricular assist devices were used in 322 cases; 159 patients were weaned off and 61 of these are still alive. Overall, 129 of the 513 patients survived and were discharged.

The current possibilities with assisted circulation are documented here in 49 articles collected in six chapters covering counterpulsation, cardiac assistance, the total artificial heart, heart transplantation, driving systems, and the outlook for the future, i.e., horizons. The papers stem from the main research groups throughout the world. The problems and efforts being made in these areas are described and summarized in the introductary chapters.

There has been fantastic progress in the past 20 years, and this has been well illustrated by the previous volumes. The transition from animal experiments clinical application is not easy, and it is necessary to understand the natural history of diseases and to balance and reflect to the cost-effectiveness.

Progress is always stimulatiny, but it should not be overestimated. A Viennese poet, Johann Nestroy, stated: "Überhaupt hat der Fortschritt das an sich, daß er noch größer ausschaut als er in Wirklichkeit ist." Realism and tenacity are the virtues of every scientist, and I am sure that the fourth volume will report as many steps forward as this third volume does in relation to the first. It is constant relativation that brings real progress to man.

2. Questions and Predictions

W. J. KOLFF

When I wrote "Questions and Predictions" for the second volume of *Assisted Circulation*, we had just had the experience with Dr. Barney Clark. Since that time there have been enormous changes, and they help to predict the near future. In the calendar year 1986, 43 patients received air-driven artificial hearts, all of them meant to be a bridge to transplantation [1]. Twenty-one of these people are still alive and apparently well with a functioning donor heart. This is a remarkable success, if one realizes that all these people were near death.

Of the first six patients who received the Jarvik type of artificial heart, five developed thromboemboli, and the lives of two long-term recipients, William C. Schroeder and Murray Haydon, were ruined by the consequences of strokes. The fear of thromboemboli is such that the average time that the artificial heart as a bridge to transplantation was left in place was less than 7 days. Indeed, many recipients of the artificial heart were taken off as soon as a donor heart became available, although it probably would have been better had they had a chance to recover from the ravages of their heart failure before being subjected to the second operation.

Dr. Mark M. Levinson [2] from Dr. Jack Copeland's group in Tucson, Arizona, and Dr. Bartley Griffith [3] in Pittsburg have clearly indicated where the thrombi originate in the Jarvik-type artificial heart. Fortunately these thrombi have not always generated emboli.

The main places where the thrombi originate are on the connectors called quick connects, between the ventricles and the atria, aorta, or pulmonary artery, and around the mechanical valves put in these connectors.

John Holfert and Pam Dew in Dr. Don Olsen's Artificial Heart Research Laboratory in Salt Lake City have redesigned the quick-connect system [4]. Dr. George Pantalos and others are using valve rings that have a straight, rather than a convex inner surface. In experimental animals, this has led to a marked reduction in localized small thrombus formation [5].

In the meantime, heart transplantation has taken a flight that was hardly imaginable a few years ago. Following the introduction of cyclosporin, the successful survival rate after heart transplantation is now between 80% and 95% in the centers that know how to do it. These transplant surgeons can, with a little practice, put in artificial ventricles, both right and left, without the help of any quick connects. Dr. Jack Kolff at Temple University in Philadelphia, Pennsylvania, and his group have implanted 20 artificial hearts without quick connects in calves [6]. Of these animals, 15 lived beyond the first operative week and some have survived

Assisted Circulation 3
F. Unger (Ed.)
© Springer-Verlag Berlin Heidelberg 1989

up to 166 days. We can now provide the heart surgeon with ventricles to which the artificial atria, artificial aorta, and pulmonary artery are already connected.

On the operating table, the surgeon can insert the valve of his choice, using the same sewing rings that are normally used to sew artificial valves in natural hearts or aortas. This makes it possible to choose the least thrombogenic artificial heart valves, which at this time seem to be tissue valves.

Since the majority of the recipients have the artificial heart only as a bridge to transplantation, we do not have to worry so much about the fact that the life expectancy of tissue valves is limited to 4–8 years; calcification will not occur before a donor heart appears.

What worries me at this time is the high cost of the tissue valves. We are therefore doing our best to create polymer tricusp semilunar valves [7, 8]. They function well and in accelerated testing they have survived up to an equivalent of 3 years. This is just a beginning.

In the very early days of work with the artificial heart, we put short, Dacron fibrils on the inside of our Silastic artificial ventricles. This led to the first survival of a calf for 1 week for Dr. Hans Zwart – an incredibly long survival period at that time [9]. Dr. Zwart opened a bottle of champagne for the occasion and received a prize of $ 1000 for his article. Unfortunately the fibrils had a tendency to come away from the Silastic, but it is now possible to anchor the fibrils on the inside of the polyurethane ventricles [10], as we have been taught to do by Dr. Robert Whalen [11].

Another possibility (now on the horizon) is to make the inner surface of hearts and valves less thrombogenic. This work has been pioneered by Dr. Sung Wan Kim at the University of Utah with heparin/prostaglandin and prostaglandin/heparin compound, and by Dr. Fazal Mohammad with albumin IgE compound.

Sorin Biomedica in Saluggia, Italy, has developed a technique by which pyrolytic carbon can be applied at low temperature to all kinds of materials, such as Dacron, polyurethane, and Silastic. This pyrolytic carbon seems to be the most inert material known to man from the point of view of thrombogenicity and from the point of view of acceptance by body tissues.

In summary, we can now foresee artificial hearts made by the vacuum-forming technique and, therefore, not very expensive. Some parts will be covered with Dacron fibrils. Other parts, particularly the moving ones, will be coated to make them less thrombogenic. These artificial hearts will not have quick connects. The surgeons will have to learn to sew them in without quick connects. This has proved to be quite possible for surgeons experienced in heart transplantation, and the surgeon in the operating room can determine which valve he wants to use and sew it into the artificial heart using the commercially available sewing ring.

With the steady increase in the transplantation programs in the civilized world, more and more patients will apply for a donor heart and not enough will be available. More and more patients will be waiting with their artificial heart until a donor heart can be found, and so the permanent artificial heart will enter quietly and unannounced through the back door.

References

1. Olsen DB, Riebman JB, De Paulis R, Durrant G, Nielsen SD (1987) Registry and tabulations of orthotopic total artificial hearts in man. ASAIO Abstracts 16:4
2. Levinson MM, Smith RG, Cork RC, Gallo J, Emery RW, Icenogle TB, Ott RA, Burns GL, Copeland JG (1986) Thromboembolic complications of the Jarvik-7 total artificial heart: case report. Artif Organs 10:236–244
3. Herlan DB, Kormos RL, Borovetz H, Griffith BP (1987) Hemodynamic and functional implications of the 100 cc vs 70 cc Jarvik-7 total artificial heart (TAH). ASAIO Abstracts 16:1
4. Holfert JH, Riebman JB, Dew PA, De Paulis R, Olsen DB (1987) Early preliminary results of a new total artificial heart connector system. ASAIO Abstracts 16:4
5. Riebman JB, De Paulis R, Deleuze P, Dew PA, Holfert J, Burns GL, Olsen DB (1987) Design and performance of a total artificial heart for smaller-sized recipients. ISAO-ESAO Abstracts (accepted for 1987 meeting) Vol. 11:4
6. Wurzel D, Kolff J, Missfeldt W, Wildevuur W, Hansen G, Brownstein L, Riebman J, De Paulis D, Kolff WJ (1988) Development of the Philadelphia heart system. ISAO-ESAO Abstracts (accepted for 1987 meeting) J artif organs 12(5):410–422
7. Pantalos G, Chiang BY, Hansen G, Perkins P, Bishop D, Jansen J, Yu L, Socha P, Burns G, Marks J, Kolff WJ (1987) Development of smaller artificial ventricles and valves made by vacuum forming. ASAIO Abstracts 16:12
8. Yu LS, Drevijn R, Kolff WJ (1987) Experimental analysis of mechanical failure of polyurethane trileaflet valve. 40th ACMB Meeting, Sept 1987
9. Zwart HHJ (1971) One week with an artificial heart. Hosp Physician Nov:2–7
10. Pantalos G, Chiang BY, Hansen G, Perkins P, Bishop D, Jansen J (1987) Artificial ventricles and valves made by vacuum forming. ASAIO Abstracts 16:12
11. Verhagen-Metman L, De Paulis R, Mohammad SF, Kolff WJ (1987) Evaluation of thrombogenesis on smooth and rough intima in artificial ventricles. ASAIO Abstracts 16:12

3. Precedents and Perspectives

P. K. GHOSH

> Those who cannot remember the past are condemned
> to repeat it.
> George Santayana, Life of Reason
>
> You can never plan the future by the past.
> Edmund Burke, Letter 1791
>
> For many were called but few were chosen.
> Sermon on the Mount, The Bible

The need for assisted circulation begins when the patient reaches the point where all standard modalities have been exhausted, when it is clear that the course is inexorably downhill from that point on [1]. Circulatory assistance becomes the alternative when the patient becomes refractory to pharmacological support. The armamentaria of assisted circulation are designed towards one specific goal – in the words of Kantrowitz – to convert the terminal heart condition into a treatable heart disease.

Historically, as in all scientific advances, research started with the *stage of concepts*, when in 1812 LeGallois [2] postulated on the complexity of replacing the heart. DeBakey's [3] design of a roller pump in 1934 formed the basic approach for left ventricular (LV) assistance.

Inevitably, soon the next *stage of experiments* followed. Venoarterial pumping with oxygenation for circulatory support of the failing heart was clinically attempted in 1954. In late valvular diseases the clinical benefits of such procedures were short-lived [4]. But its use in 1957 on a patient in myocardial infarction (MI) and shock in King's County Hospital led to his survival. Despite early scepticism, these initial clinical adventures and laboratory experiments [5] indicated that the reduction in myocardial oxygen consumption is accomplished either by reduction in end-ventricular pressure or by reduction in end-diastolic myocardial fiber length or by a combination of both.

In 1961 Dennis et al. [6] demonstrated left heart bypass by inserting an inflow cannula into the left atrium (LA) through the atrial septum and returning blood through femoral artery. In February and May 1966 Kantrowitz and his group [7] implanted U-shaped avalvular auxiliary ventricles for permanent cardiac assistance in two patients in Brooklyn. The first patient was a 33-year-old man in LV failure of 3 years' duration. He died 20 h after surgery from uncontrollable bleeding. The second patient was a 63-year-old woman suffering from chronic heart failure for 3 years. She had improved hemodynamically and clinically after implantation but on the 10th postoperative day suffered a cerebrovascular accident (CVA) and expired on the 12th day. In August 1966 DeBakey [8] successfully used an LV bypass pump for temporary circulatory assistance in a 37-year-old man for failure to wean from cardiopulmonary bypass (CPB). The inlet and the outlet tubes passed through the chest wall to a valved pumping chamber positioned outside the chest. It was used for 10 days and then removed. The patient recovered and went home.

Assisted Circulation 3
F. Unger (Ed.)
© Springer-Verlag Berlin Heidelberg 1989

At the same time, other modalities of circulatory assistance were attempted by different groups. LV assist systems were developed for both in-series support and parallel support. In 1961 Kolff and Moulopoulos [9] developed their intra-aortic balloon pump (IABP). W. C. Birtwell's dream of in-series support by counterpulsation was translated into clinical reality first by Kantrowitz et al. [10] in 1967. The clinical use of a parallel assist device was reported in 1963 by Liotta et al. [11].

Hardy and Chavez [12] attempted to transplant a chimpanzee heart into a man in 1964. In December 1967 the first successful allotransplantation of a human heart was performed by Barnard [13].

All these initial sporadic anecdotal experiences stimulated intensive research and development which has blossomed today into the clinical *stage of applications*. Assisted circulation in 1987 can be considered in six often interrelated overlapping categories:

1. In-series mechanical ventricular assistance: counterpulsation with IABP, dynamic aortic patch, etc.
2. Parallel mechanical ventricular assistance: ventricular assist devices (VADs); artificial heart as piggyback or adapted as VADs
3. Mechanical replacement: total artificial heart (TAH) for total or partial replacement
4. Bridges: VADs or TAHs as bridges to HTx for staged cardiac replacement
5. Biological replacement/assist: heart transplantation (HTx), heterotopic or orthotopic; heart-lung transplantation (HLTx)
6. Biomechanical assistance: dynamic cardiomyoplasty, counterpulsation.

In-series Mechanical Ventricular Assistance

These systems work where the entire LV output is delivered to the aorta. They reduce the end-systolic ventricular pressure and augment the aortic diastolic pressure by counterpulsation (Fig. 1). It was Harken who coined the term counterpulsation in 1958 [14]. These systems may be temporary or permanent.

Noninvasive modes are not efficient hemodynamically. Body accelerated synchronous heartbeat is a crude maneuver of the whole body [15]. The body is moved caudally in systole to help the heart eject. It is moved cranially in diastole to augment the diastolic blood pressure. External compression (ECP) was a step further and worked on the principle that intravascular pressure reflects the transmural pressure. It is effected by ECG-synchronized compression of legs by pneumatic sleeves. Soroff et al. [16], in a multihospital clinical study of ECP, reported a survival rate of 45%. Their group, as well as Shumakov from Moscow [27], had used mobile ECP units. ECP is easy to apply and it augments diastolic pressure. However, it increases venous return to the heart, increasing preload, and may precipitate pulmonary edema by quick elevation of pulmonary artery wedge pressure [27]. There is low reduction of afterload. Moreover the efficacy of the whole system is dependent on the state of constriction of the peripheral vessels and the degree of the cardiogenic shock.

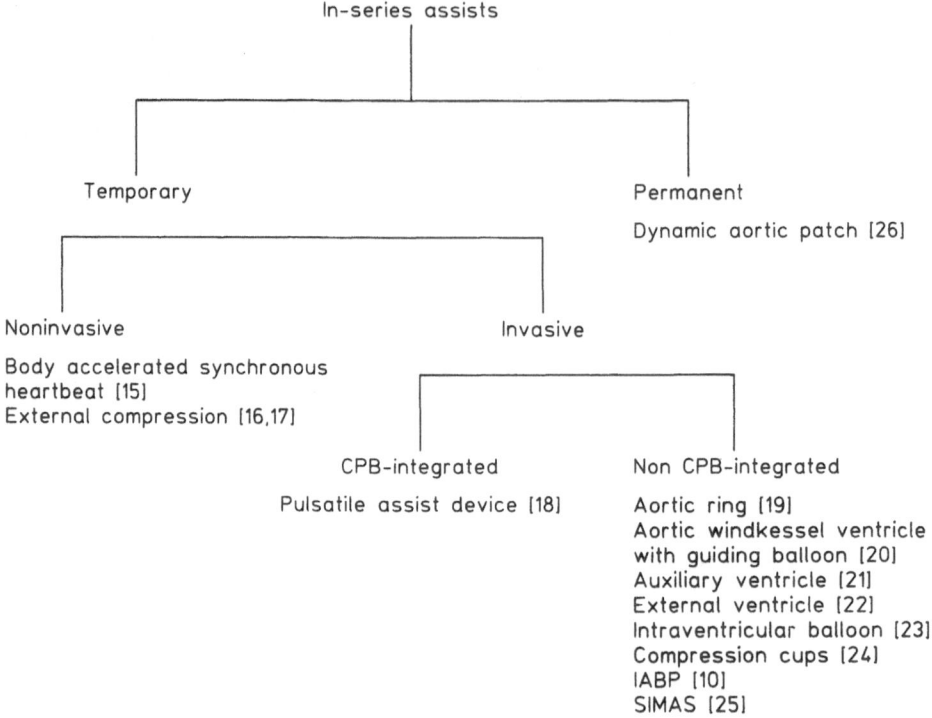

Fig. 1. Modes of in-series mechanical assistance

Among the invasive devices, the pulsatile assist device (PAD) is a plastic disposable pneumatically driven device inserted in the arterial line during CPB to produce synchronous pulsatile flow [18]. Its use usually obviates the need for intraoperative IABP. It is claimed to offer greater protection to the myocardium during CPB. The aortic ring [19] was a double-walled pneumatic sleeve wrapped around the descending thoracic aorta for 5–8 cm. It was driven by compressed air triggered by R waves. Alternate inflation and deflation led to circumaortal compression to secure diastolic augmentation. Hemodynamically it proved to be inefficient. The aortic windkessel ventricle (AWK; [20]) works on an ingenious principle by sucking up the systolic stroke volume of the LV as a guiding balloon (introduced perfemorally and positioned in the aortic arch distal to the AWK channel) occludes the periphery. In diastole the balloon collapses and the AWK discharges all the blood to the periphery. A single bidirectional channel of the AWK is implanted on the ascending aorta. The AWK reduces LV work and LV pressure.

Auxiliary ventricles [21] work on a similar principle to the AWK but have two conduits to the aorta – an inflow and an outflow – and do not need a guiding balloon. The external ventricle [22] similarly works on counterpulsation by systolic indrawing from and diastolic return of blood to the femoral arteries. The intraventricular balloon (IVB; [23]) was another spin-off from the IABP which proved to be counterproductive as the balloon increased the LV end-diastolic volume and the heart's systolic work increased to overcome the inflation pressure of the IVB. Bencini and Parola [24] had attempted to assist the mechanical work of the heart by filling the pericardial sac with air. The sac was periodically inflated and deflated to pulsate the heart. This technique of pneumatic cardiac massage led to development of massager compression cups which were double-walled sacs with rigid outer and soft inner walls [28]. Successful clinical applications also outlined the limitations and disadvantages of these devices, namely the need for a thoracotomy. A decade after the first clinical use, similar cups were implanted again by Shumakov in Moscow [29]. SIMAS is a computer-automated servomechanism developed and clinically used in cardiogenic shock, hemorrhagic shock, and circulatory support in poor risk patients [25]. Transfemoral short catheters were used in this form of myocardial augmentation.

The IABP remains the most commonly clinically used mechanical assist device for patients in acute LV failure in post-MI rhythm disorders, in cardiogenic shock, and after cardiac surgery. It has been used extensively pre-, intra-, and postoperatively in patients with poor LV function but with a prospect of reversibility. A salvage rate of 20%–30% is usually expected [30]. The ease and promptness of insertion was enhanced by the introduction of percutaneous IABPs in 1979 [31], though vascular complications and balloon failure due to unwrapping are more frequent with this technique. Moreover a percutaneous approach cannot be used in patients with access arterial calcification or kinking. Though usually surgically approached through the femoral arteries, IABPs have variously been inserted through the brachial artery or through the Dacron grafts sutured to the ascending aorta when the balloon is placed in the descending aorta.

The IABP unloads the left heart by up to 25%. It reduces afterload, augments diastolic pressure, increases myocardial perfusion, decreases myocardial oxygen consumption, increases stroke volume index, and decreases pulmonary capillary wedge pressure and pulmonary total vascular resistance. Right ventricles have been additionally supported with an IABP inserted into the pulmonary artery [32].

Permanent in-series assistance in the form of an aortic patch has been reported by Kantrowitz's group [26]. This is a balloon pump-like prosthesis driven by a transcutaneous pneumatic system (or an electric system, as in the earlier prototype). By suturing the device into a portion of the aorta, the elasticity of the descending aorta is retained and the compliance of the aorta is not altered appreciably. Thus the impedance to the outflow of LV is not inhibited. The advantages of the aortic patch are: (a) the heart remains in place and continues to do some work, (b) it is nonobligatory – it may be turned off at will for hours, (c) no anticoagulation is necessary, and (d) it is designed for a larger stroke volume than the IABP, whose diameter is limited by the internal diameter of the aorta. In a patient in chronic LV failure with cardiac output less than 2 l/min/m^2 it took over more than half of the LV work. Its disadvantages are: (a) it needs transcutaneous transfer of power for the pneumatically driven system, and (b) it cannot take over 100% of the LV work. Aortic patches have been successfully implanted in patients.

Parallel Mechanical Ventricular Assistance

Ventricular assist devices (VADs) work in parallel with the ventricle in situ, with input either from the atrium or the ventricle and output returned to the great vessels (aorta or pulmonary artery). Ventricular assist pumping can support both systemic and pulmonary circulations or either one individually. At the same time it unloads the failing ventricle, decreases myocardial oxygen demand and consumption, and allows metabolic recovery of the "stunned" myocardium [33]. Short-term survival rates of 35%–45% have been reported after the use of (VADs) for postcardiotomy cardiogenic shock [34–37].

Parallel ventricular assistance can be considered as:

1. Isolated right ventricular assist devices (RVADs)
2. Isolated left ventricular assist devices (LVADs)
3. Combined biventricular assist devices (BVADs).

All VADs basically have (a) the conduits (or cannulas – inflow and outflow) and (b) the pump.

Unger [38] had earlier discussed all the inflow and outflow cannulation sites in his lucidly illustrated review (Table 1).

When the input to the LVAD comes from LA (designated as LA bypass or left heart bypass), pulmonary artery (PA) pressure as well as LA pressure and LV flow are reduced but LV tension or work is not relieved [8]. Occasional sudden deterioration on LA bypass has been reported when extra load is added to the aorta, thus increasing tension and myocardial oxygen consumption [55]. Dennis et al. [5] had indicated that LA bypass reduces oxygen consumption by 20% but Lefemine and associates [55] consider that observation to be related to the degree of failure, as they found the solitary use of LA bypass ineffective for the support of severe LV failure. In fact it produced immediate circulatory collapse and ven-

Table 1. Cannulation sites

RVADs	LVADs		BVADs
RA → PA [39]	a) Draining LV		RA → PA
	LV apex → Asc Th Aorta	[40, 41]	+
	→ Carotid artery	[40]	LV apex → Asc Ao [53, 54]
	→ Abdomen Aorta	[40, 42]	
	→ Desc Th Aorta	[43, 44]	
	→ Femoral artery	[45]	
	Trans LA → Asc Ao	[46, 47]	
	Trans Ao → Femoral artery	[48]	
	Trans Ao → Asc Aorta	[49]	
	→ Asc Ao via graft	[50]	
	b) Draining LA		
	LA → Asc Ao	[51, 11]	
	→ Femoral a	[5]	
	Trans septal → Femoral a	[52]	

tricular failure when used for severe failure. Thus LA bypass is more applicable to right heart failure (because of direct reduction of PA pressure) than to left heart failure (because the diastolic volume and LV wall tension are not reduced). Moreover in LA bypass, the LA with its low pressures (not exceeding 20 mmHg) cannot pump blood by itself into the aorta, where the mean pressure is around 80 or 90 mmHg. Stopping LVADs with input from the LA runs the risk of total trapping of an immobile column of blood.

Theoretically these problems can be circumvented with input to an LVAD from the LV apex (designated as LV bypass). LV bypass is effective for relieving LV work and pressure and for reducing LA pressure. The LV is postulated to eject some blood through the natural aortic valve and some through the LVAD even after inactivating the parallel system. In reality, two mechanical valves in the parallel circuit have a significant gradient from 5 to 10 mmHg and higher resistance to flow than the natural aortic valve. So a smaller percentage would be pushed through the LVAD circuit than the theoretical maximum of 50% at the inactivated state of the LVAD. Moreover, the LV will have to accelerate a substantial volume of blood to move it through the rigid outlet from the LV apex. The natural aorta, being elastic, will minimize impedance to entire LV stroke volume by expanding. Secondly, as Pierce observed [56], it is counterproductive to remove a segment of functioning – albeit below par – LV myocardium when the major problem is a compromised LV. If a plug about 2 cm in diameter is removed to accept the input cannula of an LVAD, then a significant portion of LV myocardium is being removed which the patient can ill afford to give away. Thirdly an input cannula implanted to the LV apex tethers the LV, which cannot contract normally by shortening the LV dimension from apex to base. For all these reasons when a parallel LVAD fails or is inactivated, about two-thirds of the blood flow will exit through the natural aortic valve. The blood pool in the LVAD circuit, though not stagnant, will be remarkably reduced in flow, requiring an immediate increase in the anticoagulant regime. Thus if some flow is maintained it will be at a cost. Fourthly, LV bypass increases RV work [57–59]. Experimental evidence of Lefemine et al. [55] indicates that RV failure or even bradycardia will drastically reduce cardiac output and blood pressure during LV bypass. Clinical experience from Hershey and Boston [60, 61] corroborates that RV failure is often the limiting factor or the final episode in LV bypass in cardiogenic shock. Theoretically the indication for LV bypass becomes limited to isolated LV failure. At present the general trend in clinical practice is to use left atrical access for input cannulas.

The search for an ideal pump for ventricular assistance has been going on for more than a century (Table 2). Against this historical backdrop the various types of contemporary clinical pump are to be considered in terms of: (a) mode of pumping, (b) direction of flow, (c) placement, (d) actuation, (e) power source, and (f) drive system (Tables 3, 4).

The LVADs are indicated:

1. In postoperative cardiac failure when it is not possible to wean from CPB even with pharmacological and IABP support
2. In cardiac failure due to cardiomyopathy

Table 2. Milestones in the development of the "pump"

Year	Investigator(s)	Reference	Events/devices
1812	Le Gallois	2	Postulated on external preservation of organs, including heart
1855	Porter and Bradley	62	First patent on a rotary pump – "for injection"
1884	von Frey and Gruber	63	Devised the first heart-lung machine
1887	Allen	62	Patent on a modified roller pump "for blood transfusion"
1891	Truax	62	Patent on adjustable roller "surgical pump"
1895	Jacobj	64	Used a rubber bulb as a pumping chamber and propelled the perfusate by compressing the bulb with two wooden boards
1903	Brodie	65	Piston pump
1905	Embly and Martin	66	Piston pump
1905	Richards and Drinker	67	Piston pump
1910	Hooker	68	Piston pump
1922	Dixon	69	Syringe piston pump with a hypodermic syringe
1924	Beck	62	A pump used for blood transfusion
1928	Dale and Shuster	70	A hydraulic pump. Water under pressure within a rigid chamber compressed an enclosed flexible tube for propulsion
1930	Gibbs	71	An artificial heart connected to intra-pericardial great vessels in cats and dogs using the animals' own lungs for oxygenation
1932	Van Allen	72	Metal roller pump – operated manually or mechanically to massage a rubber tube for propulsion
1933	Barcroft	73	Electrically driven rotary pump for propulsion. Used centrifugal pump for perfusion in dogs by cannulation of great vessels
1934	De Bakey	3	Roller pump for continuous flow of perfusate
1935	Lindbergh	74	Pulsatile perfusion of whole organs
1937	Gibbon	75	Roller pump for extracorporeal circulation
1948	Bjork	76	Roller pump with artificial oxygenation
1950	Sewell and Glenn	77	Functional replacement of canine right heart with a roller pump with maximum minute volume of 4.7 l
1953	Gibbon	78	First successful clinical cardiopulmonary bypass
1957	Stuckey et al.	79	Use of CPB in massive MI and cardiogenic shock
1958	Kusserow	80	First experimental RVAD
1960	Saxton and Andrews	81	Experimental use of centrifugal pump
1963	Liotta et al.	11	First clinical implantation of a pulsatile LVAD
1978	Turina et al.	53	First successful clinical use of a BVAD
1978	Norman et al.	82	First use of an LVAD as a bridge to transplantation

Table 3. Classes of pump, according to characteristics

Mode of pumping	Flow direction	Placement
I. Nonpulsatile flow		
1. Sigma motor pump	I. U-shaped flow	I. Intrathoracic
2. Roller pump – Taguchi	Akutsu + Kolff	CCF LVAD (parathoracic actuator)
Litwak	Pierce-Donachy (Thoratec)	Avco
Peters	CCF LVAD	Andros
De Bakey (rotary pump)	Unger	Thoratec VIC
		Nombus
3. Centrifugal pump	II. Axiosymmetric flow	II. Parathoracic
a) Impeller pump – Biomedicus, Medtronic, Utah I	Bernhard	Turina – Biventricular
b) Propeller pump – Bernstein	Turina	TECO PVAD
		Pierce-Donachy (Thoratec)
4. Electromagnet-suspended impeller – Olsen and Brown	III. Unidirectional flow	III. Extrathoracic
a) Vortex pump – Biomedicus (demand-responsive, Vienna vaneless)	Medtronic	Litwak
		Peters
b) Teaspoon pump – Baumgartner		Bernhard (Boston Childrens)
c) Vanepump – Osaka (direct drive)		
d) Spindle pump – Hager		
5. Axial flow Pump – Schistek	IV. Axial flow – Schistek	IV. Abdominal – Portner
6. Nutational pump (Berlin)		
II. Pulsatile flow – on membrane-pump design		
1. Bellows pump		
2. Piston (pusher-plate) pump – diaphragm pump		
CCF – LVAD		
THI – E – ALVAD		
TECO 12C PVAD		
Thoratec VIC		
Aerojet MK IV		
Andros II A		
EH – LVAD		
3. Ventricle Sac pump – Kwan-Gett		
Pierce-Donachy		
AVCO		
Jarvik 7		
Unger		

Table 4. Classes of pump, according to characteristics

Drive system	Power source	Actuations
1. Pneumatic – Pierce-Donachy Bernhard Turina THI E-ALVAD Unger E-LVAD	1. Pneumatic – Pierce-Donachy Bernhard A-LVAD	1. Pneumatic – AVCO CCF LVAD
		2. Electrohydraulic – Nimbus Abiomed AVCO Aerojet E 3 Utah I
	2. Electrical – Nimbus	Jarvik
2. Electrical		3. Electromechanical a) Low speed torque motor – Thermedic b) High speed torque motor – Gould convertor in THI-E-ALVAD
	3. Thermal – Nimbus	c) Solenoid – Novaeor Andros Mk 22 Utah (Peters)
3. Mechanical – Medtronic		Hiroshima (Toguchi)
	4. Nuclear – from plutonium	4. Nuclear-thermal-hydraulic – Aerojet Mk 8 Univ. of Washington System 7

3. In acute MI with cardiogenic shock when an IABP fails to support
4. In acute viral myocarditis
5. As a support during post-transplant acute failure of donor heart, as in ischemic injury, hyperacute rejection, positive cross-match, etc.
6. As a bridge towards transplantation.

RVADs are indicated when RV failure syndrome occurs alone or combined with LV failure. Implantation of an RVAD is analogous to that of an LVAD [39]. The use of BVADs [54, 83] has been clinically established, with more than 400 documented cases. Nonpulsatile pumps have also been used for biventricular assistance [84].

Since 1975 mor than 300 patients worldwide have received LVADs. The cumulative clinical experience indicates that LVADs can support the circulation partially or totally. Myocardial function can improve after 48–96 h of LVAD support and can be assessed noninvasively during the support period. LVADs are claimed to support the circulation fully even through the episodes of supraventricular and ventricular arrhythmias, including fibrillation and asystole [85]. It may be roughly stated that about one-third of the patients with LVADs can be weaned off successfully. In one-third of patients LVADs are inadequate, usually due to additional RV failure, and the remaining third of patients remain dependent on LVAD, ultimately requiring a transplant [86, 87]. In a retrospective analysis of clinical practice at Texas Heart Institute, McGee et al. [88] indicated that

0.7% of all patients following CPB demonstrated inadequate response to conventional pharmacological and IABP support and were therefore candidates for more profound mechanical ventricular assistance. Usually, with VAD support, RV recovery takes 3–5 days while LV recovery may take 5–7 days. Progressive reduction of myocardial edema and coronary artery spasm and rebuilding of high energy phosphate content contribute to recovery.

The advantages of the VADs are:

1. The natural heart remains in situ with the potentiality of recovery
2. They are useful in large numbers of near-terminal LV failures
3. Effectively they provide functional ventricular replacement.

The disadvantages of the VADs are:
1. The obligatory nature of the system
2. The need for transcutaneous passage of cannulas or drive lines
3. The need for anticoagulant therapy
4. Potential hazards of inactivation or failure
5. Possibility of disuse atrophy of myocardium [89].

The optimal volume of flow through the parallel circuit of the VAD required for ideal circulatory assistance is not known. Flow capacity of different designs of assist pumps varies from 3.5 l/min (Utah pump of Peters) to 14 l/min (Thoratec Model VIC). Most pumps allow a normal cardiac output with a spare of more than 50%. Though a near complete takeover by VADs is possible, decompression of the failed ventricle to a normal pressure level and the reduction of wall tension and diastolic volume to normal are preferable to an empty heart [55]. In addition to decompression of the failed ventricle, maintenance of a sinus or regular ventricular rhythm is important for recovery and survival [11]. Both overdistention and negative pressure can provoke arrhythmia. Moreover an empty nonfunctioning heart recovers slower that a functioning heart. Thus theoretically, an amount of bypass from 30% to 70% may be expedient, depending on the degree of failure and the diastolic volume.

At present various VADs are available commercially, viz. Biomedicus (Biopump), Centrimed, Novacor, Thoratec (Pierce-Donachy), and other roller pumps. An international combined registry for the clinical use of mechanical ventricular assist pumps and the total artificial hearts (TAHs) has been set up [90] to consolidate data from many centers, to compare clinical results, and for computerized analysis of the data base.

Parallel assistance can also be provided with an artificial heart adapted as an LVAD [46] or implanted in piggyback fashion like the heterotopic heart transplantation [91].

The current trend in research and development of VADs overlaps in many respects with that of TAHs in terms of goal and applications. Both intermediate- (1 month–1 year) and long-term (>1 year) implantation of VADs are being tried experimentally for the treatment of postcardiotomy and postinfarction myocardial failure. If the goal of a totally implantable long-term LVAD is achieved, it may be used as an alternative in some patients in whom HTx is contraindicated. Compliance sacs have been designed for both TAH and totally implantable closed system VADs. As the actuation system and the blood pump are contained within the body with no direct communication to the outside, these compliance sacs accommodate the volume changes in the blood side of the pump. A Dacron velour textured surface of the compliance sacs as fabricated in Cleveland Clinic Laboratory has been shown to function for many years without changing compliance.

Mechanical Replacement

Reportedly V. P. Demikhov in 1937 replaced a dog's heart with two diaphragm pumps actuated by an extracorporeal electric motor [92]. The greatest contribution in the development and application of a TAH for mechanical replacement came from Willem J. Kolff and his associates – first from the Cleveland Clinic in the 1950s and 1960s, and later from Salt Lake City, Utah. Akutsu and Kolff reported in 1958 orthotopic replacement of the heart in a dog with a TAH made of polyvinylchloride and powered with a compressed air source located externally [93]. Several devices of different sizes, shapes, and power sources were described subsequently in that period. These included electromagnetic TAHs (totally implantable and consisting of solenoids) [94, 95], electromotor roller pumps [96–98], an electromotor pendulum [99], electrohydraulic TAHs [100, 101], a piezoelectric TAH [102], and an electromotor cam-driven piston TAH [103]. The design of these devices was equally varied, e.g., bellow [97, 99], membrane [98], and sac [97, 104]. After initial experiments, Kolff's group concentrated on developing pneumatic TAH technology, which set the subsequent general trend.

In that era, the initial problems were manifold, including suitability of animal model, biomaterial, power source, drive units, energy transmission, and control mechanisms. The first animal survival with a TAH for more than a day was reported from Cleveland in 1962 [105]. By 1966 the Cleveland group achieved animal survival for 2 days [106]. Within the next 5 years the animal survival was extended to more than a week [107, 108]. In retrospect it is interesting to note that the first orthotopic human implantation of a TAH as an emergency measure was performed by Cooley in 1969 before animal survival for 100 h was reported in 1971. The Liotta-Hall pneumatic TAH supported the first human recipient for 64 h prior to subsequent cardiac transplantation. Similarly, it is worth observing that the longest animal survival achieved to date is 344 days in a goat [109], which is less than the longest survival achieved in the human recipient William Schroeder [620 days]. Perhaps the qualitative difference in postoperative care explains this apparent anomaly.

In the 1970s many problems of an implantable TAH were solved to a great extent. The first TAH of Akutsu and Kolff was made of polyvinylchloride. Most initial TAH models were fabricated with silicone rubber, which had the dominant problems of thrombogenicity and limited flexion life. Texturized Dacron-flecked surfaces were introduced subsequently when the problems of hemolysis, pseudo-neointima, and calcification were recognized. Silicone-based smooth elastomers, polyurethanes, pyrolytic carbons, polyethylene, Biomer, Avcothane 51, etc. showed good blood compatibility, with minimal thrombosis and fibrin deposition. Calcification was noticed in long-term implantation of both smooth and rough materials. The Cleveland Clinic evolved the concept of biolization to refer to either the chemical or the thermal treatment of natural tissue or protein (natural tissue derivatives) by either coating or blending protein with other polymers [110, 111]. Segmented polyurethane, recognized for its durability and very low thrombogenicity, allowed fabrication of flexible, smooth seamless blood sacs with long functional life. However, later polyurethanes have been detected to be susceptible to aging on the shelf and after implantation. Dystrophic calcification of the blood pump was noticed to cause stiffening, flexion failure, and perforation [112]. Inhibition of such calcification with warfarin sodium was reported by Pierce and co-workers [113]. The problem of pannus formation at the junction of atrial sewing cuff and inlet valve was overcome by using smooth elastomer-covered atrial cuffs for connection with native atria [114]. Thromboembolism continues to be a persistent problem in all TAHs in experimental and clinical experience. A rolling diaphragmatic housing junction was devised to reduce thromboembolism (Ellipsoid heart, Pierce). Levinson et al. [115] have recently indicated various locations of origin of thrombi in areas of turbulence and stasis in the Jarvik-7 TAH.

Dependable pneumatic power units were devised by 1970 to develop controllable diastolic vacuum and systolic pressure and to regulate systolic and diastolic duration. But the early power units were bulky and stationary and such an immobile unit was used in the first human permanent TAH recipient, Dr. Barney Clark, in 1982. Heimes and Klasen reported in 1982 a compact portable wearable battery-powered pneumatic TAH-drive unit housed in a small 4.76-l case [116]. These external drivers are easy to control but require percutaneous exit tubes and continuous monitoring. Heimes further modified the portable driver, with a reduction in size and weight (about 3 kg) and a recharging interval of 6–8 h, which greatly enhanced mobility and quality of life in TAH human recipients. The Swedish patient Leif Sternberg could travel 30 km out of Karolinska carrying his Heimes portable driver. Another variety of portable pneumatic TAH-drive unit was developed in Berlin [117].

Various modes of control system were developed to regulate pump output in response to changes in venous return, peripheral resistance, etc. and to balance the output of both pumps. Kwan-Gett et al. in 1969 [118] indicated that inherent regulation of cardiac output may be based on baseline incomplete pump filling but complete emptying. Subsequently the Utah and the Cleveland groups developed the intrinsic control system obeying Starling's law. The Penn State group developed the automatic control system [119]. The Berlin group [120] and Thoma [121] also developed their own control systems. In the intrinsic control system, pneumatic power units allow only incomplete filling of right and left pumps at baseline condition. Then, the increases in atrial pressure increase ventricular filling and cardiac output while the decreases in atrial pressure decrease ventricular filling and cardiac output. The intrinsic control system is inadequate for proper cardiac output response to exercise. In the automatic control system the output of each ventricular pump is controlled by a negative feedback loop. The right side is set to maintain a definite range of LA pressure. When the LA pressure exceeds the limit, the right pump rate decreases, less blood is pumped into the pulmonary circulation, and LA return is reduced, thereby reducing LA pressure. The left pump is set to maintain a range of aortic pressure. When the peripheral resistance drops and consequently the aortic pressure falls, as in exercise, the left pump rate increases. The left pump rate is decreased in response to vasoconstriction. This system utilizes the pressure in the left pneumatic drive line to derive analogs of the aortic pressure and LA pressure and requires no implanted transducer. This automatic control system requires only an initial setup during the first few postoperative days. In the Berlin control system, the changes in RA pressure via a negative feedback loop modify the outputs of both right and left pumps. The Vienna group (Thoma) developed first the optimum control system and then a new drive system with a hot-wire thermistor probe anemometer in the pneumatic power line to recognize total filling and total ejection. These signals initiate the systole and the diastole.

As of June 1987, only pneumatic TAHs have been implanted in men for both temporary and permanent use. The first human implantation of a TAH as a bridge to transplantation was performed by Cooley in 1969. The second implantation was also performed by him in 1981 as a bridge. The current era of TAH implantation started in December 1982, when DeVries implanted the first permanent TAH in Dr. Barney Clark in Salt Lake City, Utah [122]. Subsequently only four more permanent human implantations have been performed – three by DeVries in the Humana Heart Institute, Louisville, Kentucky, USA (in Bill Schroeder in November 1984, Murray Haydon in February 1985, and Jack Burcham in April 1985) and one by Semb in the Karolinska Institute, Stockholm (Leif Sternberg in April 1985). None of the human permanent recipients is still alive. Survival was 10 days in Burcham, 112 days in Clark, 229 days in Sternberg, 488 days in Haydon, and 620 days in Schroeder. All permanent recipients received the Jarvik-7 100-ml pneumatic TAH. Eight other models of pneumatic TAH have been implanted in humans as a temporary bridge to transplantation. Each of them consists of two implantable pumps – one for the systemic and one for the pulmonary circulation. Both pumps produce pulsatile flow. Each individual pump has an elastomer blood sac housed within a rigid case. Each pump has a unidirectional flow ensured by an inlet and an outlet valve. Transcutaneous drive lines transmit air pulses between the blood sac and the rigid housing which generate the pumping action. Clinical behavior of all models of TAH has been more or less similar.

Numerous complications plague clinical implantation of pneumatic TAHs. They include hemorrhage, thromboembolism, sepsis, and CVAs. Prolonged CPB time, long atrial and great vessel anastomoses, and hepatic dysfunction predispose towards postoperative bleeding. Significant morbidities ensuing from bleeding are: (a) bleeding, (b) possible secondary immunosuppression with increased risk of infection, and (c) hypersensitization with transfusion-induced cytotoxic antibodies severely limiting transplantability. Periprosthetic infection is a time-related phenomenon and is diagnosed by:
1. Stroke
2. Drainage and poor healing around the drive lines
3. Chronic leukocytosis
4. Unexplained fever

5. Positive blood cultures for recurring organisms
6. Gastrointestinal intolerance
7. Periprosthetic gas on CAT scan.

Reverse isolation, intravenous antibiotics, pulmonary, toilet, aseptic handling of lines and cathetors, coverage of the drive lines with velour at exit sites, and cleaning the exit sites with hydrogen peroxide and povidone-iodine are suggested measures to avoid sepsis. In all five patients with permanent TAH implants, sepsis played a role in their postoperative course.

Cerebrovascular accidents are noticeably very frequent in both permanent and temporary pneumatic TAH recipients. In the immediate postimplant period, high cardiac outputs ($CI \geq 3$ l/min/m^2) are to be avoided to prevent potential cerebral reperfusion injury. Even subsequently the thromboemboli from pneumatic TAHs contribute to CVAs, as has been clinically noticed. Pannus formation, which was overcome in animal trials, has been seen again in two long-term human survivors with the Jarvik-7 TAH. Kolff [123] postulated that this pannus may be a consequence of the abrupt change in direction of flow when the blood goes from the atrium into the inflow orifice. Moreover it may grow as a sequel to endothelialization of thrombi formed on imperfect junctions.

The advantages of TAHs are (a) they are available off-the-shelf in various sizes, (b) they are available in different models and makes and in large enough numbers to meet the requirement, and (c) they are relatively inexpensive. The disadvantages are (a) they are obligatory, (b) the power source – whether pneumatic or electrical – is external, and (c) device failure or inadvertent interruption is a potential hazard.

Current experience indicates that the absolute requirements for a TAH [124] are:

1. The quality of life of the recipient must be acceptable, with adequate independence and no risk of infection by transcutaneous tubes or wires.
2. The biomaterial used must be biocompatible and hemocompatible and must last for more than 2 years without degradation or aging after implantation.
3. Calcification of membranes, pannus formation, thromboembolism, and resultant CVAs and the potential for bacterial endocarditis must be prevented.
4. The pump must automatically adapt to the flow requirements in different physiological stages.
5. The device must fit within the chest without compression of intrathoracic structures.
6. If contingency arises, the device must be able to be replaced quickly.
7. Controls must be incorporated to indicate good function of various components and to allow appropriate corrective measures for component failures.

All these constraints, the predominant clinical complications of thromboembolism and CVAs, and legal restrictions (at present in the United States only Dr. DeVries is permitted to implant seven permanent TAH) have led to highly selective application of TAHs after the initial flurry of activity in the early 1980s. No permanent implantation of TAH has been performed in the world wide since April 1985. However, pneumatic TAH has found a place in clinical practice as a bridge to heart transplantation.

The current trends in further development of TAHs are proceeding in several directions. Kolff opines [123] that a TAH with rough Dacron fibril intimas, with tissue valves, and without quick connects is probably safest – at least for the short run. The quest for a totally implantable TAH has regenerated interest in the development of the electric heart – the first prototype of which was described as early as 1959 [94]. A totally implantable TAH requires intracorporeal implantation of the pump, the compliance chambers, the energy converter, the internal batteries, the diagnostic device, and the secondary transformers as a power transmitter. Inductive coupling through the intact skin will power such a device, obviating the need for external lines, increasing patient mobility, and decreasing the risk of infection. Shuder et al. [125] in 1968 demonstrated the feasibility of such transcutaneous transmission of 50 W power through intact skin for more than 5 years.

Radionuclides such as plutonium 238 had been considered in the 1970s as an implantable power source in the United States and in Europe. Devices were built which had driven experimental TAHs in animals [126–130]. In the contemporary sociopolitical milieu, radioisotopes are unlikely to be used as a definitive energy source for totally implantable TAHs. Current work centers on electrical systems, heat engine systems, and biological energy sources.

The electrically actuated TAH (e-TAH) developed at Penn State University uses either a cam or a roller screw motion translator, positioned between two blood sacs which alternately compress the sacs by way of pusher plates [131]. A similar roller screw pusher plate e-TAH has been developed in Switzerland [132]. Other varieties of electromechanical e-TAH have been developed by THI-Gould, Novacor-Stanford, Thermomedic-Boston Children's Hospital groups, etc.

The electrohydraulic e-TAH developed at the University of Utah-Symbion employs a Jarvik-7-like heart powered by an electric motor-driven high-speed turbine between the two ventricles. The actuation fluid is a low viscosity silicone oil which is pumped back and forth from one pump housing to another – alternately compressing the two blood sacs [133]. Abiomed-MGH has a similar electrohydraulic e-TAH. The CCF-Nimbus electrohydraulic system is somewhat different [134]. The University of Tokyo group has developed an implantable e-TAH with sac and diaphragm types of blood pump without a compliance chamber, using the wireless electromagnetic coupling method for energy transmission. They have used artificial intelligence in the e-TAH control software to regulate multiple parameters [135].

Heat engine systems using lithium salt batteries are still in the R&D stage. Thermoelectropneumatic and thermoelectrohydraulic TAHs are being developed at the Cleveland Clinic and the University of Washington [134]. The use of an electrostimulated skeletal muscle, i.e., psoas muscle, as an internal source of energy for the TAH drive has also been proposed [136, 137].

Experimental attempts have also been made to obviate the "fit" problem of the mechanical right ventricle by only replacing the left ventricle with a single-chambered artificial pump [138, 139]. In selected patients such partial mechanical replacement with a univentricular TAH will have the further advantage of preservation of the native right ventricle, adequate pulmonary flow, and resultant filling of the left pump [139]. In future the concept of a univentricular TAH may be extended to permanent or temporary isolated replacement or assistance of the right heart too.

Bridges

Interim support with a TAH or another assist device with subsequent HTx was popularly christened in 1983 as the Bridge to Transplantation. The concept was originally advanced by the pioneering adventures of Cooley, who in 1969 had called the procedure "staged cardiac replacement" [140]. A diaphragm-type TAH designed by Liotta was implanted in a 47-year-old man after resection of an LV aneurysm because of failure to wean from CPB. The TAH sustained the patient for 64 h before the subsequent cardiac transplantation. The patient succumbed to *Pseudomonas* pneumonia 32 h after HTx. In the second bridge to transplantation in 1978 [82], an intracorporeal ALVAD was used for unresponsive ischemic contracture of the heart (stone heart) in a 21-year-old man who had undergone aortic and mitral valve replacement (AVR, MVR) with porcine bioprostheses and a repair of a fistula from the sinus aortae to the RV. After 5 days of support with ALVAD, cardiac and renal allografting were performed. This patient died from acute tubular necrosis of the renal allograft and multiple ileal perforations on the 14th day after transplantations. In the next bridge to transplantation in 1981, Cooley implanted a pneumatically driven Akutsu III TAH in a 36-year-old man for severe biventricular failure following aortocoronary triple bypass. After 26 h of implantation of the TAH, additional venovenous extracorporeal membrane oxygenation was initiated and continued for next 27 h before the HTx. This patient died 7½ days later from gram-negative and fungal septicemia and multiple organ failure [141].

Despite these three sporadic heroic attempts by the same group, spanning a period of 12 years, no other group at that time attempted this staged approach to HTx. Following further developments in pneumatic TAH technology and permanent implantation of a TAH in Dr. Barney Clark by De Vries in 1982 [122], several centers adopted the bridge concept to sustain their patients awaiting transplantation, as an alternative to impending death from terminal heart disease. In March 1985 Copeland and Vaughn implanted the pneumatically driven Phoenix heart (designed by Kevin Cheng) as a bridge to transplantation in a 33-year-old man for hyperacute rejection of the original allograft [142]. After 11 h of support with the TAH, the second allografting was performed. The patient died 48 h later of right ventricular failure of the second donor heart. This patient became the first human in history to live with four hearts. The first successful use of a TAH as a bridge was achieved by the same group in August 1985 [143]. A 25-year-old man awaiting a transplant for end-stage dilated idiopathic cardiomyopathy developed cardiogenic shock and a Jarvik-7 TAH was implanted. The patient sustained a nonfatal cerebral embolus on the 7th day. After 9½ days support with the TAH he underwent successful cardiac transplantation and returned to full-time work in due course. The first use of a bridge in Europe was in Salzburg in March 1986 [144]. An ellipsoid heart TAH was used in a young woman undergoing AVR who developed intractable ventricular fibrillation in the ICU. HTx followed after 24 h use of the TAH. In the University of Arizona a 40-year-old woman was the first patient in the world to be bridged twice. She was on the bridge the first time with a Jarvik-7-70 ml for 3 days, and after acute rejection of the first allograft for a second time with another Jarvik-7-70 ml for 243 days before the second allograft. She died of acute rejection of the second allograft in October 1986. To date more than 70 bridges with TAHs have been performed worldwide in 16 centers. The models of TAH implanted include the Jarvik-7-100 ml, Jarvik-7-70 ml, Akutsu, Liotta, Penn State, Unger-Ellipsoid, and Berlin hearts.

The therapeutic advantages of bridges are:

1. They provide an "off-the-shelf" solution to support circulation, preserve life, and restore normal circulatory dynamics in patients who cannot survive the waiting period before HTx.
2. A period of stable physiological support on the bridge allows resolution of organ dysfunctions caused by terminal cardiac failure. This improves the chance of success of subsequent HTx.
3. They help in removal of medical contraindications in initially nontransplant-worthy patients with reversible acute organ failure, i.e., hepatic or renal insufficiency. Such patients can be markedly improved following removal of the diseased native heart and with bridge support of circulation can be restored to the acceptable status of candidacy for HTx.
4. In emergency postcardiotomy irreversible total cardiac failure, a bridge may become the only option if the patient is to survive.
5. As emergency management of rejection of the cardiac allograft, bridges can sustain patients.

The possible options for the bridges are: (a) IABP [148], (b) LVAD, (c) BVAD, (d) orthotopic or heterotopic TAH, (e) the biological bridge [145], and (f) partial cardiac replacement [146]. Reemstma et al. [147] were the first to report the use of an IABP as a bridge. Peric et al. [148] reported successful use of IABP support for 1–37 days as a bridge to subsequent HTx in 14 patients. Zumbro and associates [149] reported the first use of successful temporary ventricular assistance of failing transplanted hearts with VADs like the Biopump and the Pierce-Donachy Thoractec pneumatic pump. Heterotopic placement of a TAH piggy-back to the native heart, as proposed by Losman and colleagues [91], may serve as a useful bridge. McKenzie and co-workers [145] provided a novel approach towards temporary bridge support by using natural donor heart unacceptable for permanent transplantation. Their patient, a 42-year-old man after an urgent quintuple aortocoronary bypass, was sustained on this orthotopic biological bridge till subsequent definitive HTx. Orthotopic mechanical replacement of a failed LV with preservation of an intact RV, as proposed by the experiments of Frazier et al. [146], may be employed as a bridge. Their strategy may possibly assure adequate pulmonary flow and resultant LA filling pressure in patients in whom the integrity of the RV has been maintained.

The criteria for the choice of device as a bridge are not well-defined at present. Though some groups, e.g., THI, University of Arizona, and Penn State, now have experience with different devices as a bridge, no scheme for the selection of devices has yet evolved. The Penn State group has indicated its preference for an

LVAD alone or for a TAH in cases where biventricular support is deemed mandatory [150]. Most patients even with biventricular failure can be supported with an LVAD alone in their experience. TAH or BVAD support is necessary if pulmonary vascular resistance is elevated to 5–10 Wood units or if postinfarction acute RV dysfunction is present. When VADs are used, the output from the pump is reduced because of the cannulas and the driving of the pump is more sensitive. A TAH is easier to drive. The Penn State group prefers a TAH to a BVAD as a TAH requires only two percutaneous tubes while a BVAD needs four. In patients with small chest an LVAD is preferred as it may not be possible to accommodate a TAH. However, with the miniJarvik-7-70 ml TAH this fit problem for small chests may be circumvented. ECMO, at present, is the only practical choice for children as the Pierce Donachy VAD is too large to be used in patients with a surface area of less than 1.0 m^2 [151]. Xenogeneic bridge with hearts from subhuman primates for use in newborns, infants, and children has been proposed by Bailey [152]. In acute rejection of cardiac transplants, a TAH, a BVAD, or an allogeneic bridge may be employed. Evidently the spectrum of patients who have been bridged so far is wide and heterogeneous, and the extent of the support required on the bridge was varied considerably. The patients satisfactorily bridged on an IABP alone are in a different category from those in whom an IABP was inadequate and a BVAD or TAH was mandated. The time has come to evolve a universal scheme of objective parameters on hemodynamic, immunological, and biological determinants.

Interim problems of the bridge, i.e., septic complications, anticoagulation need, regimens and complications, hemolysis, potential for device failure, and CVAs, will constitute some of these determinants. CVA, which plagues TAH implantations has not been observed with VADs when used as a bridge [150]. The possible causes for this observation may be:

1. VAD implantations are usually for shorter periods (<21 days) while TAH support is usually for longer periods (10 to >110 days).
2. For TAH implantation, the native heart is excised at the atrioventricular groove, leaving a denervated and partially devascularized atrial remnant to which the atrial connectors are sewn. This suture line is a potential source of thrombus formation and embolization.
3. Remaining atrial appendages become nidi for thrombus formation because of poor washout from these areas.
4. Sudden change from very low cardiac output (1 l/min) to very high cardiac output (12 l/min in the first TAH recipient, Dr. Barney Clark) can give rise to convulsions.

Favorable prognosis on a bridge may be anticipated in patients with myopathy and deteriorating congestive cardiac failure. The University of Arizona group has observed that poorer prognosis is associated with acute viral myocarditis, acute rejection of allograft, failure to wean from CPB or prolonged CPB of more than 5 h duration, fixed organ failure, hyperactive immune states, and the presence of preimplant established infection, especially pneumonia [153].

Many gray areas remain at present in the clinical application of bridges to transplantation. Future cooperative experience will help determine the proper interval on bridge prior to HTx, patient-tailored criteria for choice of device, and strategies to minimize the interim problems.

Biological Replacement/Assist

The mythological tales of all ancient civilizations indicate the age-old fascination for human HTx. In the modern era, the experiments started with the first attempt of Carrel and Gutherie [154] to transplant the heart of a small dog as a passive neutral organ in the neck of a larger dog. That transplanted heart beat at the rate of 88 per minute. Coagulation occurred in the cavities of the heart after about 2 h and the experiment was terminated. For the next half a century experiments were performed in which hearts were transplanted as auxiliary organs in various heterotopic sites. In 1933 Mann et al. [155] transplanted a denervated heterotopic cervical allograft into the carotid-jugular circulation of a dog to produce an 8-day survival. The importance of prevention of coronary air embolism and LV distention was recognized by them (Table 5). Early researchers mostly attempted cervical and abdominal heterotopic HTx [174–178].

The immunological aspects of failure of HTx were recognized early by the researchers. Mann and colleagues [155] had observed a dense infiltration of the myocardium with lymphocytes, mononuclear cells, and polymorphonuclear granulocytes and speculated in 1933 about "some biological factor which is probably identical to that which prevents survival of other homotransplanted tissues and organs." The approach of Sayegh and Creech [157] was to use donor hearts from unborn and newborn puppies but their average survival remained 3 days, the longest being 10 days. Reemtsma et al. [162] succeeded in prolonging the survival of cervical allotransplants to 26 days by using folic acid antagonists.

The most elaborate experiments in early research were done by Demikhov [156, 179]. From 1940 to 1957 he performed more than 250 heart and heart-lung transplants (HLTx). In 1949 he achieved successful orthotopic HLTx in animals. He described 24 variations in intrathoracic auxiliary HTx and auxiliary HTx in the neck and the groin. In 1956 he produced a 32-day survival with an intrathoracic heterotopic graft. He also transplanted auxiliary heart in parallel with the recipient's heart and subsequently excluded the native heart from the circulation; with this procedure the longest period for which the transplanted heart supported the entire circulation was 15 h.

In 1953 Neptune and co-workers [180] reported 6-h survival after HLTx using hypothermia in dogs. Experimental HLTx using CPB with short survival for a few hours was reported in the late 1950s [158, 181, 182]. During the same period, the attempts at orthotopic HTx in the laboratories also achieved survival for a few hours only [159, 160, 178]. Webb and Howard [158] in 1957 established hypothermic preservation of excised heart at 4 °C to achieve acceptable mechanical function on transplantation after ischemic intervals up to 6 h. In 1960 Lower and Shumway in their landmark paper [161] described their surgical technique, which was to become the basis of many subsequent procedures. They achieved a maximal survival of 21 days. They had used donor heart preservation with cold saline. They established for the first time that a mammal could return to normal activity

Table 5. Milestones in heart transplantation

Year	Author(s)	Reference	Achievement
1905	Carrel and Gutherie	154	First cervical auxiliary HTx in dogs
1933	Mann et al.	155	First recognition of cardiac allograft rejection
1949	Demikhov	156	Orthotopic HLTx in dogs
1957	Sayegh and Creech	157	Attempts in immunomodulation by using donor hearts from unborn and newborn puppies
1957	Webb and Howard	158	Hypothermic preservation of donor hearts
1958	Goldberg et al.	159	First animal orthotopic HTx on CPB
1959	Cass and Brock	160	Introduction of atrial anastomoses and other technical innovations
1960	Lower and Shumway	161	Introduced the surgical technique and reported survival for days in dogs
1962	Reemtsma et al.	162	Pharmacological immunomodulation with amethopterin after cervical HTx
1964	Hardy et al.	163	First clinical attempt with chimpanzee xenograft
1966	Lower and Cleveland	164	First HTx of human heart into a baboon
1967	Barnard	165	First successful clinical orthotopic allotransplantation
1968	Cooley et al.	166	First clinical HLTx
1969	Cooley et al.	140	First staged HTx (bridge) with TAH
1972	Castaneda et al.	167	First successful experimental auto-HLTx in baboons
1972	Marcial et al.	168	Experimental auxiliary HTx for circulatory assist
1973	Caves et al.	169	Introduction of endomyocardial biopsy for detection of rejection
1975	Barnard and Losman	170	First successful clinical heterotopic auxiliary permanent HTx
1977	Barnard et al.	171	First heterotopic baboon xenogeneic bridge for parallel assistance
1978	Norman et al.	82	First bridge to HTx with ALVAD
1980	Stanford group	172	Introduction of cyclosporin in clinical HTx
1984	Bailey et al.	173	First successful orthotopic HTx with a baboon xenograft in a neonate
1985	Copeland and co-workers	143	First successful bridge to HTx with TAH

with a transplanted heart [183]. Kondo et al. reported the use of profound hypothermia without CPB for HTx with long survival without immunosuppression [184, 185]. Various techniques and aspects of experimental auxiliary intrathoracic HTx on CPB were described around that period [186–189].

Meanwhile Hardy et al. [163] in Jackson, Mississippi, inspired by Reemtsma's chimpanzee-to-man renal xenotransplants, attempted HTx with a chimpanzee xenograft in January 1964 in a semicomatose 68-year-old man in cardiogenic shock. Although the transplanted heart functioned initially, the patient could not be weaned off CPB. The failure was attributed to the smaller size of the chimpanzee heart and its consequent inability to accept large venous return. Christiaan Barnard [165] first successfully performed a human orthotopic allotransplant in a 54-year-old truck driver, Washkansky, with end-stage ischemic heart disease in Groote Schuur Hospital, Cape Town, South Africa on 3 December 1967. The donor heart was harvested 5 min after a young man, dying of severe brain injury, was certified dead by the absence of electrocardiographic activity. This recipient lived for 18 days before succumbing to a gram-negative pneumonia. The second clinical HTx using deep hypothermia followed 3 days later in New York in an 18-day-old neonate who had failed to improve after a Waterston shunt [190]. In 1968 Cooley and colleagues [166] performed the first clinical HLTx in a 2-month-old female infant with complete atrioventricular canal defect. In 1969 the same group carried out the first staged HTx with TAH as a bridge [140].

The electrifying event of Barnard's operation had grabbed the headlines all over the world and caused a storm over moral, ethical, legal, and political issues. Soon it led to the first international forum on the definition of death. It also triggered off a global race among the cardiac surgeons. This was the most pronounced phase of the "me-too syndrome" in the sphere of cardiac surgery. HTx were performed all over the world – even in centers not fully organized for such an elaborate enterprise. By the end of 1968, 102 HTx were performed in 17 countries. However, the early wild enthusiasm soon gave in to a sane realization that the technical success of HTx was not the panacea it had been predicted to be. The limitations of available immunosuppressive regimens also became apparent. It is worthwhile to note that at the time the clinical adventures of HLTx started, only one experimental animal had survived HLTx for 10 days [191].

That the primates are different from the dogs and that the primates can have normal respiratory patterns after denervation was amply established by successful heart-lung autotransplantation in baboons by Castaneda et al. [167]. Normal cardiopulmonary functions for over 2 years after surgery were demonstrated by their experiments.

Around the same period, the group from Brazil [168] reported an experimental study on assisted circulation with auxiliary HTx. Suros and Woods [192] reported an experimental model of synchronous intrathoracic auxiliary HTx in parallel. In 1975 Barnard and Losman [170] reported the first successful clinical auxiliary permanent cardiac allotransplant in patients as biological assist devices. Subsequently the same group performed the first clinical temporary auxiliary allotransplant for parallel circulatory assist for the intermediate term [193].

Following the introduction of cyclosporin in immunosuppression in 1980, 1-year survival now exceeds 80% in some centers. Reichart's group in Cape Town has achieved a 94% 1-year survival following emergency HTx. The longest reported patient survival has now been 16 years. About 120 centers all over the world have adopted a clinical program of HTx. Several patients in various centers have successfully undergone retransplantation. Even in the elderly group above the age of 60 years, the results of HTx have been shown to comparable to those in the younger cohorts. An international registry today [194] maintains global records of all HTx and analyzes cumulative experience. In addition to endomyocardial biopsy, several noninvasive tools, e.g., high-frequency surface electrocardiogram, directional Doppler 2D echocardiography, cytoimmunological monitoring, radionuclide angiography, the first pass technique, and biochemical markers (plasma prolactin, urinary polyamines) are used in the follow-up protocol to assess the transplanted heart performance and to detect rejection. However, many problems remain unsolved in HTx. Development of coronary artery disease in grafted hearts is seen on angiography in 40% of patients by 5 years after HTx [195], which in many instances brings back the original problem. Limitations of heterotopic auxiliary HTx in recovery of the native heart are becoming apparent [196, 197]. The donor hearts may not become effective assists for the native right heart in the presence of end-stage right heart failure and high pulmonary vascular resistance even when the donor heart can function as an effective left heart bypass. Moreover, multicenter data evaluation [198] – though indicating a rapid increase in HTx in infants and children especially since the introduction of cyclosporin – has not yielded information on the effects of immunosuppresive regimens on growth and skeletal development and the possible long-term adverse effects such as hypertension, renal toxicity, and malignant neoplasms.

Organ procurement has remained another crucial problem for most clinical HTx programs. Several national and international computerized organ-sharing registries (Eurotransplant, Skandiatransplant, SEOPF, UNOS, NATCO) have been set up in Europe and America for long-distance procurement. Despite such measures, donor organ shortage continues as several new clinical HTx programs have been started during the last 4 years. The supply of suitable available donor hearts (from young brain-dead donors with no clinically evident disease) is extremely small. In the United States alone, a maximum of 9500 hearts may be available annually against an annual need for 15000 transplants. The hearts of anencephalic infants have been suggested as a substantial pool of readily available donor organs [199]. In the United States, the national "Required Request" law became operative from October 1987 in the hospitals participating in the Medicare-Medicaid Program, enabling the families of brain-dead cadavers to donate organs. Xenografts have been considered as a potential pool. Historically five xenotransplants – three orthotopic and two heterotopic grafts – have been attempted in humans. In 1964 Hardy [163] transplanted a chimpanzee heart, in 1968 Cooley [200] grafted a sheep heart, and in 1984 Bailey [173] used a baboon heart. In 1977 Barnard [171] twice used xenografts – a baboon heart and a chimpanzee heart – as parallel biological assists on a bridge in patients with postcardiotomy failure. However, the present state of immunomodulation precludes regular clinical use of xenografts. So the demand outruns the supply – even if the utilitarian futuristic sci-fi visions of mandatory scavenging of cadaveric organs can ever be made to work in a changed sociopolitical milieu. Thus heart transplantation will remain a modality available to a select group of patients in the foreseeable future.

Biomechanical Assistance

The concept of biomechanical assistance dates back more than 50 years. In this mode of biological replacement or augmentation of the failing or the insufficient myocardium, a functional autologous mitochondria-powered skeletal muscle is utilized as the energy source and thus is completely implantable and needs no

transcutaneous transfer of energy or conduits nor any immunological intervention. R. C. J. Chiu introduced the term biomechanical assistance.

In 1933 Leriche and Fontaine [201] introduced the idea of using a skeletal
muscle for actively assisting the heart. In their experiments one dog survived with
a graft of pectoralis major after a 2 cm × 4 cm excision of the LV wall. They aimed
to use skeletal muscle to replace infarcted myocardium in humans. Weinstein and
colleagues [202] in 1946 successfully sutured free grafts, averaging 28 cm^2, of vas-
tus lateralis and internal oblique muscles around two canine hearts; the grafts
showed good fixation to underlying myocardium, normal muscle histology, no
shrinkage, and a rich vascular network from underlying thickened epicardium. In
1959 Kantrowitz and McKinnon [203] reported their method of wrapping
diaphragm around the heart and the aorta to compress them, with synchronous
stimulation of the phrenic nerve in each systole. They could improve canine LV
function but the changes were not significant. Shepherd [204, 205] studied inlay
and onlay grafts of diaphragm to enlarge the RV. The muscle atrophied when left
unstimulated, but the paced grafts maintained good contractions and increased
in thickness, indicating a possible myotropic effect of electrical stimulation. However, the denervated inlay grafts showed a motion paradoxical to that of the heart.
Similar experiments with diaphragmatic grafts to the ventricle were conducted in
the 1960s by Phillips et al. [206] and Nakamura and Glenn [207]. Diaphragmatic
grafts were induced to contract by stimulation of the phrenic nerve synchronously
with each cardiac cycle. Nakamura and Glenn [207] reported the hemodynamic
efficacy of such an in vivo graft in one dog, indicated by a short-term rise in aortic
pressure. Termet and co-workers [208] had also observed similar short-term hemodynamic benefits with paced skeletal muscle. They were the first group to use
pedicled latissimus dorsi (LD) muscle flap and to indicate its advantages.

In the next decade, Kusaba [209], Spotnitz [210], von Recum [211], Vachon
[212], and their colleagues experimented with diaphragm or rectus abdominis as
pouches or onlay grafts. Each group recognized the potential of these skeletal
muscles for cardiac assistance. Kantrowitz's group showed [209, 211] that the
graft could generate 57% of the force of normal LV contraction. Spotnitz et al.
[210] demonstrated that the rectus abdominis performed poorly when applied as
a pedicle graft (swung on the internal mammary vessels) to the dog heart, but the
performance was excellent when a composite ventricle was grafted to the abdominal aorta for the high filling pressure. They achieved a maximal systolic pressure
of 600 mmHg during isovolumic contractions. A pressure of 300 mmHg in ejecting beats with a stroke volume of 50 ml could be obtained with a skeletal muscle
mass of 80–150 g. With tetanic electrical stimulations, ejection fractions of up to
50% were achieved. Vachon et al. [212] noted similar length–tension correlations
in their study of mechanical properties of canine denervated diaphragmatic
muscle pouches. In their pouch model, diaphragm tolerated transmural pressure
of 82 mmHg without evidence of ischemia and could be made to contrast at rapid
rates. However, all these investigators found muscle fatigue on repetitive stimulation and high resting stiffness to be insuperable hindrances.

Around the same time some major basic physiological concepts emerged
which influenced the whole approach of biomechanical assistance. Salomons and
co-workers [213–215] reported on the nature of skeletal muscle plasticity and

adaptive changes. In 1972 Katz [216] compared the molecular weights of myosin, actin, troponin, and tropomyosin in cardiac and slow skeletal muscles and noted several biochemical similarities. In 1979 the similarity between the subcellular structures, i.e., mitochondria, sarcoplasmic reticulum, and transverse tubules of cardiac and skeletal muscles, was pointed out by Van Winkle and Entman [217]. Lutz et al. [218] reported the coexistence of fast and slow myosin within a muscle fiber under conditions of long-term electrical stimulations.

In 1981 and 1982 the concept of electrical induction of fatigue resistance in skeletal muscles for use in cardiac reconstruction was advanced [219, 220]. Since that time, the research groups in Montreal, Philadelphia, Stanford, and Seattle have successfully conditioned the skeletal muscles to become fatigue resistant by using rates as low as 2 Hz for as few as 6 weeks by direct muscle or nerve stimulation and for as long as 1 year without adverse effects [221]. Although the transformation was not total, the histochemical conversion of fast-twitch fatigable type II fibers to aerobic slow-twitch fatigue-resistant type I fibers was documented [220]. Such converted muscles are physiologically slower, rich in mitochondria, and more durable when stressed with tetanic stimuli [215]. Their metabolism is shifted from glycolic to aerobic oxidative metabolism because of increased capillaries and mitochondria. However, there is no morphological metamorphosis, and the syncytial arrangement (as seen in myocardium) is not seen in skeletal muscles after electrical conditioning [221].

In experimental models, sternohyoid, sternocleidomastoid, serratus anterior, gracilis, and the intercostals have also been used for onlay enlargement of ventricles or counterpulsation. Recently skeletal muscle ventricles constructed as a cone [222], neoventricle [221], and extra-aortic balloon assists [223] have been tried. Skeletal muscle conditioning has been accomplished by both neural stimulation [221] and multiphasic direct muscle stimulation with multiple leads and higher stimulation energies [224]. Most of the experimental studies have been modeled for augmenting impaired LV function. RV preparations have been studied in Stanford and Seattle with a view to reconstructing RV in congenital lesions characterized by deficiency of the ventricular mass (hypoplastic right heart) or where the ventricular mass is better utilized – at present times – for maintaining the systemic circulation, as in Fontan procedures. Gaines and associates [225] in Baltimore first reported the use of free grafts of gracilis with microvascular anastomosis to the internal mammary vessels to reconstruct the RV outflow tract in infant pigs. Recent developments in microchip electronics have contributed to the development of miniature implantable and synchronized pulse train (burst) stimulators for summating skeletal muscle contractions analogous to myocardial contractions.

In humans, the myocardial force in the cardiac wall required for generating the systolic arterial pressure is about 500 g/cm^2. This is much less than the typical skeletal muscle force of 2 kg/cm^2 [226]. Moreover, the skeletal muscle powered devices for augmentation of LV function need not necessarily be required to assume the entire LV function, but rather only a fraction of the entire cardiac output [223]. A skeletal muscle powered assist device that can generate 20%–25% of cardiac output may be adequately effective for circulatory assistance in most circumstances. In the human heart the RV is basically a bellows pump where the free wall contracts against a relatively less mobile septum. This is an efficient volume pump operating at a lower pressure. The LV is a muscular cone. The thickest part of its wall is at its widest part and the thinnest at its apex. The LV ejects by circumferential shortening around the short axis. This is a reciprocating pump operating at a higher pressure. Thus the requisites for biomechanical assistance of RV with conditioned skeletal muscle may be different from those for LV assistance.

Biomechanical assistance for circulation may be employed in one of four directions: (a) muscle patch enlargement with growth potential of the cardiac chamber, (b) dynamic cardiomyoplasty with contractile function for regional loss of myocardial mass, (c) counterpulsation or for powering cardiac assist devices, and (d) as an energy source for the TAHs.

In 1964 Kusserow and Clapp attempted to power biologically a blood pump [227]. They used quadriceps femoris to power a small spring-loaded unidirectional-flow diaphragm pump by repetitive nerve stimulation in four dogs and achieved an output of 600–720 ml/min with the pump rate of 60 per minute. Fifteen years later, Ugolini and associates applied the same concept [137, 228, 229]. First they used a linear setup with triceps tendon to generate 2 W/kg at 2 Hz motor nerve stimulation. The use of the conditioned psoas muscle as an energy source for fully implantable artificial hearts has also been conceptualized [136, 137].

The muscle grafts than can be used in cardioplasty may be classified as free, pedicled, or free graft with microvascular anastomoses that are innervated, denervated, paced, or unpaced. The vascularized graft poses little risk of infection and no potential for rejection. In time, it develops a smooth endothelial-like surface and does not develop pseudointimal overgrowth. It survives well in the ventricles, grows into the myocardium, and grows along with the changes in ventricular size. Carpentier and Chachques introduced the term "dynamic cardiomyoplasty" for cardiac reconstruction with skeletal muscles. There are three basic techniques for cardiomyoplasty: (a) full thickness excision of the myocardium and substitution myoplasty, (b) partial thickness excision of the myocardium, leaving intact endocardium, and (c) onlay reinforcement, leaving the myocardium completely intact. The advantages of a dynamic cardiomyoplasty [230] are:

1. Prevention of formation or recurrence of ventricular aneurysms
2. Prevention of cardiac rupture following ischemia, a frequent cause of sudden death
3. Prevention or correction of paradoxical movements in dyskinetic ischemic or dysplastic ventricular walls to improve cardiac output in fibrofatty dysplasia of ventricles, postinfarct ventricular wall hypokinesia, postinfarct VSD with apical infarct, etc.
4. By a less extended ventricular aneurysm resection, it allows a sizeable residual chamber to remain
5. Improvement of hemostasis and results of myocardial suture by application and suturing of a biological autologous tissue
6. Reinforcement or substitution of ventricular walls with a conditioned fatigue-resistant biocompatible skeletal muscle and a possible supplementary source of neovascularization for the heart. Applicable in Uhl's anomaly, Ebstein's

anomaly, Chaga's cardiomyopathy, and reconstruction of right or left ventricular outflow tracts
7. Increased atrial output in children undergoing atriopulmonary connections (Fontan/Kreutzer procedures) in tricuspid atresia or univentricular hearts.

A myriad of problems such as graft fibrosis, denervation atrophy, fibrotic electrical exit block, growth of the graft, blood-muscle interface, and thromboembolism will have to be solved before dynamic cardiomyoplasty can be evolved into a widely practised regular clinical modality. The present trend favors the use of LD muscle because of its location, mass, mode of neurovascular supply, noncritical function, and familiarity in other reconstructive procedures.

Clinical attempts at biomechanical assistance with skeletal muscles started in 1931 (Table 6). Early attempts primarily entailed the prosthetic use of skeletal

Table 6. Landmarks in biomechanical assistance

Year	Author(s)	Reference	Event
1931	Jesus	231	Skeletal muscle repair of human LV after trauma
1933	Leriche and Fontaine	201	Free muscle graft replacement of canine LV wall
1938	Griffith and Bates	232	Repair of iatrogenic hole in human RV with pedicled pectoralis after Beck's operation
1946	Weinstein et al.	202	Free graft replacement of canine LV
1948	Petrovsky	233	Proposed use of free or pedicled diaphragmatic graft to close cardiac wounds or aneurysms
1959	Kantrowitz and McKinnon	203	Stimulation of diaphragm pedicle wrap around the canine heart
1964	Kusserow and Clapp	227	Skeletal muscle powered blood pump
1964	Nakamura and Glenn	207	First report of hemodynamic efficacy of skeletal muscle graft
1966	Termet et al.	208	First proposal for using LD muscle
1966	Petrovsky	234	The largest clinical series of use of skeletal muscle on human heart
1967	Salomons et al.	213	Physiology of muscle transformation
1968	Shepherd et al.	204	Paced muscle graft enlargement of canine ventricle
1976	Kopytov	235	Free muscle graft patch replacement of partial thickness cardiac defects in humans
1979	Ugolini	228	Proposal for muscle-powered implantable TAH
1982	Macoviak et al.	220	First direct electrical conditioning of skeletal muscle
1982	Schaff et al.	236	Pectoralis flap repair of infected false aneurysm of LV
1985	Gaines et al.	225	Microvascular myocardioplasty of RV outflow tract in pigs
1985	Chiu's group	223	Extra-aortic balloon pump
1985	Chachques and Carpentier	237	First human dynamic cardiomyoplasty for cardiac tumor
1985	Magovern et al.	238	Dynamic cardiomyoplasty in human after LV aneurysm repair

muscles to repair traumatic injuries or to reinforce the repair of cardiac aneurysms. In 1966 Petrovsky [234] reported the largest clinical series (100 cases) of the use of skeletal muscle grafts on the heart. Kopytov in 1976 [235] reported the use of unpaced grafts of diaphragm and pericardium to close 2- to 4-cm ventricular defects. No aneurysm formation was noted but shrinkage and fibrosis were observed 1–4 months after surgery. Schaff et al. [236] extended the use of unpaced pectoralis major flaps to repair infected false aneurysms following repair of LV aneurysms with Teflon felt.

On 24 January 1985, Carpentier and Chachques [237] ushered in the clinical era of dynamic cardiomyoplasty. They removed at $28 \times 20 \times 10$ cm, 1.4-kg biventricular fibroma from a 37-year-old woman and reinforced the residual thin multiperforated posterior muscular wall of both ventricles with a pedicled left LD muscle graft brought into the thorax through a window created by resection of a 3-cm segment of the lateral arc of the second rib. Synchronous muscle graft stimulation was initiated from the 5th postoperative day. Postoperative 2D echocardiography showed a 31% increase in inferior wall motion. One year postoperatively heart scans showed an increase in ejection fraction from 53% to 62% with stimulation of LD muscle graft. Magovern and associates [238] similarly reported the use of paced LD muscle graft as a functioning segmental overlay in the repair of an LV aneurysm in a 45-year-old woman. They also had utilized the fibrous endocardial flap to circumvent the problem of blood–muscle interface and paced the muscle graft synchronously with the heart with a bipolar AV sequential Symbiosis pacer. At a 13-month follow-up with Doppler echocardiography and MUGA Tc-99 scan, this patient showed evidence of continuous function of the LD muscle graft. During exercise, ejection fraction improved from 28% to 48% with synchronous pacing of the graft. Interestingly, at rest there was no apparent difference, the ejection fraction remaining at approximately 42% [239]. Both in Paris and in Pittsburgh several patients have since been treated with dynamic cardiomyoplasty.

The modality of biomechanical assistance today stands at the threshold of wider clinical application and possibly in the coming decade will be employed in a larger share of cases in which assisted circulation is employed.

Epilogue

The global magnitude of the potential patient pool in need of circulatory asssistance is staggering. In the United States alone there are 2.3 million patients with chronic heart failure, with the annual addition of 400 000 new cases. The estimated number of patients likely to benefit from cardiac assist or replacement ranges from 35 000 per year according to the NIH to 165 000 per year according to the Heart Failure Study Group. About 15 000 patients per year can benefit from a heart transplantation. Every year 12 000–15 000 babies are born with congenital heart defects and a sizeable proportion of them may require some modality of assisted circulation. In Europe the annual mortality from end-stage ischemic heart disease ranges from 2000 to 4000 per million – making an annual loss of 1.27–2.5 million lives. In Argentina and Brazil nearly 2 million people suffer from a severe from of Chaga's cardiomyopathy for which no therapeutic alternative exists. About 15%–20% of the patients admitted for MI sustain functional loss of 40% or more of LV muscle mass, leading to a mortality of 65%–90%. The incidence of severe postcardiotomy failure requiring more profound assistance than IABP or pharmacological support is estimated to be 0.7% of all cases done on CPB. It is in this light that the need for the development of a cost-effective, patient-tailored modality of circulatory assistance is best appreciated.

To salvage the heart from the cruel chronology of age, ailments, and anomalies, the research has been long and diverse. The centers today are spread over all the continents. In an earlier era, the United States provided the pioneering leadership in technological developments and applications. Given the current stringency of FDA regulations in human applications, the soaring cost of product liability in the United States, and the growth of the technology base in Japan and Europe, perhaps the epicenter of the developments will move elsewhere. That may be irrelevant so long as the corporate and the geopolitical manipulations do not jeopardize the universal secularity of science and technology. In the final analysis, there lies a very sick cardiac patient for whom all these years of research and clinical experience must offer new hopes.

References

1. Kantrowitz A (1986) The spectrum. The ninth Hastings lecture. Artif Organs 10:497–510
2. LeGallois CJJ (1813) Experiences on the principle of life. Thomas, Philadelphia. Translation of: LeGallois CJJ (1812) Experiences sur le principe de la vie. Paris
3. DeBakey ME (1934) A simple continuous flow blood transfusion instrument. New Orleans Med Surg J 87:386–389
4. Dennis C (1979) Historical background. In: Unger F (ed) Assisted circulation. Springer, Berlin Heidelberg New York, pp 1–2
5. Dennis C, Hall DP, Moreno JR, Senning A (1962) Reduction of the oxygen utilisation of the heart by left heart bypass. Circ Res 10:298–305
6. Dennis C, Hall DP, Moreno JR, Senning A (1962) Left atrial cannulation without thoracotomy for total left heart bypass. Acta Chir Scand 123:267–279
7. Kantrowitz A, Krakauer J, Sherman JL (1968) A permanent mechanical auxiliary ventricle. J Cardiovasc Surg (Torino) 9:1
8. DeBakey ME (1971) Left ventricular bypass pump for cardiac assistance. Am J Cardiol 27:3–11
9. Moulopoulos SD, Topaz SR, Kolff WJ (1962) Extracorporeal assistance to the circulation and intraaortic balloon pumping. Trans Am Soc Artif Intern Organs 8:86–88
10. Kantrowitz A, Tjønneland S, Freed PS, Phillips SJ, Butner AN, Sherman JL (1968) Initial clinical experience with intraaortic balloon pumping in cardiogenic shock. JAMA 203:113–118
11. Liotta D, Hall CW, Walter SH, Cooley DA, Crawford ES, DeBakey ME (1963) Prolonged assisted circulation during and after cardiac and aortic surgery. Prolonged partial left ventricular bypass by means of intracorporeal circulation. Am J Cardiol 12:399–405
12. Hardy JD, Chavez CM (1968) The first heart transplant in man: developmental animal investigations with analysis of 1964 case in the light of current clinical experience. Am J Cardiol 22:772–781
13. Barnard CN (1968) Human cardiac transplantation. Am J Cardiol 22:584
14. Harken DE (1979) Counterpulsation: foundation and future. In: Unger F (ed) Assisted circulation. Springer, Berlin Heidelberg New York, pp 20–23
15. Ware RW, Hall CW, Fogwell JW, Gerlach CR, Schuhmann RE, Ross JR, DeBakey ME (1971) Inertial cardiac resistance. Trans Am Soc Artif Intern Organs 17:211–212

16. Soroff HS, Birtwell WC, Giron F, Collins JA, Deterling RA (1965) Support of systemic circulation and left ventricular assist by synchronous pulsation of extramural pressure. Surg Forum 16:148–150
17. Soroff HS, Cloutier CT, Birtwell WC, Begley LA, Messer JV (1974) External counterpulsation: management of cardiogenic shock after myocardial infarction. JAMA 229:1441–1450
18. Bregman D, Goetz RH (1971) Clinical experience with a new cardiac assist device – the dual chambered intraaortic balloon assist. J Thorac Cardiovasc Surg 62:577
19. Liotta D, Hall CW, Henly WS, Beall AC, Cooley DA, DeBakey ME (1963) Prolonged assisted circulation during and after heart or aortic surgery. Trans Am Soc Artif Intern Organs 9:182–185
20. Fasching W, Deutsch M, Enenkel W, Losert U, Stellwag F, Thoma H, Unger F, Wolner E, Polzer K, Navratil J (1974) A new concept in assisted circulation: the aortic windkessel-ventricle with balloon valve. Trans Am Soc Artif Intern Organs 3:22
21. Gradel F, Akutsu T, Chaptal PA, Kantrowitz A (1965) Successful hemodynamic results with a new U-shaped auxiliary ventricle. Trans Am Soc Artif Intern Organs 11:277–283
22. Unger F (1979) Introduction. In: Unger F (ed) Assisted circulation. Springer, Berlin Heidelberg New York, pp 15–19
23. Unger F (1979) Introduction. In: Unger F (ed) Assisted circulation. Springer, Berlin Heidelberg New York, pp 87–95
24. Bencini A, Parola LP (1956) The pneumomassage of the heart. Surgery 39:375
25. Callaghan PB, Chestnut MG, Watkins DH (1965) A computer-automated servomechanism for assisted circulation. Trans Am Soc Artif Intern Organs 11:36–42
26. Kantrowitz A, Krakauer JS, Zorzi G, Rubenfire M, Freed PS, Phillips S, Lipsius M, Titinec C, Jaron D (1971) Current status of intraaortic balloon pump and clinical experience with aortic patch mechanical auxiliary ventricle. Transplant Proc III 4:1459–1472
27. Shumakov V (1979) The state of assisted circulation in USSR. In: Unger F (ed) Assisted circulation 2. Springer, Berlin Heidelberg New York Tokyo, pp 67–70
28. Kolobow T, Bowman RL (1965) Biventricular cardiac assistance energised by suction actuated recoil of a single constricting rubber ventricle. Trans Am Soc Artif Intern Organs 12:57–64
29. Shumakov V (1978) International symposium on artificial heart and artificial kidney. Brno, 1978
30. Kantrowitz A, Wasfie T, Freed PS, Rubenfire M, Wajszuck W, Schosk MA (1986) Intraaortic balloon pumping 1967–1982: analysis of complications in 733 patients. Am J Cardiol 57:976–983
31. Bregman D, Casarella WJ (1980) Percutaneous intraaortic balloon pumping: initial clinical experience. Ann Thorac Surg 29:153–155
32. Symbas PN, McKeown PP, Santora AH, Vlasis SE (1985) Pulmonary artery balloon counterpulsation for treatment of intraoperative right ventricular failure. Ann Thorac Surg 39:437–440
33. Pencock JL, Pierce WS, Wisman CB, Bull AP, Waldhausen JA (1983) Survival and complication following ventricular assist pumping for cardiogenic shock. Ann Surg 198:469–478
34. Rose DM, Lascinger J, Grossi E, Krieger KH, Cunningham JN, Spencer FC (1985) Experimental and clinical results with a simplified left heart assist device for treatment of profound left ventricular dysfunction. World J Surg 9:11–17
35. Litwak RS, Koffsky RM, Juardo RA, Mitchell BA, King P (1985) A decade of experience with a left heart assist device in patients undergoing open intracardiac operation. World J Surg 9:18–24
36. Magovern GJ, Park SB, Maher TD (1985) Use of a centrifugal pump without anticoagulants for postoperative left ventricular assist. World J Surg 9:25–36
37. Pennington DC, Samuels LD, Williams G, Palmer D, Schwartz MT, Codd JE, Merjavy JP, Lagunoff D, Joist HC (1985) Experience with the Pierce-Donachy ventricular assist device in postcardiotomy patients with cardiogenic shock. World J Surg 9:37–46
38. Unger F (1979) Introduction. Left ventricular assist devices. In: Unger F (ed) Assisted circulation. Springer, Berlin Heidelberg New York, pp 87–95

39. O'Neill MJ, Pierce WS, Wisman CB, Osbakken MD, Parr GVS, Waldhausen JA (1984) Successful management of right ventricular failure with the ventricular assist pump following aortic valve replacement and coronary bypass grafting. J Thorac Cardiovasc Surg 87:106–111

40. Taguchi K, Murashita J, Nakagaki M, Mochizuki T (1980) Transapical left ventricular bypass with local heparinisation for prolonged circulatory support. World J Surg 4:251

41. Bernhard WF, LaFarge CG, Carr JG, Keiser JT (1979) A left ventricular aortic blood pump for circulatory support in postoperative patients with acute left ventricular failure. In: Unger F (ed) Assisted circulation. Springer, Berlin Heidelberg New York, pp 96–106

42. Norman JC (1976) An intracorporeal abdominal left ventricular assist device (A-LVAD): clinical readiness and initial trials in man. Cardiovasc Dis Bull Tex Heart Inst 3:249–288

43. Oyer PE, Stinson EB, Portner PM, Ream AK, Shumway NE (1980) Development of a totally implantable electrically actuated left ventricular assist system. Am J Surg 140:17

44. Washizu T, Whalen R, Morinaga N, Harasaki H, Tsushima N, Ouchi K, Hayashi K, Snow J, Sukalac R, Jacobs G, Kiraly R, Nosé Y (1977) Parathoracic left ventricular assist device. Trans Am Soc Artif Intern Organs 23:301–308

45. Peters JL, McRea JC, Fukumasu H, Mochizuki T, Daitoh N, McGough E, Pearce M, Fee H, Rich G (1980) Recovery of cardiac function with total transapical left ventricular bypass. Trans Am Soc Artif Intern Organs 26:262–267

46. Deutsch M (1979) The ellipsoid left ventricular assist device: experimental and clinical results. In: Unger F (ed) Assisted circulation. Springer, Berlin Heidelberg New York, pp 127–137

47. Olsen EK, Pierce WS, Donachy JH, Landis DL, Rosenberg G, Phillips WM, Prophet GA, O'Neill MJ, Waldhausen JA (1979) A two and one half years clinical experience with a mechanical left ventricular assist pump in the treatment of profound postoperative failure. Int J Artif Organs 2:197–206

48. Zwart HH, Kralios AC, Kwan-Gett CS, Backman DK, Foote FM, Schoemaker F, Kolff WJ (1970) First clinical application of transarterial closed-chest left ventricular (TaCLV) bypass. Trans Am Soc Artif Intern Organs 16:386–391

49. Norman JC (1981) Mechanical ventricular assistance: a review. Artif Organs 5:103–117

50. Golding LR, Groves LK, Peter M, Jacob G, Sukalac R, Nosé Y, Loop FD (1980) Initial clinical experience with a new temporary left ventricular assist device. Ann Thorac Surg 29:66–69

51. Litwak RS, Koffsky RM, Juardo RA, Lubkan SB, Oritz AF, Fischer AP, Sherman JJ, Silvay G, Lajam FA (1976) Use of a left heart assist device after intracardiac surgery: technique and clinical experience. Ann Thorac Surg 21:191–202

52. Dennis C, Carlens E, Senning A, Hall DP, Moreno JR, Cappelletti RR, Weslowski SA (1962) Clinical use of a cannula for left heart bypass without thoracotomy. Ann Surg 156:623–637

53. Turina MT, Bosio R, Senning A (1978) Paracorporeal artificial heart in postoperative heart failure. Artif Organs 2:273–276

54. Pennington DG, Mejavy JP, Swartz MT, Codd JE, Barner HB, Lagunoff D, Bashiti H, Kaiser GC, Willman VL (1985) The importance of biventricular failure in patients with postoperative cardiogenic shock. Ann Thorac Surg 39:16–27

55. Lefemine AA, Dunbar J, DeLucia A (1986) Concepts in assisted circulation. Tex Heart Inst J 13:23–37

56. Pierce WS (1985) Letter (Reply). Ann Thorac Surg 40:524

57. Schuhmann RE, Geddes LA, Hoff HE (1970) Prolonged left ventricular bypass by a transvalvular aortic catheterisation. I. Physiologic effects and rationale of surgical concept. Surgery 67:957–968

58. Zwart HH, Kralios AC, Eastwood N, Kolff WJ (1972) Effects of partial and complete unloading of the failing left ventricle by transarterial left heart bypass. J Thorac Cardiovasc Surg 63:856–872

59. Lefemine AA (1977) Left ventricular bypass: an experimental and clinical experience. Trans Am Soc Artif Intern Organs 23:326–330

60. Bernhard WF, Berger RL, Stetz JP, Carr JG, Colo NA, McCormick JR, Fishbein MC (1979) Temporary left ventricular bypass: factors affecting patient survival. Circulation 60:131–141

61. Pae WE, Rosenberg G, Donachy JH, Landis DL, Phillips WM, Parr GV, Prophet GA, Pierce WS (1980) Mechanical circulatory assistance for postoperative cardiogenic shock: a three year experience. Trans Am Soc Artif Intern Organs 26:256–261
62. Cooley DA (1987) Development of roller pump for use in the cardiopulmonary bypass circuit. Texas Heart Inst J 14:113–118
63. von Frey M, Graber M (1885) Untersuchungen über den Stoffwechsel isolierter Organe. Ein Respirationsapparat für isolierte Organe. Virchows Arch Physic 9:519
64. Jacobi C (1895) Ein Beitrag zur Technik der künstlichen Durchblutung überlebender Organe. Arch Exp Pathol Pharmakol 36:330–348
65. Brodie TC (1903) The perfusion of surviving organs. J Physiol 29:266–275
66. Embly EH, Martin CJ (1905) The action of anaesthetic quantities chloroform upon the blood vessels of the bowel and kidney with an account of an artificial circulation apparatus. J Physiol (Lond) 32:147–158
67. Richards AN, Drinker CK (1915) An apparatus for the perfusion of isolated organs. J Pharmacol Exp Ther 7:467–483
68. Hooker DR (1910) A study of isolated kidney: the influence of pulse pressure upon renal function. Am J Physiol 27:24–44
69. Dixon WE (1922) A simple perfusion pump. J Physiol (Lond) 56:Proc XL–XLII
70. Dale HH, Shuster EHJ (1928) A double perfusion pump. J Physiol (Lond) 64:356–364
71. Gibbs OS (1930) An aritificial heart. J Pharmacol Exp Ther 38:197–215
72. Van Allen CM (1932) A pump for clinical and laboratory purposes which employs the milking principle. JAMA 98:1805–1806
73. Barcroft H (1933) Observations on the pumping action of the heart. J Physiol (Lond) 78:186–195
74. Lindberg CA (1935) An apparatus for the culture of whole organs. J Exp Med 62:409–432
75. Gibbon JH (1937) Artificial maintenance of circulation during experimental occlusion of the pulmonary artery. Arch Surg 34:1105–1131
76. Bjork VO (1948) Brain perfusion in dogs with artificially oxygenated blood. Acta Chir Scand (Suppl 137) 96:1–122
77. Sewell WH, Glenn WWL (1950) Experimental cardiac surgery. Surgery 28:474–494
78. Gibbon JH (1954) Application of a mechanical heart and lung apparatus to cardiac surgery. Minn Med 37:171
79. Stuckey JH, Newman MM, Dennis C, Burg EH, Goodman SE, Fries CC, Karlson KE, Blumenfield M, Weitzner SW, Binder LS, Winston A (1957) The use of the heart-lung machine in selected cases of acute massive myocardial infarction. Surg Forum 3:342–344
80. Kusserow BK (1958) A permanently indwelling intracorporeal blood pump to substitute for cardiac function. Trans Am Soc Artif Intern Organs 4:227
81. Saxton GA, Andrews CB (1960) An ideal heart pump with hydrodynamic characteristics analogous to the mammalian heart. Trans Am Soc Artif Intern Organs 6:288–291
82. Norman JC, Cooley DA, Kahan BD, Keats AS, Massin EK, Solis RT, Luper WE, Brook MI, Klima T, Frazier OH, Hacker J, Duncan JM, Dasco CC, Winston DS, Reul GH (1978) Total support of the circulation of a patient with postcardiotomy stone heart syndrome by a partial artificial heart (ALVAD) for 5 days followed by heart and kidney transplantation. Lancet 1:1125–1127
83. Richenbacher WE, Wisman WE, Rosenberg G, Donachy JH, Landis DL, Pierce WS (1984) Ventricular assistance: clinical experience at the Pennsylvania State University. In: Unger F (ed) Assisted circulation 2. Springer, Berlin Heidelberg New York Tokyo, pp 70–84
84. Zumbro GL, Kitchen WR, Galloway RF (1985) Mechanical assistance for biventricular failure following coronary bypass operations and heart transplantation. Heart Transplant 4:348–352
85. Norman JC (1977) Intracorporeal partial artificial hearts: initial results in ten patients. Artif Organs 1:41–52
86. Unger F (1986) Current status and use of artificial hearts and circulatory assist devices. Perfusion 1:155–163
87. Cooley DA (1984) Staged cardiac replacement: clinical experience at the Texas Heart Institute. In: Unger F (ed) Assisted circulation 2. Springer, Berlin Heidelberg New York Tokyo, pp 186–196

88. McGee MG, Zillgitt SL, Trono SA, Davis Gl, Fuqua JM, Edelman SK, Norman JC (1980) Retrospective analyses of the need for mechanical circulatory support (intraaortic balloon pump/abdominal left left ventricular assist devices or partial artificial heart) following cardiopulmonary bypass: a 44-month study of 14 168 patients. Am J Cardiol 46:135

89. Harashaki HK, Zheng Z, Morimoto T, McMohon J, Golding L, Nosé Y (1985) Morphometric studies of chronic fibrillating heart. Trans Am Soc Artif Intern Organs 31:73–78

90. Pae WE, Pierce WS (1986) Combined registry for the clinical use of mechanical ventricular assist pumps and the total artificial heart. Heart Transplant 5:6–7

91. Losman JG, Replogle RL, Kolff WJ (1982) An alternative to the orthotopic artificial heart: a point of view. Artif Organs 6:319–324

92. Shumakov VI (1975) Iskusstvennoje serdce. Moscow, Izd Znanie

93. Akutsu T, Kolff WJ (1958) Permanent substitutes for valves and heart. Trans Am Soc Artif Intern Organs 4:230–235

94. Kolff WJ, Akutsu T, Dreyer B, Norton H (1959) Artificial hearts in the chest and the use of polyurethane for making hearts, valves and aortas. Trans Am Soc Artif Intern Organs 5:298–300

95. Freebairn D, Heggs T (1964) Solenoid design for a prosthetic heart. Trans Am Soc Artif Intern Organs 10:166–170

96. Akutsu T, Houston CS, Kolff WJ (1960) Artificial hearts inside the chest using small electromotors. Trans Am Soc Artif Intern Organs 6:299–302

97. Atsumi K, Hori M, Ikeda S, Sakurai Y, Fujimori Y, Kimoto S (1963) Artificial heart incorporated in the chest. Trans Am Soc Artif Intern Organs 9:292–298

98. Liotta D, Taliani T, Giffoniello AH, Dehaza FS, Liotta S, Lizarraga R, Tolocka L, Pananao J, Bianciotti E (1961) Artificial heart in the chest: preliminary report. Trans Am Soc Artif Intern Organs 7:318–322

99. Houston CS, Akutsu T, Kolff WJ (1960) Pendulum types of artificial heart within the chest. Preliminary report. Am Heart J 59:723

100. Hastings FW, Potter WH, Holter JW (1961) Artificial intracorporeal heart. Trans Am Soc Artif Intern Organs 7:323–326

101. Burns WH, Loubier R, Bergstedt R (1965) The development of an electrohydraulic implantable artificial heart. Trans Am Soc Artif Intern Organs 11:265–268

102. Loehr ML, Kosch WF, Singer M, Pierce WS, Kirby CK (1964) The piezoelectric artificial heart. Trans Am Soc Artif Intern Organs 10:147–150

103. Pierce WS, Burney RG, Boyer MH, Driskoll RW, Kirby CK (1962) Problems encountered in experiments during the development of our artificial intrathoracic heart. Trans Am Soc Artif Intern Organs 8:118–122

104. Seidel W, Akutsu T, Mirkovitch V, Brown F, Kolff WJ (1961) Air-driven artificial hearts inside the chest. Trans Am Soc Artif Intern Organs 7:378–385

105. Akutsu T, Mirkovitch V, Topaz SR, Kolff WJ (1963) Silastic type of artificial heart and its use in calves. Trans Am Soc Artif Intern Organs 9:281–285

106. Nosé Y, Sarin CL, Klain M, Leitz KH, Tesny TJ, Phillips PM, Rose FL, Kolff WJ (1966) Elimination of some problems encountered in total replacement of the heart with an intrathoracic mechanical pump: venous return. Trans Am Soc Artif Intern Organs 12:301–311

107. Akutsu T, Takano H, Takagi H, Turner MD, Henson EC, Crowell JW (1972) Pathophysiology and new problems in total artificial heart. J Thorac Cardiovasc Surg 64:762–771

108. Hershgold EJ, Kwan-Gett CS, Kawai J, Rowley K (1972) Hemostasis, coagulation and the total artificial heart. Trans Am Soc Artif Intern Organs 18:181–185

109. Atsumi K, Fujimasa I, Imachi K, Nakajima M, Tsukagoshi S, Mabuchi K, Motomura K, Kuono A, Ono T, Miyamoto A, Takido N, Inou N (1985) Longterm substitution with an artificial heart in goats. Trans Am Soc Artif Intern Organs 8:155–165

110. Kambic H, Barenburg S, Harasaki H, Gibbons D, Kiraly R, Nosé Y (1978) Glutaraldehyde-protein complexes as blood-compatible coatings. Trans Am Soc Artif Intern Organs 24:426–438

111. Imai Y, Tajima K, Nosé Y (1971) Biolised materials for cardiovascular prosthesis. Trans Am Soc Artif Intern Organs 17:6–9

112. Harasaki H, Gerrity R, Kiraly R, Jacobs G, Nosé Y (1979) Calcification in blood pumps. Trans Am Soc Artif Intern Organs 25:305–310

113. Pierce WS, Donachy JH, Rosenberg G, Baier E (1980) Calcification: inhibition by warfarin-sodium. Science 208:601–603
114. Jarvik RK, Kessler TR, McGill LD, McGill DB, Olsen DB, DeVries WC, Deneris J, Blaylock JT, Kolff WJ (1981) Determinants of pannus formation in long-surviving artificial heart calves and its prevention. Trans Am Soc Artif Intern Organs 27:90–96
115. Levinson MM, Smith RG, Cork RC, Gallo J, Emery RW, Icenogle TB, Ott RA, Burns GL, Copeland JG (1986) Thromboembolic complications of Jarvik 7 total artificial heart: case report. Artif Organs 10:236–244
116. Heimes HP, Klasen F (1982) Completely integrated wearable TAH-drive unit. Int J Artif Organs 5:157–159
117. Affeld K, Frank J, Baer P, Bücherl ES (1978) A new portable driving unit for implantable blood pumps. Trans Am Soc Artif Intern Organs 24:600–605
118. Kwan-Gett CS, Wu Y, Collan R, Jacobsen S, Kolff WJ (1969) Total replacement artificial heart and driving system with inherent regulation of cardiac output. Trans Am Soc Artif Intern Organs 15:245–250
119. Landis DL, Rosenberg G, Donachy H, Pierce WS (1980) Automatic control for the artificial heart. In: IEEE Frontiers of engineering in health care, pp 305–310
120. Henning C, Grosse-Siestrup C, Krantznerger W, Kless H, Bücherl ES (1978) The relationship of cardiac output and venous pressure in long surviving calves with total artificial hearts. Trans Am Soc Artif Intern Organs 24:616–624
121. Thoma H (1984) Drive and management of circulation support system. In: Unger F (ed) Assisted circulation 2. Springer, Berlin Heidelberg New York Tokyo, pp 339–366
122. DeVries WC, Anderson JL, Joyce LD, Anderson FL, Hammond EL, Jarvik RK, Kolff WJ (1984) Clinical use of the total artificial heart. N Engl J Med 310:273–278
123. Kolff WJ (1988) Experiences and practical considerations for the future of artificial hearts and of mankind: the 10th Hastings lecture, 1986. Artif Organs 12:89–111
124. Hahn C (1985) Replacement of the heart. Heart Transplant 4:494–495
125. Schuder JC, Owens J, Stephenson H, Mackenzie J (1968) Response of dogs and mice to longterm exposure to the electromagnetic field required to power an artificial heart. Trans Am Soc Artif Intern Organs 14:291–295
126. Kantrowitz A, Altieri F, Beall A, Blackshear PL, Goldenberg N, Gorlin R et al. (1976) ERDA artificial heart program workshop. US Energy Research and Development Administration
127. Cole DW, Holman WS, Mott WE (1973) Status of the USAEC's nuclear powered artificial heart. Trans Am Soc Artif Intern Organs 19:537–541
128. (1973) The totally implantable artificial heart: economic, legal, medical, psychiatric and social implications. Washington DC Government Printing Office. (DHEW publication No NIH 74–191)
129. Bevilacqua S, Famulari A, Cucchiara G, Cortesini R (1975) Electrically driven nuclear artificial heart. II Congress of the ESAO, Berlin, 1975
130. Cortesini R, Cucchiara G (1979) Total artificial heart replacement with consecutive heart transplantation. In: Unger F (ed) Assisted circulation. Springer, Berlin Heidelberg New York, pp 385–393
131. Rosenberg G, Snyder AJ, Landis DL, Geslowitz DB, Donachy JH, Pierce WS (1984) An electric motor-driven total artificial heart: seven months survival in the calf. Trans Am Soc Artif Intern Organs 30:69–73
132. Jufer M (1985) A totally implantable electrical heart. Heart Transplant 4:496–498
133. Jarvik RK (1981) The total artificial heart. Sci Am 244:74–80
134. Nosé Y (1986) Totally implantable artificial organ: cardiac prosthesis. Artif Organs 10:102–113
135. Atsumi K, Fujimasa I, Imachi K, Mabuchi K, Maeda K, Abe Y, Chinzei T (1987) Fundamental studies on implantable total artificial heart in University of Tokyo. Abstracts, p 40. International meeting on heart transplantation, total artificial heart and assist devices. Brussels, 1987
136. Frey M, Thoma H, Gruber H, Stöhr H, Havel M (1986) The chronically stimulated psoas muscle as an energy source for artificial organs: an experimental study in sheep. In: Chiu RCJ (ed) Biomechanical cardiac assist. Futura, Mount Kisco, NY, pp 179–191

137. Ugolini F (1986) Skeletal muscle for artificial heart drive: theory and in vivo experiments. In: Chiu RCJ (ed) Biomechanical cardiac assist. Futura, Mount Kisco NY, pp 193–210
138. Pierce WS, Morris L, Gardiner BN, Burney RG, Leppik I, Madmud L, Danielson GK (1965) Experimental use of a single mechanical ventricle to replace the dog's heart. Trans Am Soc Artif Intern Organs 11:271–276
139. Frazier OH, Colon R, Taenaka Y, Igo S, Fuqua J (1986) Replacement of the left ventricle with a single-chambered artificial pump. J Heart Transplant 5:286–290
140. Cooley DA, Liotta D, Hallman GL, Bloodwell RD, Leachman RD, Millam JD (1969) Orthotopic cardiac prosthesis for two staged cardiac replacement. Am J Cardiol 24:723–730
141. Cooley DA, Akutsu T, Norman JC, Serrato MA, Frazier OH (1981) Total artificial heart in two staged cardiac transplantation. Cardiovasc Dis Bull Texas Heart Inst 8:305–319
142. Vaughn CC, Copeland JG, Cheng K, Austin J, Levinson M, Emery RW (1986) Interim cardiac replacement with a mechanical heart: staged cardiac transplantation. Texas Heart Inst J 13:45–52
143. Emery RW, Levinson MM, Icenogle TB, Carrier M, Ott RA, Copeland J, McAller-Rhenman MJ, Nicholson SM (1987) Selection of patients for cardiac transplantation. Circulation 75:2–9
144. Unger F, Chmelizek F, Jungwirth W, Koller I, Laczkovics A, Lehner I, Lexer G, Olsen DB, Pohla G, Schistek R, Wolner E (1988) Artificial heart and cardiac transplantation: report on the first European combined procedure. Artif Organs 12:51–55
145. McKenzie FN, Menkis AH, Grant DR, Keown PA, Stiller CR, Kostuk WJ (1986) Bridge to heart transplantation: the biologic option. J Heart Transplant 5:365
146. Frazier OH, Colon R, Taenaka Y (1986) Surgical technique and hemodynamic characteristics of partial cardiac replacement with an artificial left ventricle. Texas Heart Inst J 13:345–351
147. Reemtsma K, Drusin R, Edie R, Bregman D, Dobelle W, Hardy M (1978) Cardiac transplantation for patients requiring mechanical circulatory support. N Engl J Med 298:670–671
148. Peric M, Frazier OH, Marcis M, Radovancevic B (1986) Intraaortic balloon pumping as a bridge to transplantation. J Heart Transplant 5:380
149. Zumbro GL, Kitchens WR, Galloway RF (1986) Mechanical assistance for bridging to heart transplantation and support of the failing transplanted heart. J Heart Transplant 5:382
150. Magovern JA, Pennock JL, Campbell DE, Pae WE, Pierce WS, Waldhausen JA (1986) Bridge to heart transplantation: the Penn State experience. J Heart Transplant 5:196–202
151. Pennington DG, Codd JE, Merjavy JP, Swartz MT, Kaiser GC, Barner HB, Willman VL (1983) The expanded use of ventricular bypass systems for severe cardiac failure and as a bridge to cardiac transplantations. Heart Transplant 3:38–46
152. Baily LL (1987) Biologic versus bionic heart substitutes: will xenotransplantation play a role? Trans Am Soc Artif Intern Organs 33:51–53
153. Levinson MM, Smith RG, Copeland JG, Icenogle TI (1987) Patient selection in early human temporary artificial heart experience. Abstracts, p 36. International meeting on heart transplantation, total artificial heart and assist devices. Brussels, 1987
154. Carrel A, Guthrie CC (1905) The transplantation of veins and organs. Am Med 10:1101
155. Mann FC, Priestlay JT, Markowits J, Yater W (1933) Transplantation of the intact mammalian heart. Arch Surg 26:219–224
156. Demikhov VP (1962) Some essential points of the techniques of transplantation of the heart, lungs and other organs. In: Experimental transplantation of vital organs. Medgiz State Press for Medical Literature, Moscow, pp 29–48
157. Sayegh SF, Creech O (1957) Transplantation of the homologous canine heart. J Thorac Surg 34:692
158. Webb WR, Howard HS (1957) Cardiopulmonary transplantation: restoration of function of the refrigerated heart. Surg Forum 8:313–317
159. Goldberg M, Berman EF, Akman OC (1958) Homologous transplantation of the canine heart. J Int Coll Surg 30:575–586
160. Cass MH, Brock R (1959) Heart excision and replacement. Guy's Hosp Rep 108:285–290

161. Lower RR, Shumway NE (1960) Studies on the orthotopic homotransplantation of the canine heart. Surg Forum 11:18–19
162. Reemtsma K, Williamson WE, Iglesias F, Pena E, Sayegh SF, Creech O (1962) Studies in homologous canine heart transplantation: prolongation of survival with a folic acid antagonist. Surgery 52:127
163. Hardy JD, Chavez CM, Kurrus FD, Neely WA, Eraslan S, Turner MD, Fabian LW, Labecki TD (1964) Heart transplantation in man: developmental studies and report of a case. JAMA 188:1132–1140
164. Griepp RB, Ergin MA (1984) The history of experimental heart transplantation. Heart Transplant 3:145–151
165. Barnard CN (1967) The operation: a human cardiac transplantation. An interim report of the successful operation performed at Groote Schuur Hospital. S Afr Med J 41:1271–1274
166. Cooley DA, Bloodwell RD, Hallman GL, Nora JJ, Harrison GM, Leachmen RD (1969) Organ transplantation for advanced cardiopulmonary disease. Ann Thorac Surg 8:30–46
167. Castaneda AR, Arnar O, Schmidt-Habelman P, Moller JH, Zamora R (1972) Cardiopulmonary autotransplantation in primates. J Cardiovasc Surg (Torino) 37:523
168. Marcial MB, Armelin E, Stolf N, Piantino PC, Marcuz R, Verginelli G, Zerbini EJ (1972) Assisted circulation with an auxiliary heart transplant. J Thorac Cardiovasc Surg 63:696
169. Caves PK, Stinson EB, Graham AE, Billingham ME, Grehl TM, Shumway NE (1973) Percutaneous transvenous endomyocardial biopsy. JAMA 225:288–291
170. Barnard CN, Losman JG (1975) Left ventricular bypass. S Afr Med J 49:303–312
171. Barnard CN, Wolpowitz A, Losman JG (1977) Heterotopic cardiac transplantation with a xenograft for assistance of the left heart in cardiogenic shock after cardiopulmonary bypass. S Afr Med J 52:1035–1038
172. Pennock JL, Oyer PE, Reitz BA, Jamieson SW, Bieber CP, Wallwork J, Stinson EB, Shumway NE (1982) Cardiac transplantation in perspective for the future: survival, complications, rehabilitation and costs. J Thorac Cardiovasc Surg 83:168–177
173. Bailey LL, Nehlsen-Cannarella SL, Concepcion W, Jolley WB (1985) Baboon-to-human cardiac xenotransplantation in a neonate. JAMA 254:3321–3329
174. Marcus E, Wong SNT, Luisada AA (1951) Homologous heart grafts: transplantation of the heart in dogs. Surg Forum 2:212–217
175. Wesolowski SA, Fennessey JF (1953) Pattern of failure of the homografted canine heart. Circulation 8:750
176. Downie HG (1953) Homotransplantation of the dog heart. AMA Arch Surg 66:624–636
177. Marcus E, Wong SNT, Luisada AA (1953) Homologous heart grafts. I. Technique of interim peribiotic perfusion. II. Transplantation of the heart in dogs. AMA Arch Surg 66:179
178. Webb WR, Howard HS, Neely WA (1959) Practical method of homologous cardiac transplantation. J Thorac Surg 37:361–366
179. Demikhov VP (1962) Experimental transplantation of vital organs. Consultants' Bureau, New York, pp 49, 126
180. Neptune WB, Cookson BA, Bailey CP, Appler R, Rajkowski F (1953) Complete homologous heart transplantation. AMA Arch Surg 66:174
181. Blanco G, Adam A, Rodriques-Perez D, Fernandes A (1958) Complete homotransplantation of a canine heart and lungs. AMA Arch Surg 76:20
182. Lower RR, Stofer RC, Hurley EJ, Shumway NE (1961) Complete homograft replacement of the heart and both lungs. Surgery 50:842–845
183. Lower RR, Stofer RC, Shumway NE (1961) Homovital transplantation of the heart. J Thorac Cardiovasc Surg 41:196–204
184. Kondo Y, Gradel FO, Chaptal P, Meier W, Cottle HR, Kantrowitz A (1965) Immediate and delayed orthotopic homotransplantation of the heart. J Thorac Cardiovasc Surg 50:781–791
185. Kondo Y, Gradel F, Kantrowitz A (1965) Heart homotransplantation in puppies: long survival without immunosuppressive therapy. Circulation 31 (Suppl 1):1181–1187
186. Sen PK, Parulkar GB, Panday SR, Kinare SG (1965) Homologous canine heart transplantation: a preliminary report of 100 experiments. Ind J Med Res 53:674

187. McGough EC, Brewer PL, Reemtsma K (1966) The parallel heart: studies on intrathoracic auxiliary cardiac transplants. Surgery 60:153
188. Barrie J, Latreille R, Vadot L, Grunwald D, Miguet B (1966) Transplantation heterotopique d'un coeur auxillaire. Ann Chir Thorac Cardiovasc 5:256
189. Johansson L, Soderlund S, William-Olsson G (1967) Left heart bypass by means of a transplanted heart: a preliminary report. Scand J Thorac Cardiovasc Surg 1:23
190. Kantrowitz A, Haller JD, Joos H, Cerruti MM, Carstensen HE (1968) Transplantation of the heart in an infant and an adult. Am J Cardiol 22:782–790
191. Jamieson SW, Stinson EB (1984) Heart-lung transplantation. In: Unger F (ed) Assisted circulation 2. Springer, Berlin Heidelberg New York, pp 298–306
192. Suros J, Woods JE (1973) A synchronised intrathoracic auxiliary heart transplant in parallel. J Thorac Cardiovasc Surg 65:415–424
193. Cooper DKC, Barnard CN (1984) Clinical application of implanted natural auxiliary hearts. In: Unger F (ed) Assisted circulation 2. Springer, Berlin Heidelberg New York Tokyo, pp 307–318
194. Solis E, Kaye MP (1986) The registry of the International society for heart transplantation: third official report – June 1986. J Heart Transplant 5:2–5
195. Nitkin RS, Hunt SA, Schroeder JS (1985) Accelerated atherosclerosis in a cardiac transplant patient. J Am Coll Cardiol 6:243
196. Allen MD, Naasz C, Popp RL, Hunt SA, Garis ML, Oyer PL, Stinson EB (1987) Noninvasive assessment of donor and native heart function after heterotopic heart transplantation. Abstracts, p 32. International meeting on heart transplantation, total artificial heart and assist devices. Brussels, 1987
197. Cham B, Bossuyt A, DeWilde P, Taeymans Y, Block P, Jonckheer MH, Welch W (1987) Scintigraphic followup of patients with a heterotopic heart transplant. Abstracts, p 33. International meeting on heart transplantation, total artificial heart and assist devices. ISAO, Brussels, 1987
198. Pennington DG, Sarafian J, Swartz M (1985) Heart transplantation in children. Heart Transplant 4:441–445
199. Cabasson J, Blanc WA, Joos HA (1969) The anencephalic infant as a possible donor for cardiac transplantation. Clin Pediatr 8:86–89
200. Cooley DA, Hallman GL, Bloodwell RD (1968) Human heart transplantation. Am J Cardiol 22:804–810
201. Leriche R, Fontaine R (1933) Essai experimental de traitment de certains infarctus du myocarde et de l'aneurisme du coeur par une greffe de muscle strie. Bull Soc Nat Chir 59:229
202. Weinstein M, Shafiroff BG (1946) Grafts of free muscle transplants upon the myocardium. Science 104:410
203. Kantrowitz A, McKinnon WMP (1959) The experimental use of the diaphragm as an auxiliary myocardium. Surg Forum 9:266–268
204. Shepherd MP, Tamaki H, Mustard WT (1968) Experimental study of the paced denervated diaphragmatic pedicle graft. Br J Surg 55:91
205. Shepherd MP (1969) Diaphragmatic muscle and cardiac surgery. Ann R Coll Surg Engl 45:212–231
206. Phillips WL, Pallin S, Crastnopol P (1969) Diaphragm transplantation. Angiology 20:628
207. Nakamura K, Glenn WWL (1964) Graft of the diaphragm as a functioning substitute for the myocardium. J Surg Res 4:435–439
208. Termet H, Chalencon JL, Estour F (1966) Transplantation sur le myocarde d'un muscle strie exciete par pacemaker. Ann Chir Thorac Cardiovasc 5:260–263
209. Kusaba E, Schraut W, Satwatani S, Jaron D, Freed P, Kantrowitz A (1973) A diaphragmatic graft for augmenting left ventricular function: a feasibility study. Trans Am Soc Artif Intern Organs 19:251–257
210. Spotnitz HM, Merker C, Malm JR (1974) Applied physiology of the canine rectus abdominis: force-length curves correlated with functional characteristics of a rectus powered "ventricle": potential for cardiac assistance. Trans Am Soc Artif Intern Organs 20:747–755
211. von Recum A, Stulc JP, Hamada O, Baba H, Kantrowitz A (1977) Long-term stimulation of a diaphragm muscle pouch. J Surg Res 23:422–427

212. Vachon BR, Kunov H, Zingg W (1975) Mechanical properties of diaphragm muscle in dogs. Med Biol Eng Comput 13:252–260
213. Salomons S, Sreter F (1967) Significance of impulse activity in transformation of skeletal muscle type. Nature 263:30–34
214. Salomons S, Vroba G (1969) The influence of activity on some contractile characteristics of mammalian fast and slow muscle. J Physiol (Lond) 210:535–549
215. Salomons S, Henriksson J (1981) The adaptive response of skeletal muscle to increased use. Muscle Nerve 4:94–105
216. Katz A (1972) Contractile proteins in normal and failing myocardium. Hosp Pract 7:10
217. Van Winkle WB, Entman ML (1979) Comparative aspects of cardiac and skeletal muscle sarcoplasmic reticulum. Life Sci 25:1189
218. Lutz H, Weber H, Billeter R, Jenny E (1979) Fast and slow myosin within single skeletal muscle fibers of adult rabbits. Nature 281:142
219. Macoviak JA, Stephenson LW, Alavi A, Kelly AM, Edmunds LH (1981) Effect of electrical stimulation on diaphragmatic muscle used to enlarge right ventricle. Surgery 90:271–277
220. Macoviak JA, Stephenson LW, Armenti F, Kelly AM, Alavi A, Mackler T, Cox J, Palatianos GM, Edmunds LH (1982) Electrical conditioning of in situ skeletal muscle for replacement of myocardium. J Surg Res 34:429–439
221. Macoviak JA, Stinson EB, Starkey TD, Hansen DE, Cahill PD, Miller DC, Shumway NE (1987) Myoventriculoplasty and neoventricle myograft cardiac augmentation to establish pulmonary blood flow. J Thorac Cardiovasc Surg 93:212–220
222. Acker MA, Hammond RL, Mannion JD, Salomons S, Stephenson LW (1986) An autologous biologic pump motor. J Thorac Cardiovasc Surg 92:733–746
223. Neilson IR, Brister SJ, Khalafalla AS, Chiu RC (1985) Left ventricular assistance in dogs using a skeletal muscle powered device for diastolic augmentation. Heart Transplant 4:343–347
224. Dewar ML, Drinkwater DC, Wittnich C, Chiu RCJ (1984) Synchronously stimulated skeletal muscle graft for myocardial repair. J Thorac Cardiovasc Surg 87:325–331
225. Gaines WE, Goldberg NH, Mergner WJ (1985) Reconstruction of the right ventricular outflow tract with a vascularised free flap of striated muscle. Surg Forum 36:250
226. Mommaerts WFHM (1964) Heart muscle. In: Fishman AP, Richard DW (eds) Circulation of blood. Men and ideas. American Physiological Society, Bethesda, p 152
227. Kusserow BK, Clapp JF III (1964) A small ventricle-type pump for prolonged perfusions: construction and initial studies including attempts to power a pump biologically with skeletal muscle. Trans Am Soc Artif Intern Organs 10:74–78
228. Guizzi GL, Ugolini F (1979) Proposal for a total orthotopic muscle powered artificial heart system for live application. 12th international conference on medicine and biological engineering, Jerusalem, 1979
229. Ugolini F, Camerini M (1985) The mechanical and energetic output of a specially stimulated insulated skeletal muscle for artificial heart drive: theory of behaviour and in vivo experimental results. Proceedings of the 14th meeting of the neuroelectric society, p 39. Greece, 1985
230. Chachques JC, Grandjean PA, Carpentier A (1986) Dynamic cardiomyoplasty: experimental cardiac wall replacement with a stimulated skeletal muscle. In: Chiu RCJ (ed) Biomechanical cardiac assist. Futura, Mount Kisco, NY, pp 59–84
231. Jesus FR de (1931) Bol Asoc Med PR 23:380
232. Griffith GC, Bates W (1938) A ventricular perforation in transplanting a new blood supply. New Int Clin NS 2:17
233. Petrovsky BV (1961) The use of diaphragm grafts for plastic operations in thoracic surgery. J Thorac Cardiovasc Surg 41:348
234. Petrovsky BV (1966) Surgical treatment of cardiac aneurysms. J Cardiovasc Surg (Torino) 7:87
235. Kopytov LF (1976) Plastic closure of myocardial defects with combined diaphragm and pericardial grafts. Eksp Khir Anesteziol 2:9
236. Schaff HV, Arnold PG, Reeder GS (1982) Late mediastinal infection and pseudoaneurysm following left ventricular aneurysmectomy repair utilising pectoralis major muscle flap. J Thorac Cardiovasc Surg 84:912–916

237. Carpentier A, Chachques JC (1985) Myocardial substitution with a stimulated skeletal muscle: first successful clinical case (Letter). Lancet 1:1267
238. Magovern GJ, Park SB, Magovern GJ, Bencart DH, Tullis G, Rozar E, Kao R, Christleib I (1986) Latissimus dorsi as a functioning synchronously paced muscle component in the repair of a left ventricular aneurysm (Letter). Ann Thorac Surg 41:116
239. Magovern GJ (1987) Reply. Letter. Ann Thorac Surg 43:687

Part I
Counterpulsation

4. Counterpulsation:
Stagnation or Evolution in Assisted Circulation?

F. UNGER

By definition, counterpulsation is a method for assisting the heart in series according to the ECG. The goal is to unload the ventricles in the ejection phase and to increase the myocardial blood supply in the filling phase of the heart. Due to the fact that counterpulsation works in series with the natural heart, the devices are up to 25% effective and are dependent on a certain moderate circulation. In cases of complete heart deterioration or fibrillation the systems do not work.

The following devices are available:

- Intra-aortic balloon pump (IABP; Fig. 1)
- Dynamic aortic patch (DAP; Fig. 2)
- Intra-aortic ventricle (IAV)
- Aortic *Windkessel* ventricle (AWK)
- External ventricle.

The indications for their use are:

1. Pump failure after open-heart surgery
2. Cardiogenic shock after myocardial infarction
3. Impending infarction and reinfarction
4. High-risk patients for general surgery
5. In connection with interventional cardiology.

The best-known established method is the IABP. For years there has been no change in indications for its use; however, application has expanded to cardiological postinfarction cases. The main benefit of the IABP inflated in diastole is an up to 60% increase in coronary artery blood flow, whereby the diastolic blood pressure increases up to 100%. The increased blood flow in the coronaries results in a diminishing of the infarction area. A deteriorated heart muscle can recover and reestablish the metabolic steady state due to the unloaded heart; the work load can be reduced by up to 25%.

Since the evaluation of the IABP by Moulopoulos and Kolff in 1962 and the first clinical implantation by Kantrowitz in 1967, the scope of applications has changed. The indication in open-heart surgery is given in only 1%–1.5% of cases. In our own experience, the indication is only 0.3%. This is the result of better monitoring of patients in ECC and of improved myocardial protection. There are four groups of patients: preoperative, perioperative, intraoperative, and post myocardial infarction. In preoperative use the survival rate is up to 75%, in intraoperative 37%. Patients with coronary artery disease respond better to IABP than patients with valve failure do.

Assisted Circulation 3
F. Unger (Ed.)
© Springer-Verlag Berlin Heidelberg 1989

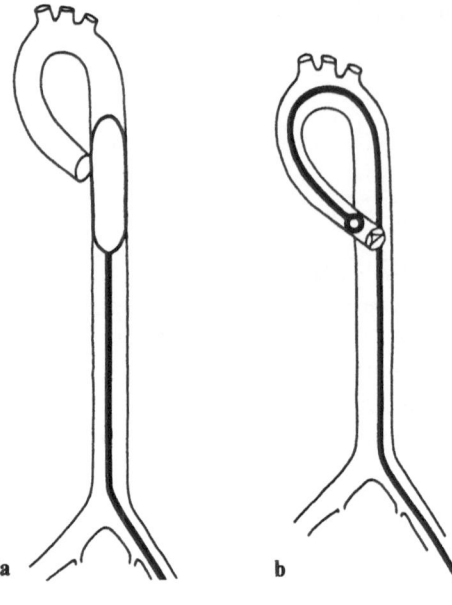

Fig. 1. a Intra-aortic balloon pump. **b** Balloon blocking ascending aorta

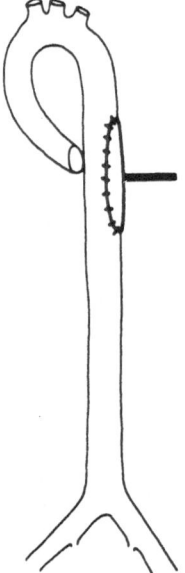

Fig. 2. Dynamic aortic patch (DAP)

Despite a well-reproducible performance, the incidence of complications varies between 10% and 22.5%, whereby ischemia of the limb is the main vascular complication in 8%–17% of cases. There are also more severe complications, leading to amputation or paraplegia. The insertion and positioning of the IABP can be complicated by severe calcification of the aortic or iliac artery. Failures of the balloon itself are also seen, such as unwrapping in 3% of cases. In my own experience, this has happened twice.

Despite the complications, the IABP is an established procedure and is regarded as standard in every case of open-heart surgery, as well as in every CCU. An estimated 50000 pumps were implanted in 1987. The devices are commercially available; four major companies share the market.

The standard technique is to insert the balloon percutaneously via the femoral artery, so that the balloon is positioned in the descending thoracic aorta. The balloon is made of smooth polyurethane, and the wire is also covered with biocompatible polyurethane. The balloon is driven pneumatically according to the ECG. In systole the balloon is collapsed, in diastole inflated; this produces the desired beneficial effect.

The devices and methods in use earlier are becoming part of history, such as the BASH method, external ventricles, external counterpulsation, and the *Windkessel* ventricle, which was very effective. However, these old methods should experience a renaissance along with the dynamic aortic patch in cases requiring long-term support. For years now, chronic implantation has been the goal for patients with cardiomyopathy. Some ideas have been investigated, particularly the dynamic aortic patch. This method could be of value in combination with a muscular power source. The implantation of the device is very difficult, especially the positioning of the guiding balloon (see *Assisted Circulation 1*).

This section includes papers by Kantrowitz, Bregman, and Moulopoulos, the pioneers in this field. Dr. Kantrowitz describes the different methods of assisting a heart synchronously, focuses on the techniques and complications of IABP, and describes the use of a dynamic aortic patch for chronic assistance.

Dr. Bregman discusses the feasibility of percutaneous implantation of the IABP. Dr. Moulopoulos describes the concept of a reduced balloon, which is implanted, in contrast to the IABP, in the ascending aorta after the aortic valves (Fig. 1 a, b). The balloon, which is implanted via the femoral artery, is inflated in systole (in contrast to diastolic augmentation with the IABP), so that the occluded part of the aorta is ventricularized and the systole will increase coronary artery perfusion. This technique has not yet been tested clinically. Further, the author brings up again the idea of an intraventricular balloon, which is, in may opinion, questionable, because it would increase the wall tension.

Nevertheless, counterpulsation by means of devices synchronous with the heart is a very well-established procedure, and the earlier concepts should have a chance to be revitalized in view of new developments. In the past 5 years there has been no great progress; perhaps the next 5 years will bring more, as devices are combined with muscular power supply.

5. Intra-aortic Balloon Pumping: Clinical Aspects and Prospects

A. KANTROWITZ

Since the introduction of the heart-lung machine, intra-aortic balloon pumping (IABP) has been the only method of temporary assisted circulation to gain acceptance as a standard therapy. IABP proved effective in stabilizing the circulation of patients with cardiogenic shock after acute myocardial infarction [1] and useful in supporting those with low cardiac output syndrome associated with cardiac surgery. Now, 20 years after the initial clinical application of balloon pumping, it may be useful to review its indications, technique, and complications, as well as to gauge the future prospects of in-series assistance delivered in the descending thoracic aorta.

Historical Overview

Investigations which followed the clinical advent of cardiac catheterization in 1940 increased the precision with which the mechanical events of the arterial pressure cycle were characterized and provided the basis for experimental therapeutic interventions. In 1951, manipulation of arterial pressure cycle parameters under laboratory conditions gave evidence of the validity of the principle of diastolic augmentation. By arranging for the arterial pressure pulse of an experimental animal to enter the coronary circulation during cardiac diastole, Kantrowitz and Kantrowitz [2] demonstrated the potential for obtaining a clinically important increase in coronary artery flow.

The following decade witnessed efforts to find a clinical implementation of this concept [3]. To meet the need for a nonsurgical, rapidly initiated form of short-term circulatory support, balloon pumping was proposed by W. Kolff and his colleagues Moulopoulos and Topaz in 1962 [4], and at about the same time by Clauss and associates [5]. Neither group, however, developed a clinically feasible procedure. It later became evident that these workers' use of latex for the balloon pump chamber assured that its inflation would occlude the aorta, compromising hemodynamic efficacy; the use of carbon dioxide as the actuating gas by Moulopoulos et al. probably contributed to failure to elicit significant circulatory improvement.

Kantrowitz and colleagues at Maimonides Medical Center (Brooklyn) were encouraged to develop IABP by their experience with a permanently implanted system for achieving diastolic augmentation. This valveless, U-shaped mechanical auxiliary ventricle (MAV) was anastomosed to the ascending and descending

Assisted Circulation 3
F. Unger (Ed.)
© Springer-Verlag Berlin Heidelberg 1989

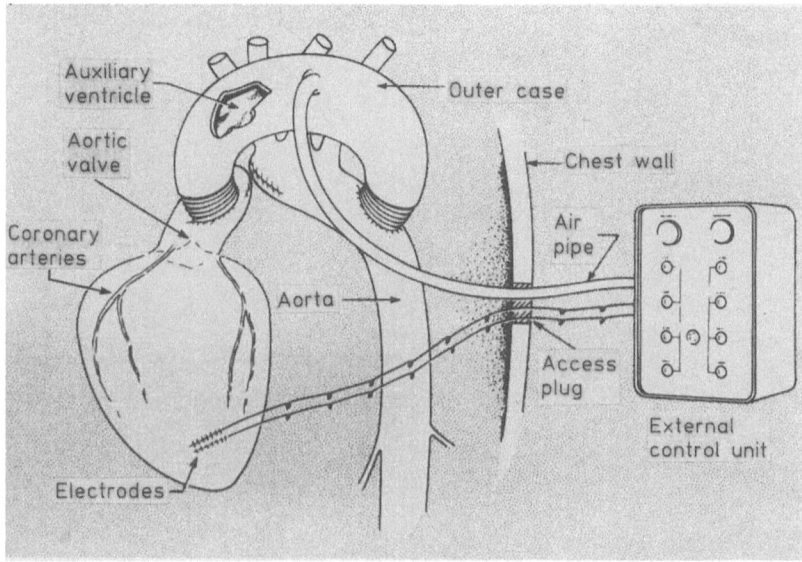

Fig. 1. Valveless U-shape MAV anastomosed to the ascending and descending portions of the thoracic aorta. This was the first device implanted in a patient with the intention for it to remain permanently in the body to assist the failing left ventricle. It was the forerunner of the intra-aortic balloon pump and the later auxiliary ventricle implanted in the aortic wall

portions of the thoracic aorta, and the aorta was transected at the level of the arch. The MAV's inner bladder served as the blood conduit. It was compressed by pressurized gas during cardiac diastole, significantly increasing coronary artery flow and cardiac output (Fig. 1). The clinical efficacy of the MAV was demonstrated in two patients with advanced, medically refractory, congestive failure [6] in 1966.

The goal in designing the balloon pump was to achieve a technique of diastolic augmentation requiring minimal surgical intervention which could be deployed rapidly for the benefit of patients in acute circulatory collapse [7]. For this purpose, catheter-mounted polyurethane balloons were fabricated for insertion into the descending thoracic aorta through a femoral arteriotomy. Pressurized helium was admitted to the balloon catheter through a solenoid valve whose operation was controlled by a modified oscilloscope. The oscilloscope provided two time delays. The first extended from the R wave of the electrocardiogram to the closure of the aortic valve. During this period the balloon was actively deflated. At the beginning of diastole, the balloon was inflated. The duration of inflation was controlled by the second time delay. The timing of balloon inflation and deflation was refined by examining the central aortic pressure waveform, as displayed on the oscilloscope, and adjusting the time delays until optimal changes in the waveform resulted.

The effect of balloon pumping (and of other types of diastolic augmentation) can be characterized in physical and in physiological terms. From the physical standpoint the technique introduces periodic pressure perturbations into the cen-

Aortic root pressure

Fundamental component of
aortic root pressure

Aortic root flow

Fundamental component of
aortic root.flow

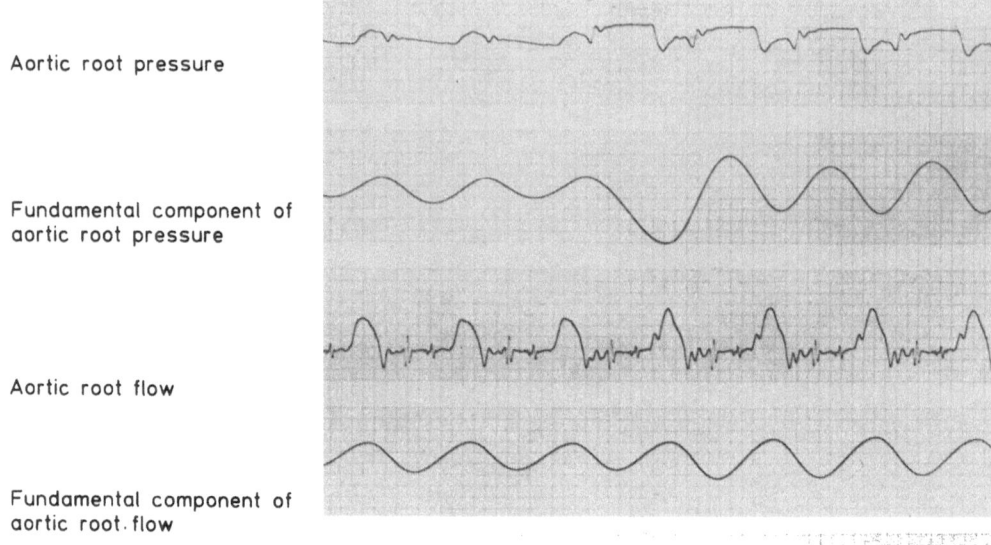

Off ◄─── ───► On

Fig. 2. Recording of central aortic pressure and flow and their fundamental components in an experimental animal. At *left*, with balloon inactive, fundamental components of pressure and flow are essentially in phase. At *right*, with balloon pumping in progress, fundamental components of pressure and flow are approximately 180° out of phase. See text

tral aorta that shift the phase relations between pressure and flow in the circulatory system (Fig. 2). Physiologically, balloon deflation at the onset of ventricular systole diminishes the afterload on the left ventricle (LV) by suddenly decreasing central aortic pressure. In effect, volume is removed from the circulation. From the standpoint of myocardial energetics, IABP adds external energy to the cardiovascular system. For a patient in circulatory collapse, whose failing myocardium cannot contract with sufficient force to maintain normal hemodynamic status, the rationale for introducing external energy into the system seems intuitively clear.

Studies on animals in induced heart failure showed that balloon pumping reduced LV end-diastolic pressure by 40%, and myocardial tension-time index by 20%. At the same time it raised cardiac output by 50%, coronary artery blood flow by 100%, and LV dp/dt by 25% (Fig. 3). Physiologically, the diminution of intracardiac peak systolic and LV end-diastolic pressures, with the decrease in tension-time index, indicated reduction in myocardial wall tension. Therefore, the heart's oxygen consumption was lessened. Reduced end-diastolic pressure also suggested reduced LV volume, connoting a trend toward reversal of compensatory LV dilatation. The reduction in systolic ejection time and myocardial wall tension, together with augmented coronary flow, implied improved myocardial oxygenation [8].

Since they were first presented, these findings have been confirmed and very substantially extended in two decades of study of IABP. But in 1967, they were sufficient, with evidence of the relative safety of the technique, to warrant clinical

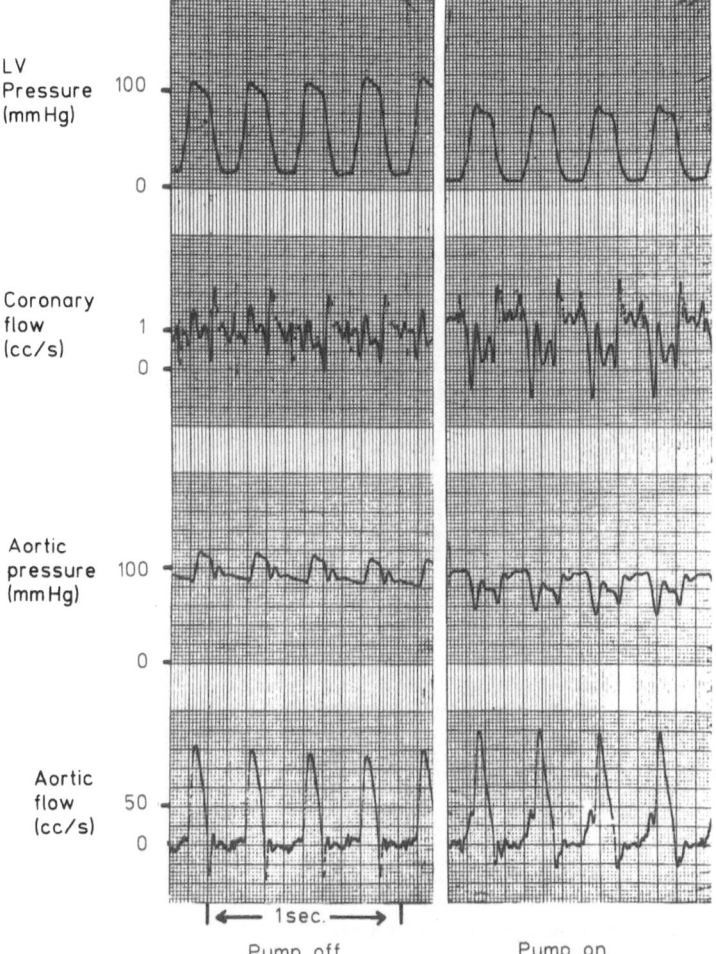

LV
Pressure
(mmHg)

Coronary
flow
(cc/s)

Aortic
pressure
(mmHg)

Aortic
flow
(cc/s)

|← 1 sec. →|

Pump off   Pump on

Fig. 3. Recording of hemodynamic parameters as measured in a canine experiment

studies in a group of patients with a hopeless prognosis. Patients in cardiogenic shock secondary to acute myocardial infarction who failed to respond to maximal application of pharmacological therapy provided such a group.

The initial clinical trials by Kantrowitz and his colleagues documented the fact that balloon pumping could restore such patients to an essentially normal hemodynamic state (Fig. 4), and that it could enable many to recover from the shock state [1, 8]. A cooperative clinical trial confirmed the safety and efficacy of IABP in cardiogenic shock [9] and gave further strong stimulus to widespread adoption of the technique. The early research on IABP is discussed comprehensively in Weber and Janicki's review [10].

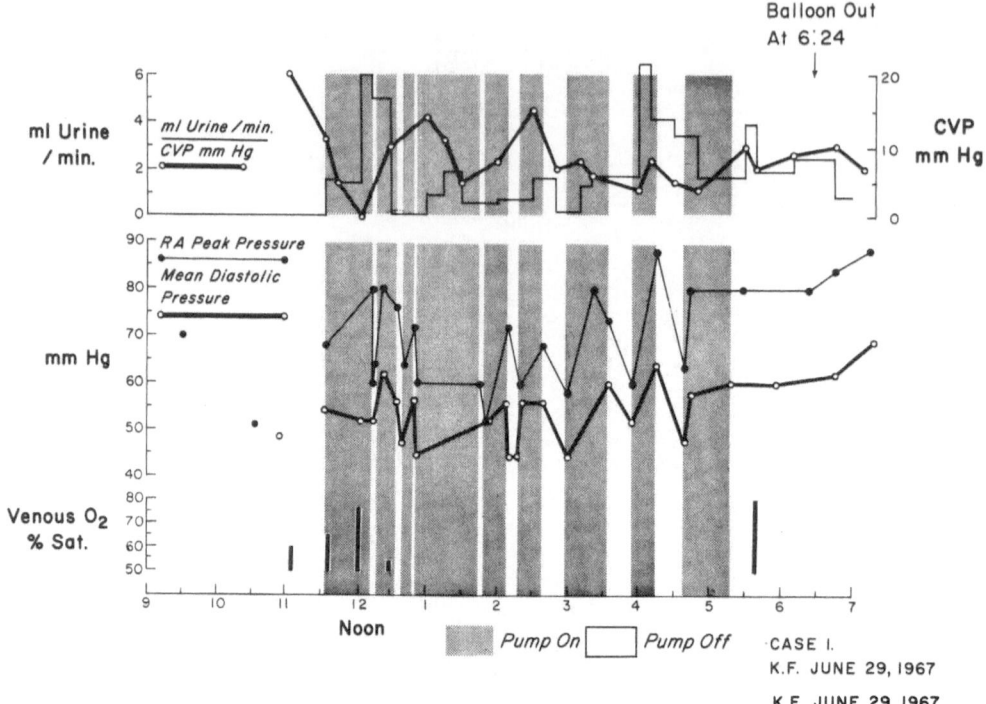

Fig. 4. Clinical source of patient in medically refractory cardiogenic shock during IABP. The treatment summarized here was given in 1967, prior to the development of current indices of cardiac performance in shock

Indications

In our view, indications for balloon pumping include:

Pump failure
1. After acute myocardial infarction with left ventricular power failure or cardiogenic shock
2. After rupture of the ventricular septum or papillary muscle
3. After onset of acute mitral regurgitation.

In association with cardiac surgery
1. Preoperative support
   a) To provide time for diagnosis and treatment planning
   b) To improve myocardial metabolism and function in anticipation of various procedures, including transplantation
2. Postoperative, for pump failure (low output syndrome)
3. Acute myocardial infarction, for prophylaxis of LV power failure or cardiogenic shock and reduction of infarct size
4. Unstable angina pectoris
5. Ventricular arrhythmias refractory to pharmacological therapy
6. Selection of treatment in chronic LV failure

7. Septic shock unresponsive to pharmacological management
8. Intraoperative support for cardiac patients undergoing noncardiac surgery.

Dispute continues about certain indications. As an example, D'Agostino and Baldwin regard IABP for prophylaxis of high-risk patients who are to undergo cardiac catheterization, cardiac surgery, or major noncardiac surgery, septic shock, and limitation of infarct size as "controversial" [11]. Our own opinion is that appropriate assessment of risks and benefits in such situations will often lead to the conclusion that IABP is strongly indicated, except in the instance of infarct limitation. In patients in whom this is a consideration, IABP may be a desirable adjunct to thrombolytic therapy and percutaneous coronary angioplasty if pronounced circulatory decompensation arises [12].

A number of workers have reported intrapulmonary artery balloon pumping, with or without synchronized IABP, in patients in whom acute right ventricular failure developed in the course of cardiac surgery [13–15]. Although this is an extension of the balloon pumping technique, it is not discussed here because of its limited application.

Contraindications

Several absolute contraindications to IABP are recognized at present. In severe insufficiency of the aortic valve, each balloon-generated increment in aortic pressure would increase the LV afterload. If aortic dissection develops during balloon pumping, the procedure should be halted immediately and the balloon removed. The presence of a prosthetic graft in the thoracic aorta is also considered a contraindication to IABP by some clinicians [11], but our group does not concur.

Commercially Available Balloon Pump Systems

At the time of writing, four manufacturers in the United States offer balloon pumping systems (Fig. 5, 6).

The manner in which such systems relate balloon action to the events of the cardiac cycle is still a critically important consideration. The newest commercially available systems, described as "automatic," assume that the time delays between the QRS wave and the opening and closing of the aortic valve are a function of the heart rate. The shape of this family of function curves has been determined statistically from a large number of patients. The operator still estimates the QRS wave-to-aortic valve opening and closing time intervals at the patient's present heart rate, but doing so selects a specific member of the family of function curves for the machine to use as the heart rate changes. Such statistically based information is, however, correct only on the average. For any specific patient, the estimates may well be wrong. Furthermore, even for one specific patient at one specific heart rate, the time intervals vary depending on the patient's hemodynamic condition. Patients in whom an intra-aortic balloon is placed are usually hemodynamically unstable.

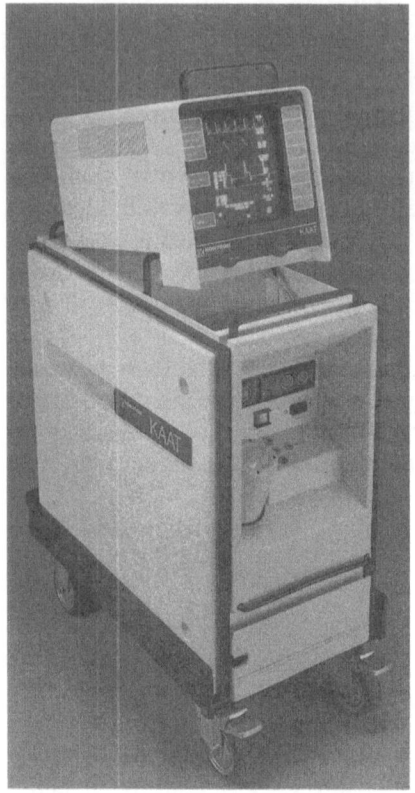

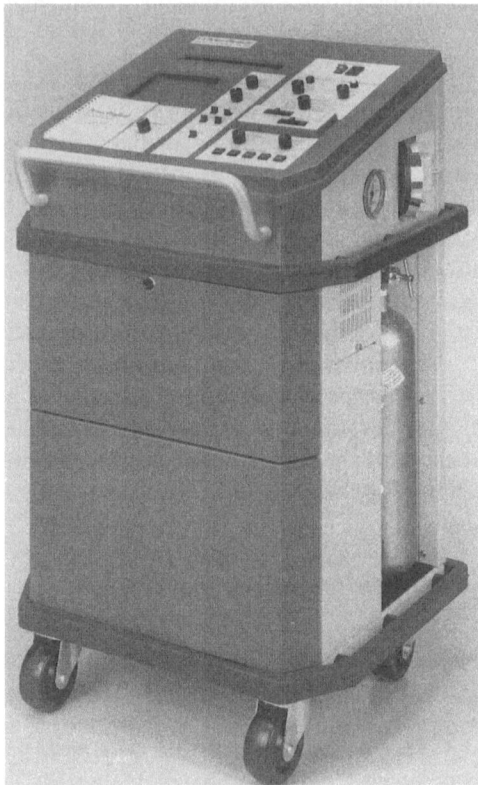

Fig. 5   **Fig. 6**

Fig. 5. Kontron Intraaortic Balloon Pump Drive Unit, one of four IABP systems sold in the United States. Others on the market are made by Aries, Datascope, and the Mansfield Scientific Company. These drive units incorporate microprocessor-based controls and offer advantages over early drive units, such as alerting operators to changes in critical patient parameters

Fig. 6. The Aries Model 900 (see legend to Fig. 5)

Thus, notwithstanding claims of automatic operation, timing of IABP inflation and deflation in the present state of the art is essentially manual, and is still the responsibility of the operator. As mentioned below, the ability to wean the patient from IABP through gradual decrease in the volume of the inflated pumping chamber is important, and not all systems permit this.

Whatever the system chosen, use of a single-chamber balloon pump is recommended (Fig. 7). Claims that multiple-chamber configurations or other deviations from the single-chamber design can augment rostral flow have not been documented. Such configurations may reduce the efficacy of IABP. Percutaneous balloons are discussed below.

Helium is recommended as the inflating gas for all balloon pump systems commercially available in the United States. As noted by our group from the ini-

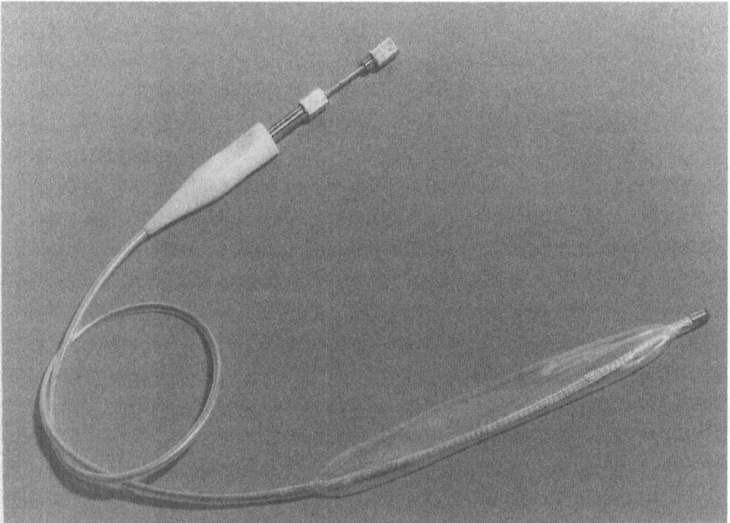

Fig. 7. Single-chamber balloon pump. Gas is transmitted through the catheter to the cylindrical polyurethane balloon, having a volume displacement of 37 cc. Volume displacement of commercially available balloon pumps range from 8 cc for pediatric use to 60 cc

tiation of its work on balloon pumping, helium has 1/20th the density of carbon dioxide and therefore affords more rapid movement of gas. As compared with carbon dioxide, helium permits more substantial diastolic augmentation or the use of a smaller catheter diameter, to lessen the risk of aortic damage and compromise of the circulation distal to the point of balloon insertion while maintaining the desired level of efficacy of assistance.

Further Considerations of Balloon Timing

It has been evident since the outset of our investigations that IABP's hemodynamic benefits are critically dependent on the temporal relationship between balloon action and the mechanical events of the cardiac cycle. This consideration, in fact, influenced our decision to use helium as the inflating gas. Although detailed discussion of this topic is beyond the scope of this chapter, several points require emphasis.

To oversimplify complex issues, optimal balloon action occurs when device inflation is initiated just before the dicrotic notch of the central aortic pressure waveform, and when deflation occurs at the end of diastole, i.e., bordering on the beginning of isovolumetric systole (Fig. 8). Under these conditions, and assuming that the balloon does not occlude the aorta and that gas transport rates and inflation pressure are appropriate, coronary flow is maximized and the left ventricle is "unloaded" to the maximal degree.

The confirmation that maximal hemodynamic benefits of assistance are being obtained requires computation of the relevant hemodynamic parameters. Facili-

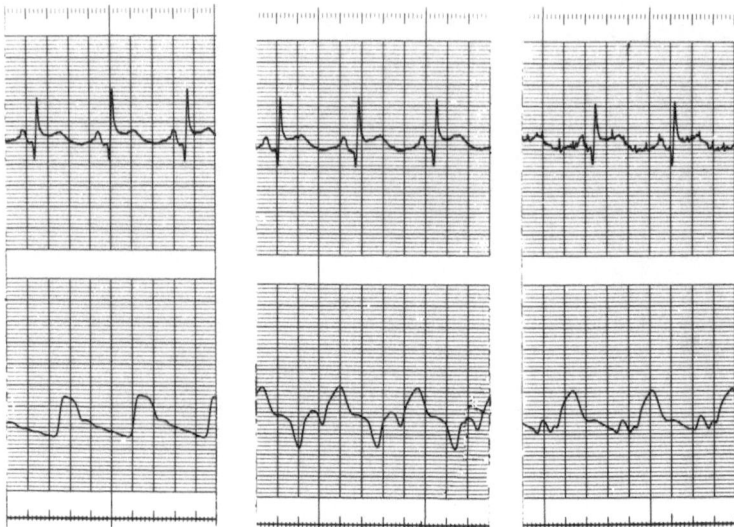

Fig. 8. Recording of hemodynamic parameters during experimental balloon pumping illustrating unassisted (*left*) correct (*middle*), and inadequate balloon pump timing settings (*right*)

ties for on-line computation are not always available in the clinical setting. Under such circumstances, certain factors which, empirically, represent necessary conditions for maximally effective assistance can be assessed by visual inspection of the central aortic pressure waveform. When timing is acceptable, the end-diastolic pressure in the central aorta is usually lower after balloon deflation than in an unassisted cycle; the peak diastolic pressure is at least as great as the unassisted peak systolic pressure; and the peak systolic pressure is lower than the unassisted peak systolic pressure. Satisfying these criteria is, of course, not sufficient to assure that balloon phasing is optimal.

Commercial balloon pump drivers, operating in the so-called "ECG collapse" or "anticipatory" mode, process the electrocardiogram to detect the R wave, as noted above. Alternatively, they use a "pulse trigger" mode, in which the increase in central aortic pressure due to cardiac systole serves as a reference for determining IABP timing. From this reference point the appropriate intervals to balloon activation and deactivation are computed. Currently available equipment deflates the balloon when a premature beat is sensed and incorporates various safety features to deal with some tachyarrhythmias and detect gross balloon "rupture." But the main point, with respect to the hemodynamic benefits of IABP, bears repetition: when the patient's heart rate varies, optimal timing cannot be maintained without the intervention of a human operator. And when the patient's heart rate changes repeatedly within a short span of time, even a highly trained operator has difficulty in securing optimal benefits of assistance. Current commercial balloon pump drivers are also limited in their ability to follow rapid heart rates and cannot implement special timing algorithms that certain patients may require, for example, optimizing coronary flow at the expense of maximal LV unloading.

Failure to achieve optimal timing may seriously compromise the benefits of IABP. A number of investigators, including members of our own group, are therefore seeking to develop improved drivers. There are grounds for optimism that the machines that will result from these efforts will be more effective than current models in meeting the needs of patients with severe ventricular arrhythmias and other conditions.

Technique

The steps in the balloon pumping technique to be described are appropriate for patients in LV power failure, cardiogenic shock, unstable angina, or low output syndrome associated with cardiac surgery. The same technique is recommended for patients at lesser risk.

1. If not already placed, a Swan-Ganz thermodilution catheter, a central venous pressure line, and a radial artery line are placed in the patient's vascular system. Fluid volume and electrolyte abnormalities, inadequate ventilation, and disorders of cardiac rhythm are corrected. If not previously verified, the absence of contraindications to IABP is investigated.

2. A balloon catheter of appropriate size is chosen. The diameter of the fully inflated balloon should be such as to assure that the balloon diameter is somewhat less than that of the aorta. Complete occlusion of the aorta must be avoided, as it diminishes the physiological effectiveness of IABP.

3. The balloon is placed within the patient's vascular system. Two techniques are available for most situations: percutaneous insertion and placement through a surgical cutdown. In either case, the balloon is inserted through the common femoral artery, unless use of this avenue is contraindicated. The femoral artery route should not be used in patients with aneurysms of the thoracic or abdominal aorta, or in those in whom a prosthetic graft has been used previously to repair the aorta.

4. The balloon is cautiously advanced into the descending thoracic aorta so that the catheter tip is just distal to the origin of the left subclavian artery. Atherosclerotic plaques in the aorta or iliofemoral system may be so extensive as to preclude use of this approach. The hazard of dislodging a fragment of atheromatous plaque is more than theoretical.

Confirmation of proper placement by means of a portable chest X-ray or fluoroscopy may be useful – although rarely required in experienced hands – to assure that neither the vessels of the aortic arch nor the renal arteries are compromised by balloon placement. In this connection, some reports indicate that patients are allowed to sit up during balloon pumping [16]. Such practices are being followed more often, particularly in the instance of those undergoing long-term pumping. Such patients need the same frequent observation that recumbent patients receive.

5. Heparin, 5000 units, is given at the onset of balloon pumping and every 4 h afterward until balloon removal. Patients who receive IABP after cardiopulmonary bypass are given low-molecular weight dextran, in a dose not to exceed

10 ml/kg per 24 h. This treatment lessens the risk of cell "sludging" and improves the microcirculation in vital organs and skeletal muscle.

6. When the balloon pump is activated, the timing of inflation and deflation is immediately checked and corrected as necessary. Assessment of balloon timing is a skill conferred only by training and experience and must never be left to incompletely trained personnel. A trained individual should reassess the appropriateness of timing adjustments whenever changes in heart rate are detected, whenever the patient's physiological state changes or adjustments in therapy are initiated, and otherwise at least at hourly intervals.

7. The patient's physiological and clinical status is monitored after the desired timing has been achieved and thereafter at regular intervals. The frequency of such monitoring depends, in general, on the urgency of the indication for IABP. Parameters to be measured include electrolyte concentrations, partial pressures of O_2 and CO_2, acid-base balance, osmolarity, plasma volume, red cell mass, cardiac output, pulmonary capillary wedge pressure, arterial and venous pressures, including the CVP, and urine output. Coagulation parameters should also be followed as necessary for prompt detection of activation of the hemostatic mechanisms.

Clinical observations of the patient's condition must be recorded regularly, the frequency again depending on the urgency of the indication for IABP. Also imperative is frequent checking of skin temperature and peripheral pulses of the extremity through which the balloon has been introduced into the vascular system.

8. If vasopressors are being administered, they are withdrawn as soon as central aortic pressures are high enough to prevent the inflated balloon from occluding the aorta.

9. The indication for discontinuing IABP depends, of course, on the indication for initiating the procedure. In patients in cardiogenic shock who recover circulatory stabilization, discontinuation comes under consideration some hours after hemodynamic parameters have become normal and all physiological derangements due to circulatory decompensation have been corrected [17]. To halt IABP, a trial of weaning is attempted. The balloon's inflated volume is reduced by approximately one-third and the patient's physiological response is observed. If the circulation remains stable, the inflated volume of the balloon is further reduced and the patient's condition observed. These steps are repeated. When turning off the balloon leads to no hemodynamic change, it can be removed. There is no satisfactory evidence that the duration of weaning should be a function of the duration of preceding IABP, as Bolooki recommends [13].

Procedures Postpumping

1. After balloon removal, it is desirable to assure that no clots remain by passing embolectomy catheters proximally and distally. The requisite enlargement of a percutaneous balloon entry site allows a nonconstricting arterial repair to be carried out. If surgical closure of a percutaneously inserted balloon is not performed, it is imperative to apply hand pressure to the groin for at least half an hour. Spe-

cial bedside clamps, sand bags, or pressure dressings can be used for this purpose. The patient should remain in bed for 8 h after balloon removal. Persistent bleeding from the insertion site or deterioration in the quality of distal pulses is an indication for operative repair, with appropriate steps to locate and remove clots.

2. The patient is followed like any other patient after a vascular procedure.

3. Partial thromboplastin or clotting times should be monitored frequently for 24–48 h.

Nonfemoral Insertion

When obstruction of the femoral or iliac arteries makes introduction of the balloon through a femoral artery impossible, insertion through an axillary artery may be successful. After cardiac surgery on patients whose aortoiliac disease makes transfemoral insertion impractical, it is possible to place the balloon catheter through the ascending aorta. An 8-mm end-to-side graft is sutured to the edges of an incision in the ascending aorta and the balloon is placed. To lessen the risk of infection and reduce the patient's exposure to anesthetic, it is recommended that the patient's chest incision be closed. The graft is brought out of the chest through an intercostal incision. When IABP has been completed, the balloon is removed and the graft closed and buried subcutaneously. The secondary small chest incision is closed under local anesthesia.

Comments on Technique

Balloon pumping has been carried out in the emergency room, the hospital room, the coronary care unit, the surgical intensive care unit, the catheterization laboratory, and the operating room. Kratz noted that in the operating room, standard leads may be incapable of obtaining electrocardiographic signals suitable for IABP. He recommended the use of temporary epicardial pacing electrodes in such instances as a source of interference-free signals [18]. Except in special situations, the intensive care setting is probably most appropriate for IABP extending beyond a few hours.

Commercial units are small enough to permit ground or air transport of patients receiving IABP. LoCicero et al. reported 50 consecutive cases of interhospital transport of stabilized patients receiving IABP [19]. They concluded that transportation was uneventful in such cases. Gottlieb et al. reached the same conclusion on the basis of results in 11 cases [20].

The performance of IABP and its adjunctive management in patients in cardiogenic shock and other forms of circulatory decompensation have been described by many authors. Aspects of technique in patients with cardiogenic shock were discussed by Kantrowitz [21]. Gafford and Ayres offered an excellent discussion of the role of balloon pumping and other therapeutic modalities in the management of cardiogenic shock [22]. A detailed approach to the correction of physiological derangements due to the shock state or its prior pharmacological management has been presented by Krakauer et al. [17].

Within the last several years substantial experience with the use of the percutaneous intra-aortic balloon pump has been accumulated [13, 23–25]. Advantages include rapidity of initiation (within 15 min) and ability of cardiologists and radiologists to undertake the procedure. The percutaneous balloon is equal in hemodynamic efficacy to the surgical balloon, but vascular complications, as noted below, are thought to be commoner after percutaneous placement.

Restrictions on the duration of IABP have not been defined but as a practical matter are of minor importance. Several authors have recorded extended periods of IABP in patients with circulatory decompensation, presumably the most severe test of the temporal boundaries of the procedure; the periods in question were 30 and 38 days [26], 49 days [27], and 327 days [28]. In our own experience, a number of patients have been assisted for periods of several weeks to months [29]. As discussed below, some evidence indicates that the frequency of certain complications is correlated with the duration of IABP. Furthermore, since the patient's mobility is restricted during assistance, and extended assistance may drain coronary care resources, prolonged pumping is highly unusual. There is, however, renewed interest in prolonged pumping in selected patients as a bridge to transplant.

As a technique of weaning the patient from IABP, some clinicians [11] recommend reducing the ratio of assisted to total heart beats. For example, in the first stage of weaning, every second heart beat might be assisted, then every third, and so on. This practice exposes the patient's myocardium to large moment-to-moment variations in afterload, and, in turn, to comparable variations in demand for external work. Indeed, the conclusion of Flaherty et al. [30] that IABP plus nitroglycerin is no more effective than "routine management" in patients with threatened or evolving infarction is more likely to reflect the use of this unphysiological approach to weaning than lack of efficacy of IABP with nitroglycerin. Weaning by gradual reduction in balloon volume is a far less risky way of proceeding. Fuchs et al. reported observations supporting this approach to weaning [31]. (Similar considerations compel rejection of the advice some workers offer about tachyarrhythmias, namely, that in such circumstances assistance should be given on alternate beats.)

Complications

Since the first clinical utilization of IABP in 1967, substantial experience has been compiled, permitting definition of the distribution of complications and determination of their frequency. Among the largest series reported to date in which complications were analyzed are those of McEnnay et al. [32] and Kantrowitz et al. [33]. McEnany et al. presented experience in 728 cases. The need for assistance after heart surgery led to 225 insertions, or 30%; angina (23%) and cardiogenic shock (20%) were the next most frequent reasons for starting IABP. Mechanical lesions associated with acute myocardial infarction, LV power failure, prophylaxis for surgery or catheterization, septic shock, and reduction of infarct size were included among other indications. Sixty-eight "major" complications occurred in 747 insertion attempts, or 8.8%. These were complications causing death, another therapeutic procedure, reduction of the anticipated duration of assistance, permanent morbidity, or death. In addition, "minor" complications developed in 96 patients (12.8%). The types and frequencies of complications were: vascular, 9.6% of all insertion attempts; bleeding, 4.1%; infection, 4.1%; wound drainage, balloon leak, and "inappropriate position," 3.8%. The procedure-associated mortality was 0.8%.

In the analysis of our own series, comprising 872 insertion attempts in 733 patients, different definitions make direct comparisons with the McEnany series impossible. We grouped IABP complications as follows:

Category I.   Spontaneous resolution without treatment, with IABP in situ (e.g., serosanguineous discharge, loss of pulse in an extremity, temperature spike)

Category II. Resolution after treatment or removal of IABP (e.g., limb ischemia, fever, bleeding from arteriotomy site, infection)

Category III. Residual deficit (e.g., amputation, ischemic neuropathy, embolization)

Category IV. Contributory cause of death (e.g., cardiac arrest during femoral artery embolectomy)

Complications in the first two categories were defined as minor, and those in the latter two categories, as major.

Complications were noted in 44.8% of the insertion attempts, of which one-third cleared spontaneously and almost two-thirds were resolved either by treatment or by IABP removal. Of all insertion attempts, 3% led to permanent impairment, and 1%, to complications classed as contributory causes of death. As in most reported series, the majority of the complications were vascular, and infectious complications occurred more frequently than bleeding. Patients with prior histories of diabetes and prolonged hypertension tended to incur a higher incidence of vascular sequelae [34]. Figure 9 shows the distribution of vascular, infectious, and bleeding complications according to age in the patients in our series.

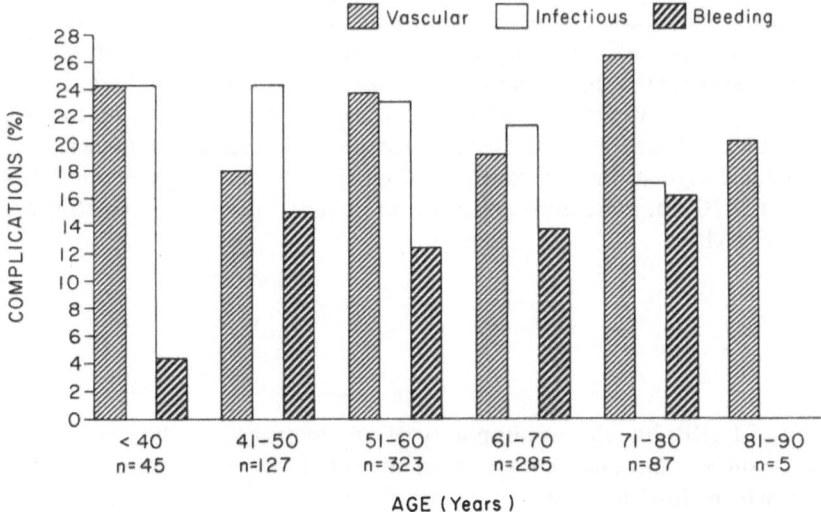

Fig. 9. Distribution of complications in Kantrowitz series according to age [33]

Observations in other reported series are, broadly speaking, consistent with our findings [23, 35–39].

Percutaneous placement of the balloon pump may result in a higher frequency of vascular sequelae [11, 13, 24, 40]. In a series of 101 comparable patients assigned randomly to surgical or to percutaneous insertion at our hospital, 22% of the latter group were complicated by vascular complications, as against only 6% of the surgical group [25]. It is logical to suppose that most workers who employ the percutaneous technique for insertion use it as well for balloon removal. As noted above, this obviates the possibility of utilizing an embolectomy catheter and may account for the greater burden of vascular insults. Gottlieb et al. [37] carried out a multivariate risk factor analysis for vascular complications of IABP in 206 consecutive patients. They found that a history of preexisting peripheral vascular disease and use of the percutaneous approach were the major risk factors.

Among the less common complications reported in the literature are the following:

1. Rupture of the balloon [32, 41]: by calcified atherosclerotic plaque with entrapment in femoral artery [42]
2. Gas embolism [32]
3. Cerebral air embolism [43]
4. Occlusion of left internal mammary artery [16]
5. Bilateral renal artery occlusion after ascending aorta insertion [44]
6. Spinal cord infarction by cholesterol emboli formed by fragmentation of atheromatous plaques [45]
7. Late paraplegia probably associated with dissection of aorta [46]
8. Ascending aorta insertion – 50% complication rate reported [47], unless a graft is used [48]
9. "Compartment syndrome" involving calf musculature [49]

Both the frequency and the severity of IABP complications depend largely on the nature of the indication for mechanical assistance. Most clinicians rely on IABP for patients with various forms of acute circulatory decompensation, evidently readily resolving the risk-benefit issue in favor of intervention. Debate persists about the appropriateness of performing IABP in patients in whom the risk of loss of circulatory function appears slight, for example, many patients with uncomplicated acute myocardial infarction or angina. Continued efforts to identify risk factors for IABP complications will allow more judicious patient selection for "prophylactic" IABP.

Discussion

The efficacy of IABP, its relative simplicity of application, and the minimal requirement for surgery have made it the treatment of choice in the wide variety of situations in which short-term or temporary mechanical cardiac assistance is indicated. The technique has been developed and routinized to the point that physicians all over the world, and not just a small group of surgeons and bioengineers, can summon up its benefits, secure as to the fundamentals of technique and adjunctive management. Nevertheless, scientifically and clinically, vigorous research, discussion, and controversy continue to surround IABP. There is still debate, for example, about the extent to which balloon phasing can be optimized and the clinical benefits of such enhancements. Disputes have been voiced about the efficacy of IABP in the aftermath of certain cardiac surgical calamities, and the appropriateness of prolonged IABP has been called into question.

In the latter connection, IABP continued over weeks or months draws heavily on hospital personnel and services. Yet observations from our laboratory's analysis of complications in 733 patients over a 16-year period do indicate that prolonged IABP can be beneficial [33]. Freed et al. found that of 27 patients from this series in whom pumping was continued for 33 days, on the average, 17 survived to leave the hospital [50]. Eight of the 17, treated in the early years of clinical IABP, went on to undergo surgical correction of anatomical lesions; they survived 2 or more years after discharge. Today, of course, patients presenting indications for surgery would be managed more aggressively, but it is noteworthy that prolonged IABP did not forestall successful surgical intervention.

But even more interesting is the group comprising seven patients with a history of congestive heart failure who were discharged from the hospital. All died within 6 months of discharge; one died of a cerebrovascular accident and six of congestive heart failure. It seems likely that after undergoing prolonged IABP and experiencing substantial improvement in cardiac function, these patients were enabled to survive for months despite the fact that they were no longer receiving mechanical cardiac assistance. It is reasonable to hypothesize that continued in-series support would have allowed long-term survival in this group. However, since prolonged IABP ist costly, as noted, patients in advanced chronic congestive failure who do not present indications for conventional cardiac surgery would appear to require some form of permanent LV support.

For the most part, indeed, the medical community is coming to recognize that permanent mechanical circulatory assistance has the potential not merely to extend life but to enable rehabilitation and return to productive activity. Among those urgently in need of such support are at least two groups of patients: (a) those, like the above-described patients, in end-stage LV failure for whom total heart replacement is either contraindicated or not specifically indicated; and (b) those with circulatory collapse after open-heart surgery who do not respond adequately to standard therapy (IABP and vasoactive medications). Common to both groups of patients is the fact that the circulatory system has reached an operating region in which available functioning myocardium and metabolic processes are insufficient, even with maximal pharmacological stimulation and support, to restore homeostasis. Therapeutic possibilities for such patients are restricted, almost by definition, to those that augment the patient's remaining cardiac function by adding additional energy to the cardiovascular system in the form of a functional equivalent of LV myocardium. Estimates of the numbers of patients who might benefit from such treatment are still imprecise, but various assessments indicate that as many as 100 000 new patients join the class of potential beneficiaries each year [51].

Several permanently implantable assist systems are in advanced stages of development, as described elsewhere in this volume. These have parallel-circuit configurations that can eject virtually the entire LV stroke volume into the systemic circulation. The trade-off for such hemodynamic capability is the requirement for obligatory function; these systems necessitate the use of relatively long conduits and artificial valves. Progress has been made in the design of both valves and intravascular surfaces within the past decade. However, more than momentary interruption of the pumping action of any of the current totally implantable, parallel-circuit, LV assist systems would create regions within the assist system of low blood flow or even stasis, in turn giving rise to an unacceptably high risk of thromboembolism. Thus, the reliability requirement for such systems is necessarily high. Clinical tests scheduled to begin soon will determine whether the required component and system reliability (particularly as applicable to valves) is within the present state of the art.

An alternative approach builds on the proved benefits of IABP in chronic congestive failure and our past successes with a permanently implanted mechanical auxiliary ventricle [52]. The advantages of IABP include simplicity with respect to both the assist system and its engineering, and the clinical procedure of cardiac assistance, relative freedom from adverse effects, and hemodynamic efficacy in the patient with profound myocardial decompensation and some remaining myocardial contractility. A permanent configuration of the balloon pump would have even greater advantages for the patient who requires long-term support.

Early work in our laboratory on the U-shaped mechanical auxiliary ventricle, a system with a large surface area of artificial material and long conduits, made evident the crucial role of interactions between the organism and the implanted assist device components, particularly the intravascular surface [6]. Comparable results have emerged in the development of other ventricular assist systems. Although both insight into blood-prosthesis interactions and the design of blood surfaces of intravascular prostheses are far more sophisticated than in those years, one generalization from that time remains valid. The risk of adverse effects of an artificial material on the hemostatic mechanisms remains approximately proportional to the surface area of artificial material implanted within the vascular system. The auxiliary ventricle now being readied for clinical evaluation by our group presents to the bloodstream the smallest surface area of artificial material of any LV assist system currently under development, since it is incorporated in the wall of the aorta (Fig. 10, 11). Because of this and because no artificial blood-carrying conduits are used, it can be deactivated without peril to the patient; when inactive, it functions like a passive aortic graft.

Our investigation of this auxiliary ventricle began in 1969. The assist device comprised a pneumatically actuated fusiform pumping bladder implanted in the wall of the descending thoracic aorta in the same operating location as the balloon pump. A gas conduit led through a percutaneous access device to an external gas supply and driver. Laboratory studies demonstrated that the aortic balloon could replicate the hemodynamic actions of IABP while averting the disturbances of the hemostatic mechanisms observed with earlier generations of the mechanical auxiliary ventricle [52]. Clinical evaluation of the system in three patients between 1971 and 1976 gave objective evidence of the ability of mechanical support

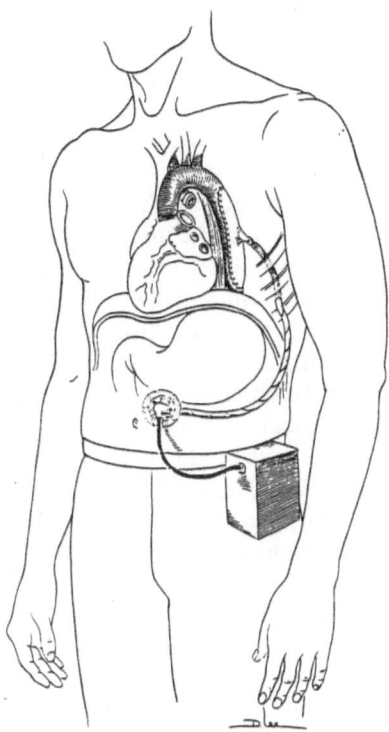

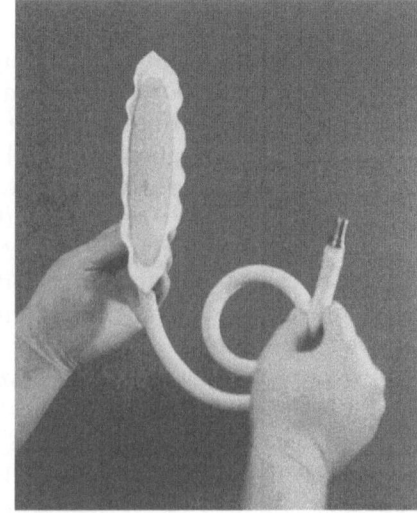

Fig. 10   **Fig. 11**

Fig. 10. Schematic of auxiliary ventricle system showing blood pump implanted in the wall of the descending thoracic aorta, percutaneous access device for transmission of pneumatic power and electrical signal, and detachable battery-powered activator-controller. (Alternative line-powered activator-controller weighing less than 50 lb not shown)

Fig. 11. Auxiliary ventricle designed for incorporation in wall of descending thoracic aorta

to reverse longstanding, pharmacologically intractable chronic congestive failure [52]. In the first patient, support during a 96-day postoperative course gave encouraging evidence of the ability of mechanical assistance to bring about cardiac rehabilitation. The patient's exercise tolerance increased markedly, pointing to improved cardiac reserve, and the transverse cardiac diameter was reduced by 15%. Comparison of findings at cardiac catheterization before and after implantation of the dynamic aortic patch, as it was then called, confirmed that several weeks' mechanical assistance had brought about substantial improvement in cardiac function. Strong evidence of hemodynamic efficacy was obtained in two subsequent clinical trials of the auxiliary ventricle.

These early implantations also demonstrated certain serious shortcomings of the system which could not be overcome with the techniques then at our disposal. We therefore suspended clinical evaluation of the system. A subtle problem, fluid migration from the bloodstream through the pumping chamber to the external aspect of the aorta, was soon resolved by establishing that a relatively impermeable material, Biomer, would be suitable for this component. More difficult was the problem of reliable, infection-free percutaneous access, long a difficulty in several areas of medicine. The propensity of epithelium to restore continuity in proximity to artificial openings in the skin leads, usually, to infection or extrusion of prostheses implanted percutaneously. This problem has been solved in cooperation with Drs. I. Bernstein, F. Vaughan, and colleagues in investigative dermatology at the University of Michigan School of Public Health. Working with them, our staff has developed a novel percutaneous access device (PAD). In tissue culture media, Lexan PADs are coated with fibroblasts from the intended recipient which form a confluent multilayer surface. The fibroblasts extend cell processes into the nanopores, creating a tight "lock." Upon implantation, the fibroblasts on the PAD surface merge with host fibroblasts, providing a biological seal and a barrier to migration of epithelial cells. An important further feature of this PAD design is a Dacron velour-covered flange into which tissue ingrowth takes place, isolating the PAD-tissue interface from mechanical stresses.

Implanted in miniature swine, PADs of this design have remained in situ with no clinical sign of infection for periods now up to 5 years [53, 54]. Thus, prolonged percutaneous access has become clinically feasible, and, in turn, use of pneumatic power for an implanted cardiac assist prosthesis is realistic. A portable power supply and actuating circuitry are well within the present state of the art.

With the identified problems of the auxiliary ventricle thus resolved, our group is proceeding to qualify the system for clinical investigation and eventual availability in the clinical setting. Our belief is that in-series assistance will be an appealing and rational solution for a considerable number of patients depending on long-term ventricular assistance for management of chronic, advanced LV failure. The patients will enjoy several advantages. In the first place, preoperative determination of the precise hemodynamic benefits of the permanently implanted system can be obtained through a trial of balloon pumping, and the amount of cardiac assistance provided can be tailored to the patient's needs. The adjunctive clinical management has been well worked out in patients receiving IABP [17, 21, 22] as well as in trials of preceding configurations of the auxiliary ventricle [52]. Finally, system failure need not be catastrophic, inasmuch as the system is nonobligatory. Since the components most susceptible to breakdown will be external, they will be readily replaceable.

Thus, the auxiliary ventricle concept appears to be a realistic approach to capturing the benefits of in-series cardiac assistance for ambulatory subjects outside the hospital setting.

References

1. Kantrowitz A, Tjønneland S, Freed PS, Phillips SJ, Butner AN, Sherman JL (1968) Initial clinical experience with intra-aortic balloon pumping in cardiogenic shock. JAMA 203:113–118
2. Kantrowitz A, Kantrowitz A (1953) Experimental augmentation of coronary flow by retardation of the arterial pressure pulse. Surgery 34:678–687
3. Kantrowitz A (1987) Moments in history: introduction of left ventricular assistance. ASAIO Trans 10:39–48

4. Moulopoulos SD, Topaz S, Kolff WJ (1962) Diastolic balloon pumping (with carbon dioxide) in the aorta – a mechanical assistance to the failing circulation. Am Heart J 63:669–675

5. Clauss RH, Missier P, Reed GE, Tice D (1962) Assisted circulation by counter-pulsation with an intra-aortic balloon. Methods and effects. In: Digest, 15th Annual Conference on Engineering in Medicine and Biology. American Institute of Electrical Engineers, Instrument Society of America, Chicago, Illinois 4:44

6. Kantrowitz A, Akutsu T, Chaptal P-A, Krakauer J, Kantrowitz A, Jones RT (1966) A clinical experience with an implanted mechanical auxiliary ventricle. JAMA 197:525–529

7. Schilt W, Freed PS, Khalil G, Kantrowitz A (1967) Temporary nonsurgical intraarterial assistance. Trans Am Soc Artif Intern Organs 13:322–328

8. Kantrowitz A, Krakauer JS, Zorzi G, Rubenfire M, Freed PS, Phillips S, Lipsius M, Titone C, Cascade P, Jaron D (1971) Current status of intraaortic balloon pump and initial clinical experience with aortic patch mechanical auxiliary ventricle. Transplant Proc 3:1459–1472

9. Scheidt S, Wilner G, Mueller H, Summers D, Lesch M, Wolff G, Krakauer J, Rubenfire M, Fleming P, Noon G, Oldham N, Killip T, Kantrowitz A (1973) Intraaortic balloon pumping in cardiogenic shock. Report of a co-operative clinical trial. N Engl J Med 288:979–984

10. Weber KT, Janicki JS (1974) Intraaortic balloon counterpulsation: a review of physiological principles, clinical results, and device safety. Ann Thorac Surg 17:602–636

11. D'Agostino RS, Baldwin JC (1986) Intra-aortic balloon counterpulsation: present status. Compr Ther 12:47–54

12. Satler LF, Rackley CE (1986) Assessment of adequate circulatory assist during intra-aortic balloon counterpulsation. Chapter 12. In: Brest AN (ed) Advances in critical care cardiology. Cardiovascular clinics. Davis, Philadelphia, pp 141–149

13. Bolooki H (1985) Current status of circulatory support with an intraaortic balloon pump. Cardiology Clin 3:123–133

14. Spence PA, Weisel RD, Easdown J, Jabr AK, Yap V, Salerno TA (1985) The hemodynamic effects and mechanism of action of pulmonary artery balloon counterpulsation in the treatment of right ventricular failure during left heart bypass. Ann Thorac Surg 39:329–335

15. Symbas PN, McKeown PP, Santora AH, Vlasis SE (1985) Pulmonary artery balloon counterpulsation for treatment of intraoperative right ventricular failure. Ann Thorac Surg 39:437–440

16. Rodigas PC, Bridges KG (1986) Occlusion of left internal mammary artery with intra-aortic balloon: clinical implications. J Thorac Cardiovasc Surg 91:142–143

17. Krakauer JS, Rosenbaum A, Freed PS, Jaron D, Kantrowitz A (1971) Clinical management ancillary to phase-shift balloon pumping in cardiogenic shock. Am J Cardiol 27:123–128

18. Kratz JM (1986) Intraaortic balloon pump timing using temporary myocardial pacing wires. Letter to the editor. Ann Thorac Surg 42:120

19. LoCicero J, Hartz RS, Sanders JH, Hireter DC, McDonough TJ, Michaelis LL (1985) Interhospital transport of patients with ongoing intraaortic balloon pumping. Am J Cardiol 56:59–61

20. Gottlieb SO, Chow PH, Chandra H, Ouyang P, Shapiro EP, Bush DE, Gottlieb SH (1986) Portable intraaortic balloon counterpulsation: clinical experience and guidelines for use. Cathet Cardiovasc Diagn 12:18–22

21. Kantrowitz A (1988) Mechanical assistance to the circulation in shock. Chapter 42. In: Hardaway RM (ed) Shock: irreversible stage of dying. PSG Publishing, Littleton, MA

22. Gafford FH, Ayres SM (1985) Shock associated with acute myocardial infarction: pathophysiology, diagnosis, treatment, and prevention. In: McIntosh HD (ed) Cardiology series, vol 8, No 1. Baylor University College of Medicine, Houston, TX, pp 853–869

23. Shahian DM, Neptune WB, Ellis FH, Maggs PR (1983) Intraaortic balloon pump morbidity: a comprehensive analysis of risk factors between percutaneous and surgical techniques. Ann Thorac Surg 36:644–651

24. Martin RS, Moncure AC, Buckley MJ et al. (1983) Complications of percutaneous intraaortic balloon insertion. J Thorac Cardiovasc Surg 85:186–190

25. Goldberg M, Kantrowitz A, Rubenfire M, Goodman G, Freed PS, Hallen L, Reiman P (1987) Intra-aortic balloon pump insertion: a randomized study comparing percutaneous and surgical techniques. J Am Coll Cardiol 3:515–523

26. Disler PB, Scott Millar RN, Obel IWP (1978) Prolonged circulatory support with the intra-aortic balloon pump after myocardial infarction. Thorax 33:504–507
27. Brantigan CO, Grow JB, Schoonmaker FW (1976) Extended use of intra-aortic balloon pumping in peripartum cardiomyopathy. Ann Surg 183:1–4
28. Ashar B, Turcotte LR (1981) Analysis of longest IAB implant in human patient (327 days). Trans Am Soc Artif Intern Organs 27:372–379
29. Rubenfire M, Krakauer J, Ciborski M, Wajszczuk W, Malinowski E, Jaron D, Freed P, Kantrowitz A (1972) Prolonged circulatory support by intraaortic balloon pumping. Circulation 45–46(2):II-214
30. Flaherty JT, Becker LC, Weiss JL, Brinker JA, Bulkley BH, Gerstenblith G, Kallman CH, Weisfeldt ML (1985) Results of a randomized prospective trial of intraaortic balloon counterpulsation and intravenous nitroglycerin in patients with acute myocardial infarction. J Am Coll Cardiol 6:434–446
31. Fuchs RM, Brin KP, Brinker JA, Guzman PA, Heuser RR, Yin FCP (1983) Augmentation of regional coronary blood flow by intraaortic balloon counterpulsation in patients with unstable angina. Circulation 68:117–123
32. McEnany MT, Kay HR, Buckley MJ, Daggett WM, Erdmann AJ, Mundth ED, Rao RS, de Toeuf J, Austen WG (1978) Clinical experience with intraaortic balloon pump support in 728 patients. Circulation 58 (Suppl 1):124–132
33. Kantrowitz A, Wasfie T, Freed PS, Rubenfire M, Wajszczuk W, Schork MA (1986) Intraaortic balloon pumping 1967 through 1982: analysis of complications in 733 patients. Am J Cardiol 57:976–983
34. Wasfie T, Freed PS, Rubenfire M, Wajszczuk W, Reimann P, Brozyna W, Schork MA, Kozlowski J, Kantrowitz A (1988) Risks associated with intraaortic balloon pumping in patients with and without diabetes mellitus. Am J Cardiol 61:558–562
35. Beckman CB, Geha AS, Hammond GL, Baue AE (1977) Results and complications of intraaortic balloon counterpulsation. Ann Thorac Surg 24:550–557
36. Downing TP, Miller DC, Stinson EB, Burton NA, Oyer PE, Reitz BA, Jamieson SW, Shumway NE (1981) Therapeutic efficacy of intraaortic balloon pump counterpulsation: analysis with concurrent "control" subjects. Circulation 64 (Suppl II/2):108–113
37. Gottlieb SO, Brinker JA, Borkon AM, Kallman CH, Potter A, Gott VL, Baughman KL (1984) Identification of patients at high risk for complications of intraaortic balloon counterpulsation: a multivariate risk factor analysis. Am J Cardiol 53:1135–1139
38. Sturm JT, McGee MT, Fuhrman TM, Davis GL, Turner SA, Edelman SK, Norman JC (1980) Treatment of postoperative low output syndrome with intraaortic balloon pumping: experience with 419 patients. Am J Cardiol 45:1033–1036
39. Sanfelippo PM, Baker NH, Ewy HG, Moore PJ, Thomas JW, Brahos GJ, McVicker RF (1986) Experience with intraaortic balloon counterpulsation. Ann Thorac Surg 41:36–41
40. Pennington DG, Swartz M, Codd JE et al. (1983) Intraaortic balloon pumping in cardiac surgical patients: a nine-year experience. Ann Thorac Surg 36:125–131
41. Rajani R, Keon WJ, Bedard P (1980) Rupture of an intra-aortic balloon. J Thorac Cardiovasc Surg 79:301–302
42. Aru GM, King JT, Hovaguimian H, Floten HS, Ahmad A, Starr A (1986) Brief communication: the entrapped balloon: report of a possibly serious complication. J Thorac Cardiovasc Surg 91:146–149
43. Haykal HA, Wang A-M (1986) CT diagnosis of delayed cerebral air embolism following intraaortic balloon pump catheter insertion. Comput Radiol 10:307–309
44. Baciewicz FA, Kaplan BM, Murphy TE, Neiman HL (1982) Bilateral renal artery thrombotic occlusion: a unique complication following removal of a transthoracic intraaortic balloon. Ann Thorac Surg 33:631–634
45. Harris RE, Reimer KA, Crain BJ, Becsey DD, Oldham HN (1986) Case report: spinal cord infarction following intraaortic balloon support. Ann Thorac Surg 42:206–207
46. Seifert PE, Silverman NA (1986) Late paraplegia resulting from intraaortic balloon pump. (Correspondence) Ann Thorac Surg 41:700
47. Meldrum-Hanna WG, Deal CW, Ross DE (1985) Complications of ascending aortic intraaortic balloon cannulation. Ann Thorac Surg 40:241–244
48. Snow N, Horrigan TP (1986) Ascending aortic IABP complications (Letter to the editor) Ann Thorac Surg 42:229

49. Glenville B, Crockett JR, Bennett JG (1986) Compartment syndrome and intraaortic balloon. Thorac Cardiovasc Surg 34:292–294
50. Freed PS, Wasfie T, Zado B, Kantrowitz A (1988) Intraaortic balloon pumping for prolonged circulatory support. Am J Cardiol 61:554–557
51. Helmus MN, Citrin DB (1987) Cardiovascular implants. In: Spectrum: diagnostics, medical equipment and supplies, and ophthalmics – products and technologies. Arthur D. Little Decision Resources, Cambridge, MA, May, pp 2–72
52. Kantrowitz A, Freed PS, Wasfie T, Kozlowski J, Rubenfire M (1985) Permanent cardiac assistance in chronic congestive failure by means of a mechanical auxiliary ventricle. In: Chang TMS, Bing-Lin-He (eds) Hemoperfusion and artificial organs. China Academic, Beijing, pp 149–165
53. Freed PS, Wasfie T, Bar-Lev A, Hagiwara K, Vemuri D, Vaughan F, Bernstam L, Gray R, Bernstein I, Kantrowitz A (1985) Long-term percutaneous access device. Trans Am Soc Artif Intern Organs 31:230–234
54. Bar-Lev A, Freed PS, Mandell G, Cardona R, Vaughan F, Bernstam L, Bernstein I, Kantrowitz A (1987) Long-term percutaneous access device. In: Advances in continuous ambulatory peritoneal dialysis. Proceedings of the seventh CAPD Conference, Kansas City, Missouri, February 1987. Peritoneal Dialysis Bull, pp 81–87

6. Clinical Experience
with Percutaneous Intra-aortic Balloon Pumping

D. Bregman

It is estimated that one and a half million Americans sustained an acute myocardial infarction in 1982 [1]. In the same year, more than 100 000 cardiac surgical procedures were performed [2]. The development of direct techniques for coronary revascularization has resulted in a multitude of critically ill patients requiring open-heart surgery. In an effort to deal with the increasing numbers of patients who present with the many complicated patterns of coronary artery or valvular heart disease, or both, and require urgent open-heart surgery, a spectrum of cardiac support measures ranging from simple pharmacological maneuvers to a variety of mechanical assist devices have been devised.

Temporary mechanical assist devices that employ the principle of arterial counterpulsation have met with the most consistent clinical success [3]. Early cardiogenic shock has been reversed, coronary catheterization and anesthetic induction have been carried out in acutely ill patients with coronary insufficiency syndromes, and patients undergoing cardiotomy have been successfully freed from the extracorporeal pump with the help of these devices.

The concept of counterpulsation, which forms the basis for intra-aortic balloon pumping (IABP), was first described by Harken in 1958 [4]. As originally proposed, blood removed from the body via the femoral artery during ventricular systole was rapidly reinfused during diastole to augment coronary perfusion pressure. By this method, in the normotensive preparation, one could decrease left ventricular work while increasing coronary blood flow. However, the prolonged use of this form of circulatory support was limited because of excessive hemolysis. Furthermore, bilateral femoral arteriotomies were required, and in the hypotensive state counterpulsation via the femoral route was shown to produce no increase in coronary blood flow [5].

In 1962, Moulopoulos et al. [6] suggested the use of an "intra-aortic" balloon positioned in the descending thoracic aorta to accomplish the same purpose as external counterpulsation, but without the drawbacks. The balloon was inflated in diastole at the closure of the aortic root, augmenting coronary perfusion. With the onset of systole the balloon collapsed, creating a "vaccum" effect which decreased left ventricular afterload. After a hiatus of 7 years, Kantrowitz et al. [7] reported the first successful clinical application of the intra-aortic balloon (IAB) in a patient with cardiogenic shock.

The finding that counterpulsation decreased the extent and severity of ischemic injury [8–11] and opened dormant coronary collateral vessels [12] was intriguing, and suggested to others that perhaps counterpulsation ought to be seriously considered, not only in patients with cardiogenic shock, but also early

Assisted Circulation 3
F. Unger (Ed.)
© Springer-Verlag Berlin Heidelberg 1989

in the course of uncomplicated infarcts, to minimize the quantity of myocardium that ultimately becomes necrotic [13].

However, in spite of its acceptance, indications for IABP remain unclear and continue to evolve as experience accumulates. Although initially employed in patients with cardiogenic shock, careful follow-up of such patients showed that mortality was largely unaltered [3]. Nevertheless, application of the IAB has expanded to prophylactic management of patients with mild-to-moderate hemodynamic decompensation. At the present time, IABP is widely used for circulatory support in patients with postoperative left ventricular failure, unstable angina refractory to medical treatment, and recurrent myocardial ischemia following acute myocardial infarction.

Conventional insertion of the IAB device requires surgical exposure of the common femoral artery and end-to-side anastomosis of a prosthetic graft to the artery with vascular surgical techniques. Subsequent removal of the balloon necessitates a second surgical procedure that requires either oversewing or removal of the graft. Most clinical series estimated that complications occurred in 20% of patients undergoing conventional IABP [14–25]. However, necropsy evaluation suggested that the actual complication rate was much higher, and that most mishaps occurred as a result of device insertion [26].

In 1979 a single-chambered 40-cc percutaneous IAB (Percor) was constructed around a central wire [27–31]. The IAB was wrapped manually, which allowed for percutaneous insertion into the femoral artery through a 12-F sheath via the modified Seldinger technique (Fig. 1). Percutaneous balloon insertion requires approximately 5–10 min and has been successfully performed in the cardiac catheterization laboratory, coronary care unit, operating suite, and recovery room. Difficulties with percutaneous insertion were encountered on advancing the IAB through tortuous and atherosclerotic vessels. In these circumstances arterial injury, dislodging of thrombus, or failure to insert the balloon often resulted. Difficulties in manually wrapping the percutaneous balloon necessitated a mechanical device to perform uniform wrapping of the balloon membrane. There have been reported instances of hand-wrapped IABs failing to unfurl at the onset of balloon pumping because of initial overwrapping.

A dual-lumen IAB (Percor DL) was developed with a flexible inner lumen that allows the balloon to be advanced over a 0.038-in. J-tip safety guidewire that has already been positioned in the descending thoracic aorta. To gain access to this central lumen, the wrapping knob with its attached support wire must be removed. When the IAB is in place, the J-tip guidewire is also removed, allowing for the monitoring of central aortic pressure through the balloon.

In a further balloon design advance, the wrapping knob has been incorporated at the base of the IAB catheter and is an integral part of the balloon. This knob rotates the inner lumen a mechanically fixed number of turns and causes the balloon membrane to wrap around the inner lumen. Access to the inner lumen now requires only removal of the support wire, and not of the wrapping knob. The sterile IAB package is designed to act as a passive wrapping guide for the balloon membrane when the wrapping knob is being rotated. The dual-lumen IAB (DL-II) which incorporates the wrapping knob is available on a 12-F catheter. A new 10.5-F single-lumen IAB with a mechanical wrapper has been developed

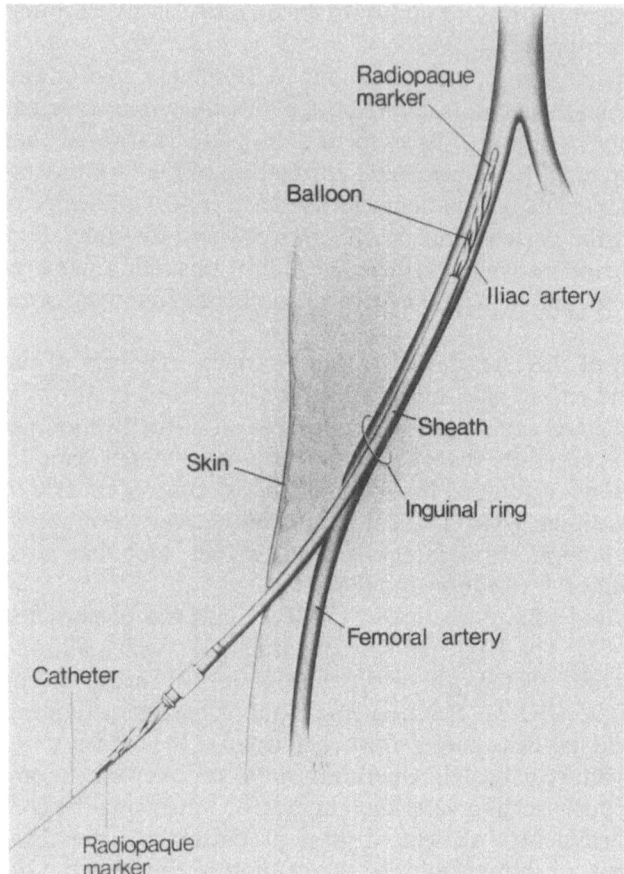

Fig. 1. Percutaneous intra-aortic balloon insertion

for patients with severe peripheral vascular disease or small femoral arteries. It is believed that the slimmer catheter will allow more blood to flow distal to the IAB and thus prevent limb ischemia.

Technique of Percutaneous Intra-aortic Balloon Insertion

Employing the modified Seldinger method [31], the percutaneous IAB is inserted by means of the following technique: After the inguinal region has been prepared and draped, the common femoral artery is punctured with a standard 18-gauge arterial needle, and a 0.038-in. (0.097-cm) J-tip guidewires is introduced through the needle. After removal of the needle, an 8-F dilator is passed over the guidewire to predilate the subcutaneous tissues and the arterial puncture site. The dilator is then exchanged for an 11-in. 12-Fi dilator–sheath combination, which is advanced over the guidewire into the artery. To control hemorrhage, 1 in. of the sheath is left exposed.

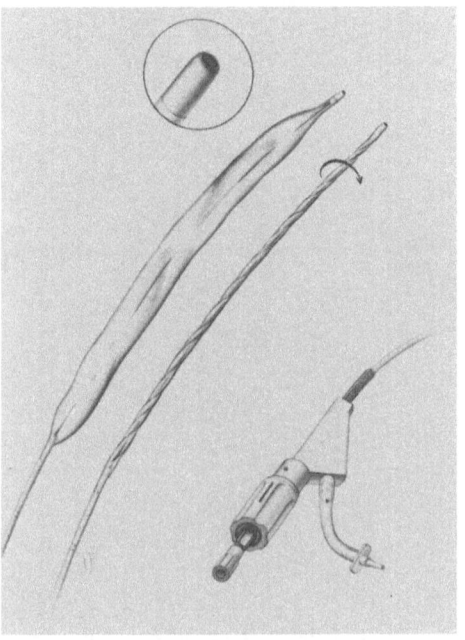 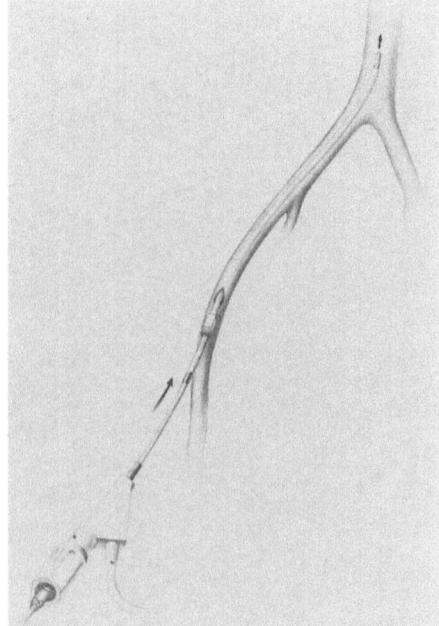

Fig. 2   **Fig. 3**

Fig. 2. The ballon is wrapped

Fig. 3. Balloon advanced through 12-F sheath in femoral artery

The percutaneous DL-II balloon should be prepared in the following manner: The inner sterile package is opened and the IAB removed, together with its protective tray. The balloon is furled by rotation of the wrapping knob clockwise (Fig. 2). The wrapping knob stops turning when the balloon is completely wrapped. The balloon is inspected to ensure that the membrane wraps evenly over the entire length. If incomplete wrapping is observed, the knob is rotated counterclockwise to unwrap the balloon, then rotated clockwise to rewrap it. The one-way valve is now connected to the IAB luer connector and aspirated a full 50 cc with a syringe to remove any air remaining in the balloon. The balloon is moistened by submerging it in sterile saline. The appropriate length of catheter to be inserted may be estimated by placing the catheter on the patient's chest with the tip 1 cm below the angle of Louis, and then noting the marking on the catheter. The guidewire and 12-F dilator are then removed, leaving the 12-F sheath in place. Bleeding is controlled by firm compression of the exposed sheath. The furled balloon is then inserted through the sheath (Fig. 3) and is positioned under fluoroscopy in the descending thoracic aorta. The sheath is pulled back prior to the initiation of IABP so that only a few inches of sheath remain in vivo. The vacuum is released by detaching the one-way valve. The balloon is unwrapped by rotation of the wrapping knob counterclockwise until it stops turning, and the balloon catheter is attached to the pumping console to initiate IABP. If a difficult insertion is expected because of tortuosity of the aorta or difficulty in passing the

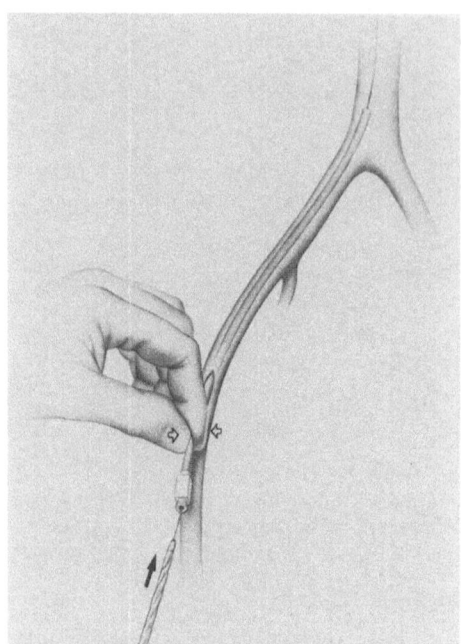

Fig. 4. Balloon advanced over J-tip guidewire through 12-F sheath

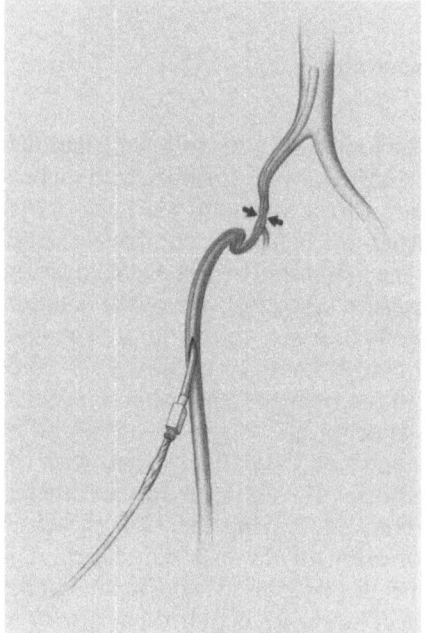

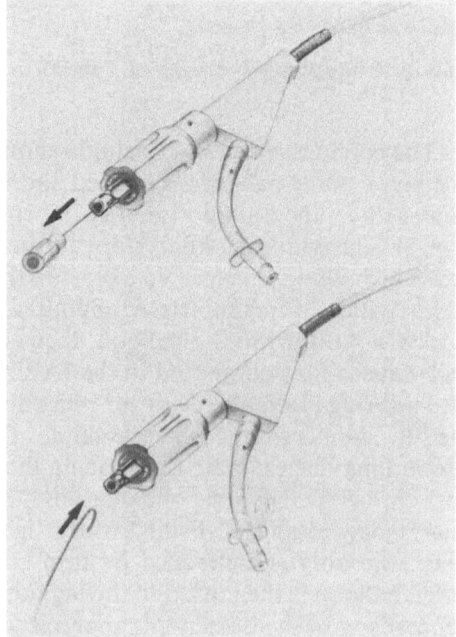

Fig. 5   **Fig. 6**

Fig. 5. Tortuosity preventing advancement of percutaneous balloon

Fig. 6. Central wire withdrawn for percutaneous balloon and J-tipped 0.035-in. guidewire passed
through balloon and into the aorta

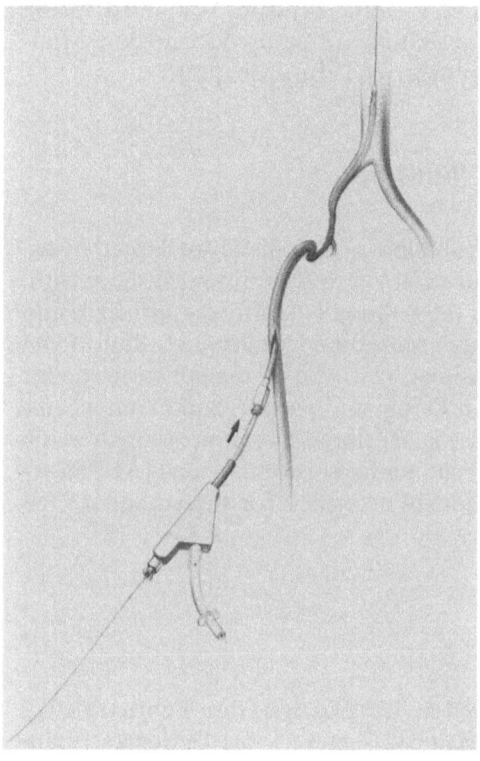

Fig. 7. Balloon advanced over guidewire through sheath and into the aorta. The flexible tip of the balloon negotiates the tortuosity by following the guidewire

initial guidewire, the IAB can be advanced over the guidewire from the beginning. Under fluoroscopic control, the guidewire is advanced until it reaches the proximal descending aorta.

The ballon is wrapped and a vacuum is created as described above. The inner stylet is removed from the balloon while the balloon is held with both hands, and while the vacuum is maintained the IAB is submerged in sterile saline to lubricate it. The dilator is removed from the dilator–sheath assembly but the guidewire is not. Bleeding can be controlled by pinching the sheath assembly. The tip of the DL-II is inserted over the safety guidewire; the balloon is then inserted into the sheath, rotating counterclockwise, which tightens the wrapping of the balloon (Fig. 4). The balloon is advanced over the guidewire, and when it is properly placed the vacuum is released and balloon pumping initiated.

If resistance is encountered in passage through the sheath or femoral artery, no force should be applied, lest dissection occur (Fig. 5). Instead, with the balloon still in the vessel, the inner stylet should be removed from the wrapping knob and the guidewire inserted through the inner lumen (Fig. 6).

The DL-II balloon is flexible and will follow the tortuous pathway of the guidewire (Fig. 7). Sometimes the tip of the catheter may be felt against the aortic arch; the catheter is then withdrawn about 1 in. outward so that the tip lies just below the left subclavian artery. Correct inflation and deflation of the balloon may be confirmed with fluoroscopic visualization. The sheath seal prevents bleeding from the sheath–catheter junction and a sterile dressing is applied to the sheath and balloon catheter assembly. The sheath seal is sutured to the skin. Management of patients on the IABP has been described elsewhere [32].

Removal of Percutaneous Intra-aortic Balloon

Before removal of the balloon catheter, the balloon is completely collapsed by aspiration with a syringe. The balloon is pulled down to (but not into) the sheath. The femoral artery immediately distal to the balloon is tightly compressed, and the balloon and sheath are then removed as a unit. Blood is allowed to spurt from the artery for a few seconds, and compression is shifted over the puncture site for 30 min. Distal pulses are monitored with a Doppler apparatus and manual compression is adjusted so that an audible pulse is registered. A compression dressing is applied to the puncture site for 24 h. Weaning from percutaneous IABP is accomplished in the same manner as previously described for the standard IAB pump [33].

Results

Percutaneous IAB insertion was attempted in 155 patients from February 1979 to June 1983 at Columbia Presbyterian Medical Center (Table 1). Successful insertion was accomplished in 149 patients (96%). In ten patients the initial inser-

Table 1. Successful insertions of percutaneous IAB at Columbia-Presbyterian Medical Center from 1979 to 1983

		CCU	Cath. lab
Preop.	Unstable angina with general surgery	1	–
	Unstable angina with cardiac surgery	13 (2)	10
	Unstable angina – treated with medication	2 (1)	1
	Postinfarction angina – treated with medication	2 (1)	4
	Postinfarction angina with surgery	10 (1)	3
	Cardiogenic shock – treated with medication	2	3 (2)
	Cardiogenic shock with surgery	1	4 (1)
	Recurrent ventricular tachycardia – medication	1	–
	Failed Grüntzig procedure with emergency surgery	–	3
	Acute VSD with surgery	1	2 (1)
	Acute VSD without surgery	–	1 (1)
	Anesthesia support for open-heart surgery	2	9 (1)
Periop.	Low output – OR	61 (38)	
Postop.	Low output	11 (6)	
	Cardia arrest	2 (1)	
Total assisted		149	
Total discharged		92 (62%)	

Parentheses indicate no. of deaths.

tion attempt failed. However, four of these ten eventually underwent successful IAB implantation by the long insertion technique.

The patients were evenly divided according to indications into a medical and a surgical group. Of the 149 patients, 74 received the IAB for a surgical indication; 61 had intraoperative low cardiac output, 11 had postoperative low output, and two had cardiac arrest. Medical indications for counterpulsation included unstable angina in 27, postinfarction angina in 19, cardiogenic shock in ten, acute ventricular septal defect (VSD) complicating myocardial infarction in four, recurrent ventricular tachycardia in one, and three unsuccessful Grüntzig procedures. When hemodynamic decompensation occurred in the three patients undergoing transluminal angioplasty the IAB was inserted and emergency coronary revascularization was carried out. The patients were subsequently discharged from the hospital. Only one patient received the IAB prophylactically for unstable angina prior to a general surgical procedure. This patient survived and the balloon was removed in the immediate postoperative period [34].

The location of balloon insertion varied. Sixty-one patients had the balloon implanted in the operating room, 13 in the open-heart surgery recovery room, 40 in the cardiac catheterization laboratory, and 35 in the cardiac care unit.

Of the 75 patients in whom the IAB was successfully inserted for a medical indication (Fig. 8), 59 (79%) eventually underwent a cardiac surgical procedure, while 16 were treated medically. Only six of the 59 patients undergoing preoperative IAB support combined with definitive surgical procedures died. In contrast, 45 of 74 patients (61%) requiring intraoperative or postoperative IAB support died.

We reviewed the first 113 consecutive patients undergoing percutaneous IAB insertion (Table 2). Complications of insertion occurred in 11 (10.1%). However,

Table 2. Complications on insertion of percutaneous IAB, 1979–1982 ($n = 113$)

Complication	No. of patients
Unable to insert in first femoral artery, successful in second	4
Unable to insert in first femoral artery, no second attempt	4
Unable to insert in both femoral arteries	6
Guidewire perforation of abdominal aorta	1
Aortic dissection	0
Uncontrolled bleeding	0
Long inserter used successfully	7

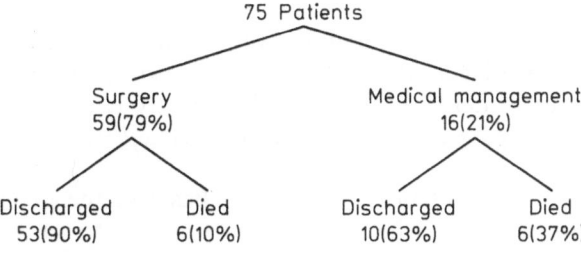

Fig. 8. Outcome for 75 patients in whom IABP insertion was successful

Table 3. Complications after insertion of percutaneous
IAB, 1979–1982 ($n = 113$)

Complication	No. of patients
Iliac occlusion (asymptomatic)	1
Femoral-popiteal artery bypass	1
Limb ischemia	2
Femoral clot after balloon removal	4
Bleeding after removal[a]	1
Weak dorsalis pedis pulse	1
Sepsis	0
False aneurysm	0

[a] Open insertion, closed removal.

only one guidewire perforation of the aorta occurred as a result of insertion of
the device. Complications related to balloon use and removal included femoral
thrombi in four patients, asymptomatic iliac occlusion in one, and one weak a.
dorsalis pedis pulse (Table 3). There were no false aneurysms, aortic dissections,
or septic complications in this series. However, extensive autopsies were not performed.

Four patients in whom percutaneous IAB insertion by the conventional approach was unsuccessful underwent successful balloon implantation by the long
inserter technique. There were no insertion-related complications in these patients. One patient had an improperly positioned IAB which intermittently occluded the origin of the superior mesenteric artery. The resulting abdominal pain
was relieved by advancing the balloon to its correct position [35].

During our first 4 years of clinical experience with percutaneous IABP at the
Columbia-Presbyterian Medical Center, certain observations were made and new
advances reduced the "hazards" associated with the technique [36].

1. The percutaneous IAB must be inserted by a physician skilled in the Seldinger technique of cardiac catheterization. Those institutions following this suggestion have clearly reduced morbidity associated with the procedure.

2. Ideally, the insertion procedure should be carried out under fluoroscopic
control.

3. The advent of the long dilator sheath has significantly increased the success
of insertion.

4. In cases of critically ill patients undergoing cardiac catheterization who
have poor ventricular function, study of the aortoiliac system is highly desirable
as a guide for subsequent balloon insertion.

5. In cases of high-risk cardiac patients undergoing open-heart surgery where
an IAB was not inserted prior to anesthetic induction, we recommend obtaining
femoral artery access with an arterial needle and then a guidewire, which are
maintained in the sterile operative field. If IABP is subsequently required for
weaning from cardiopulmonary bypass, arterial access is then already established
for IAB insertion.

6. A major advance in percutaneous balloon technology has been the advent
of the dual-lumen percutaneous balloon, which can follow a guidewire into the

aorta, virtually eliminating aortic dissection. In addition, arterial pressure monitoring can be performed directly through the balloon.

7. Utilizing the technique of balloon removal described earlier, we have occasionally retrieved specimens of thrombus which emerged from the femoral artery and therefore have not embolized distally.

It is clear from these remarks that attention to detail will significantly reduce the potential morbidity associated with percutaneous IABP. If these guidelines are followed, the system will remain the mechanical assist treatment of choice for the temporary management of medically refractory left ventricular power failure and other ischemic cardiovascular states.

Recent Advances

Percutaneous balloon technology was advanced once again in 1985 by the introduction of the Datascope prewrapped IABs, the PERCOR-STAT and PERCOR STAT-DL. The balloons are prewrapped during manufacturing and packaged in that condition so that the physician needs merely to apply a vacuum to the balloon and remove it from its package, once the introducer sheath has been placed. The balloon is then ready for insertion. The oblique spiral wrapping of the previous generation of balloons has been replaced with long parallel folds that make easier insertion into the sheath possible. The prewrapped balloons continue to have a volume of 40 cc but they are also now available with 10.5-F, 9.5-F, and 8.5-F catheter diameters. The 10.5-F balloon is a dual-lumen device, continuing the advantages of guidewire insertion and pressure monitoring through the balloon. The 9.5- and 8.5-F balloons are single-lumen balloons which allow maximum peripheral perfusion in the small patient or the patient with significant peripheral vascular disease.

Except for the ease of insertion and the elimination of the need to wrap or unwrap the prewrapped balloon, IABP parameters and methods of removal remain the same. The diameters of the introducer sheaths have been reduced commensurate with the reduction in balloon catheter diameter. The 10.5-F balloons require an 11.5-F dilator and the smaller, single-lumen balloons require the 10-F introducer. The introducer sheath lengths remain the same. A sheath remover is now also available to enable the physician to take full advantage of the smaller French size balloon catheters by allowing removal of a conventional sheath from the artery without endangering the balloon catheter. The sheath removers are color coded to match the color of the hub of the French size introducer sheath for which they are intended.

References

1. American Heart Association (1982) Heart facts, PR8. American Heart Association, New York
2. American Heart Association (1982) Heart facts, PR9. American Heart Association, New York

3. Bregman D, Bailin M, Bowman FO, Parodi EN, Baubert SM, Edie RN, Spotnitz HM, Reemtsma K, Malm G (1977) A pulsatile assist device (PAD) for improved myocardial protection during cardiopulmonary bypass. Ann Thorac Surg 24:547–627

4. Harken DE (1958) Presentation at the International College of Cardiology meeting, Brussels, Belgium

5. Dormandy JA, Goetz RH, Dripke DC (1969) Hemodynamics and coronary blood flow with counterpulsation. Surgery 65:311

6. Moulopoulos SD, Topaz S, Kolff WF (1962) Diastolic balloon pumping (with carbon dioxide) in the aorta – a mechanical assist to the failing circulation. Am Heart J 63:669

7. Kantrowitz A, Tjonneland F, Freed PS, Phillips SJ, Butner AN, Sherman JF (1968) Initial clinical experience with intra-aortic balloon pumping in cardiogenic shock. JAMA 203:135

8. Nachlas MM, Sieband MP (1967) The influence of diastolic augmentation on infarct size following coronary artery ligation. J Thorac Cardiovasc Surg 53:698

9. Feola M, Limet RR, Glick G (1971) Direct and reflex vascular effects of intra-aortic balloon counterpulsation in dogs at four levels of aortic pressure. Clin Res 19:313

10. Haddy FJ (1970) Pathophysiology and therapy of the shock of myocardial infarction. Ann Intern Med 73:809

11. Johnson SA, Scanlon PJ, Loeb HS, Moran JM, Pifarre R, Gunnar RM (1977) Treatment of cardiogenic shock in myocardial infarction by intra-aortic counterpulsation and surgery. Am J Med 62:687–692

12. Gold HK, Leinbach RC, Buckley MJ, Mundth E, Daggett WM, Austen WG (1976) Refractory angina pectoris: follow-up after intra-aortic balloon pumping and surgery. Circulation 54 [Suppl 3]:41–46

13. Levine FH, Gold HK, Leinbach RC, Daggett WM, Austen WG, Buckley MJ (1979) Safe early revascularization for continuing ischemia after acute myocardial infarction. Circulation 60 [Suppl 1]:1–5

14. McEnany MT, Kay HR, Buckley MJ, Daggett WM, Erdmann AJ, Mundth ED, Rao RS, DeTeouf J, Austen WG (1978) Clinical experience with intra-aortic balloon pump support in 728 patients. Circulation 58 [Suppl 1]:1–124–32

15. Gunstensen J, Goldman BS, Scully HE, Huckell VF, Adelman AG (1976) Evolving indications for preoperative intra-aortic balloon pump assistance. Ann Thorac Surg 22:535–543

16. Cooper GN, Singh AK, Christian FC, Cashman C, Vargas L, Karlson KE (1977) Preoperative intra-aortic balloon support in surgery for left main coronary stenosis. Ann Surg 185:242–246

17. Scheidt S, Wilner G, Mueller H, Summers D, Lesch M, Wolff G, Drakauer J, Rubenfire M, Fleming P, Noon G, Oldham N, Killip T, Kantrowitz A (1973) Intra-aortic balloon counterpulsation in cardiogenic shock: report of a cooperative clinical trial. N Engl J Med 288:979–984

18. LaFemine AA, Kosowshi B, Madoff I, Black H, Lewis M (1977) Results and complications of intra-aortic balloon pumping in surgical and medical patients. Am J Cardiol 40:416–420

19. Beckman CB, Geha AS, Hammond GL, Barre AE (1977) Results and complications of intra-aortic balloon counterpulsation. Ann Thorac Surg 24:550–557

20. Cleveland JC, LeFemine AA, Madoff I, Black H, Amato J, Sewell DH, Rheinlander HF, Cleveland RJ (1975) The role of intra-aortic balloon counterpulsation in patients undergoing cardiac operations. Ann Thorac Surg 20:652–658

21. Dunkman WB, Steinbach RC, Buckly MJ, Mundth ED, Kantrowitz AR, Austen WG, Sanders CA (1972) Clinical and hemodynamic results of intra-aortic balloon pumping in surgery and cardiogenic shock. Circulation 46:465–477

22. Leinbach RC, Gold HK, Kinsmore RE, Mundth ED, Buckley MJ, Austen WG, Sanders CA (1973) The role of angiography in cardiogenic shock. Circulation 47, 48 [Suppl III]:III-95–98

23. Wolfson K, Karsh DL, Langou RA, Geha AS, Hammond GL, Cohen LS (1978) Modifications of intra-aortic balloon catheter to permit introduction by cardiac catheterization techniques. Am J Cardiol 41:733–738

24. Gold HK, Leinbach RC, Buckley MJ, Mundth ED, Daggett WM, Austen WG (1976) Refractory angina pectoris: follow-up after intra-aortic balloon pumping and surgery. Circulation 54 [Suppl III]:III-41–46

25. Willerson JT, Curry GC, Watson JT, Leshin SJ, Ecker RR, Mullins CB, Platt MR, Sugg WL (1975) Intra-aortic balloon counterpulsation in patients in cardiogenic shock, medically refractory left ventricular failure and/or recurrent ventricular tachycardia. Am J Med 58:183–191
26. Isner JM, Cohen SR, Virmani R, Lawrinson W, Roberts WC (1980) Complications of the intra-aortic balloon counterpulsation device; clinical and morphological observations in 45 necropsy patients. Am J Cardiol 45:260–267
27. Bregman D, Casarella WJ (1980) Percutaneous intra-aortic balloon pumping: initial clinical experience. Ann Thorac Surg 29:153–155
28. Bregman D (1980) Intra-aortic balloon counterpulsation. Circulatory assistance and the artificial heart. In: Pierce WS (ed) USA-USSR joint symposium, Tbilisi, USSR, Sept 20–22 1979, US Dept of Health and Human Services, PHS, NIH, pp 155–165
29. Bregman D, Cohen SR (1983) Mechanical techniques of circulation support: a percutaneous intra-aortic balloon device. Artif Organs 7:38–48
30. Bregman D, Nichols AB, Weiss MB, Powers ER, Martin EC, Casarella WF (1980) Percutaneous intra-aortic balloon insertion. Am J Cardiol 46:261–264
31. Seldinger SI (1953) Catheter replacement of the needle in percutaneous arteriography: a new technique. Acta Radiol (Stockh) 39:368
32. Bregman D (1974) Management of patients undergoing intra-aortic balloon pumping. Heart Lung 3:916
33. Bregman D (1976) Mechanical support of the failing heart. Curr Probl Surg 13(12)
34. Nichols AB, Weiss MB, Bregman D, Casarella WJ (1981) Percutaneous intra-aortic balloon insertion in patients with aorto-iliac disease. Cathet Cardiovasc Diagn 7:443–449
35. Karlson SB, Martin EC, Bregman D, Fankuchen EI, Casarella WJ (1981) Superior mesenteric artery obstruction by intra-aortic balloon simulating embolism. Cardiovasc Intervent Radiol 4:236
36. Bregman D (1982) Percutaneous intra-aortic balloon pumping. A time for reflection. Chest 82:397

7. Systolic Counterpulsation

S. D. MOULOPOULOS

The Terms and Principles

Mechanical assistance to the failing circulation can be effected by following two principles:

1. An external or internally implanted energy source may provide the circulatory system with the missing power to achieve adequate flow to the peripheral organs.
2. A mechanical device can be used to affect hemodynamic parameters within the two phases of each cardiac circulatory cycle, in order to increase peripheral flow to normal values.

It should be noted however, that if the heart is contracting, even if output is reduced, the application of an additional energy source will have to be "positioned" within one or both phases of the cycle. As a consequence, the use of an auxiliary energy source will necessarily involve not only the first but the second principle too. Therefore, analysis of the assistance techniques used should proceed according to the phase – systolic or diastolic – during which they are applied. Figure 1 indicates the "positioning" of the assistance techniques used until now.

Helping the heart during cardiac systole first occurred to researchers and was attempted under the term *systolic copulsation* techniques. Pumping air during systole within the pericardium [1], inflating a left intraventricular balloon during systole, and engulfing the heart in a rigid cup and pumping between heart and cup [2] were some of the techniques tried.

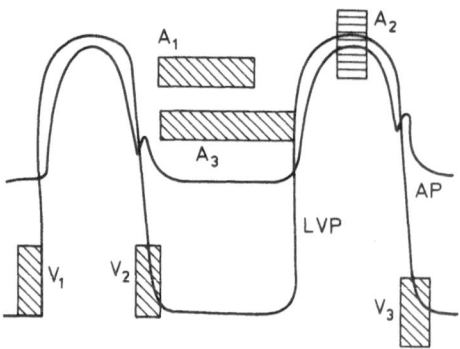

Fig. 1. Positioning of the assistance interventions within the two phases of the cardiac cycle. V_1, end-diastolic intraventricular pumping; A_2, mid-systolic intra-aortic or intraventricular pumping; V_2, end-systolic intraventricular pumping; V_3, end-systolic–metadiastolic left ventricular peripheral vein shunt; A_1, intra-aortic diastolic pumping; A_3, intra-aortic diastolic pumping continued into the isometric phase of the next systole

Assisted Circulation 3
F. Unger (Ed.)
© Springer-Verlag Berlin Heidelberg 1989

Pumping in the aorta during diastole had been termed *counterpulsation* [3]. The term was coined with the idea that a pump would propel the blood in a "countercurrent" way, from the descending aorta toward the ascending aorta and the coronary arteries. In fact, counterpulsation promotes blood flow during diastole toward the periphery, in the same sense that the heart directs the flow during systole. The diastolic phase is thus used to apply an energy source. A further advantage of counterpulsation is that it would not interfere with the activity of the left ventricle during systole, if it were not for the reduction of the resistance met by the next cardiac systole (1962).

The utilization of assistance techniques during systole would involve counterpulsation in a literal sense. At first sight, it is inconceivable that any interference should counteract the ventricular action during systole. However, *systolic counterpulsation* under specific conditions has proved experimentally to be helpful to the failing heart.

Systolic Counterpulsation with a Small Balloon in the Ascending Aorta

A spherical balloon, with a diameter equal to that of the ascending aorta (Fig. 2), is inflated for 60–80 ms during the middle third of the ejection phase of the left ventricular contraction [4]. The relatively brief pulse does not produce a significant increase in peripheral resistance or in left ventricular end-diastolic pressure in an animal cardiogenic shock model, neither does it affect myocardial oxygen consumption. It significantly increases the peak systolic left ventricular-aortic pressure gradient, by 7.9 ± 1.3 mmHg. The beneficial effects consist in significant increases in aortic flow ($9.9\% \pm 1.38\%$) and in coronary flow ($35.97\% \pm 10.93\%$) (Fig. 3).

The increase in coronary arterial flow with this technique is probably due to a systolic diversion of additional flow toward the coronary arteries. The increase in aortic flow may reflect an improvement of left ventricular contractility due to

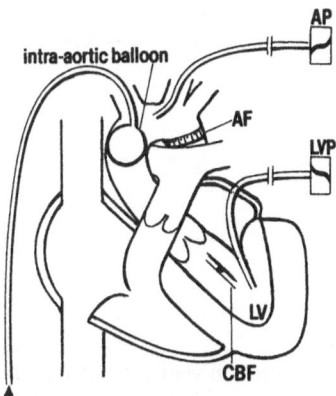

R-triggered pumping apparatus   Fig. 2. Small spherical balloon in the ascending aorta

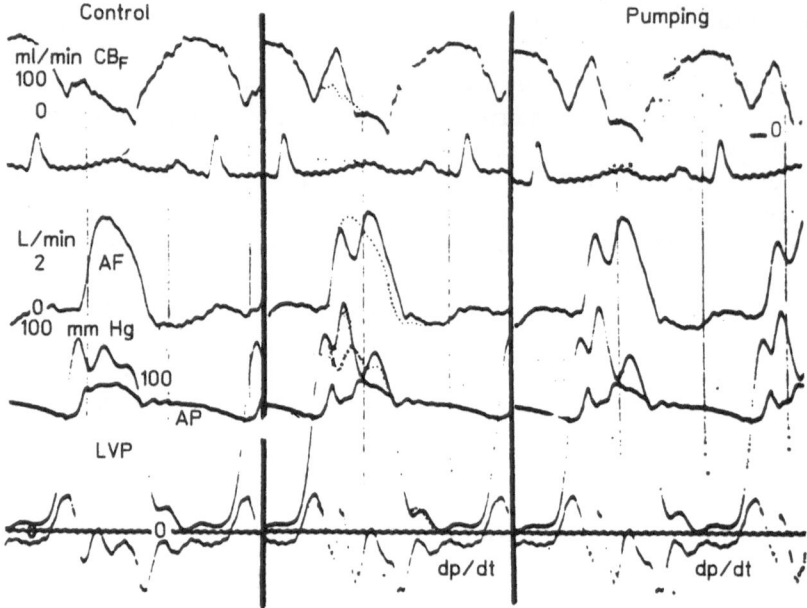

Fig. 3. Brief mid-systolic intra-aortic balloon inflation (*right column*) in comparison to control values (*left column*). *CSF*, coronary sinus flow; *AF*, aortic flow; *AP*, aortic pressure; *LVP*, left ventricular pressure

either the increase in coronary perfusion or to a "fake" increase in peripheral resistance, probably stimulating the ventricle to a stronger contraction.

Systolic Counterpulsation with a Balloon or a Catheter in the Left Ventricle

If systolic counterpulsation of brief duration (90 ms) is effected in the same cardiogenic shock model within the left ventricle (Fig. 4) during the middle third of the ejection phase of left ventricular contraction, similar results are obtained. Coronary flow increases by 18.8% ± 3.7% and aortic flow by 18% ± 4.9%. It is

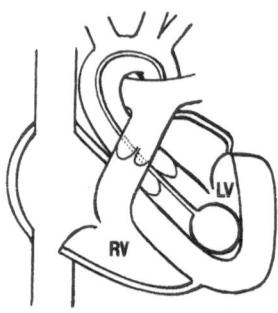

Fig. 4. Small spherical balloon in the left ventricle (*LV*). *RV*, right ventricle

noticeable that intraventricular systolic pumping increases coronary flow to a lesser degree than does intra-aortic systolic pumping, but increases aortic flow more than the latter. The difference in coronary flow increase can be understood from the different position of the balloons, the aortic one inducing a systolic diversion of the flow to the coronary arteries. The difference in aortic flow increase can possibly be attributed to the interference of the intraventricular balloon with other parameters, such as left ventricular ejection fraction and ventricular chamber compliance (see below).

In systolic intraventricular counterpulsation one would be tempted to attribute the results in general to a copulsation effect. It is of particular interest that better results were obtained during brief duration pumping in the middle third of systole than during pumping in the two other thirds or over the whole systole. This indicates that other effects besides mechanical copulsation are responsible for the result and that one can change ventricular output by modifying hemodynamic parameters within the systolic phase.

Left Intraventricular Pumping in Late Systole

Several assistance techniques tried in the past have been aiming at improving the peripheral circulation by increasing contractility or reducing peripheral resistance. Another important factor affecting manifestations of cardiac failure is ventricular compliance. Low ventricular compliance cannot be easily affected by any means. Mechanical techniques can modify compliance by changing the dv/dp relation at the end of systole.

A low chamber compliance animal model was produced by placing an elastic net around the ventricles (Fig. 5). Systolic pumping into the left ventricle was achieved by placing in it a spherical balloon with a capacity of 5 ml and inflating the balloon for 100 ms at late systole. The end-systolic intraventricular pumping induced a reduction of left ventricular end-diastolic pressure by 5.3 ± 0.1 mmHg, an increase in systolic aortic pressure by 20.7 ± 0.3 mmHg, an increase in aortic flow by 377 ± 29 ml/min, and an increase in left ventricular dp/dt by 8.5 ± 1 mmHg $\cdot$ s^{-1} (Fig. 6).

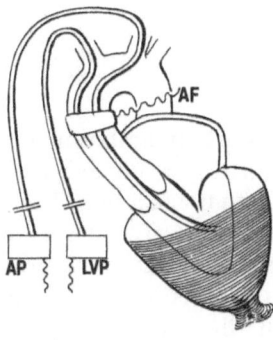

Fig. 5. Reduced ventricular compliance animal model. An elastic net is placed around the ventricles. *AF*, aortic flow; *AP*, aortic pressure; *LVP*, left ventricular pressure

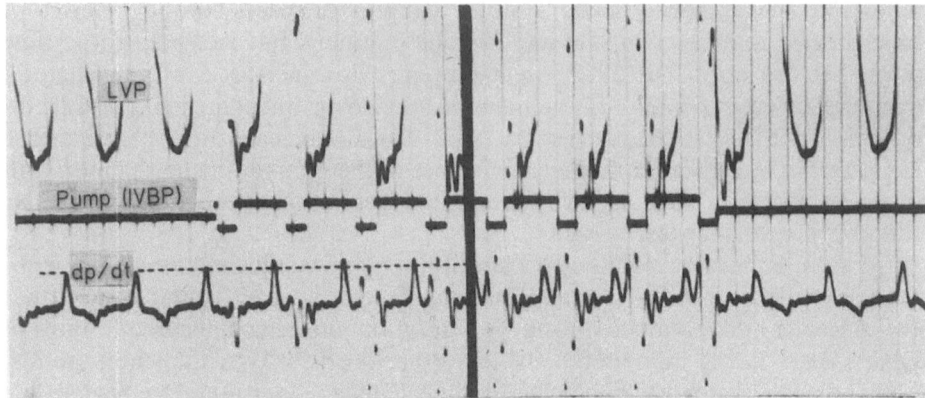

Fig. 6. Effect of end-systolic intraventricular balloon pumping (*IVBP*) on left ventricular end-diastolic pressure (*LVP*) and dp/dt

The technique increases left ventricular chamber compliance not by increasing the left ventricular end-diastolic dimensions but by reducing the end-systolic blood volume in the ventricle and therefore increasing the available ventricular filling space for the next diastolic phase. The data indicate the importance of the compliance factor for the effects of an assistance technique. While in a low contractility model mid-systolic brief intraventricular pumping may be more beneficial, in a low compliance model end-diastolic pumping is the method of choice.

The results of brief end-systolic intraventricular pumping may also be of theoretical interest. An increase in aortic flow is obtained, while the left ventricular end-diastolic pressure is actually reduced. This is not affected by lowering the peripheral resistance. Thinking in pressure-flow terms, a peculiar situation is found here, in which the proto-diastolic pressure is lowered by end-systolic pumping. Hence the intraventricular proto-to-end diastolic pressure gradient and not the end-diastolic pressure is increasing in parallel to the aortic flow. It is of interest that left ventricular contractility (dp/dt) and aortic flow may increase without an increase in left ventricular end-diastolic pressure, as one would assume to be necessary according to the Frank-Starling law, but following a steeper slope of the left ventricular diastolic pressure.

Systolic Counterpulsation in a "Ventricularized" Aorta

Classical diastolic intra-aortic counterpulsation has an important limitation: it is not effective when the heart is not beating or even when aortic pressure drops below a certain level (usually 60 mmHg systolic). This is due to the fact that the intra-aortic balloon operates in a chamber, the aorta, with an inlet valve (the aortic valve) only. The lack of an outlet valve can only be insignificant if the aortic pressure does not drop when the balloon is deflated, so that the blood pushed by the balloon toward the periphery does not regurgitate back into the aorta and prevent the balloon from sucking blood from the very weak left ventricle. This disadvantage limits the application of the technique to cases with a systolic aortic pressure above 60 mmHg.

A new technique has been tried in a cardiogenic shock animal model [6]. Two balloons were inserted in the aorta (Fig. 7). The proximal one was used as a di-

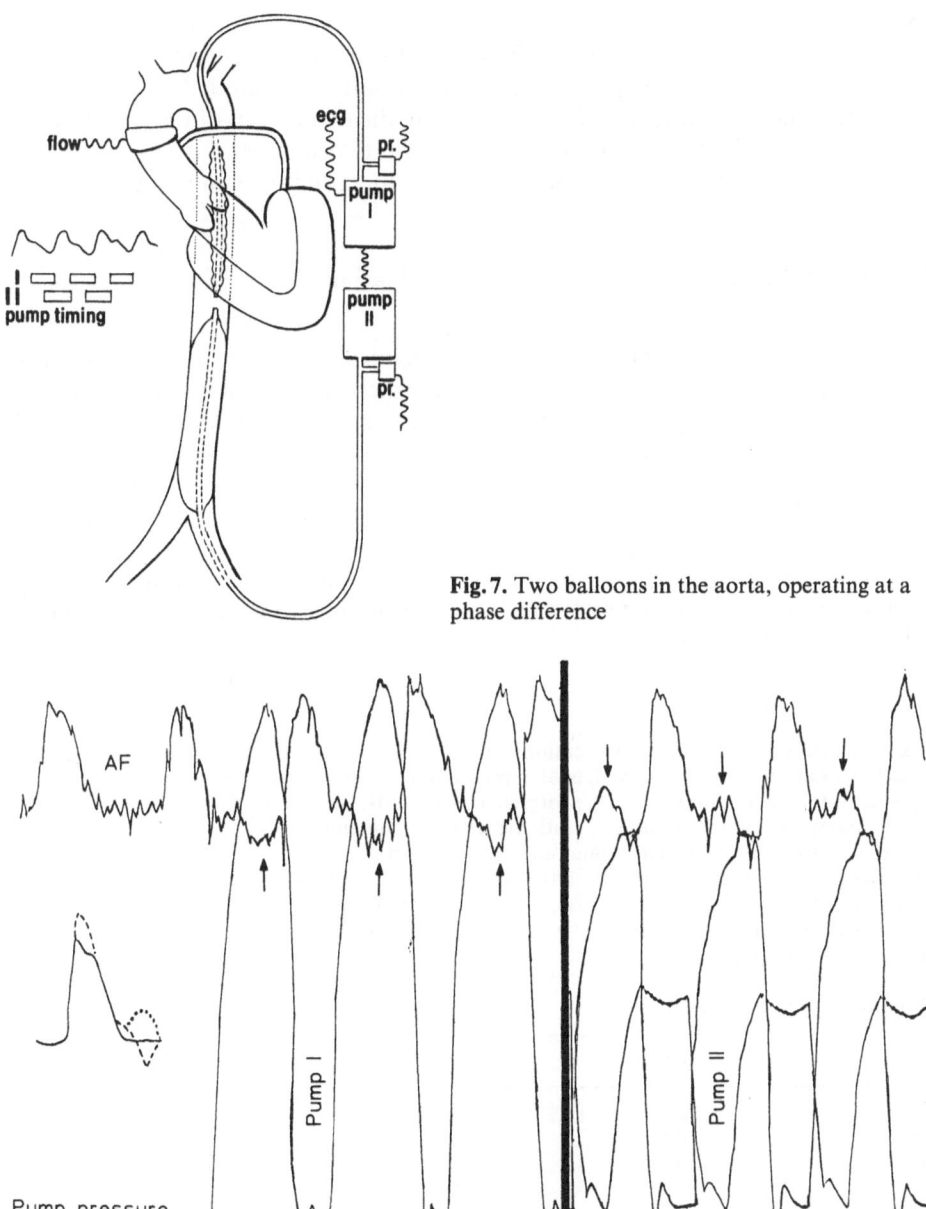

Fig. 7. Two balloons in the aorta, operating at a phase difference

Fig. 8. Effect of two intra-aortic balloons, pumping at a phase difference, on aortic flow (*AF*)

astolic counterpulsation balloon. The distal one was inflated during systole. In that way it acted as an outlet valve for the proximal balloon, the latter thus operating in a "ventricularized" aorta with two valves, one being the aortic valve and one, the distal balloon, inflating during systole. Using this technique the aortic flow increased by 31.6% ± 8.73% (Fig. 8). When the heart was fibrillated the two-balloon system could maintain an aortic flow of 400 ml/min in a 22-kg dog.

Research efforts are aiming to find ways to provide assistance to cases with severe reduction of aortic pressure or with a nonfunctioning left ventricle. Current attempts in this direction involve utilizing the two phases of the cardiac cycle when the heart is functioning or imitating the two phases in a ventricularized aorta with two balloons when the heart is not functioning adequately.

Specific Indications of Systolic Counterpulsation

The experimental application of several mechanical assistance techniques during the systolic phase of the cardiac circulatory cycle indicates their potential usefulness in the treatment of low contractility and/or low compliance conditions. It also illustrates the complexity of the circulatory assistance problem and the need for careful evaluation of the heart's condition before the application of a specific technique. The nature of the preponderant abnormality, i.e., whether it is low contractility or low compliance, should be assigned an important role in the selection of the technique for a functioning heart. Tables 1 and 2 summarize the effects of the techniques used on the experimental models of prevailing low contractility or low compliance.

Table 1. Effect of assistance interventions on an experimental shock model. A_1, intra-aortic diastolic pumping; A_2, midsystolic intra-aortic pumping; A_3, protracted intra-aortic diastolic pumping; V_1, end-diastolic intraventricular pumping; V_2, end-systolic intraventricular pumping; V_3, end-systolic left ventricular–peripheral vein shunt; IAB, intra-aortic diastolic balloon without a pump; AP, aortic pressure; LVEDP, left ventricular end-diastolic pressure; AF, aortic flow; mVO_2, minute volume oxygen

Method	Severe shock				
	AP	LVEDP	AF	dp/dt	mVO_2
A_1	↓	↓	↑	NS	↓
A_2	↑	NS	↑	NS	NS
A_3	↑	NS	↑	↑	NS
V_1	↑	↑	↑	↑	NS
V_2	NS	NS	↓	NS	NS
V_3	–	–	–	–	–
IAB	↑	NS	↑	NS	–

Table 2. Effect of assistance interventions on an experimental low compliance model. Symbols as in Table 1

Method	Low compliance state				
	AP	LVEDP	AF	dp/dt	mVO_2
A_1	↑	↓	↑	NS	NS
A_2	↑	↓	↓	↑	↑
A_3	–	–	–	–	–
V_1	↑	↑	↓	↑	↑
V_2	↑	↓	↑	↑	NS
V_3	NS	↓	NS	↑	↓
IAB	↑	NS	↑	↓	NS

References

1. Benzini A, Parda P (1956) The pneumomassage of the heart. Surgery 39:375
2. Anstadt G, Blakemore W, Baue A (1965) A new instrument for prolonged mechanical cardiac massage. Circulation 32 (Suppl 2):43
3. Claus R, Birtwell W, Albertal G (1961) Assisted circulation: I. The counterpulsator. Cardiovasc Surg 41:447
4. Moulopoulos S (1984) Systolic counterpulsation with a small balloon to increase coronary flow. In: Unger F (ed) Assisted circulation 2. Springer, Berlin Heidelberg New York Tokyo, p 38
5. Moulopoulos S, Stamatelopoulos S, Ekonomidis K, Adamopoulos S, Saridakis N, Antoniou A, Haniotis F (1984) A new technique to increase reduced left ventricular compliance. Eur Heart J 5:331
6. Moulopoulos S, Stamatelopoulos S, Ekonomidis K, Saridakis N, Tsoutsos D, Adraktas A (1987) "Ventricularization" of the aorta. A new method of support to the severely failing circulation. VIIth Congr. International Society for Artificial Organs, Munich 1987, Sept
7. Moulopoulos S (1983) Mechanical cardiac assistance. In: Hurst J (ed) Clinical assays on the heart. McGraw-Hill, New York, p 233

Part II
Cardiac Assistance

8. Ventricular Assist Devices: Possibilities and Limits

F. Unger

It is now 25 years ago that Dennis designed systems to assist a failing heart after open cardiac surgery, at a time when an open-heart case was a real hazard and the operative mortality was as high as 10%. The early concept has since been modified. Zwart and Litwak proposed systems to assist a failing heart via a trans-aortic access to the left ventricle; this concept is being discussed again, with implantation of a catheter in the left ventricle. Frazier now proposes unloading the left ventricle by means of a small rotary pump integrated in the catheter, which can handle an afterload of 100 mmHg.

The "classical" devices are pulsatile, pneumatically driven ventricles driven synchronously and asynchronously with the natural ECG. These devices work parallel to and replace the function of the heart. Devices that work in series with the natural heart are the IABP, intra-aortic ventricles, and the *Windkessel* ventricle.

There are two methods of implantation, with access via the left atrium (Fig. 1) or via the left ventricle (Fig. 2). The disadvantage of the first method is that the left ventricle is not unloaded properly and remains under tension up to the point of overtension. A left atrio-aortic is sufficient only for partial support of the heart.

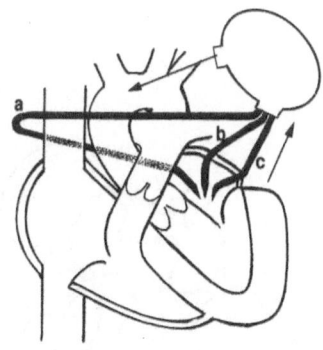

Fig. 1

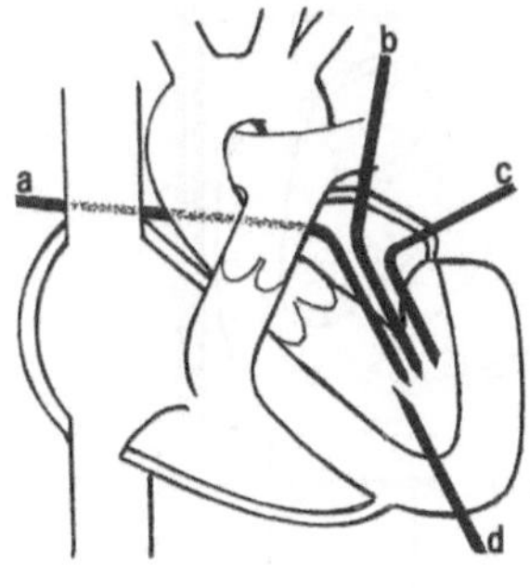

Fig. 1

Fig. 2

Fig. 2

Fig. 1. Left atrio-aortic left ventricular assist device (LAA-LVAD). Sites of cannulation: *a*, right superior pulmonary vein; *b*, roof of the atrium; *c*, via left auricle

Fig. 2. Implantation sites for left-ventricle access for the LVAD: *a*, via right pulmonary vein; *b*, via roof of the left atrium; *c*, via the left auricle; *d*, via the apex

Assisted Circulation 3
F. Unger (Ed.)
© Springer-Verlag Berlin Heidelberg 1989

As mentioned an LVAD can take over the work of the left ventricle entirely, due its parallelism. The main requirement is a working right ventricle. If the right ventricle fails an additional device on the right (an RVAD) side is necessary.

Access to the left ventricle for parallel-working devices can be achieved via the left atrium or via the left ventricle. The left-atrial access is always indicated when a temporary implantation is planned. For a permanent implantation or for bridging to transplantation a transapical left ventricular acces can be used.

The arterial return with both methods is to the ascending or descending aorta or the abdominal aorta (Fig. 3). The route depends mainly on the type of device used: for a temporary device with a paracorporeal position on access to the ascending aorta is most feasible; for a permanent device with a transapico-aortic bypass access to the abdominal aorta is preferable.

In cases of an isolated right ventricular failure syndrome a right ventricular assist device is necessary. The RVAD is implanted in the right ventricle via the right atrial appendage and the pulmonary artery. In cases where the LVAD is not working adequately due to a right heart failure syndrome the RVAD and LVAD are combined in a biventricular assist device (BVAD); (Fig. 4) which totally replaces the function.

We differentiate between *pulsatile* devices with artificial heart chambers (De Bakey, Kantrowitz, Bernhard, Gredel, Kwan-Gett, Pierce, Portner, Hill, Unger, Jarvik) which are driven pneumatically or electrically (Portner, Frazier, Whalen) and *nonpulsatile* blood pumps (Rollerpump, Centrimed, Biomedicus, Affeld, Bramm, Schistek, Hager, Quian).

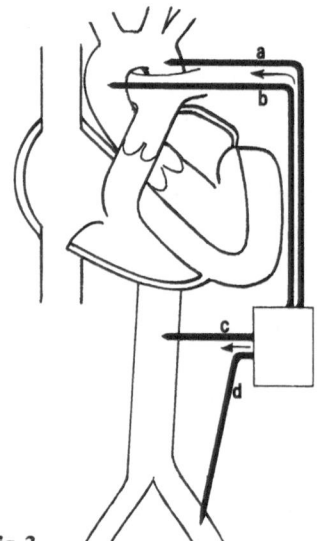

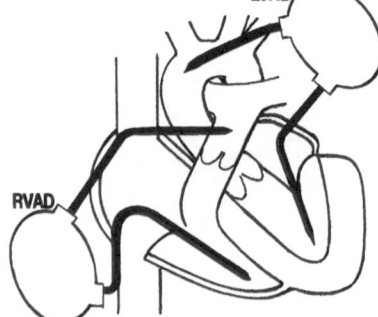

Fig. 3   **Fig. 4**

Fig. 3. Arterial return with an LVAD: *a*, to the ascending aorta; *b*, to the descending aorta; *c*, to the abdominal aorta; *d*, to the iliac artery

Fig. 4. Implantation site of a biventricular assist device (BVAD). *RVAD*, right ventricular assist device; *LVAD*, left ventricular assist device

An LVAD is indicated (a) in postoperative cardiac failure after open-heart surgery, (b) as a bridge to transplantation, and (c) possibly in cardiogenic shock after an acute myocardial infarction. An RVAD is indicated in isolated right ventricular failure after open-heart surgery. The BVAD is indicated (a) when an LVAD is not working properly due to right heart failure, (b) in cases of severe left and right heart failure after open-heart surgery or myocardial infarction, and (c) as a bridge to transplantation.

The pumps in clinical use are designed only for temporary support. A permanent substitute requires another design on a mechanical basis, such as those that are in construction by Portner, Whalen, or Frazier. Temporary mechanical pumps are driven electrically. These components are sources of failure in the long term. The problem of energy transmission is diminished, but the pumps require a compliance chamber with the same volume as that which is displaced. For temporary support the paracorporeal position is sufficient; for permanent support implantation in the abdominal cavity is necessary, but this requires extensive surgery, which is an additional trauma. Also, the perfusion to the heart is diminished in direct proportion to the distance of the site of return from the heart. The VADs can be driven synchronously or asynchronously to the ECG, but to avoid thromboemboli they must be driven at the maximal stroke.

In addition to the pulsatile blood pumps, nonpulsatile impeller pumps (Medtronic) and rotex pumps (Biomedicus) are in use with IABP to achieve pulsation. The nonpulsatile blood pumps are for very short-term use only. Heparinization, thrombus formation, and hemolysis are limiting factors. A fascinating new idea is the implantion of an open pump in the left ventricle to overcome shock after an acute myocardial infarction. The disadvantages of the nonpulsatile pumps are compensated by the low costs – at a time when budgets are being out the commercially available pulsatile blood pumps do not seem to be affordable. The actual number of clinical applications nonpulsatile pumps is not known, as registry of such implantations exists. Reports on unsuccessful attempts sometimes appear, but these do not give a picture of the real extent of use.

From 1962 to the present, 396 VADs using pulsatile pneumatically driven pumps have been employed. In 74 cases the VAD served as a bridge to cardiac transplantation (Fig. 5, Table 1). In 322 patients cardiogenic shock after open-

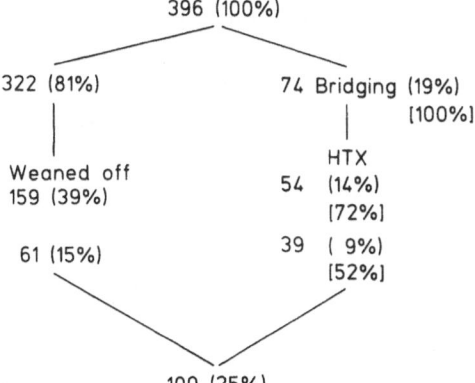

Fig. 5. Number of patients using assist devices who were discharged between 1962 and 1988

Table 1. Clinical implantations of ventricular assist devices 1962–1988

A

Device	No. of patients	Weaned off	Discharged
LVAD	221	88	39
RVAD	53	21	10
BVAD	122	48	12
Total	396	157 (39%)	61 (15%)

B

Device	No. of patients with bridging	HTX	Discharged
LVAD	29	22	17
RVAD	1	1	1
BVAD	44	31	21
	74 (19%) [100%]	54 (14%) [72%]	39 (14%) [52%]

Table 2. Bridging with assist devices versus TAH 1962–1988

	VAD	TAH	Total
Total no. of patients	74 (100%)	111 (100%)	185 (100%)
No. undergoing HTX	54 (72%)	72 (64%)	126 (68%)
No. survived	39 (52%)	29 (26%)	68 (36%)

heart surgery was the indication. From this pool of 396 patients, 25% were discharged, whereby the far better clinical outcome was in the group of bridging cases (52% versus 15% in the shock group). The absolute numbers are low, but we must consider that these patients had literally no other hope of survival. In a comparison between the VAD and the TAH the rate of outcome is similar: a total of 36% of the patients survived and were able to be discharged (Table 2).

Twenty-seven centers (18 of them within the United States) have clinical experience VADs. Seventy percent of the patients are men, 30% are women, with an average age of 56 years. In the bridging group the mean age is 34 years. The mean duration of circulatory support is 1.5 days with LVADs, 9 days with BVADs. In the bridging group the support lasts for a mean of 8 days. Complications encountered are:

- Bleeding, 45%
- Irreversible cardiac failure, 37%
- Renal failure, 32%
- Infection, 24%
- Respiratory failure, 22%
- Thrombus formation, 8%

- Mechanical failure, 2%
- Inadequate output, 2%

The list of complications makes evident how severely ill the patients are prior to the use of an assist device.

In this chapter, ten papers cover the problems encountered with VADs and the progress which has been achieved within the past few years.

Dr. Schoen, of the Boston group, and Dr. Bernhard discuss the pathological findings in 41 patients who received assist devices. The mean duration of support was 62 h. The blood pump they used was axisymmetrical and pneumatically driven. In 24 cases the bladder was textured, in 17 smooth. Thirty-nine patients had suffered postoperative cardiac failure, two cardiopulmonary failure. Nineteen were able to be weaned off, and six patients (14%) were discharged. Dr. Schoen evaluates the pathology of cardiac failure after cardiac surgery and after an acute myocardial infarction in contrast to cardiomyopathy and graft rejection. The causes of death are analyzed in detail.

Dr. Pae, of the Hershey group headed by Dr. Pierce, describes their 25 patients. Dr. Pae is also involved in the international registry, and I thank him very much for providing me with brand new data. The Hershey group uses the Pierce-Conachy heart, a lens-type ventricle without stagnation areas inside the blood chamber, which is driven pneumatically. This pump is commercially available. Of the 25 patients in whom it was applied, 13 were weaned off and nine survived. Six patients received the LVAD as a bridge to transplantation. Complications they report are bleeding and neurological problems.

Dr. Swartz, of Dr. Pennington's group in St. Louis, reports on clinical experience with 148 patients. They used various devices, such as the Medtronic pump, the membrane oxygenator ECMO (Scimed), the Thoratec pump, the Portner-Novacor, and the Jarvik TAH. This is the largest comparative group worldwide. They discuss the indications in postoperative cardiac failure, after acute myocardial infarction, and for bridging. Overall, there are 32 surviving patients (23%), whereby the outcome with the nonpulsatile pumps is not as good as that the pulsatile Thoratec blood pump. The complications they have encountered are bleeding (77%), biventricular failure (54%), infection (27%), mediastinitis (13.5%), thrombus formation (23%, mostly in the group of patients with nonpulsatile blood pumps), and hemolysis (38%). This paper depicts very well the limitations of assisted circulation. The authors conclude that the salvage rate is only 21%. For bridging they recommend the totally implantable Novacor system or a TAH.

Dr. Atsumi, of the Tokyo group, describes his 85 cases; 46 patients could be weaned off and 18 discharged (21%). Atsumi's group uses a sac-type pneumatically driven heart made of smooth polyurethane with integrated valves. This device is also commercially available. Complications seen are bleeding, renal insufficiency, and infection in 22 cases.

For many years, Dr. Golding, of the Cleveland Clinic, has used nonpulsatile blood pumps in postoperative heart patients and as a bridge to transplantation. In 51 cases Medtronic and Biomedicus pumps were used, whereby 25 patients could be weaned off and 11 discharged (21%). The author mentions bleeding, cardiac failure, infection, and stroke as complications. The hemolysis is up to 1500 mg. In six cases nonpulsatile blood pumps were used as a bridge, and three of the patients survived.

Dr. Campbell, of the Chicago group, follows the same concept as Dr. Golding. In 20 cases nonpulsatile blood pumps (Biomedicus) were used; 12 patients could be weaned off and eight discharged (40%). To achieve a pulsatile blood flow an intra-aortic balloon pump is inserted. Dr. Campbell performs a left atrial aortic bypass.

Dr. Rose, from New York, describes his experience in 82 cases where roller pumps were used as the VAD with a left atrio-aortic bypass. Thirty-two patients were weaned off and 21 discharged (25%). At the end of the article the author states some of the financial implications and points out the costs of nonpulsatile blood pumps.

Dr. Lawson, from the Thoratec company, reports on worldwide experience with the Pierce-Conachy pump. In 6 years, 164 cases of clinical application have been registered; it was used is a bridge in 68 cases and was successful in 43.

Dr. Quian, from Shanghai, presents his concept of a nonpulsatile blood pump with theoretical considerations. The first design has been tested with a mock circulation and in a goat.

Dr. Bramm, in cooperation with Dr. Olsen, relates his progress in developing a nonpulsatile blood pump in which the impeller is suspended in a magnetic field.

Dr. Hager, of the Salzburg group, presents an alternative blood pump: the spindle pump. The impeller is removed and replaced by a spindle. This spindle is sufficient to maintain a nonpulsatile blood flow in animal experiments, but the hemolysis is still high. This device is being tested as an LVAD.

Dr. Schistek, from Salzburg, describes two different nonpulsatile blood pumps. He has designed another impeller within the pump and inserts the impellers in a U-shaped ventricle. The devices can be used as an LVAD or a BVAD and are sufficient to obtain nonpulsatile flow. The two pumps can also function as a TAH.

In general, assisted circulation by means of pneumatically driven blood pumps has a definite place in the treatment of cardiac failure and postoperative cardiac failure, and possibly after myocardial infarction.

At present, the outcome is encouraging, measured against the indications given in patients who are severely ill and have literally no other hope of survival. The success rate for cases of bridging to transplantation is 50%. This is not yet acceptable for the manufacturers, who hesitate to produce in series and to develop new designs. The presently available devices are working well, however, and the potential market is large, especially among patients who suffer cardiac failure after myocardial infarction. The first step toward a totally implantable artificial heart will be a mechanical LVAD for patients with a cardiomyopathy. Within the next 5 years we hope to see permanent implants. Today, the mechanical blood pumps work well for temporary use. The nonpulsatile blood pumps are also acceptable, but only for the short term as well, due to the danger of embolization and hemolysis. The scope of indications needs to be enlarged, as cardiological problems affect a large population.

9. Pathological Considerations in Temporary Cardiac Assistance

F. J. SCHOEN and W. F. BERNHARD

Short-term circulatory support has been provided successfully with both ventricular assist devices (VADs) and total artificial hearts (TAHs). Of the approximately 1% of adult patients who develop severe cardiogenic shock following otherwise uncomplicated cardiac surgery, ventricular recovery (and hospital discharge) has been reported in as many as 40%–45% of those treated by aggressive temporary mechanical support [1]. Cardiac function and quality of life are excellent in long-term survivors [2, 3]. Due to the limited availability of donor organs for cardiac transplantation, many candidates succumb before a suitable donor organ becomes available. A number of these severely ill patients have survived until (and following) their transplants with the aid of a mechanical support device implanted in the face of precipitous hemodynamic decline [4, 5]. Thus, experience with temporary cardiac assistance (TCA) has accumulated in two groups of patients: (a) those in postcardiotomy cardiogenic shock, in whom the objective is ventricular recovery; and (b) those needing a "bridge" to transplantation, when no ventricular recovery is expected; in this situation, the goal is hemodynamic support of the patient until cardiac replacement may be done with a donor heart. Although there is a potential role of temporary ventricular support in patients with cardiogenic shock due to acute myocardial infarction, clinical experience with TCA done for this indication is extremely limited.

This paper reviews the pathological considerations in temporary mechanical cardiac assistance. The objective is to enhance the rational clinical use and further development of mechanical devices for both transient and permanent circulatory support. In particular, we summarize (a) the morphology and pathophysiology of substrate lesions for which cardiac assistance may be indicated, (b) the devices and their previous use, (c) the mechanistic basis for functional myocardial recovery during cardiac assistance, and (d) the patient pathology and device complications encountered and anticipated.

Pathology of Cardiac Failure

Acute Myocardial Ischemia and Infarction

Classical acute myocardial infarction occurs when the perfusion of the myocardium is reduced severely below its needs, causing profound *ischemia* (i.e., imbalance of blood supply and demand). Prolonged ischemia results in permanent loss of function through cell death by coagulation necrosis. Under typical conditions,

Assisted Circulation 3
F. Unger (Ed.)
© Springer-Verlag Berlin Heidelberg 1989

irreversibly injured (i.e., necrotic) cardiac myocytes cannot regenerate; death of these cells is generally followed by their removal and subsequent replacement by fibrous connective tissue. Thus, necrosis elicits edema within hours, an acute inflammatory response within the first day, phagocytosis of necrotic cells after several days, neovascularization and formation of collagen after 1–2 weeks, and the development of a dense collagenized scar after 4–6 weeks [6].

The outcome of ischemia is largely dependent on the severity and duration of flow deprivation [7]. Experimental studies have elucidated the progressive biochemical, functional, and morphological changes which occur in acutely ischemic myocardium [8]. Despite rapid onset of biochemical abnormalities and profound functional derangement, including loss of contractility, within 60 s of onset of severe ischemia, cell death is not immediate but occurs only following 20–40 min. Thus, viable but severely ischemic myocardium can be dysfunctional.

As demonstrated experimentally in the dog – and the situation is presumably similar in humans – severe ischemia lasting approximately 20–40 min or longer leads to irreversible damage to cardiac myocytes [8]. In contrast, when restoration by reperfusion of myocardial blood follows briefer periods of flow deprivation (less than 20 min), loss of cell viability generally does not result [9, 10]. Indeed, following short-term transient ischemia and subsequent reperfusion, biochemical and functional recovery generally occurs. However, return of a normal biochemical and functional state does not necessarily occur immediately but rather can be delayed as long as several days (i.e., prolonged postischemic ventricular dysfunction, or the "stunned myocardium" [11]).

With more extended ischemia, a wavefront of cell death moves through the myocardium to involve progressively more of the transmural thickness of the ischemic zone [8]. Although the extent of necrosis is largely complete within 3–6 h in experimental models, progression of necrosis frequently follows a more protracted course in humans, largely due to a well-developed coronary arterial collateral system in man. Early alleviation of ischemia results in myocardial salvage peripheral to already necrotic zones, and thus, reperfusion salvages reversibly injured cells. This can occur following global ischemia (as in cardiac surgery) or regional ischemia (as in coronary thrombolysis during an evolving acute myocardial infarct). Other effects of reperfusion include accelerated destruction of cells that are already lethally injured, leading to a morphological pattern often called "contraction band necrosis" [11].

Cardiac Failure Following Open-Heart Surgery

Recent technical advances have enhanced myocardial preservation, including limitation of operative duration, widespread effective use of hypothermia, and induced hyperkalemic cardioplegia. Nevertheless, a small percentage of patients undergoing cardiac surgery cannot be weaned from intraoperative cardiopulmonary bypass (CPB) using conventional pharmacological therapy and volume loading. Approximately half of these patients respond to counterpulsation with the intra-aortic balloon pump (IABP), but the remainder, approximately 1% of patients undergoing open-heart surgical procedures [12], require more profound cardiac assistance.

Individuals who die shortly following various cardiac surgical procedures or patients who have had clinical TCA frequently have myocardial necrosis, with or without hemorrhage and edema [7, 13]. Necrosis with contraction bands is frequently observed. Acute myocardial injury occurring during open-heart surgery has some pathophysiological features analogous to those described above for acute myocardial infarction. Biochemical and morphological changes secondary to global ischemia (occurring during ischemic arrest with CPB) are qualitatively similar to those noted during regional ischemia; however, they generally develop more slowly [14, 15].

Myocardial Disease: Cardiomyopathy, Myocarditis, Cardiac Transplant Candidates, Graft Rejection

The term *cardiomyopathy* describes heart disease in which the pathology originates within the myocardium [16–18]. According to the World Health Organization, *cardiomyopathy* is heart muscle disease of unknown cause; *specific heart muscle disease* is heart muscle disease of known cause or associated with disorders of other systems [19]. Myocardial diseases attributable to coronary artery disease, systemic or pulmonary hypertension, valvular heart disease, or congenital cardiovascular malformations (whether in the heart or circulation) are excluded. Thus, patients having heart failure with nonspecific pathological findings are said to have *idiopathic* cardiomyopathy, while cardiac failure in patients with severe coronary atherosclerosis and secondary myocardial damage have "heart failure due to coronary heart disease" (often called "ischemic cardiomyopathy" [20]). The prognosis of either idiopathic dilated cardiomyopathy or heart failure due to coronary artery disease is poor, with less than 50% of patients surviving 2 years [21]. Most candidates for heart transplantation have idiopathic cardiomyopathy or end-stage coronary heart disease. Of the first 288 patients undergoing transplantation at Stanford, 46% suffered from coronary disease, 45% from cardiomyopathy, and the remainder from congenital or valvular heart disease [22].

Myocarditis, a relatively uncommon cause of heart failure, is an inflammatory process of the heart muscle due to known or unknown causes [23, 24]. Myocarditis is commonly associated with viral infections, either as a direct infection or as a result of a postviral immunological reaction against the heart (myocytes, interstitial cells, or noncellular components). The outcome of myocardial inflammatory destruction varies widely, ranging from rapidly progressive acute cardiac failure (weeks or months), to chronic congestive heart failure (dilated cardiomyopathy) occurring over many years, or probably, to complete resolution without functional sequelae [17, 23]. Percutaneous transvenous endomyocardial biopsy has enhanced the ability to identify this condition [25]. Although some studies suggest that patients with myocarditis may respond favorably to administration of anti-inflammatory and immunosuppressive agents, use of such therapy in myocarditis is controversial.

Approximately one-fourth of patients awaiting transplantation succumb prior to the location of a suitable donor organ [26]. Deterioration is frequently precipitous. TCA may serve as a bridge to transplantation in these circumstances, as well as potentially supporting patients having myocarditis or those having acute cardiac rejection following transplantation. Acute rejection is a potentially reversible inflammatory process in many respects analogous to idiopathic myocarditis [27]. Circulatory support could provide the time for effective mitigation of the process with immunosuppressive agents. Furthermore, coronary arteriosclerosis developing in the transplanted heart (chronic rejection), often with myocardial infarcts, is a major course of late death following allograft transplantation [28]. Although timely identification of patients with cardiac graft arteriosclerosis is difficult, since in the denervated heart ischemic damage is not heralded by chest pain, some such patients may benefit from cardiac assistance during preparation for retransplantation.

Clinical Temporary Cardiac Assistance

Devices Used

The IABP is now the most widely used temporary mechanical aid to circulation [29]. Although all cardiac output passes through the patient's own ventricles, the IABP adds volume to the aorta during diastole, augmenting coronary arterial perfusion, and removes it during systole. Most other assist devices direct at least a portion of circulation through the device itself, producing pulsatile or nonpulsatile flow. Nonpulsatile devices employ roller pumps or centrifugal pumps with or without extracorporeal perfusion. Heart-lung machines and extracorporeal membrane oxygenators (ECMOs) are representative of nonpulsatile assist devices. Heart-lung machines are used almost exclusively during open-heart surgery because of the acquired defects in hemostasis which result from their extended use [30–32]. Though patients can be supported considerably longer on an ECMO, it is used chiefly for rapid resuscitation, with the advantage that a thoracotomy is not require [33, 34].

Pulsatile VADs deployed for temporary support have a flexible polymeric blood sac enclosed in a rigid chamber. For left ventricular assistance, blood in the left atrium or left ventricle enters a cannula and passes through an inlet valve into the sac and then through an outlet valve into the thoracic or abdominal aorta. For right ventricular assistance, the right atrium and pulmonary artery are the inflow and outflow cannulation sites, respectively. Bilaterally placed individual pumps can be used for biventricular support. Usually, for TCA, the pump case itself, depending on the model, is placed paracorporeally against the chest or intra-abdominally. Contemporary pulsatile pumps are pneumatically driven by external air pulses directed through a hose into the rigid case, where the blood sac is compressed. All pneumatic devices necessitate percutaneous conduits.

The pulsatile pumps most widely used include the Pierce-Donachy pneumatic device with a blood sac made of a smooth-surfaced polyurethane (Biomer) and Björk-Shiley tilting disk valves, and the Bernhard-Thermedics VAD, which employs a polyurethane blood sac and porcine bioprosthetic valves. The most recent model of the latter has a blood sac made of an integrally textured surface designed to promote formation of a controlled pseudointimal lining [35]. The TAHs that have been used clinically are pneumatically driven [4, 5]. They contain two implantable pumps similar in basic design to those of the VADs: flexible sacs in rigid cases with attached percutaneous air conduits. A TAH is anastomosed to the atria and great vessels after removal of the patient's ventricles; one pump supports the systemic circulation while the other supports the pulmonary circulation. The Jarvik-7, with its smooth polyurethane bladder and Metronic-Hall tilting disk valves, has been the most frequently used TAH device for bridging to transplantation [4, 5, 36].

Temporary Ventricular Support: Results and Complications

Ventricular assist devices have aided patients who cannot be weaned from extracorporeal circulation following cardiotomy and, to a lesser extent, patients with acute myocardial infarction who have some degree of potentially reversible ventricular dysfunction. Experience is growing with use of the TAH and pulsatile VADs to provide interim support prior to cardiac transplantation in patients suffering from various forms of myocardial disease, acute cardiac transplant rejection, and postmyocardial infarction cardiogenic shock.

Postcardiotomy Cardiogenic Shock

Clinical experience in the management of postcardiotomy cardiogenic shock has been obtained using three types of VAD: (a) roller pumps, (b) centrifugal (vortex) pumps, and (c) pneumatic pulsatile pumps. Regardless of the system used, the goal is to diminish myocardial oxygen consumption and work, while allowing time for recovery of a metabolically deranged myocardium. Left atrial to aortic TCA with roller pumps has been employed with varied results by many investigators. Two recent reports illustrate the results that can be achieved with these systems [37, 38]. In one study, 18 of 27 patients (67%) were weaned from the device, nine were discharged from the hospital, and seven were well long-term [35]. In the other, 21 of 46 patients (46%) were successfully weaned from the device and 16 were discharged; most had excellent late cardiac function [36].

Complications encountered in the above studies included severe coagulopathy, which was a direct cause of death in nine patients, and neurological injury, which occurred in two. In some patients who did not survive, there may have been progressive right heart failure, which probably resulted from right heart ischemia because of inadequate left heart bypass flows – a potential limitation of any system based on cannula size. Nevertheless, roller pumps have the advantage of simplicity, availability, and low cost, despite the disadvantages of potential for thromboembolism, the need for anticoagulation therapy, flow limitations, blood trauma, and nonpulsatility.

The advantages of modern vortex pumps are simplicity, availability, relatively low cost, minimal blood trauma, and little or no need to use systemic anticoagulants. Left atrial to aortic bypass with a centrifugal pump has been reported in 21 patients, with ten patients (48%) having been weaned and five of them (24%) having been discharged from the hospital and surviving 1–3 years after surgery [39]. A major factor limiting success was the inability to maintain adequate flow with left heart assistance alone when there was associated severe right ventricular failure. Complications were not specifically addressed in that study. In contrast, another study found that hemorrhage necessitating reoperation, hemolysis, and thrombi in the pump were common [40]. One patient had an arterial embolus. Thus, heparin therapy was recommended with such pumps.

Pneumatic pulsatile VADs eliminate the need for systemic anticoagulation therapy, minimize blood trauma and the potential for thromboembolism, and provide complete physiological support of the systemic and pulmonary circulations, either together or individually. In one study, the Pierce-Donachy VAD was used in 21 patients who could not be weaned from CPB with conventional techniques [41]. Eleven patients (52%) were ultimately weaned from ventricular support. The overall hospital discharge rate was 43%. Nine long-term survivors followed up to 60 months after hospital discharge had good cardiac status and quality of life. Complications occurred in nearly half of the 21 patients and included respiratory insufficiency and bleeding that required reoperation in one-third of the patients, despite the fact that no anticoagulation therapy was used. Hemolysis, infection, and thromboembolism were absent, as were neurological events attributable to assist pumping. Similar experiences were reported in another 17 patients having TCA for postcardiotomy cardiogenic shock [42]. Overall survival and hospital discharge rates were 41%, while long-term survival and quality of life were reported as excellent. The most common complication was bleeding; three of the eight patients who were weaned required exploration for hemorrhage. Thromboembolism and hemolysis could not be attributed to ventricular assist pumping, and neurological events were absent.

We recently reported a study of 41 patients distributed among four centers with left (33 patients), right (5), or biventricular (3) temporary ventricular assistance with textured (24) or smooth (17) surfaced diaphragm pumps, during an evaluation supported by the National Institute of Health [13]. Cardiac failure had occurred in 39 postoperative patients with a mean total CPB time of 306 min (range 69–600). Two patients had cardiomyopathy. Mean duration of support in all patients was 62 h. In 16 patients (40%) whose condition improved, mean duration of TCA was 127 h (range 48–264), compared with a mean of 19 h (range 1–120) in 25 patients whose condition did not improve. Of 17 patients in whom duration of support exceeded 72 h, 15 (88%) improved, 11 were weaned, and 6 survived long-term. Tissue examination (in 33 patients) by biopsy at pump implantation or autopsy revealed coagulation or contraction band myocyte necrosis, with or without hemorrhage, in 26 patients. Of these, ten improved and six were long-term survivors. Pump-related complications included pulmonary embolism, most likely related to a right atrial cannulation site thrombus, and an aortic cannulation site infection in one patient each.

Bridge to Transplantation
In the last several years, over 50 patients have received temporary ventricular support or a pneumatic TAH as a bridge to transplantation. Many have subsequently received successful transplants and are alive. In a representative study, the Jarvik-7 TAH was implanted into six moribund patients awaiting cardiac transplantation. Four of these patients were reported well and at home after implantation

of the device and subsequent allograft transplantation [5]. One patient died following transplantation owing to sepsis and multiorgan failure that preceded artificial heart implantation. Another patient died with acute allograft rejection 60 days postoperatively. Fifty days of total mechanical support with the artificial heart were accumulated in these six patients, who collectively with other patients so treated demonstrate the ability of both the paracorporeal assist pump and the TAH to provide temporary circulatory support to patients who decompensate hemodynamically while awaiting a donor organ for orthotopic heart transplantation, and to patients who reject a donor heart after transplantation. However, although clinically apparent thromboembolic events were infrequent, each artificial heart contained areas of macroscopic aggregations of platelets and thrombi. It is important that systems designed and used for bridging procedures minimize the likelihood of device-related complications (infection, thromboembolism) that might contraindicate subsequent transplantation.

Pathology and Physiology of Temporary Cardiac Assistance

Causes of Death

In our study of 41 patients receiving TCA, death of 35 nonsurvivors was due to myocardial necrosis (14), hemorrhage (9), cerebrovascular accident (3), and other causes (9) [13]. The three instances of cerebrovascular accident were each hemorrhagic and were not considered to have an embolic etiology on the basis of detailed pathological examination.

Multiple reasons for failure of TCA in postcardiotomy cardiogenic shock have been noted. Improvement can be obviated by the use of the devices at a sufficiently late stage to prevent deterioration. In our study, patients who were assisted less than 2–3 days died predominantly of abnormalities likely existing before initiation of cardiac assistance, particularly hemorrhage. Uncontrollable hemorrhage, a major cause of death after TCA in most studies, is considered to be largely a result of the hemostatic abnormalities induced by the extended duration of CPB necessary for the operative procedure [30–32], resuscitation attempts, and pump implantation, and is thus to a large extent present before insertion of the assist device. Multiple system failure, an important compromising factor after TCA, probably relates to the prolonged low output state before pump implantation.

Cardiac Pathology: Mechanisms of Reversible Cardiac Dysfunction

The pathogenesis of the specific myocardial abnormality in reversible cardiac dysfunction is unknown. Acute myocardial injury existing prior to TCA is clearly an important limiting factor to the success of TCA in postcardiotomy and post-myocardial infarct patients. However, although perioperative myocardial infarction is considered to have an important negative influence on prognosis, four of the 15 long-term survivors reported by Pennington and colleagues had perioperative infarcts [43]. The acute cardiac changes found in patients who have had TCA are nonspecific, and likely to have arisen largely, if not completey, before implantation of the assist device. Although the early mortality of most cardiac operations is low, acute myocardial damage is an important complication of these procedures. Pathological studies show a high frequency of myocardial necrosis in nonsurvivors of cardiac operation [44, 45]. Nevertheless, many patients who cannot be weaned from extracorporeal circulation or who die early postoperatively show no damage observable by gross inspection or light microscopic analysis. There are three possible explanations for this lack of correlation of structure with function. Firstly, in some of these patients, the lesions may have had insufficient time to develop recognizable morphological manifestations. Secondly, the pathological changes may be limited to the ultrastructural level, and ultrastrutural studies cannot be done reliably on autopsy specimens. Finally, it is likely that there are no morphological correlates to certain states of functional myocardial impairment.

Assist devices decompress the failing ventricle, thereby decreasing myocardial work and oxygen demand while maintaining coronary blood flow and systemic tissue perfusion [7]. The benefit permitted by pump support could be based within either necrotic myocardium or viable myocardium or both. However, since established myocardial necrosis cannot undergo functionally significant improvement during the short duration of TCA, and the performance of nonviable myocardium is essentially unaffected by enhanced flows and perfusion pressures, the reversible functional abnormality must primarily involve factors other than modification of prior necrosis. Rather, such necrosis may serve as a morphological marker that a potentially large volume of adjacent myocardium is functionally and biochemically deranged, but reversibly, so perhaps out of proportion to the extent of necrosis [7]. Thus, TCA not only facilitates myocardial salvage through reduction of myocardial oxygen utilization, thereby inhibiting the effects of myocardial ischemia and the extent of evolving infarction, but also permits the biochemical and functional recovery of viable but injured myocardium by supporting systemic perfusion during this critical period. The most likely processes which could account for reversibility of dysfunction include resolution of intracellular or interstitial myocardial edema or hemorrhage in injured but viable myocardium, and the recovery of contractility to myocardium with prolonged but reversible ischemic dysfunction.

Reperfusion of temporarily ischemic myocardium, such as occurs following CPB or coronary thrombolysis, has several consequences, including salvage of reversibly injured myocytes and acceleration and modification of morphological changes produced by the degeneration of dead myocytes (e.g., contraction bands) [11]. Furthermore, reperfusion of severely ischemic myocardium is followed by striking increases in tissue water and electrolytes [9]. Significant intracellular (largely mitochondrial) edema occurs in hearts after the global ischemia encountered during cardiac operations [46]. Resolution of edema could potentially be accomplished within several days and contribute to recovery of cardiac function.

Despite only sublethal damage to myocardial cells suffering ischemia of short duration followed by reperfusion (i.e., no necrosis), return of normal myocardial metabolism and function (both sensitive measures of myocardial injury) may be delayed, perhaps as long as several days (i.e., the myocardium is viable but "stunned"). Most patients who improve during TCA have been supported for 48–72 h or more [13]. The time course of return of normal myocardial metabolism and contractility after restoration of adequate circulation, determined experimentally, is compatible with the observed several days of TCA before weaning is possible [7, 9, 10]. It is likely that recovery of reversibly injured myocardium from prolonged ischemic dysfunction is the major pathophysiological mechanism responsible for the efficacy of TCA in reversing postcardiotomy (or post-myocardial infarction) cardiac failure [7].

Furthermore, in most studies, right ventricular failure is an important factor compromising success in some patients [13, 35]. The significance and mechanism of right ventricular processes in acute myocardial failure and its potential recovery are not clear. Reversible right ventricular dysfunction in the early postoperative period could relate to multifactorial acute right-sided myocardial injury or perhaps to the effects of complement-mediated, polymorphonuclear leukocyte activation, demonstrated to occur after cardiac operations [47]. The resultant stasis of polymorphonuclear leukocytes in lung capillaries and arterioles could cause obstruction leading to acute pulmonary hypertension. Irrespective of cause, some patients with right ventricular failure may be salvaged with appropriate pharmacological and mechanical support.

Patient/Device Interactions

During the early years of experiments with the cardiac assist device and TAH implantations, many animals died of technical or mechanical failures. As design and techniques improved, animal survivals were prolonged and the causes of death were usually related to pulmonary insufficiency, low cardiac output, and thromboembolism [48–51]. Biomaterial emboli were noted occasionally. More recently, during extended experiments of 3–6 months, device failure modes and related pathological processes frequently have included dysfunction caused by fracture of mechanical prosthetic valves [52], and calcification of bioprosthetic valves [53] and pumping bladders [54–57].

Studies of clinical TCA have shown rare embolic sequelae. In our study, no patient had a documented pump-related systemic embolus, despite absence of anticoagulation through most of the course of TCA [13]. The most significant thrombi were noted in association with connections of conduits to the heart and in a pump in which the weaning procedure included prolonged cross-clamping of pump conduits. In those cases, thrombi appeared related to details of conduit placement and weaning technique rather than to specific deficiencies of assist pump design. Although pump-related thromboemboli have been uncommon in patients with paracorporeal or implanted temporary assist devices (in this and other studies), close attention to each of these potential problems is justified in future investigations of both short-term and long-term mechanical cardiac assistance.

In contrast, patients who have long-term TAH implantations with the Jarvik-7 and other replacement pumps have almost uniformly experienced serious thromboembolic sequelae [4, 5, 58, 59]. These pumps, used either transiently or long-term, frequently show small thrombi at the junctions of various components of the pump and of the pump with conduits. In patients with circulatory assist devices in general, the appropriate management of anticoagulation and the potential efficacy of adjunctive antiplatelet agents remains to be determined.

The use of transcutaneous conduits in desperately ill patients may predispose to infection at the sites of skin penetration. However, serious infection has been only an occasional problem in temporary ventricular assistance and total heart implantation [13, 60]. Nevertheless, the potential risk of infection, particularly with opportunistic organism, should be carefully considered, especially when temporary assist devices are used in patients who are or are soon likely to be immunosuppressed, particularly heart transplant candidates (awaiting hearts) or recipients (being treated for rejection). Fracture of a Björk-Shiley valve necessitated replacement of the inflow valve in a clinical TAH implantation [58]. Hemolysis has not been a clinically significant problem.

Calcification of pumping bladders and valves is a major limiting factor in the long-term investigation of blood pumps of all types in animals. Microscopic (but not gross) calcific deposits were recently noted on the pumping diaphragms of two clinical Jarvik-7 TAHs implanted for 488 and 621 days [61]. However, calcification of the pumping bladder or valves has not been noted during short-term clinical ventricular assistance in this or other series, and is not anticipated in short-term TCA. Nevertheless, mineral deposits can form rapidly under certain circumstances in humans. For example, extrinsic calcification of a superficial thrombus on a bioprosthetic heart valve was observed 3 days postoperatively in a patient with postoperative renal failure [62].

References

1. Pae WE (1987) Temporary ventricular support. Current indications and results. Trans Am Soc Artif Intern Organs 33:4–7
2. Rose DM, Laschinger J, Grossi E et al. (1985) Experimental and clinical results with a simplified left heart assist device for treatment of profound left ventricular dysfunction. World J Surg 9:11–17
3. Pennington DC, Bernhard WF, Golding LR et al. (1985) Long-term follow-up of postcardiotomy patients with profound cardiogenic shock treated with ventricular assist devices. Circulation 72 (Suppl II):II-216-226
4. Joyce LD, Johnson KE, Pierce WS et al. (1986) Summary of the world experience with clinical use of total artificial hearts as heart support devices. J Heart Transplant 5:229–235
5. Griffith BP, Hardesty RL, Kormos RL et al. (1987) Temporary use of the Jarvik-7 total artificial heart before transplantation. N Engl J Med 316:130–134
6. Fishbein MC, MacLean D, Maroko PR (1978) The histopathologic evolution of myocardial infarction. Chest 73:843
7. Schoen FJ, LaFarge CG, Bernhard WF (1985) Pathology and pathophysiology of temporary cardiac assist. Am Soc Artif Intern Organs J 8:174–181
8. Reimer KA, Jennings RB, Tatum AH (1983) Pathobiology of acute myocardial ischemia: metabolic, functional and ultrastructural studies. Am J Cardiol 52:72A–81A
9. Jennings RB, Reimer KA (1983) Factors involved in salvaging ischemic myocardium: effect of reperfusion of arterial blood. Circulation 68 (Suppl I):I-25-I-36
10. Kloner RA, Ellis SG, Lange R, Braunwald E (1983) Studies of experimental coronary artery reperfusion. Effects on infarct size, myocardial function, biochemistry, ultrastructure and microvascular damage. Circulation 68 (Suppl I):8–15
11. Braunwald E, Kloner RA (1985) Myocardial reperfusion: a double-edged sword? J Clin Invest 76:1713–1719

12. McGee MG, Zillgitt SL, Trono R et al. (1980) Retrospective analyses of the need for mechanical circulatory support (intraaortic balloon pump/abdominal left ventricular assist device or partial artificial heart) after cardiopulmonary bypass. A 44-month study of 14168 patients. Am J Cardiol 46:135–142

13. Schoen FJ, Palmer DC, Bernhard WF (1986) Clinical temporary ventricular assist. Pathologic findings and their implications in a multi-institutional study of 41 patients. J Thorac Cardiovasc Surg 92:1071–1081

14. Jennings RB, Reimer KA, Hill ML, Mayer SE (1981) Total ischemia in dog hearts, in vitro. I. Comparison of high energy phosphate production, utilization, and depletion, and of adenine nucleotide catabolism in total ischemia in vitro vs. severe ischemia in vivo. Circ Res 49:892–900

15. Schaper J, Schwarz F, Kittstein H et al. (1982) The effects of global ischemia and reperfusion on human myocardium: quantitative evaluation by electron microscopic morphometry. Ann Thorac Surg 33:116–122

16. Johnson RA, Palacios L (1982) Dilated cardiomyopathies of the adult. N Engl J Med 307:1051–1058, 1119–1120

17. Abelmann WH (1984) Classification and the natural history of primary myocardial disease. Prog Cardiovasc Dis 27:73–94

18. Davies MJ (1984) The cardiomyopathies: a review of terminology, pathology and pathogenesis. Histopathology 8:363–393

19. Brandenburg RO, Chazou E, Cherian G et al. WHO (1980) Report of the WHO/ISFC Task Force on definition and classification of cardiomyopathies. Br Heart J 44:672–673

20. Pantely GA, Bristow JD (1984) Ischemic cardiomyopathy. Prog Cardiovasc Dis 27:95–114

21. Franciosa JA, Wilen M, Ziesche S, Cohn JN (1983) Survival in men with severe chronic left ventricular failure due to either coronary heart disease or idiopathic dilated cardiomyopathy. Am J Cardiol 51:831–836

22. Jamieson SW, Oyer P, Baldwin J et al. (1984) Heart transplantation for end-stage ischemic heart disease: the Stanford experience. Heart Transplant 3:224–228

23. Kereiakes DJ, Parmley WW (1984) Myocarditis and cardiomyopathy. Am Heart J 108:1318–1326

24. Weinstein C, Fenoglio JJ (1987) Myocarditis. Hum Pathol 18:613–618

25. Aretz HT (1987) Myocarditis: the Dallas criteria. Hum Pathol 18:619–624

26. Copeland JG, Emery RW, Levinson MM et al. (1987) Selection of patients for cardiac transplantation. Circulation 75:2–9

27. Bieber CP, Stinson EB, Shumway NE et al. (1970) Cardiac transplantation in man. VII. Cardiac allograft pathology. Circulation 41:753–772

28. Hess ML, Hastillo A, Mohanakumar T et al. (1983) Accelerated atherosclerosis in cardiac transplantation: role of cytotoxic B-cell antibodies and hyperlipidemia. Circulation 68 (Suppl II):II-94–II-101

29. Bolooki H (1985) Current status of circulatory support with an intra-aortic balloon pump. Cardiol Clin 3:123–133

30. Harker LA (1986) Bleeding after cardiopulmonary bypass. N Engl J Med 314:1446–1448

31. Addonizio VP, Colman RW (1982) Platelets and extracorporeal circulation. Biomaterials 3:9–15

32. Bick RL (1985) Hemostasis defects associated with cardiac surgery, prosthetic devices, and other extracorporeal circuits. Semin Thromb Hemost 11:249–280

33. Bartlett RH, Toomasian J, Roloff D et al. (1986) Extracorporeal membrane oxygenation (ECMO) in neonatal respiratory failure. Ann Surg 204:236–245

34. Sell LL, Cullen ML, Whittlesey GC et al. (1986) Hemorrhagic complications during extracorporeal membrane oxygenation: prevention and treatment. J Pediatr Surg 21:1087–1091

35. Szycher M, Poirier V, Franzblau C et al. (1981) Biochemical, histological, and ultrastructural assessments of pseudoneointimal linings derived from fibroblast-seeded integrally textured polymeric surfaces. J Biomed Mater Res 15:247–265

36. Yared SF, Johnson GS, DeVries WC (1986) Results of artificial heart implantation in man. Transplant Proc 18 (Suppl 2):69–74

37. Litwak RS, Koffsky RM, Jurado RA et al. (1985) A decade of experience with a left heart assist device in patients undergoing open intracardiac operation. World J Surg 9:18–24

38. Rose DM, Laschinger J, Grossi E et al. (1985) Experimental and clinical results with a simplified left heart assist device for treatment of profound left ventricular dysfunction. World J Surg 9:11–17

39. Magovern GJ, Park SB, Maher TD (1985) Use of a centrifugal pump without anticoagulants for postoperative left ventricular assist. World J Surg 9:25–36

40. Pennington DG, Merjavy JP, Swartz MT et al. (1985) The importance of biventricular failure in patients with postoperative cardiogenic shock. Ann Thorac Surg 39:16–26

41. Pae WE, Pierce WS, Pennock JL et al. (1987) Long-term results of ventricular assist pumping in postcardiotomy cardiogenic shock. J Thorac Cardiovasc Surg 93:434–441

42. Pennington DG, Samuels LD, Williams G et al. (1985) Experience with the Pierce-Donachy ventricular assist device in postcardiotomy patients with cardiogenic shock. World J Surg 9:37–46

43. Pennington DC, Bernhard WF, Golding LR et al. (1985) Long-term follow-up of postcardiotomy patients with profound cardiogenic shock salvaged by ventricular assist devices. Circulation 72 (Suppl 2):216–226

44. Bulkley BH, Hutchins GM (1977) Myocardial consequences of coronary artery bypass graft surgery. The paradox of necrosis in areas of revascularization. Circulation 56:906–913

45. Schoen FJ, Titus JL, Lawrie GM (1983) Autopsy-determined causes of death after cardiac valve replacement. JAMA 249:899–902

46. Schaper J, Schwarz F, Kittstein H et al. (1982) The effects of global ischemia and reperfusion on human myocardium. Quantitative evaluation by electron microscopic morphometry. Ann Thorac Surg 33:116–122

47. Kirklin JK, Westaby S, Blackstone EH et al. (1983) Complement and the damaging effects of cardiopulmonary bypass. J Thorac Cardiovasc Surg 86:845–856

48. Olsen D, Van Kampen K, Volder J, Kolff WJ (1973) Pulmonary, hepatic and renal pathology associated with an artificial heart. Trans Am Soc Artif Intern Organs 19:578–582

49. Kawai J, Volder J, Donovan FM, Kolff WJ (1974) Long-term effects of the artificial heart. Ann Surg 179:362–371

50. Akutsu T (1974) Results of 70 experiments in calves with total artificial hearts. Causes of death and problems. In: Huang NHC, Normann N (eds) Cardiovascular flow dynamics and measurements. University Park Press, Baltimore, pp 941–956

51. Pierce WS, Brishron JA, Donnelly JH et al. (1977) The artificial heart. Progress and promise. Arch Surg 112:1430–1438

52. Taenaka Y, Olsen DB, Nielson SD et al. (1985) Diagnosis of mechanical failures of total artificial hearts. Trans Am Soc Artif Intern Organs 31:79–82

53. Harasaki H, McMahon JT, Nose Y (1985) Pathogenesis of valve calcification. Comparison of three tissue valves. In: Rubin RP, Weiss GB, Putney JW (eds) Calcium in biological systems. Plenum, New York, pp 669–675

54. Bernhard WF, LaFarge CG, Liss RH et al. (1978) An appraisal of blood trauma and the blood-prosthetic interface during left ventricular bypass in the calf and humans. Ann Thorac Surg 26:427–436

55. Harasaki H, Gerrity R, Kiraly R et al. (1979) Calcification in blood pumps. Trans Am Soc Artif Intern Organs 25:305–310

56. Pierce WS, Donachy JL, Rosenberg G (1980) Calcification inside artificial hearts. Inhibition by warfarin-sodium. Science 208:601–603

57. Coleman DL, Lim D, Kessler T et al. (1981) Calcification of nontextured implantable blood pumps. Trans Am Soc Artif Intern Organs 27:97–104

58. DeVries WC, Anderson JL, Joyce LD et al. (1984) Clinical use of the total artificial heart. N Engl J Med 310:273–278

59. Copeland JC, Levinson MM, Smith R et al. (1986) The total artificial heart as a bridge to transplantation. A report of two cases. JAMA 256:2991–2995

60. Murray-Leisure KA, Aber RC, Rowley JL et al. (1986) Disseminated *Trichosporon beigelii* (*cutaneum*) infection in an artificial heart recipient. JAMA 256:2995–2998

61. Taylor KD, Goldthorpe SH, Topaz SR, Jarvik RK (1987) Analysis of blood diaphragms from three long term clinical Jarvik-7 total artificial heart implants. Trans Soc Biomater 10:243

62. Ishihara T, Ferrans VJ, Jones M et al. (1981) Calcific deposits developing in a bovine pericardial bioprosthetic valve 3 days after implantation. Circulation 63:718–723

10. Ventricular Assistance:
The Pennsylvania State University Experience

W. E. Pae Jr., G. Rosenberg, and W. S. Pierce

Introduction

Profound ventricular failure after cardiac operations occurs in nearly 4% of patients [1]. Fortunately, with the appropriate use of volume loading, inotropic, vasodilator, and intra-aortic balloon support, about 70% of these patients can be weaned from cardiopulmonary bypass. A small percentage, however, are unresponsive to this conventional therapy and will die in the operating theater unless a more aggressive form of circulatory support is available. During the last decade, the relative safety and efficacy of temporary mechanical ventricular support for postcardiotomy cardiogenic shock has been demonstrated by investigators using various ventricular support systems. Ventricular recovery and hospital discharge have been reported in as many as 35%–45% of those patients who, otherwise, would have been expected to die [2–9]. Even more encouraging are recent reports that cardiac function and quality of life are excellent in long-term survivors following their hospital discharge [3, 4, 6, 8–10]. During the same 10-year period, there has been renewed interest in cardiac transplantation, which considerably prolongs the lives of patients with end-stage cardiomyopathy. This interest and these improved results, however, have increased the number of centers and procedures, so that donor organs have become less available. Since the prognosis for survival of these patients without transplantation is less than 1 year, the arrival of a suitable donor organ before the patient's demise is of obvious importance. The role of temporary ventricular support and transplantation seem to be complementary as clinical evidence accumulates indicating that temporary ventricular support is a safe method of maintaining the systemic and at times the pulmonary circulation in patients whose hemodynamic condition deteriorates while awaiting cardiac transplantation [11–16]. At present, temporary ventricular support is appropriate in two broad groups of patients: (a) those with postcardiotomy cardiogenic shock and whose ventricular function is expected to recover, and (b) those requiring a bridge to transplantation, when no ventricular recovery is expected and the goal is hemodynamic support until a suitable donor organ is located. It is possible that an undefined number of patients in the former group might be reclassified into the latter group if ventricular function is not recovered and the patient is otherwise a suitable candidate for cardiac transplantation. The exact role of ventricular support in acute myocardial infarction and cardiogenic shock remains to be defined. Therapeutic protocols have been suggested but clinical experiences in this area are few [17, 18]. However, application of temporary support under these conditions can be understood in the terms of the categories encom-

Assisted Circulation 3
F. Unger (Ed.)
© Springer-Verlag Berlin Heidelberg 1989

passing expectation of ventricular recovery and suitability for orthotopic cardiac transplantation. This report describes our experience with the use of ventricular assistance in both postcardiotomy cardiogenic shock and bridge to cardiac transplantation from June of 1979 to June of 1987.

Ventricular Assist Device

The ventricular assist device that was designed and manufactured by our group was employed in all cases [17, 19]. The paracorporeal placed pneumatic pump is composed of a flexible blood sac of segmented polyurethane, which is seam free and has a highly polished surface, enclosed within a rigid polysulfone case (Fig. 1). The inner chamber of the case is oblate spheroid; a flexible diaphragm transects the frontal plane of the outer case and separates the air port from the thin-walled blood sac. Björk-Shiley 70 ° concavo-convex Delrin inlet and outlet valves provide unidirectional flow. The pumping action is created by pulses of air introduced between the pump housing and the flexible sac, which periodically compress the valved blood sac. For left ventricular assistance, blood is removed from the left atrial appendage using a curved, segmented polyurethane-coated 51-F light-house tipped cannula. Blood is returned to the ascending aorta by way of

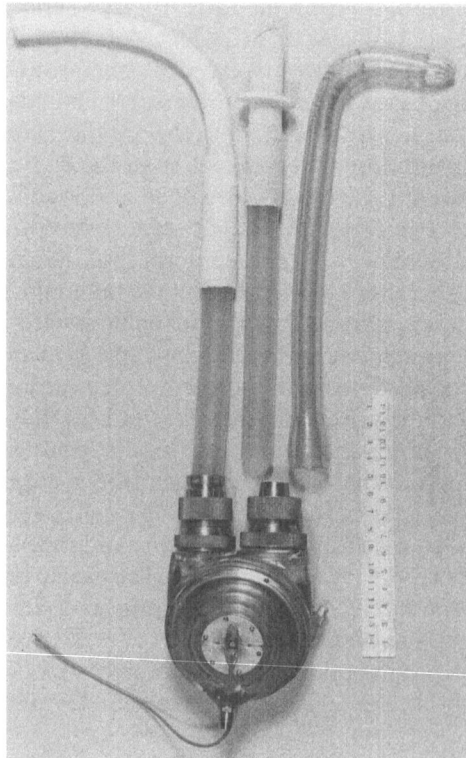

Fig. 1. The Pennsylvania State University sac-type pneumatic ventricular assist device. The segmented polyurethane sac is enclosed within a rigid polysulfone case. The wire exiting the case is attached to a Hall effect switch. The outflow composite cannula (*left*) and the atrial inflow cannula (*right*) can be utilized in either left or right ventricular assistance. The cannula in the middle is used for apical left ventricular inflow in bridge to transplant applications

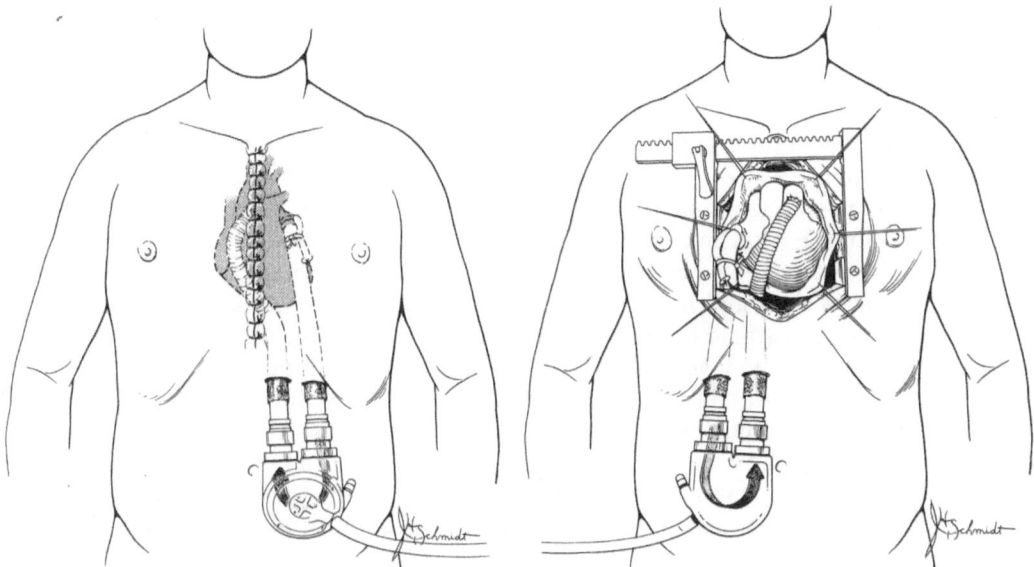

Fig. 2. The Pennsylvania State University sac-type ventricular assist device as it appears following implantation for postcardiotomy cardiogenic shock. Blood is withdrawn from the left atrium into the assist device and returned to the ascending aorta

Fig. 3. The Pennsylvania State University sac-type ventricular assist device as it appears following implantation for right ventricular failure. Blood is withdrawn from the right atrium and returned to the pulmonary artery

a composite, segmented polyurethane-woven 14-mm Dacron cannula (Fig. 2). We believe that left atrial drainage is the method of choice in patients with postcardiotomy cardiogenic shock. This method simplifies insertion and prevents further myocardial damage. Alternatively, blood can be removed from the left ventricular apex utilizing a straight inflow cannula if left atrial cannulation is not feasible for technical reasons, or in the case of bridge to cardiac transplantation, where our experience would indicate that this method is superior. Right ventricular assistance is provided by right atrial inflow cannulation, while the outflow conduit is anastomosed pulmonary artery (Fig. 3). Two pumps can be implanted when biventricular assistance is required. The inflow and outflow cannulas exit the chest below the costal margin, while the pump lies on the anterior abdominal wall. The pump is tethered to the control console by a 2-m polyvinylchloride tube.

Usually the pump is run in a full-to-empty mode, in which complete pump filling is detected by a Hall effect switch in the pump case. Observation of the pump or analysis of the air line pressure curve reveals complete emptying. The full-to-empty mode provides maximum washout of the blood sac and thereby decreases the possibility of thrombus formation. The pneumatic drive unit is also capable of functioning in a synchronous mode coupled to the electrocardiogram signal, or in an asynchronous fixed rate mode. The pump output is the product of the stroke volume (70 ml) and the pumping rate. Maximum output is approximately 7 l/min.

Postcardiotomy Cardiogenic Shock

Indications and Implant Techniques

In patients undergoing cardiac surgery who we feel are high risk, we have found it prudent to place a femoral arterial catheter prior to the initiation of cardiopulmonary bypass to facilitate rapid insertion of the percutaneous intra-aortic balloon. Following a technically satisfactory procedure, a patient who cannot be weaned is first treated by conventional medical therapy. Accurate hemodynamic monitoring of right and left atrial pressures, pulmonary artery and aortic pressures, as well as cardiac output is necessary to make intelligent and rational decisions in patient management. Patients with a cardiac output index of <1.8 l/min/m^2, a left atrial pressure of >18–25 mmHg, a right atrial pressure of <15 mmHg, and a peak systolic aortic pressure of <90 mmHg who are unable to be weaned from cardiopulmonary bypass using conventional therapy, including the intra-aortic balloon, are candidates for left ventricular assistance. Right ventricular failure is manifested by a cardiac output index of <1.8 l/min/m^2, a peak systolic aortic pressure of <90 mmHg, and a left atrial pressure of <15 mmHg, despite volume loading to a right atrial pressure of 25 mmHg with a competent tricuspid valve. Right ventricular failure results in a pulmonary blood flow that is inadequate to provide sufficient preload to the left ventricle. This may occur as an isolated event, but also may occur and not be apparent until left ventricular assist pumping is instituted. Medical treatment of right ventricular failure includes correction of acidosis, hypoxia, hypercarbia, and infusion of isoproterenol to lower the pulmonary vascular resistance and improve right ventricular contractility [20–22]. Additionally, the infusion of prostaglandin E$_1$ into the right atrium coupled with norepinephrine infusion into the left atrium has recently been reported to be a reasonable and beneficial adjunct under these circumstances [23]. When these methods of supporting the pulmonary circulation are unsuccessful, mechanical support is indicated and a right ventricular assist device should be inserted.

Prior to institution of circulatory support, we have routinely searched for a patent foramen ovale, present in approximately in 25% of adult patients [24]. Closure is mandatory prior to circulatory support, particularly in the case of right ventricular failure, to eliminate right to left shunting at the atrial level and subsequent hypoxia. Although theoretically, left ventricular decompression by apical ventricular inflow cannulation may be more efficacious in lowering myocardial oxygen consumption and left ventricular work, our clinical experience suggests that the risk of apical inflow cannulation outweighs the theoretical benefit when ventricular recovery might be expected [25]. For left ventricular assistance, the pump inflow cannula is generally inserted into the left atrial appendage through concentrically placed pursestring sutures. These are snared with rubber keepers which remain in the chest and allow easy removal. Inflow for right ventricular assistance is accomplished in a similar fashion through pursestring sutures placed in the midbody of the right atrium. The composite outflow cannula is anastomosed end to side to the aorta for left ventricular support and the main pulmonary artery for right ventricular support. Once the inflow and outflow cannulas are brought out below the sp-costal margin, air is evacuated from the system and the cannulas connected to the assist device. Cardiopulmonary bypass is then gradually reduced as ventricular assistance is initiated. When assist pump output index (stroke volume × pump rate divided by body surface area) exceeds 2.0 l/min/m^2, bypass is discontinued.

Implantation of an assist device should not be considered in a postcardiotomy patient who has a technically imperfect procedure. For instance, a ventricular assist device should not be used if a patient has a residual hemodynamically significant lesion, such as a paravalvular leak or a residual ventricular septal defect, or has had incomplete myocardial revascularization. Moreover, a successful outcome is unlikely in a patient who has well documented preoperative organ dysfunction such as renal failure or an intracurrent condition such as bacterial endocarditis. Evidence suggests that advanced age serves as a relative contraindication, with most series reporting no survivors in patients over 70 [3–5, 10, 21, 26]. Prolonged cardiopulmonary bypass prior to the initiation of ventricular assist pumping sets the stage for significant problems. Most investigators feel that the sequelae of a protracted period of cardiopulmonary bypass, specifically elevated plasma hemoglobin levels and bleeding diathesis secondary to damaged blood components, significantly reduce survival with ventricular assistance but do not serve as definite contraindications [27].

Postoperative Management and the Weaning Process

We generally discontinue assist pumping daily for periods up to 60 s in order to permit a sequential evaluation of ventricular function [28]. When the patient's left ventricle is capable of maintaining a left atrial pressure of < 20 mmHg, a systolic aortic pressure of > 100 mmHg, and a cardiac output index of > 2.0 l/min/m^2 with the pump off for 60 s, the assist pump output is progressively decreased at 6-h intervals to permit the patient's left ventricle gradually to assume complete circulatory support. Adequate left ventricular function as defined by the criteria above, must be demonstrated at least four times over 24 h prior to assist pump removal. Importantly, to insure good washing of the prosthetic blood sac, the pump rate is not decreased below 30 beats per minute. Additionally patients are maintained on low molecular weight dextran (40000 daltons), which is begun when chest tube drainage is less than 50 cc/h and is discontinued approximately 6–8 h prior to anticipated removal. Ventricular assist device removal is accomplished in the operating room with the patient under general anesthesia. Repeat sternotomy is performed and the cannulas are clamped and final hemodynamic measurements obtained. If the cardiac output index is adequate with suitable filling pressures, the atrial cannula is removed and the previously placed pursestring sutures tied. The outflow cannula is removed by dividing the Dacron graft just proximal to its anastomosis to the aorta or pulmonary artery and oversewing the stump. Management thereafter is conventional.

Patient Experience

During this 8-year period, 25 patients required ventricular assist pumping. The types of ventricular assist pumping employed and the clinical outcomes are summarized in Table 1. Nine patients were long-term survivors. Three of these patients were women and six were men; their ages ranged from 39 to 69 years (mean = 54.6). The preoperative diagnosis, left ventricular function, and New York Heart Association (NYHA) cardiac classification are tabulated in Table 2. All nine patients were NYHA class IV because of disabling angina pectoris, which occurred alone or in conjunction with congestive heart failure resulting from ischemic or valvular heart disease. Only three patients had normal ejection fractions and two of these had associated severe mitral regurgitation, which led to overestimation of the ejection fractions from the cineangiograms.

The intraoperative and postoperative events that led to the use of the ventricular assist pump are noted in Table 3. Myocardial preservation was accomplished with the use of multidose asanguinous crystalloid potassium cardioplegia, as well as systemic and topical hypothermia during a single period of aortic cross-clamping. Three patients required emergency operation: patient 5, for unstable angina refractory to medical therapy and intra-aortic balloon counterpulsation; patient 1, for unstable angina, hypotension, and intractable ventricular tachycardia; and patient 4 for cardiogenic shock caused by ischemic mitral regurgitation after an acute myocardial infarction. Two patients were initially weaned from cardiopulmonary bypass, but refractory cardiogenic shock developed in the intensive care unit 12–14 h postoperatively. The origin of cardiac decomposition could not be defined in most cases. Only in patient 3 did a perioperative infarction occur, and the induction of anesthesia, even in the emergency cases, was uneventful. The prosthetic valves in patients who underwent valve replacement functioned satisfactorily.

For the seven patients who could not be weaned from the initial period of cardiopulmonary bypass, the delay to institution of circulatory support ranged from 10 to 84 min (mean = 45 min) and was not considered excessive. Times from the start of cardiopulmonary bypass to the first attempt at weaning ranged from 97 to 300 min (mean = 158 min). Times from the start of cardiopulmonary bypass to the insertion of the ventricular assist pump ranged from 127 to 330 min (mean =

Table 1. Types and results of ventricular assist pumping (Pae et al. [10])

	No. of patients	Weaned	Long-term survivors
LVAD	18	10 (55.6%)	7 (38.9%)
RVAD	3	3 (100%)	2 (66.7%)
BVAD	4	0 (0%)	0 (0%)
	25	13 (52%)	9 (36%)

LVAD, left ventricular assist device; RVAD, right ventricular assist device; BVAD, biventricular assist device

Table 2. Preoperative characteristics of long-term survivors of ventricular assistance (Pae et al. [10])

Pa-tient	Age	Sex	Diagnosis	EF	LVEDP (mmHg)	NYHA	Other
1	53	M	LV aneurysm, 100% LAD, 70% CX, 100% RCA	<0.20	28	IV	Previous MI, CHF, recurrent ventricular tachycardia, refractory hypotension prior to the induction of anesthesia
2	53	F	MR, AR	0.56	14	IV	Previous OMC
3	52	M	TR, 60% LM, 70% CX, 100% RCA	0.18	–	IV	Previous MI and CVA
4	40	M	Acute MR, 60% LM, 90% LAD, 100% RCA	0.37	35	IV	Previous MI
5	60	M	80% LAD, 95% CX, 100% RCA	0.25	17	IV	Previous MI, AODM
6	64	M	AS, AR, 90% CX, 100% RCA	0.39	22	IV	Previous MI
7	69	M	MR, 70% CX, 70% RCA	0.53	10	IV	Previous TIA
8	61	F	MR, 90% LM, 90% LAD, 90% CX, 80% RCA	0.45	20	IV	Recent MI
9	39	F	MS, 95% LAD, 95% LADD	0.66	6	IV	Hypertension

EF, ejection fraction; LVEDP, left ventricular end-diastolic pressure; NYHA, New York Heart Association class; M, male; F, female; LV, left ventricular; LAD, left anterior descending coronary artery; CX, circumflex coronary artery; RCA, right coronary artery; MR, mitral regurgitation; LM, left main coronary artery; AR, aortic regurgitation; TR, tricuspid regurgitation; AS, aortic stenosis; MS, mitral stenosis; LADD, left anterior descending diagonal branch coronary artery; MI, myocardial infarction; CHF, congestive heart failure; OMC, open mitral commissurotomy; CVA, cerebrovascular accident; AODM, adult onset diabetes mellitus; TIA, transient ischemic attack

203 min). Total bypass times in these patients ranged from 167 to 384 min (mean = 279 min).

Seven of the nine patients required only left ventricular assist pumping, but in three patients concomitant right ventricular failure necessitated right ventricular support with isoproterenol. Two patients had predominant right ventricular failure and required right ventricular assist pumping, but their less severe left ventricular failure was treated with the intra-aortic balloon. In our series, there were no survivors among the patients who underwent biventricular assist pumping.

Results

Of the initial group of 25 patients who required ventricular assist pumping, 18 (72%) required the left ventricular assist pump, 10 of the 18 (55.6%) were weaned, and 7 (38.9%) survived. One-third of these patients had right ventricular failure which was responsive to drug therapy. The right ventricular assist pump and an intra-aortic balloon were used in three patients; all were weaned and two patients

Table 3. Intraoperative and postoperative events leading to the use of the ventricular assist pump (Pae et al. [10])

Patient	Age/sex	Procedure	Aortic cross-clamp time (min)	Start CPB to 1st wean (min)	Start CPB to IABP (min)	Start CPB to VAP (min)	CPB (min)	Elective or emergency	Events
1	53/M	LV aneurysm-ectomy SVG	53	100	115	127	167	Emergency	Intractable VT
2	53/F	AVR/MVR	190	300	NA	330	384	Elective	No ejection post-CPB No IABP
3	52/M	TA/DVG	52	97	NA	136	187	Elective	Preoperative cardiogenic shock
4	40/M	MVR/TVG	100	130	IABP – preop	140	225	Emergency	
5	60/M	TVG	45	NA	IABP – inserted postop in ICU	Second CPB 127	77+127	Emergency	Postcardiotomy cardiogenic shock 12 h post-TVG
6	64/M	AVR/DVG	127	203	214	244	287	Elective	
7	69/M	MVR/DVG	83	NA	IABP – inserted postop in ICU	Second CPB 58	117+58	Elective	Postcardiotomy cardiogenic shock 14 h post-MVR, DVG
8	61/F	MVR/QVG	93 (QVG) 76 (SUB MVR)	126	140	250	374	Elective	Unable to wean CPB QVG Severe MR Immediate MVR
9	38/F	OMC/SVG	53	108	151	192	326	Elective	

LV, left ventricular; CPB, cardiopulmonary bypass; IABP, intra-aortic balloon pumping; VAP, ventricular assist pumping; VT, ventricular tachycardia; M, male; F, female; AVR, aortic valve replacement; MVR, mitral valve replacement; NA, not applicable; TA, tricuspid annuloplasty; ICU, intensive care unit; OMC, open mitral commissurotomy; SUB, subsequent; MR, mitral regurgitation; SVG, single aortocoronary bypass grafting; DVG, double aortocoronary bypass grafting; TVG, triple aortocoronary bypass grafting; QVG, quintuple aortocoronary bypass grafting

Table 4. Assist pump perfusion data (Pae et al. [10])

Patient	Age/sex	Bypass	Flow rate (l/min/m²)	RHF	Time of VAP (h)	Time to discharge after VAD removal (days)
1	53/M	RA–PA	2.9	P	72	23
2	53/F	LV–AO	2.7	–	192	59
3	52/M	LA–AO	3.4	–	216	20
4	40/M	LA–AO	2.7	D	120	31
5	60/M	LA–AO	3.8	D	100	56
6	64/M	RA–PA	2.8	P	116	22
7	69/M	LA–AO	4.0	D	154	39
8	61/F	LA–AO	3.4	–	288	86
9	38/F	LA–AO	4.0	–	168	29

M, male; F, female; VAP, ventricular assist pumping; RHF, right heart failure; RA, right atrial; PA, pulmonary artery; LV, left ventricular; AO, aortic; P, profound, requiring right ventricular assist device; D, drug-responsive right ventricular failure; VAD, ventricular assist device

Table 5. Complications following ventricular assist pumping (Pae et al. [10])

Mechanical failure	0
Perioperative myocardial infarction	1
Renal failure	1
Bleeding	3
Respiratory insufficiency	4
Neurological	2
Infection	0
Hemolysis	0

survived (66.7%). Biventricular assist pumping was used in four patients, none of whom was weaned from support (Table 1). In the nine long-term survivors, peak device flows ranged from 2.7 to 4.0 l/min/m² (mean = 3.3) and the total ventricular assist perfusion times from 72 to 288 h (mean = 158 h) (Table 4). Neither infection nor hemolysis was seen. The most frequent complication was respiratory insufficiency, which occurred in four of nine patients who required prolonged ventilatory support (Table 5). Postoperative bleeding was the second most frequent complication, and three of the nine patients required exploration. Although no patient required long-term dialysis, temporary dialysis for renal failure, which subsequently resolved, was used for patient 4. Only patient 3 had enzymatic and electrocardiographic criteria for perioperative infarction; the bypass graft to the circumflex marginal coronary artery was noted to be occluded when the assist pump was removed. Definite enzymatic and electrocardiographic criteria for perioperative infarction were absent in the remaining patients. Last, neurological events were evident in two patients. Patient 2 was lethargic for nearly 3 weeks but, at the time of hospital discharge, had no residual neurological deficit.

In patient 5, a left hemiparesis was seen; its cause could not be directly attributed to assist pumping, as there was no evidence of thrombus in the pump or in the cannulas. However, prolonged hypotension before reoperation to begin mechanical circulatory assist pumping may have been the etiology.

Patients surviving remained in the hospital after the assist pump was removed from 20 to 86 days (mean = 41 days). All patients were discharged to their homes. The follow-up period ranged from 30 to 68 months (mean = 39 months) (Table 6). Five late deaths have occurred among these nine patients (patients 1, 2, 3, 7, and 8). Patient 1 died of a pulmonary embolus 18 months after hospital discharge. An autopsy revealed extensive mural thrombus in the right ventricle and it is thought to have been the origin of the pulmonary embolus. Patient 2 died while sleeping, presumably of an arrhythmia, 38 months after returning home. Until her death, she was employed full time and had no cardiac disability. Patient 3 died of a cardiac arrest 25 months after discharge; before his death, he had no limitation to his activity. Patient 7 died 30 months after discharge. The cause is unknown, but follow-up information suggested very mild congestive heart failure and poor compliance with medical treatment. Patient 8, who preoperatively had diminished left ventricular function with ischemic mitral regurgitation and multivessel coronary artery disease resulting in class IV symptoms of congestive heart failure and angina pectoris, remained in compensated congestive heart failure. However, her angina was relieved and she was able to resume limited activity as a housewife.

Table 6. Postoperative characteristics of long-term survivors (Pae et al. [10])

Patient	Age/sex	Time of survival to June 1987 (months)	NYHA class	EF	Life-style
1	53/M	18	II	N/A	Disabled due to sympathetic reflex dystrophy. Died due to pulmonary embolus
2	53/F	38	I	0.44	Employed full-time, cafeteria worker. Died suddenly, probable arrhythmia
3	52/M	25	II	N/A	Retired engineer, no activity limitation. Died; etiology unknown
4	40/M	73	I–II	0.29	Full activity, retired (volunteer worker)
5	60/M	68	II	0.45	No cardiac disability. Residual left hemiparesis
6	64/M	64	I–II	0.34	Full activity, employed part-time as carpenter
7	69/M	30	II	N/A	Retired bartender. Died; etiology unknown
8	61/F	12	III–IV	0.15	Housewife, compensated CHF, died
9	39/F	30	I	0.45	Full-time employment as manager

M, male; F, female; NYHA, New York Heart Association; EF, ejection fraction; CHF, congestive heart failure; N/A, not available

She died of congestive heart failure 1 year after being discharged from the hospital. Other than this patient, the improvement in NYHA classification in these patients after operation was remarkable. Before operation, all nine patients were in NYHA class IV; postoperatively all were in NYHA class I or II, except for patient 8. Although postoperative cardiac catheterizations were not performed, ventricular function was evaluated by radionuclide angiography in the six of the nine patients (Table 6). The ejection fraction improved or remained essentially the same in four of the six patients and was greatly improved in one of them. Only in patient 8 did the ejection fraction fall markedly, and she had continued to have symptoms of congestive heart failure.

Except for patient 8, whose cardiac disability limited her physical activity, quality of life among the survivors was satisfactory. The patients who were previously employed (patients 2, 6, and 10) returned to work and had no health-related absences. The retired individuals (patients 3, 4, and 7) had no cardiac disability and resumed fairly vigorous physical activity. Patient 1 was partially disabled because of a sympathetic reflex dystrophy (an unrelated previous problem), and patient 5, in whom left hemiparesis developed perioperatively, was partially limited by his neurological defect but remained active with no demonstrable cardiac disability.

Discussion

The precise etiology of postcardiotomy ventricular failure is often unknown, but it is thought to be multifactorial. Certainly postcardiotomy cardiogenic shock appears to occur more often in patients with abnormal preoperative ventricular function. Despite technically successful operative procedures to relieve the hemodynamic burden of valvular heart disease or to revascularize jeopardized myocardium, additional ventricular impairment may result from inadequate myocardial protection. The cumulative effects may lead to cardiogenic shock. Nevertheless, these results clearly show that many patients, with what would have previously been lethal ventricular failure, can have progressive recovery of ventricular function and survive [28]. The mechanisms of ventricular recovery are not entirely understood. Many studies have shown that an ischemic myocardial injury is characterized, on an ultrastructural level, by intermyofibrillar edema and mitochondrial swelling [29]. Myocardial edema reduces ventricular compliance and contractility and, if progressive, can lead to ventricular failure [30]. These changes are potentially reversible, provided they are not permitted to progress to infarction. Additionally, following a sublethal ischemic insult, myocardial adenosine triphosphate (ATP) concentrations fall, and nucleotide metabolites accumulate and are subsequently washed out of the ischemic myocardium during reperfusion. Myocardial ATP is resynthesized from these nucleotide precursors, and their loss results in a prolonged period of ATP depletion [29]. In the event of reversible myocardial injury, ventricular assistance provides time required to permit resorption of both intercellular and interstitial water from the injured myocardium as well as repletion of ATP stores. Additionally, ventricular assist pumping has been demonstrated to improve the distribution of blood flow between the endocardium and epicardium as well as perhaps open up collateral channels [31]. Ventricular unloading produces a favorable oxygen demand to supply ratio while at the same time providing for systemic and/or pulmonary support until reversible injury subsides [32, 33]. Regardless of the precise etiology, these results would indicate that following reversible ischemic injury the "stunned" myocardium may require 7 or more days of ventricular support prior to recovery.

Although a number of well described problems have been associated with the utilization of ventricular assistance, of paramount importance is diffuse postoperative bleeding. Our experience suggests that cardiopulmonary bypass times exceeding 4 h lead to the well recognized sequelae of platelet destruction as well as platelet dysfunction. To avoid this problem, efforts must be made to prevent delay in institution of circulatory support. Additionally, our data would suggest that systems which are designed to minimize blood trauma and thromboembolism without the use of systemic anticoagulation have distinct advantages.

Regardless of the etiology of right ventricular failure, its presence requires particular attention first with medical therapy and then the prompt institution of right ventricular support. Certainly pharmacologically resistant right ventricular failure will lead to an unsuccessful outcome in these patients unless there is prompt institution of right ventricular support.

Current data therefore indicate that temporary ventricular support in patients who cannot be weaned from cardiopulmonary bypass is reasonable and therapeutic treatment to extend life [16]. Ventricular recovery and quality of life are satisfactory and in long-term hospital survivors cardiac and noncardiac disability is rare [6, 10]. The future accomplishments must include identification of perioperative factors that indicate which patients will benefit from the assist devices and simplification of implantation techniques.

Staged Cardiac Transplantation

Indications, Techniques, and Results

Circulatory support with the intra-aortic balloon, followed by cardiac transplantation, was first reported by Reemtsma et al. [34]. More recently, Hardesty et al. [35] have reported that their results compare favorably with the results obtained with patients who are not as ill and who do not require aggressive hemodynamic support. For patients who are transplant candidates and who may initially respond to the intra-aortic balloon, but whose conditions then further deteriorate, more aggressive ventricular support may be desirable [11]. The absolute number of patients who might require such therapy remains to be defined. In our institution, since February of 1984, 52 patients have been accepted for orthotopic heart transplantation. Eight of the 52 patients died while waiting cardiac transplantation because of donor organ unavailability. Because of this significant problem with donor availability, in July of 1985 we began utilizing temporary left ventricular support as a bridging procedure in cardiac transplantation.

Hemodynamic criterion for assist pump insertion include systolic arterial blood pressure of less than 90 mmHg, a cardiac output index of $<1.8 \text{ l/min/m}^2$,

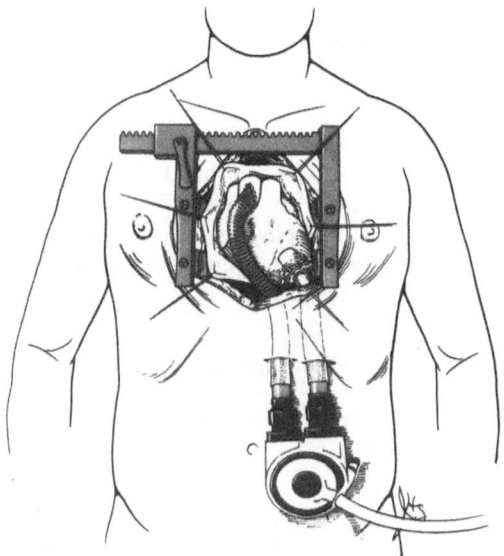

Fig. 4. The Pennsylvania State University sac-type ventricular assist device as it appears following implantation for bridge to transplant. Note that in this application, blood is withdrawn from the left ventricular apex into the device and returned to the ascending aorta

a pulmonary capillary wedge pressure >25 mmHg, and a reduced renal blood flow as evidenced by urine output of <20 cc per hour in a patient with maximal inotropic as well as intra-aortic balloon support. When a patient's hemodynamic status deteriorates the patient is taken to the operating theater and placed on cardiopulmonary bypass in a standard fashion utilizing bicaval cannulation. A patent foramen ovale is searched for and, if present, closed. Following this we elect to utilize apical ventricular cannulation in an effort to provide complete ventricular decompression and maximum lowering of atrial pressures as well as to avoid injury to the atrial remnants [11]. It is unnecessary to utilize aortic cross-clamping. Support is instituted from the ventricular apex to the ascending aorta (Fig. 4). The outflow graft is sutured as low as possible to the ascending aorta in order to allow its excision with recipient cardiectomy. The pump is positioned paracorporeally as previously described for use in postcardiotomy cardiogenic shock. The patient is weaned from cardiopulmonary bypass, and management thereafter is conventional until a donor organ is located. Invasive monitoring and mechanical ventilation are discontinued as soon as practical to minimize sources of sepsis. It is our opinion that the patients who receive this device should not be listed for cardiac transplantation until they have recovered all organ function and are then medically acceptable for transplantation, using criteria similar to those required prior to assist pump use. If a contraindication were to develop, such as infection and/or organ failure, we would not proceed to an allograft procedure. Additionally, although these patients are listed as highest priority, we would not deny an organ to another equally ill patient who did not have an assist device in his chest. We believe out patients are stable and can wait longer.

At present the optimum form of anticoagulation after temporary implantation of artificial devices is not known. Although warfarin is the logical choice for these devices, and most long-term animal experiments have used warfarin anticoagulation, the use of warfarin while awaiting a donor organ is impractical. We currently use dipyridamole to inhibit platelet function and after chest drainage has ceased we begin therapy which intravenous heparin, maintaining the whole blood activated clotting time at approximately 150 s.

Since July of 1985 six patients have undergone apical ventricular to aortic assist pumping for bridge to cardiac transplantation. The clinical characteristics and hemodynamic indices of these patients are listed in Tables 7 and 8, respectively. Two patients died prior to receiving an orthotopic transplant and four patients were transplanted after 3, 11, 21, and 31 days of support. One patient died

Table 7. Clinical characteristics of patients undergoing bridge to transplant

Patient	Age/ sex	Cardiac pathology	Support device	Duration of support	Antiplatelet or anti-coagulation therapy
BP	25/F	Idiopathic CMP	LVAD	21 days	LMD
EA	21/M	Viral CMP	LVAD	11 days	LMD
SS	26/M	Idiopathic CMP	LVAD	31 days	LMD + dipyridamole Heparin (after 14 days)
RG	25/M	Idiopathic CMP	LVAD	3 days	LMD + dipyridamole Heparin (after 2 days)
CP	48/M	Ischemic CMP	LVAD	7 h	None
PD	48/M	Postinfarction cardiogenic shock	BVAD	12 days	LMD

CMP, cardiomyopathy; LVAD, left ventricular assist device; BVAD, biventricular assist device; LMD, low molecular weight dextran

Table 8. Hemodynamic indices prior to and following implantation of the ventricular assist device for bridge to transplant[a]

Patient	Preimplant					Postimplant			
	BP	CVP	LAP	CI	IS	BP	CVP	LAP	CI
BP	89/63	21	32	1.7	DB-50	112/60	17	14	2.7
EA	105/55	N/A	21	2.4	D-2 DB-13	140/65	16	10	2.8
SS	90/70	7	30	1.2	D-5 DB-10	135/85	6	4	2.7
RG	90/50	18	30	N/A	D-10 DB-16	128/76	13	15	3.0
CP	96/59	11	27	2.0	D-3 DB-15	N/A	N/A	N/A	N/A
PD	100/50	10	25	1.6	DB-5	110/40	7	12	2.5

BP, arterial blood pressure (mmHg); CVP, central venous pressure (mmHg); LAP, left atrial pressure (mmHg); CI, cardiac index (l/min/m^2); IS, inotropic support; D, dopamine (µg/kg/min); DB, dobutamine (µg/kg/min); N/A, not available
[a] All patients received inotropic and intra-aortic balloon support prior to implantation of the ventricular assist device.

Table 9. Complications and clinical outcome in patients undergoing bridge to transplant

Patient	Complications	Transplanted	Outcome
BP	Superficial wound infection around cannulas	Yes	Alive and well (19 months)
EA	Urinary tract infection, catheter sepsis	Yes	Died 27 days post-transplantation
SS	Cerebrovascular accident, *Candida albicans* endocarditis/aortitis	Yes	Alive and well (3 months)
RG	None	Yes	Alive and well (3 months)
CP	Apex infarct resulted in bleeding	No	Died
PD	Pneumonia, sepsis	No	Died

of systemic sepsis 27 days following orthotopic heart transplantation. The three remaining patienst are alive and well at the time of writing (Table 9).

These results demonstrate the ability of a paracorporeal assist pump to provide temporary circulatory support in patients who decompensate hemodynamically while awaiting a donor organ for orthotopic cardiac transplantation. It is important, however, that systems designed and utilized for bridging procedures minimize the likelihood of device-related complications (infection, thromboembolism) that will lead to absolute contraindications to transplantation. The decision as to which system to employ is difficult because there is little experience to aid the surgeon in determining whether a patient needs univentricular support or biventricular support prospectively. If biventricular support is necessary, it is still unclear whether the total artificial heart, except in the circumstance of acute rejection, offers superior therapy to two externally placed ventricular assist devices. Although more experience is necessary in order to define the precise indications and contraindications of applying the various support systems, it is our feeling that the single left ventricular assist device forms a third line of circulatory support for the patient with normal pulmonary vascular resistance who requires a bridging procedure [11]. Our experience with several patients who have required bridging procedures has shown that left ventricular decompression and associated lowering of atrial pressure has promoted satisfactory improvement of right heart function.

In summary, a period of clinical investigations is needed to demonstrate whether or not critically ill patients will achieve short- and long-term survival and rehabilitation that are equivalent to current survival rates and rehabilitation of patients undergoing orthotopic cardiac transplantation alone. If such results are achieved, ethical questions must be answered as to whether bridging procedures are justifiable in our current status in which the potential recipients far outnumber the donor hearts available. Certainly bridging procedures would not increase the total number of transplants performed but they may change the identity of the individuals who receive them [36, 37].

References

1. McEnany MT, Kay HR, Buckley MR et al. (1978) Clinical experience with intra-aortic balloon pump support in 728 patients. Circulation 58:122–132
2. Pennock JL, Pierce WS, Wisman CB, Bull AP, Waldhausen JA (1983) Survival and complications following ventricular assist pumping for cardiogenic shock. Ann Surg 198:469–478
3. Rose DM, Colvin JB, Culliford AT et al. (1982) Long-term survival with partial left heart bypass following perioperative myocardial infarction and shock. J Thorac Cardiovasc Surg 83:483–492
4. Pennington DG, Samuels LD, Williams G et al. (1985) Experience with the Pierce-Donachy ventricular assist device in postcardiotomy patients with cardiogenic shock. World J Surg 9:37–46
5. Gaines WE, Pierce WS, Donachy JH et al. (1985) The Pennsylvania State University paracorporeal ventricular assist pump: optimal methods of use. World J Surg 9:47–53
6. Pennington DC, Bernhard WF, Golding LR, Berger RL, Khuri SF, Watson JT (1985) Long-term follow-up of postcardiotomy patients with profound cardiogenic shock treated with ventricular assist device. Circulation 72:216–226
7. Magovern GJ, Park SB, Maher TD (1985) Use of a centrifugal pump without anticoagulants for postoperative left ventricular assist. World J Surg 9:25–36
8. Rose DM, Laschinger J, Grossi E, Krieger KH, Cunningham JN, Spencer FC (1985) Experimental and clinical results with a simplified left heart assist device for treatment of profound left ventricular dysfunction. World J Surg 9:11–17
9. Litwak RS, Koffsky RM, Jurado RA, Mitchell BA, King P (1985) A decade of experience with a left heart assist device in patients undergoing open intra-cardiac operation. World J Surg 9:18–24
10. Pae WE, Pierce WS, Penncok JL, Campbell DB, Waldhausen JA (1987) Long-term results of ventricular assist pumping in postcardiotomy cardiogenic shock. J Thorac Cardiovasc Surg 93:434–441
11. Pennock JL, Pierce WS, Campbell DB et al. (1986) Mechanical support of the circulation followed by cardiac transplantation. J Thorac Cardiovasc Surg 92:994–1004
12. Hill JD, Farrar DJ, Hershon JJ et al. (1986) Use of a prosthetic ventricle as a bridge to cardiac transplantation for postinfarction cardiogenic shock. N Engl J Med 314:626–628
13. Phillips SJ, Kongtahworn C, Zeff RH et al. (1986) Heart transplantation and left ventricular support: experience with 12 patients (Abstract). J Heart Transplant 5:366
14. Bolman RM, Spray TL, Canle C et al. (1986) Heart transplantation in patients requiring preoperative mechanical support (Abstract). J Heart Transplant 5:374
15. Pae WE, Pierce WS (1987) Combined registry (ISHT-ASAIO) for the clinical use of mechanical ventricular assist pumps and the total artificial heart: first official report – 1986. J Heart Transplant (in press)
16. Pae WE (1987) Temporary ventricular support: current indication and results. ASAIO Trans 10:4–7
17. Pae WE, Pierce WS (1980) Mechanical left ventricular assistance: current devices, future prospects. In: Moran JM, Michaelis LL (eds) Surgery for the complications of myocardial infarction. Grune Stratton, New York, pp 411–426
18. Pae WE, Pierce WS (1981) Temporary left ventricular assistance in acute myocardial infarction and cardiogenic shock: rationale and criteria for utilization. Chest 79:692–695
19. Pierce WS, Donachy JH, Landis DL et al. (1978) Prolonged mechanical support of the left ventricle. Circulation 58:133–146
20. Parr GVS, Pierce WS, Rosenberg G et al. (1980) Right ventricular failure after repair of left ventricular aneurysm. J Thorac Cardiovasc Surg 80:79
21. Bernhard WF, Berger RL, Stetz JP et al. (1979) Temporary left ventricular bypass. Factors affecting patient survival. Circulation 60 (Suppl 2):131
22. O'Neill MJ, Pierce WS, Wisman CB et al. (1984) Successful management of right ventricular failure with the ventricular assist pump following aortic valve replacement and coronary bypass grafting. J Thorac Cardiovasc Surg 87:106
23. D'Ambra MN, LaRara PJ, Philbin DM et al. (1985) Prostaglandin E1: a new therapy for refractory right heart failure and pulmonary hypertension after mitral valve replacement. J Thorac Cardiovasc Surg 89:567

24. Magovern JA, Pae WE, Richenbacher WE et al. (1986) The importance of a patent foramen ovale in left ventricular assist pumping. Trans Am Soc Artif Intern Organs 32:449
25. Pierce WS (1979) Clinical left ventricular bypass: problems of pump inflow osbtruction and right ventricular failure. ASAIO Trans 2:1
26. Pierce WS, Parr GVS, Myers JL et al. (1981) Ventricular-assist pumping in patients with cardiogenic shock after cardiac operations. N Engl J Med 305:1606
27. Pierce WS (1980) Panel conference, cardiac support. Trans Am Soc Artif Intern Organs 26:625
28. Myers JL, Parr GVS, Pae WE et al. (1981) The role of the ventricular assist pump for post-cardiotomy cardiogenic shock: a four and one-half year experience. Artif Organs 5 (Suppl):244
29. Sturm JT, Bossart MI, Holob DA, Milam JD, Norman JC (1979) Ultrastructural analysis of stone heart syndrome at onset and six days later following, total support of circulation with a partial artificial heart or left ventricular assist device (ALVAD). Cardiovasc Dis Bull Texas Heart Inst 6:29–41
30. Foglia RP, Lazar HL, Steed DL et al. (1978) Iatrogenic myocardial edema with crystalloid primes: effects on left ventricular compliance, performance, and perfusion. Surg Forum 29:312–315
31. Axelrod HI, Galloway AC, Murphy MS et al. (1987) Percutaneous cardiopulmonary bypass with a synchronous pulsatile pump combines effective unloading with ease of application. J Thorac Cardiovasc Surg 93:358–365
32. Pennock JL, Pierce WS, Waldhausen JA (1976) Quantitative evaluation of left ventricular bypass in reducing myocardial ischemia. Surgery 79:523–533
33. Pennock JL, Pae WE, Waldhausen JA (1979) Reduction of myocardial infarct size: comparison between left atrial and left ventricular bypass. Circulation 59:275–279
34. Reemstsma K, Drusin R, Edie R, Bregman D, Dobelle W, Hardy M (1978) Cardiac transplantation for patients requiring mechanical circulatory support. N Engl J Med 298:670–671
35. Hardesty RL, Griffith BP, Trento A, Thompson ME, Ferson PF, Bahnson HT (1986) Mortally ill patients and excellent survival following cardiac transplantation. Ann Thorac Surg 41:126–129
36. Relman AS (1986) Artificial hearts – permanent and temporary. N Engl J Med 314:644–645
37. Annas GJ (1985) No cheers for temporary artificial hearts. Hastings Cent Rep 15(5):27–28

11. Temporary Mechanical Circulatory Support: Clinical Experience with 148 Patients

M. T. SWARTZ, D. G. PENNINGTON, L. R. McBRIDE, L. W. MILLER, J. E. REEDY, K. R. KANTER, and J. TAUB

Introduction

Acute cardiogenic shock remains one of the major causes of death in patients with heart disease. Some patients who develop cardiogenic shock can be effectively supported with pharmacological therapy and an intra-aortic balloon pump (IABP). However, other patients have ventricular failure refractory to drugs and IABP and require a more complete form of mechanical support. These patients' long-term prognoses are poor unless they undergo corrective surgery, percutaneous transluminal coronary angioplasty (PTCA), insertion of an assist device, cardiac transplantation, or some combination of these procedures prior to the development of major organ failure. Considerable progress has been made over the past decade in the development of mechanical circulatory support devices. These devices range from short-term partial support systems to devices which can completely support the circulation for months. While most of our clinical experience with circulatory support systems has been obtained with patients during or immediately following cardiac surgery [1, 2], we have also encountered several patients under different circumstances who required circulatory support for cardiogenic shock. Our experience has recently been expanded to include patients with acute myocardial infarction shock, patients with cardiomyopathy whose condition suddenly deteriorated, and patients with acute cardiorespiratory insults who were treated with circulatory support devices in order to provide stabilization prior to, during, or after cardiac catheterization, cardiac surgery, or cardiac transplantation [3–6].

Since 1978, we have used six different circulatory support systems: the Medtronic centrifugal pump (Medtronic Corp., Minneapolis, Minn), the Pierce-Donachy Thoratec pump (Thoratec Corp., Berkeley, Calif), the Scimed membrane oxygenator (ECMO; Scimed Inc., Minneapolis, Minn), with a centrifugal or roller pump, the Biomedicus centrifugal pump (Biomedicus Inc., Eden Prairie, Minn), the Novacor left ventricular assist system (LVAS; Novacor Corp., Oakland, Calif), and the Jarvik-7 total artificial heart (TAH; Symbion Inc., Salt Lake City, Utah). Our experiences are summarized according to the type of device employed, but it should be made clear that these methods are not mutually exclusive; in six patients, two of the systems were used in sequence. For each device the patients are divided into four categories: postcardiotomy ventricular failure, acute deterioration, bridge to transplantation, and post cardiac transplantation cardiogenic shock (Table 1). Furthermore, the hemodynamic criteria for ventricular failure were the same for all patients, regardless of the type of device. These cri-

Assisted Circulation 3
F. Unger (Ed.)
© Springer-Verlag Berlin Heidelberg 1989

Table 1. Indications for support in 148 patients with 154 devices

Type of device	Number of devices per patient group			
	Post-cardiotomy	Acute deterioration	Bridge to transplant	Post transplant
Thoratec	28	2	10	4
Centrifugal (Medtronic or Biomedicus)	36	0	0	1
ECMO	45	18	3	3
Implantable (Novacor or Jarvik)	0	0	4	0
Total	109	20	17	8

teria are similar to those outlined by Norman et al. [7] for patients with IABP support and optimal preload levels: cardiac output index less than $2.0 \ l/min/m^2$, systemic vascular resistance greater than 2100 dynes-s/cm^5, left and/or right atrial pressure greater than 20 mmHg, and urine output less than 20 cc/h, in spite of optimal inotropic and vasodilator drug support. Although some of the patients treated with ECMO also had severe respiratory insufficiency, the primary indication was cardiac failure; no patients who had primary respiratory failure with mild or moderate cardiac failure are included in this report.

Methods/Results

Nonpulsatile Ventricular Assist Devices

From 1978 until 1986, 37 patients were supported with nonpulsatile pumps. Twenty-two patients had the Medtronic pump and 15 patients received the Biomedicus pump. There were 28 male and nine female patients ranging in age from 1 year to 84 years (mean 54.4 years). The duration of support ranged from 2 h to 16 days, with a mean of 2.3 days. Thirty-six patients (22 Medtronic, 14 Biomedicus) had postcardiotomy cardiogenic shock and one patient received a Biomedicus for right ventricular failure following cardiac transplantation.

The Medtronic pump propels blood by imparting kinetic energy from a rotating impellor, the only moving part, which is magnetically coupled to an external drive unit. The Medtronic unit was connected to the patient by thin-walled cannulae constructed of polyurethane and reinforced with stainless-steel filament windings. All blood-contacting surfaces except that of the pyrolitic carbon impellor were coated with biocompatible polyurethane. The cannula design allowed considerable versatility in obtaining vascular access. Since these pumps produce only nonpulsatile flow, pulsatility was provided in 34 patients by an IABP. The Biomedicus centrifugal pump (Fig. 1) utilizes rotating cones to generate energy, which is recovered in the form of pressure flow work. While operating at a given constant speed, the pump generates nearly constant pressure over a wide range of flow rates. The pumping action is transmitted by magnetic coupling to the

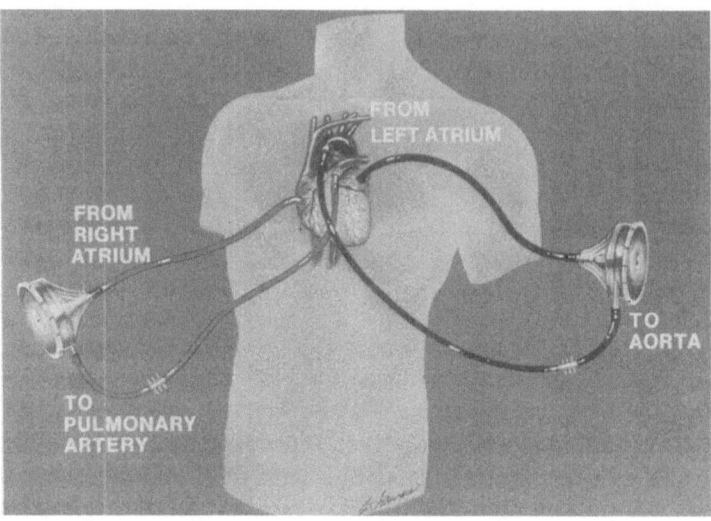

Fig. 1. Biventricular support with Biomedicus centrifugal pumps utilizing atrial pump inflow

mated drive magnet. Although there are no specific cannulae designed for the Biomedicus pump, investigators have been able to adapt standard cardiopulmonary bypass cannulae and tubing to contrive a system.

Among the 32 patients undergoing left ventricular bypass, the withdrawal catheter was placed in the left ventricle in nine and the left atrium in 23. The reinfusion cannula was placed into the ascending aorta through a dacron or PTFE graft (12 Medtronic patients) or directly into the ascending aorta through a purse-string suture. In patients undergoing right ventricular bypass, the withdrawal cannula was inserted into the right atrium and the infusion cannula was placed into the right ventricle, across the pulmonary valve into the pulmonary artery in three patients and directly into the pulmonary artery through a dacron graft in ten additional patients. No attempt was made to remove the cannula without re-operation, and repeat sternotomy was agreed upon by the patient and/or family prior to centrifugal pump placement.

Heparinization was not part of our original protocol. However, after the first two Medtronic patients developed severe thromboemboli, we elected to begin continuous intravenous heparin in order to maintain the activated partial thromboplastin time (APTT) at twice the preoperative value as soon as bleeding was controlled. In most cases, this was 36–48 h following pump insertion. All but one patient had cold blood potassium cardioplegic arrest during aortic clamping. One patient, the post cardiac transplant recipient, did not have his aorta clamped since the right ventricular assist device was inserted in the intensive care unit (ICU) without cardiopulmonary bypass. The aortic clamp times in 35 patients ranged from 26 to 250 min (mean 117 min) and were less than 2 h in all but four patients and greater than 3 h in two patients. Thirty-four patients had the centrifugal pump inserted during the initial operation in order to wean them from cardiopulmonary bypass. However, delays in the decision to implant the pump often led

Table 2. Complications in 148 patients with 154 devices

Complication	Type of device							
	Thoratec		Centrifugal		ECMO		Implantable	
	$n=44$	%	$n=37$	%	$n=69$	%	$n=4$	%
Bleeding	32	73	30	81	51	73	1	25
Biventricular failure	30	68	28	76	50	72	3	75
Renal failure-	16	36	12	32	21	30	2	50
dailysis	12	27	4	11	14	20	2	50
Infection-	15	34	7	19	15	22	4	100
mediastinitis	5	11	2	6	6	8	2	50
Neurological deficit	7	16	5	14	9	13	1	25
Thrombus-	9	20	9	23	5	7	1	25
embolus	4	9	4	11	0	0	1	25
Hemolysis	7	16	14	38	11	16	0	0
Respiratory failure	6	14	2	6	8	12	1	25
Limb ischemia (IABP)	1	3	3	9	3	4	0	0
Cannulation problems	1	3	2	6	2	3	0	0
Mechanical failure	3	7	1	3	0	0	0	0

to prolonged total bypass time, which ranged from 132 to 488 min (mean 261 min). Two patients were returned to the operating room several hours after cardiac operations for placement of the centrifugal pump as a result of hemodynamic deterioration.

Although the number of long-term survivors was low, eight patients demonstrated significant improvement in ventricular function. Five of them improved sufficiently to allow for centrifugal pump removal; two of these five died of renal and/or cerebral failure. Three patients are long-term survivors for 16–85 months. One patient died at 46 months of cancer. The complications occurring in these patients are shown in Table 2. Errors in cannulation probably contributed to an unsuccessful outcome in two patients; in one, the aortic graft was partially obstructed, in the other, the withdrawal cannula was placed into an infarcted apex and inadvertently into the right ventricle, resulting in severe hypoxemia. In another patient, the withdrawal cannula was properly positioned within the left atrium, but hypoxia resulted from right-to-left shunting through a patent foramen ovale (PFO). In subsequent cases with left atrial cannulation, the right atrium was explored if hypoxia developed shortly after left assistance was initiated.

Bleeding was the most frequent as well as the most damaging complication, occurring in 30 of the 37 patients. Twenty-one patients were reexplored for bleeding postoperatively, and in nine additional patients bleeding was a major factor contributing to their deaths in the operating room. Almost all patients had mild derangement of the coagulation profiles, but no consistent pattern of coagulation abnormalities was noted. Hemolysis occurred in 14 patients. Thrombi developed in the Medtronic pump in the first two patients, both of whom had been perfused for several days without heparin. At autopsy, small thrombi were found in the cannulae and behind the rotor impellors of both patients, one of whom had extensive coagulation disorders, diffuse bleeding, and multiple organ failure. Following the institution of a program of heparinization after 36–48 h, no instances of cannula thrombosis or systemic embolization were detected with a Medtronic pump. However, in a few patients, a small adherent fibrin clot was noted behind the rotor impellor in spite of heparin therapy. Four patients with Biomedicus pumps developed thrombi within the pump. These thrombi were of various sizes and were located in different areas throughout the pumphead. In addition, since there were no specific cannulae designed for the Biomedicus pump, it was not unusual to see circular thrombus formation at the point at which the cannula was attached to the tubing by a connector or at the point where the tubing was connected to the pumphead. These thrombi occurred despite the fact that the patients had been on continuous heparin since the postoperative bleeding had subsided. Two of these four patients suffered from embolization of thrombi to the brain and/or kidneys.

Thirteen patients had biventricular failure, which was treated either with biventricular assist devices (BVAD) (eight patients) or with an RVAD and IABP (five patients). Fifteen additional patients developed right ventricular failure, which was inadequately treated with increasing doses of inotropic drugs. In our early experience, we did not recognize the full importance of biventricular failure and the necessity to treat it with biventricular support. For the past several years, we have treated biventricular failure more aggressively with the use of either BVADs or RVAD and IABP. As a result, we have had improving success with postcardiotomy patients.

Twelve patients developed renal failure, four of whom were dialyzed. Dialysis, however, did not prevent their ultimate demise. A recent review of VAD patients who developed renal failure [8] has shown that the chances of survival are low once the serum creatinine has risen above 2.0 mg/dl, despite the fact that the patients were aggressively treated in the early stages of renal insufficiency. Five patients had diffuse cerebral ischemia, probably resulting from prolonged periods of hypoperfusion. Seven patients suffered from infections, none of which could be directly attributed to the centrifugal VAD. Most of the infections were pneumonias which developed as a result of the patients' being immobilized in bed. Four patients suffered complications of the IABP, two had leg ischemia, one had leg necrosis, and one bled excessively following IABP rupture of the abdominal aorta.

The centrifugal pumps proved effective in restoring circulatory support in postcardiotomy patients with severe ventricular failure. Five of the 37 patients were weaned, three of whom are long-term survivors. Failures due to biventricular failure, bleeding, renal failure, complications with an IABP, and multiple organ failure were common. Left atrial cannulation proved more successful than left ventricular cannulation. The Medtronic system has the advantage of incorporating the cannulae with the blood pump in a one-piece unit, whereas the Biomedicus pump requires the investigator to construct a cannula system with in-line connectors which increase the tendency for thrombus formation. Both systems are relatively simple to insert; however, the fact that both require continuous heparinization is a distinct disadvantage. Postoperative bleeding often is a devastating complication. The period of hypoperfusion while the patient is bleeding often leads to multiorgan failure several days later. Finally, the current centrifugal pump systems render the patient virtually immobile, limiting the pump's use to a duration of probably less than 1 week.

Pierce-Donachy Thoratec Pump

In February 1981, we began laboratory experiments with a paracorporeal pneumatic, sac-type ventricular assist device designed by Pierce and Donachy at Pennsylvania State University. Although extensive animal experiments and human experience with this VAD had demonstrated its effectiveness, it appeared that pump inflow was limited in some patients by left ventricular cannula obstruction. Since our experience with the Medtronic pump had also demonstrated better results with left atrial than with left ventricular cannulation, we preferred the left atrium as the pump inflow cannulation site. We performed acute and chronic experiments in calves with left atrial cannulation and demonstrated the effectiveness of the Pierce-Donachy pump in this configuration [9].

The Pierce-Donachy VAD is constructed of a machined polycarbonate housing with an angle port design [10] which contains a flexible seam-free, segmented polyurethane sac (Fig. 2). The assist device utilizes Björk-Shiley inlet and outlet valves and has a stroke volume of 65 ml with a dynamic ejection fraction of approximately 0.75. Inlet cannulae for the atria or left ventricle and outlet cannulae which can be used for the aorta or pulmonary artery are available. The left ven-

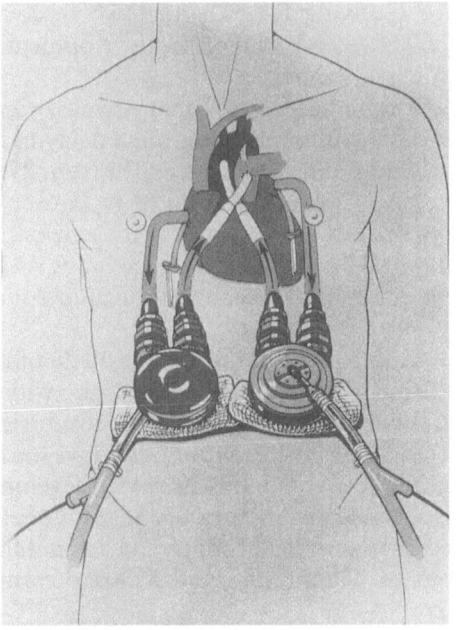

Fig. 2. Biventricular support with Pierce-Donachy Thoratec VADs; atrial cannulation

tricular apex cannula and the aortic cannula are large-bore, wire-wound, segmented polyurethane tubes with extremely smooth internal blood-contacting surfaces. The atrial cannula is a 51-French Sarns venous drainage cannula which has been coated with segmented polyurethane and shaped to a right-angle configuration. A dacron graft forms the end of the aortic cannula, permitting a standard vascular anastomosis to the aorta or pulmonary artery. The ventricular cannula is fitted with a felt washer to permit fixation to the ventricular myocardium. This cannula system allows cannulation of the left ventricle, the left or right atrium, the aorta, or the pulmonary artery. The pneumatic-power units employed in these studies were produced by Vitamek Incorporated (Vitamek Inc. Houston, Texas) or Thoratec Incorporated. The control console is capable of functioning in three modes: a manual set-rate mode, a synchronized mode which detects the R-wave of the electrocardiogram, or a fill-to-empty mode which operates by activating a hall-effect switch when the blood sac is full, thus initiating the emptying cycle. When the VAD is operating in the fill-to-empty mode, the rate times the stroke volume (65 cc) equals VAD flow. Heparin was not used in our clinical series until the patient was being weaned from the VAD or had been on the VAD for at least 1 week. At this time heparin was given continuously to maintain the APTT at 1.5 times normal. Long-term patients were switched to oral warfarin and dipyridamole if possible.

From February 1982 to November 1987, we encountered 44 patients with ventricular failure refractory to drugs and IABP who were selected for the insertion of a Thoratec VAD. They ranged in age from 15 to 72 years (mean − 49.2 years). There were 34 men and ten women. Twenty-eight patients were unable to be weaned from cardiopulmonary bypass following cardiac operations. Another ten patients received Thoratec VADs when their condition deteriorated while they were awaiting cardiac transplantation. Four patients developed cardiogenic shock after cardiac transplantation (two receiving RVADs and two receiving BVADs). Two patients had insertion of a Thoratec VAD for the development of acute myocardial infarction-induced cardiogenic shock.

In the 28 postcardiotomy patients, the total cardiopulmonary bypass times ranged from 90 to 528 min with a mean of 263 min, reflecting some delay in insertion of the VAD. However, the aortic clamp times, which ranged from 27 to 156 min (mean − 80 min), were not excessive. The recognition of biventricular failure [11] in these patients was greater than in our centrifugal VAD series, with 13 patients receiving LVADs, nine receiving BVADs, and six receiving RVADs (with IABP to support the left ventricle). All 28 patients had atrial cannulation for pump inflow.

The VAD mean flows ranged from 1.12 to 3.09 l/min/m^2. While all 28 of the postcardiotomy patients were weaned from cardiopulmonary bypass with a VAD, nine of them died in the operating room of severe bleeding and biventricular failure. The other 19 patients underwent VAD perfusion for 2–13 days (mean 4.5 days) and 16 of them were weaned after between 5 and 12 days. Eleven patients were discharged from the hospital; one died at 6 months of congestive heart failure and cardiomyopathy and one died at 54 months of cancer. The remaining nine patients have been followed up from 1 to 53 months, and six are presently New York Heart Association Class I [12].

Ten patients with cardiomyopathy received Thoratec VADs as bridges to cardiac transplantation. The seven men and three women ranged in age from 24 to 56 years, with a mean age of 41.9 years. The duration of support ranged from 12 h to 75 days, with a mean of 16 days. Five patients underwent transplantation and were discharged from the hospital, one of whom died at 6 months due to accelerated rejection as a result of noncompliance with the proper medication protocol. The other five patients were rejected as candidates for cardiac transplantation on the basis of renal failure, sepsis, or bleeding.

Four patients received Thoratec VADs due to the development of cardiogenic shock after cardiac transplantation. Three men and one woman ranging in age from 40 to 56 years (mean – 45 years) were supported for from 12 h to 5 days. The first two patients appeared to have predominantly right ventricular failure and were supported with a RVAD and an IABP. However, both developed progressive left heart failure and sepsis, which eventually led to their deaths. The remaining two patients had BVADs inserted; however, they developed renal failure and infectious complications. None of these patients improved enough to be weaned, and their complications were so severe that retransplantation was not a consideration.

Two additional patients had Thoratec VADs inserted for acute myocardial infarction shock. A 48-year-old man who was 4 days post anterolateral myocardial infarction was placed on a Thoratec LVAD and a Biomedicus RVAD. At the time of insertion of the BVADs his serum creatinine was 5.0, but he was still producing small amounts of urine. It was our hope that restoration of renal perfusion by use of VAD support might allow his kidneys to recover. Unfortunately, this was not the case, and his renal failure continued to worsen. In addition, he developed severe bleeding complications which further excluded him as a candidate for cardiac transplantation. The other patient, a 51-year-old man, suffered an acute myocardial infarction with sudden deterioration in the coronary care unit. He was placed on femoro-femoral ECMO and stabilized. He was then transferred to the operating room for placement of a Thoratec LVAD using a ventricular cannula. Initially, we thought his heart was irreversibly damaged, and that he would require cardiac transplantation. Over the next 6 days, however, his heart recovered to the point that the LVAD was removed. However, he also developed severe renal failure which did not improve after 3 months of hemodialysis. Three months after VAD removal, he died of renal failure and arrhythmias.

Complications in the Thoratec patients were similar to those which occurred in the centrifugal pump patients (Table 2). Bleeding was a common problem, occurring in 73% of the patients. Thirty patients had biventricular failure, and 27 of them received support with either BVADs or an RVAD and IABP. Sixteen patients developed renal failure, 12 of whom were dialyzed; none of those 12 survived. Fifteen patients developed infectious complications, which were usually pneumonia or intravascular line sepsis [13]. Three patients developed infections related to the cannulae of the VAD. Two patients who had their devices for 24 and 75 days developed superficial staphylococcal skin infections at the cannulation exit sites. The third patient developed mediastinitis from an infected cannula tract 5 days after the device was removed.

Seven patients developed neurological complications. Three patients had diffuse ischemia due to hypoperfusion prior to insertion of the assist device and four patients suffered from cerebrovascular accidents (CVAs) diagnosed by CT scan or at postmortem examination. One was the result of a mechanical failure of the console. The second patient suffered a CVA during the weaning period when flow was at its lowest. Both patients recovered full neurological and motor function. The third patient had evidence of an embolic stroke shortly after insertion of the VAD. It was never conclusively proven whether this was the result of an embolic shower of air or clot. The fourth patient was maintained on a BVAD for 28 days. For 10 days, she did not receive any anticoagulation due to retroperitoneal bleeding. At autopsy, thromboemboli were found in the brain and kidneys. Both VADs had clots on the valves and in the blood sacs. Pulmonary edema occurred in five patients, but was most severe in two patients with biventricular failure who received RVADs and IABPs. In these two cases, the left ventricular function was worse than suspected, so when pulmonary artery flow was increased by the RVAD, markedly elevated left atrial pressures and massive pulmonary edema resulted. The resulting hypoxia was so severe that there was insufficient time to insert an LVAD prior to the development of irreversible cerebral injury.

Fifteen patients underwent repeat sternotomy for VAD removal without the need for cardiopulmonary bypass. One patient in whom a left atrial cannula had been inserted from the right side near to the entrance of the left superior pulmonary vein was placed on cardiopulmonary bypass for approximately 10 min during the removal of the left atrial cannula. The VADs were usually removed by ligating the atrial appendage and oversewing the small cuff of dacron graft left on the aorta or pulmonary artery. We are not aware of any complications related to this technique, and there has been no necropsy evidence of infection related to leaving a portion of graft behind. Five patients had VADs removed while on cardiopulmonary bypass at the time of orthotopic cardiac transplantation. In these five patients all remnants of the aortic and pulmonary artery grafts were removed in order to reduce the possibility of infection, which might have been increased by the use of immunosuppresive drugs.

Extracorporeal Membrane Oxygenation (ECMO)

From February 1982 to November 1987, we employed ECMO in 69 patients (aged 1 day to 74 years) with severe cardiac failure due to diverse causes. Our initial case was a 17-year-old girl with postcardiotomy syndrome who developed severe cardiopulmonary failure after a cardiac arrest. Since she had pulmonary edema, hypoxemia, acidosis, and biventricular failure, we believed the VAD would not provide sufficient support. Since there was some evidence in the literature [14–16] that ECMO was helpful in cardiac as well as in pulmonary insufficiency, we instituted femoro-femoral ECMO under emergency conditions while intermittently performing external cardiac massage. Her recovery was dramatic, allowing her to be weaned from ECMO within 24 h, and she subsequently did well.

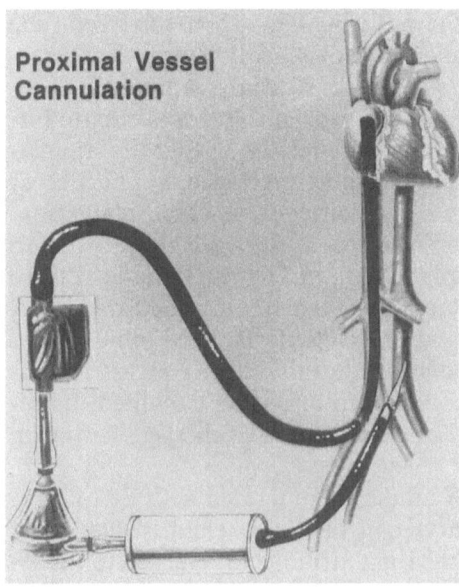

Proximal Vessel Cannulation

Fig. 3. Femoro-femoral ECMO circuit with a Biomedicus pump and Scimed oxygenator

In adults, the perfusion circuit consisted of a Scimed membrane lung and a Biomedicus or Centrimed centrifugal pump connected to the patient by Tygon tubing and leading to standard (USCI) femoral cannulae. Proximal femoral arterial and venous cannulae were placed in some (Fig. 3). Initially, we attempted to use centrifugal pumps in pediatric patients; however, hemolysis and thrombus formation within the pump often developed. We attributed these complications to low flows through large-volume pumpheads and to the inability of the Biomedicus pump to dissipate heat during perfusion. Subsequently, we have used roller pumps in the pediatric ECMO circuits, which are otherwise identical to the adult version. All patients received continuous intravenous heparin to maintain the activated clotting time (ACT) at between 150 and 200 s. For patients who required ECMO to be weaned from conventional cardiopulmonary bypass, the membrane oxygenation circuit used during the cardiac operation could be converted to the femoro-femoral position without changing the membrane or the tubing.

The complications with this group of patients can be seen in Table 2. Biventricular failure was present in 50 of the 69 patients (72%). Bleeding occurred in 51 patients because of the need for continuous heparinization and was a major factor contributing to the death of many of these patients. Since many of them bled at a rate which made it virtually impossible to keep their volume stable, their hemodynamic status continued to deteriorate throughout the time they were on ECMO. Even though the heparin dose was maintained at the lowest possible levels, the effects of blood contact with such large areas of artificial surface also contributed to the bleeding complications. As a result of complement activation, thrombocytopenia, and hemolysis, simple surgical bleeding often advanced to a coagulopathy.

Twenty-one patients developed renal failure, 14 of whom were dialyzed. The results in this group of patients were similar to those mentioned in the Pierce-Donachy Thoratec and centrifugal pump groups. Early dialysis did little to reverse the renal failure, and there was only one survivor of this complication. Fifteen patients developed infections, six of which were related to ECMO cannulation. Five children developed mediastinitis. One adult developed an infection at the femoral cannulation site approximately 2 weeks after cardiac transplantation. Nine patients developed neurological complications, most of which were due to the shock state which occurred prior to replacement on ECMO. In none of these patients could the neurological deficits be attributed to embolization from a portion of the perfusion circuit. Two adults and one child developed limb ischemia associated with the use of an IABP to provide pulsatility during ECMO perfusion. Cannula obstruction in two acutely deteriorating patients limited the resuscitation attempts because of low flows; both patients died shortly after being placed on bypass.

Forty-five patients, 31 children and 14 adults, were treated with ECMO for postcardiotomy cardiogenic shock. Twenty-eight of the 31 children had chest cannulation, with blood withdrawn from the right atrium and returned to the ascending aorta, and three children had the iliac vessels cannulated. In the adult population, two patients had chest cannulation and twelve had the site of cannulation switched to the femoral vessels in order to allow closure of the chest and reduce the chance of infection and bleeding.

Thirteen of the 31 children had improvement in ventricular function sufficient to allow them to be weaned from ECMO, and nine were long-term survivors. Of the 16 adult patients, however, only one was successfully weaned and survived. This patient was a 54-year-old woman who suffered hemodynamic deterioration and refractory ventricular arrhythmias approximately 2 h after replacement of her aortic valve. She was placed on femoro-femoral ECMO in the ICU and supported for 3 days, after which time she was successfully weaned. Retrospectively, it appears that this patient did not suffer an acute myocardial infarction and that her deterioration was attributable to the arrhythmias. While on ECMO she was able to tolerate treatment with antiarrhythmic drugs, allowing her rhythm to stabilize.

Eighteen other adult patients were placed on ECMO for acute deterioration in either the ICU or the cardiac catheterization laboratory. Duration of support ranged from 1 to 122 h with a mean of 28.3 h. Of these 18 patients, one refused further treatment, nine were weaned, six died after being weaned, and three are long-term survivors. Two of the three survivors had suffered cardiac arrest during PTCA and were placed immediately on femoro-femoral ECMO. They were rushed to the operating room, where they underwent successful coronary artery bypass grafting. The third survivor was the 17-year-old girl previously described in this section.

Three patients were placed on ECMO as a "bridge to cardiac transplantation." One patient was no longer suitable for transplantation and died after 2 days, when attempts to wean him from ECMO were unsuccessful. Two patients were maintained on ECMO for 5 and 3 days before undergoing orthotopic cardiac transplantation. One died approximately 16 h after transplantation of pulmonary embolism, sepsis, and acute right heart failure. The second patient died 1 month post transplantation of sepsis and multiorgan failure.

Three patients were placed on ECMO after cardiac transplantation. A 1-week-old infant with a hypoplastic left ventricle suffered hemodynamic deterioration shortly after cardiac transplantation and was supported on ECMO for 8 days before dying of fungal sepsis. The second patient, a 29-year-old woman, developed biventricular failure approximately 4 days after cardiac transplantation. She was supported on ECMO for 6 days and weaned, but she died of severe biventricular failure several hours later. Approximately 8 h after cardiac transplantation, a 10-year-old boy received oral cyclosporin intravenously and suffered a massive fat embolism resulting in severe biventricular failure and hypoxemia. He was placed on femoro-femoral ECMO for 24 h with dramatic improvement and was weaned. He is alive 6 years post ECMO and recently underwent successful retransplantation.

Peak ECMO flows ranging from 0.6 to 3.0 l/min/m^2 (mean 2.37) promptly restored hemodynamics in all but two patients. ECMO perfusion was maintained for 30 min to 18 days (mean – 51.7 h). Nineteen patients were weaned from ECMO with the use of inotropic drugs and/or an IABP. Six patients were weaned from ECMO with ventricular assist devices and two patients underwent transplantation. Fourteen patients are long-term survivors, survival ranging in duration from 6 to 69 months, with a mean of 32.6 months.

Implantable Devices

Four men, aged 27, 47, 48, and 59 years, who were potential cardiac transplant recipients underwent insertion of implantable devices. Three had the Novacor Model 100 left ventricular assist system (LVAS) inserted. The LVAS (Fig. 4) consists of a balanced solenoid energy converter, dual pusher-plate, sac-type blood pump, and a microprocessor-based control and monitoring console. The energy converter and blood pump are encapsulated in a fiberglass/polyester resin shell,

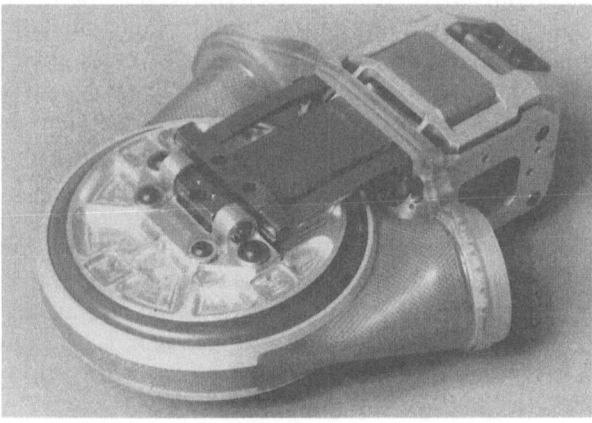

Fig. 4. Unencapsulated Novacor LVAS

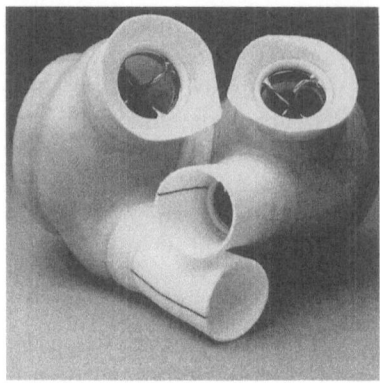

Fig. 5. Symbion Jarvik-7 TAH

with dacron conduits connecting the pump to the left ventricular apex and the ascending aorta. A percutaneous extension cable connects the energy converter to an extracorporeal control console. Twenty-one-millimeter Carpentier-Edwards pericardial bioprosthesic valves are used to allow unidirectional blood flow through the pump. Electrical energy supplied by the control console is converted into hydraulic work by the energy converter, which is then used to eject blood from the pump. The control console is also used to continuously monitor both the LVAS and patient parameters. Synchronous counterpulsation is achieved by sensing pump fill and ejection rates, based upon signals from displacement transducers within the energy converter. The system can also be operated in a mode synchronized to the patient's ECG, as well as in a fixed-rate asynchronous mode.

One patient had a Jarvik 7-70 total artificial heart (TAH). The two ventricles of the Jarvik-7 are made of polyurethane supported on polyurethane bases (Fig. 5). Rings of polycarbonate support Medtronic disc valves. The diaphragm consists of three layers of Avcothane with graphite between the blood-contacting layer and the intermediate layer and a dacron mesh between the intermediate layer and the air-contacting layer. Connections to the natural atria and great vessels are made with a "quick-connect" system. There have been some recent modifications. These changes include fabrication of the pump casing from polyurethane instead of aluminium, changing the connectors from polycarbonate to polyurethane, and a 40% decrease in the dp/dt of the pneumatic drive system.

Duration of support ranged from 27 to 91 days. One Novacor patient and the Jarvik TAH patient developed sepsis and renal failure, which excluded them as candidates for cardiac transplantation. The second and third Novacor patients were perfused for 91 and 52 days before successful orthotopic cardiac transplantation. Both are presently doing well 1 year and 4 months post transplantation. Three patients had some degree of biventricular failure. The patient who received the Jarvik 7-70 TAH had severe biventricular failure, which was the primary reason for our selection of the TAH. Two patients with the Novacor LVAS had moderate right ventricular failure which was managed effectively with isoproterenol and epinephrine for the first 3–4 days post implantation. The two patients who were excluded from transplantation developed severe renal failure and were dialyzed without success. Although all four patients developed infectious complications, the two nonsurvivors had sepsis and mediastinitis. One surviving Novacor patient had an infection of the drive line of the LVAS which was treated with antibiotics. At the time of transplantation, the drive-line tract was found to be infected with staphylococcus, but it had not entered the mediastinum. After cardiac transplantation, the tract was opened for drainage and healed without any further problems. The second Novacor survivor developed an infection of the drive line and pump pocket. The abdominal pump pocket was left open to drain and was treated with systemic and topical antibiotics. This patient also developed positive blood cultures of the same organism as the pump pocket (*S. aureus*). Cultures of both these sites were negative after 3 weeks of treatment. After cardiac transplantation, a large accumulation of *Candida albicans* was found in the LVAS outflow graft. Post-transplant fungal blood cultures were negative during the entire postoperative period. However, the patient received amphotericin for 6 weeks after transplantation and is presently doing well.

Discussion

Table 2 shows the complications in this series. It is interesting to note that the three major complications – bleeding, biventricular failure, and renal failure – occurred with similar percentages in the Thoratec, centrifugal VAD, and ECMO patient groups. Bleeding was the most frequent complication, occurring in 70% –80% of all patients, regardless of which device was implanted. Similarly, biventricular failure occurred in 70% of the patients. Renal failure, which was almost uniformly fatal, occurred in 30%–36% of the patients. The increased incidence of infectious complications in the Thoratec-VAD group and the implantable-device group can be attributed to the increased length of time that these devices were in place. Table 3 shows a breakdown of patient characteristics according to the type of device. Centrifugal VAD patients had the lowest incidence of infection (19%) but were on the assist devices for a mean of only 2.3 days. The Thoratec-VAD patients had a 34% infectious complication rate with a mean duration on the assist device of 8.5 days. All four of the patients in the implantable-device group had infectious complications which probably can be explained by their mean duration of support of 50 days.

Table 3. Patient characteristics by device

Type of device	No. of patients	Sex M/F	Age (mean years)	Duration of support (mean days)
Centrifugal	37	28/9	54.4	2.3
Thoratec	44	34/10	49.2	8.5
ECMO	69	43/26	Range 1 day–74 years 14 < 1 year	3.4
Implantable	4	4/0	45.2	50

Embolic complications were as high in the centrifugal pump group as in the Thoratec group, despite the fact that the centrifugal-VAD patients received continuous heparinization within 24 h of device insertion. However, the Thoratec group was on the device nearly four times as long. The frequency of thrombus formation and embolization was low in the ECMO group, undoubtedly due to the moderate levels of anticoagulation which were started as soon as the device was inserted. The incidence of hemolysis was twice as great in the centrifugal-VAD patients as the Thoratec and ECMO patients. Furthermore, hemolysis in Thoratec and ECMO patients decreased over time. However, in many centrifugal pump patients, hemolysis increased progressively with their length of time on the pump.

Although the incidence of leg ischemia was relatively low, it was of such a severe nature that it contributed significantly to the patients' demise. Cannula obstruction has been virtually eliminated as we have gained experience in cannulation techniques and in choosing the proper sites for each individual patient. Mechanical failure, although worrisome, never resulted in irreversible damage to a patient, because backup consoles were always available.

From our review of this series of patients, it seems apparent that life-threatening complications are likely to be encountered no matter which currently available assist device one uses. These critically ill patients are particularly susceptible to complications. Until more reliable predictors for determining the reversibility of myocardial injury are developed, it is unlikely that survival rates will exceed 50% in the myocardial recovery group. Renal failure alone, which is almost always fatal, accounts for 30%–40% of the total mortality. It is difficult to determine how much of a detrimental effect bleeding has on overall survival, although it was a significant factor in many of our patients. Hopefully, the incidence of bleeding can be further reduced by judicious administration of blood products, meticulous surgical technique, and closure of the sternum when possible. Once diagnosed, severe biventricular failure can be treated readily with Thoratec VADs, centrifugal pumps, ECMO, and total artificial hearts. Only the implantable LVAS cannot provide biventricular support. For this reason, patients who are to undergo insertion of an LVAS should have a thorough evaluation of their right ventricular function, including echocardiography and right heart catheterization when possible.

The outcome in these 148 patients is outlined in Table 4. The highest percentage of survival was in the Thoratec-VAD group, at 36%. This was more than twice as high as in the ECMO group, which had a 16% survival, and four times as high as in the centrifugal-VAD patient group, which had an 8% survival. Since there were only four patients who had implantable devices, with a 50% survival, it is difficult to project the outcome for larger patient groups. Part of the reason for the better overall results with the Thoratec pump is the fact that it was designed specifically as a VAD to be used for periods of 1 day to several months. Other advantages of this system are that it does not require continuous anticoagulation and has a versatile cannulation system which can be used for left or right ventricular support. These characteristics make it an excellent device for postcardiotomy or bridge-to-transplant patients. In spite of the superior technical characteristics of the Thoratec VAD, there may have been other factors which ac-

Table 4. Results in 148 patients with 154 devices

	Thoratec	Centrifugal	ECMO	Implantable
Number of patients	44	37	69	4
Number weaned	16	5	27	0
Number survived	11	3	14	–
Number transplanted	5	0	2	2
Number survived	5	–	0	2
Total survivors	16	3	14	2

counted for the different survival rates. For example, some patients were excluded from the Thoratec study according to rather strict NHLBI criteria, while exclusion criteria were not as stringent for ECMO and centrifugal-pump patients.

In spite of our attempts to avoid selecting patients who had suffered irreversible organ damage, some of those selected undoubtedly had irreversible renal, cerebral, or cardiac injury which was not apparent at the time of the insertion of the assist system. Retrospectively, 45 patients had such a severe cardiac injury that recovery was very unlikely. Sixteen patients died in the operating room within a few hours of device insertion due to massive bleeding and/or biventricular failure. Therefore, of the 148 patients studied, 49 showed evidence of improved myocardial function and 45 were weaned from the devices, with 28 long-term survivors. In addition, nine patients received cardiac transplants, of whom seven were long-term survivors.

In almost all cases, initial circulatory support was sufficient to allow weaning from cardiopulmonary bypass or resuscitation from cardiogenic shock. However, adequate flow levels could not be maintained in some patients, including a centrifugal-pump patient with stenosis of an aortic VAD graft, two ECMO patients on femoro-femoral bypass, and several patients with severe biventricular failure who had insertion of single assist devices. Right ventricular failure was recognized and treated with support devices more often in the Thoratec and Biomedicus patients than in the Medtronic-pump patients. Between 1982 and 1984, several patients with severe biventricular failure were treated with ECMO, although this may have been unwise in the immediate postcardiotomy adult patients.

Bleeding was severe in 114 of 148 patients, particularly immediately postoperatively. However, some patients who survived the immediate postoperative period later developed severe bleeding due to coagulopathy or thrombocytopenia. The need for continuous heparinization limited the effectiveness of ECMO in the immediate postoperative period. Thromboemboli which occurred in the first two Medtronic patients led us to begin heparin in all subsequent centrifugal-pump recipients as soon as the initial bleeding was controlled. Thrombocytopenia occurred frequently in the centrifugal-pump patients and may have been related to continued use of the IABP. Unfortunately, bleeding problems were not eliminated for the Thoratec-VAD patients, none of whom received heparin until they were ready to be weaned from the device, or in the bridge-to-transplant group until after they had been on the device for a minimum of 1 week.

Hemolysis was often related to events occurring prior to insertion of the assist system; however, it persisted longer and was more severe in patients treated with centrifugal pumps and ECMO. Renal failure was fatal in 50/52 patients in spite of dialysis in 32. Infectious complications could rarely be attributed directly to the assist system. They were more commonly the result of having numerous intravenous catheters and prolonged ventilator support. In addition, patients with bleeding complications who required reexploration for bleeding or tamponade had a high risk of infection. Thirty-one patients suffered neurological complications, probably attributable to hypoperfusion prior to placement of the assist system in 22 cases. Nine patients suffered embolization of a thrombus which had formed in some component of the assist device system.

Between 1978 and 1985, our efforts were concentrated on patients with postcardiotomy ventricular failure. Since 1985, we have expanded our program to include patients who develop cardiogenic shock following acute myocardial infarction (MI), prior to cardiac transplantation, and after cardiac transplantation. Patients who develop cardiogenic shock after acute MI are the largest potential group of candidates for mechanical circulatory support. Up to this time, we have primarily used femoral ECMO to treat these patients in the acute setting. However, we have converted six patients to VADs in an attempt to bridge them to cardiac transplantation, since we believed that the extent of their myocardial damage was severe enough to preclude survival. Two of these six patients were eventually weaned from the assist devices and able to maintain near normal ejection fractions. Unfortunately, both of these patients died due to multiorgan failure as a result of prolonged periods of hypoperfusion prior to implantation of the VADs. Eleven of the 17 patients whom we attempted to bridge to cardiac transplantation suffered acute MIs and cardiogenic shock prior to placement of mechanical circulatory support. This information, along with the data from a recent report [17] showing the relationship of acute MI to survival in postcardiotomy patients, suggests that acute MI shock severe enough to require more than IABP for mechanical circulatory support may be irreversible in a large percentage of the patients. However, the current experience with acute MI patients trreated with VADs is inadequate for drawing conclusions. It is not known whether prolonged mechanical support for 3–4 weeks may allow for myocardial recovery which is not possible using present therapy. Patients could have assist devices inserted after the acute event, be stabilized, and undergo cardiac operations within a few weeks. These patients then undergo operation in more stable condition than if they had been rushed to the operating room in a state of shock with the hope that their hearts would recover. Our experience shows that ECMO is not an acceptable method for prolonged treatment of cardiogenic shock. It should be used only as a palliative measure to stabilize the patient until other procedures can be performed [18].

Nationwide, the bridge-to-cardiac transplantation group is the largest, due in part to the large number of centers performing cardiac transplantation, the shortage of donor organs, and the popularity of the procedure because of a relatively high survival rate.

Post-cardiac transplant patients requiring mechanical circulatory support represent the smallest group of patients [6, 19]. It appears that with most of these patients, the chances of myocardial recovery are relatively low, so that most of them will require retransplantation. However, retransplantation is difficult in this group of patients because of the high rate of complications. Chronically ill immunosuppressed patients with end-stage heart disease are not ideal candidates for insertion of assist devices. Although pulmonary hypertension and right heart failure after cardiac transplantation might be expected to resolve with temporary ventricular support, our experience has been discouraging. Most of our patients have developed renal failure and infections after 4 or 5 days of support. Seven of our eight patients who were supported after cardiac transplantation received biventricular support with ECMO, BVADs, or RVAD and IABP. In the two patients who received RVADs and IABP, left ventricular function eventually deteriorated to the point that even with an IABP acceptable support could not be maintained. For that reason, in our two most recently operated patients we implanted BVADs at the outset.

The Thoratec VAD seems preferable in patients with postcardiotomy ventricular failure since it has a large margin of safety, is virtually self-regulating, provides pulsatile flow, and does not require continuous heparinization. Its disadvantages are related to the more tedious and time-consuming insertion techniques. The centrifugal pumps are easier to insert but require continuous heparinization as soon as the initial bleeding episode has subsided and do not provide pulsatile flow. There is a higher incidence of hemolysis with the centrifugal pumps than with the Thoratec VADs. The Thoratec VAD has also proven to be an excellent device for use in the bridge-to-transplant category [20]. Not only does it have the capability to provide biventricular support but it also allows patients to be more mobile than they would be with centrifugal pumps or ECMO [21]. As opposed to a TAH, the Thoratec VAD does not require that the heart be removed, so the patient can be weaned from the devices if the heart unexpectedly recovers. ECMO is least desirable during the immediate postoperative period because of the need for continuous anticoagulation. For the patient who has not previously undergone a sternotomy and requires rapid hemodynamic stabilization, ECMO seems to be the method of choice. Femoro-femoral cannulation and initiation of ECMO can be quickly accomplished in an ICU or cardiac catheterization laboratory by use of a portable ECMO system, while insertion of a Thoratec or centrifugal pump requires a sternotomy. Therefore, ECMO is useful in patients who develop cardiogenic shock during cardiac catheterization or following acute myocardial infarction [18]. It is then possible to transfer patients on ECMO to the operating room for definitive surgery or for insertion of a more sophisticated assist device. Patients with combined respiratory and cardiac failure may benefit most from ECMO, particularly when the respiratory failure is due to an acute insult which is likely to be reversible.

Implantable systems such as the Novacor LVAS or Jarvik-7 TAH are best suited for patients who are awaiting cardiac transplantation. Since these devices are implantable, it was thought that the incidence of infection would be reduced. However, recent data from the University of Pittsburgh [22] have shown a high incidence of mediastinal infections with the use of the Jarvik TAH. All three of our patients with the Novacor LVAS eventually developed infections, although in our two survivors the infections never involved the mediastinum. It seems that current systems which require drive lines to traverse the body wall will have an increased risk of infection, related in part to the length of time the device is in place. The Novacor LVAS is probably not an ideal device for postcardiotomy cardiac failure, since its insertion requires replacement of a large cannula into the left ventricular apex. In addition, the Novacor LVAS provides only left ventricular support, which may not be adequate in postcardiotomy patients due to the high incidence of right ventricular failure [11]. Currently, the Novacor LVAS is our first choice of a device for bridge to transplantation.

Conclusion

Ventricular support systems have assumed an increasingly important role in our care of patients with cardiogenic shock. Although the current overall salvage rate is only 24%, all the patients mentioned in this review were certain to die without the use of these devices. Further work is needed to improve our accuracy in patient selection, to determine the reversibility of myocardial injury in acute settings (such as the operating room), to simplify devices and thereby reduce the time required for insertion, to control bleeding before and after insertion of the device, and to evaluate more patients with nonoperative cardiogenic shock. As we attempt to resolve these questions, we can use the experience and data being acquired on these temporary support device patients to answer questions which will arise when permanent implantable systems are developed. Issues such as immunological effects of the pump, blood-surface interactions, control mechanisms, and anticoagulation protocols can all be studied in these temporary device patients.

References

1. Pennington DG, Merjavy JP, Swartz MT, Willman VL (1982) Clinical experience with a centrifugal pump ventricular assist device. Trans Am Soc Artif Intern Organs 28:93–99
2. Pennington DG, Samuels LD, Williams GA, Palmer D, Swartz MT, Codd JE, Merjavy JP, Lagunoff D, Joist JH (1985) Experience with the Pierce-Donachy ventricular assist device in postcardiotomy patients with cardiogenic shock. World J Surg 9:37–46
3. Pennington DG, Merjavy JP, Codd JE, Swartz MT, Miller LW, Williams GA (1984) Extracorporeal membrane oxygenation for patients with cardiogenic shock. Circ Supp I Cardiovasc Surg 70:130–137
4. Pennington DG, Codd JE, Merjavy JP, Codd JE, Swartz MT, Willman VL (1984) Temporary mechanical support of patients with profound ventricular failure. In: Unger F (ed) Assisted circulation 2. Springer, Berlin Heidelberg New York Tokyo, pp 85–99
5. Kanter KR, McBride LR, Pennington DG, Swartz MT, Ruzevich SA, Miller LW, Willman LV (1988) Bridging to cardiac transplantation with pulsatile ventricular assist devices. Ann Thorac Surg 46:124–140
6. Pennington DG (1989) Circulatory support before transplantation. In: Wallwork J (ed) Heart and heart lung transplantation. Saunders, Philadelphia, pp 41–86
7. Norman JC, Cooley DA, Igo SR, Hibbs CW, Johnson MD, Bennett JG, Fuqua JM, Trono R, Edmonds CH (1977) Prognostic indices for survival during postcardiotomy intra-aortic balloon pumping. J Thorac Cardiovasc Surg 74:709–720

8. Kanter KR, Swartz MT, Pennington DG, Madden M, McBride LR, Ruzevich SA, Termuhlen DF (1987) Renal failure in patients with ventricular assist devices. Trans Am Soc Artif Intern Organs 33:426–428
9. Pennington DG, McBride LR, Swartz MR, Bashiti H, Hahn J, Pierce WS (1982) Left atrial-aortic (LA-Ao) perfusion with a ventricular assist device (VAD). Trans Am Soc Artif Intern Organs 28:579–582
10. Donachy JH, Landis DL, Rosenberg G, Prophet GA, Ferrari O, Pierce WS (1979) Design and evaluation of a left ventricular assist device: the angle port pump. In: Unger F (ed) Assisted circulation 2. Springer, Berlin Heidelberg New York Tokyo, pp 138–146
11. Pennington DG, Merjavy JP, Swartz MT, Codd JE, Barner HB, Lagunoff D, Bashiti H, Kaiser GC, Willman VL (1985) The importance of biventricular failure in patients with postoperative cardiogenic shock. Ann Thorac Surg 39:16–26
12. Ruzevich SA, Kanter KR, Pennington DG, Swartz MT, McBride LR, Termuhlen DF (1988) Long-term follow-up of survivors of postcardiotomy circulatory support. Trans Am Soc Artif Intern Organs 34:116
13. McBride LR, Ruzevich SA, Pennington DG, Kennedy DJ, Kanter KR, Miller LW, Swartz MT, Termuhlen DF (1987) Infectious complications associated with ventricular assist device support. Trans Am Soc Artif Intern Organs 33:201–202
14. Bartlett RH, Gazzaniga AB, Fong SW, Jeffries MR, Roohk HV, Haiduc N (1977) Extracorporeal membrane oxygenator support for cardiopulmonary failure: experience in 28 cases. J Thorac Cardiovasc Surg 73:375–386
15. Hill JD, DeLeval MR, Fallat RJ, Bramson ML, Eberhart RC, Schulte HD, Osborn JJ, Barber R, Gerbode F (1972) Acute respiratory insufficiency: treatment with prolonged extracorporeal oxygenation. J Thorac Cardiovasc Surg 64:551–562
16. Weiss M (1982) Cardiopulmonary assistance with membrane oxygenation in a case of acute heart failure following drug intoxication. ASAIO J 5:27–37
17. Pennington DG, McBride LR, Kanter KR, Swartz MT, Miller LW (1988) The effect of perioperative myocardial infarction on survival of postcardiotomy patients supported with ventricular assist devices. Circ Supp III Cardiovasc Surg 78:110–115
18. Kanter KR, Swartz MT, Pennington DG, McBride LR, Miller LW, Ruzevich SA (1988) Emergency extracorporeal membrane oxygenation (ECMO) for cardiopulmonary resuscitation (abstract). J Heart Transplantation 7:75
19. Zumbro GL, Shearer G, Kitchens WR, Galloway RF (1985) Mechanical assistance for biventricular failure following coronary bypass operation and heart transplantation. J Heart Transplantation 4:348–352
20. Farrar DJ, Hill JD, Gray LA, Pennington DG, McBride LR, Pierce WS, Pae WE, Glenville B, Ross D, Galbraith TA, Zumbro GL (1988) Heterotopic prosthetic ventricles as a bridge to cardiac transplantation. N Engl J Med 318:333–340
21. Pennington DG, Kanter KR, McBride LR et al. (1988) Seven year's experience with the Pierce-Donzchy ventricular assist device. J Thorac Cardiovasc Surg 96:901–911
22. Griffith BP, Kormos RL, Hardesty RL, Armitage JM, Dummer JS (1988) The artifical heart: infection-related morbidity and its effect on transplantation. Ann Thorac Surg 45:409–414

12. Current Status of Clinical Application of Ventricular Assist Devices in Japan

K. Atsumi, Y. Sezai, T. Fujita, S. Nitta, N. Sato, and T. Horiuchi

Introduction

The first clinical case of ventricular assistance by means of a pulsatile pump (To-kyo University type) in Japan occurred in Mitsui Memorial Hospital in 1980. The clinical application of ventricular assist devices (VADs) was performed very infrequently in Japan until 1983; however, since 1984 the number of cases has been increasing year by year, as shown in Fig. 1.

In 1984, the VAD Registry Committee was organized in Japan; Dr. T. Horiuchi (Tohoku University) and Dr. Y. Sezai (Nihon University) were appointed as the chairman and the vice-chairman respectively, and the author was appointed as the consultant. In 1988, Dr. Y. Sezai was appointed as the chairman and Dr. T. Fujita (National Cardiovascular Center) as the vice-chairman.

By the end of 1987, 86 clinical cases (53 males and 33 females) of VAD use had been registered. In this paper, the data of the VAD Registry are reported.

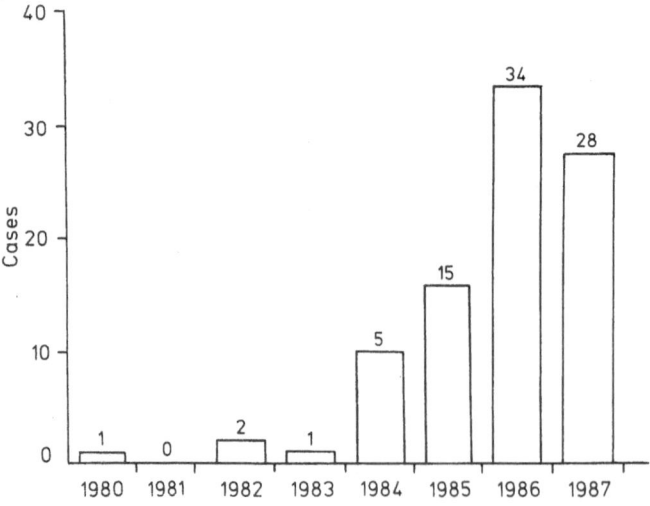

Fig. 1. Number of patients receiving VAD support in Japan, according to year

Assisted Circulation 3
F. Unger (Ed.)
© Springer-Verlag Berlin Heidelberg 1989

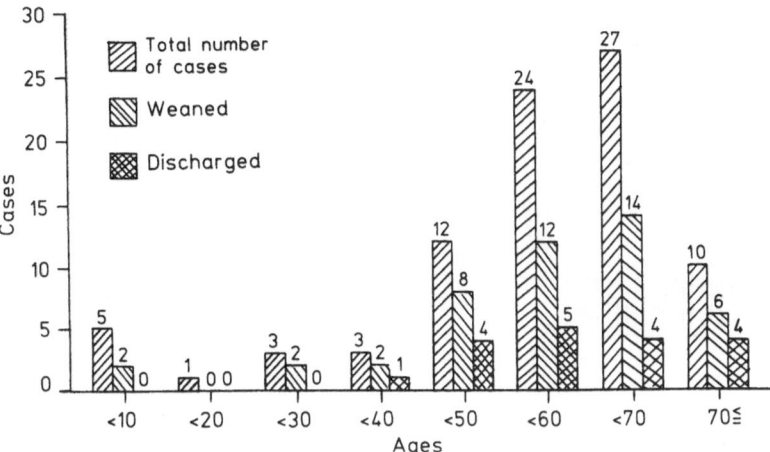

Fig. 2. Clinical results according to age group

Age of Patients

The ages of the VAD patients in Japan are shown in Fig. 2, together with clinical results. The largest group is the 60- to 70-year-olds, followed by the 50- to 60-year-olds. Ten patients were over 70 years old: not such a small number.

Cardiac Diseases in the VAD Patients

Of the 86 patients who received VADs, 43 had ischemic heart disease (IHD), 28 heart valve replacement (VHD), 10 congenital heart disease (CHD), and 5 miscellaneous diseases (OTH), as shown in Fig. 3. In the valve replacement group, fe-

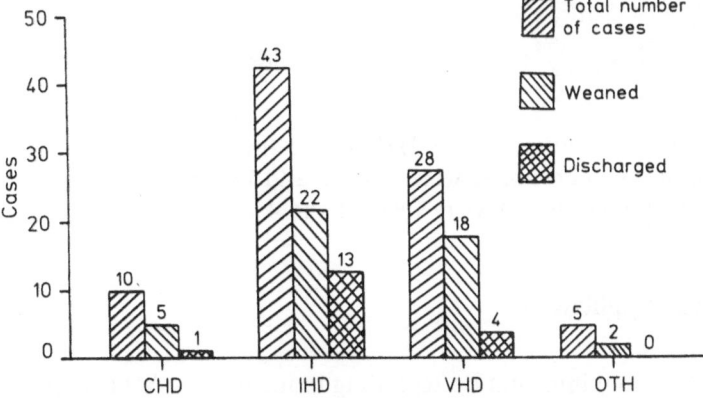

Fig. 3. Clinical results according to heart disease. *CHD*, congenital heart disease; *IHD*, ischemic heart disease; *VHD*, heart valve replacement; *OTH*, others

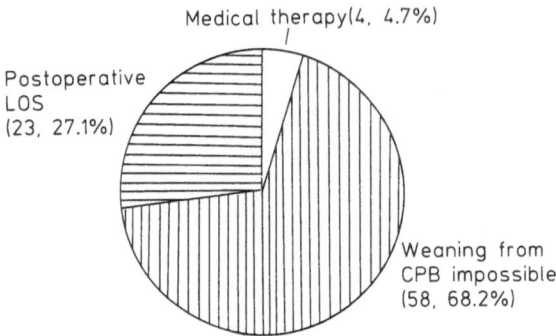

Fig. 4. Indications for VAD application

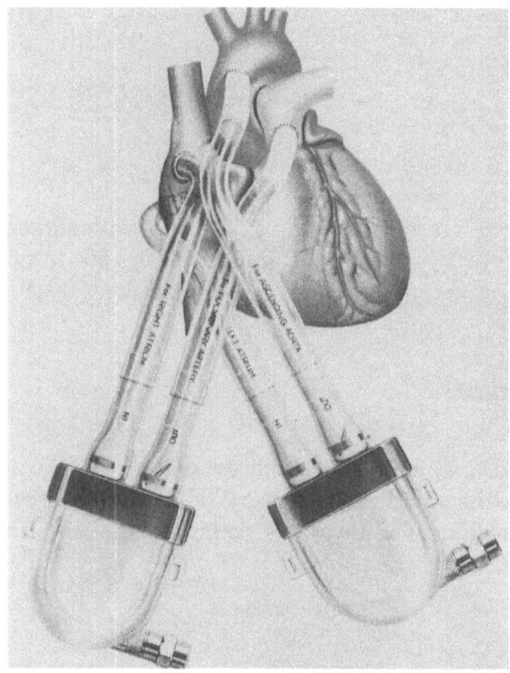

Fig. 5. Biventricular assistance

males outnumbered males; however, in the IHD group the reverse was the case. Of the 43 patients in the IHD group, 22 were weaned and 13 were discharged. Of the 28 patients in the VHD group, 18 were weaned and 4 were discharged.

Indications for VAD Application

Of the 86 patients for whom information regarding indication for VAD application is available, 58 (68.2%) could not be weaned from extracorporeal circulation and 23 (27.1%) were low cardiac output patients who suffered acute myocardial

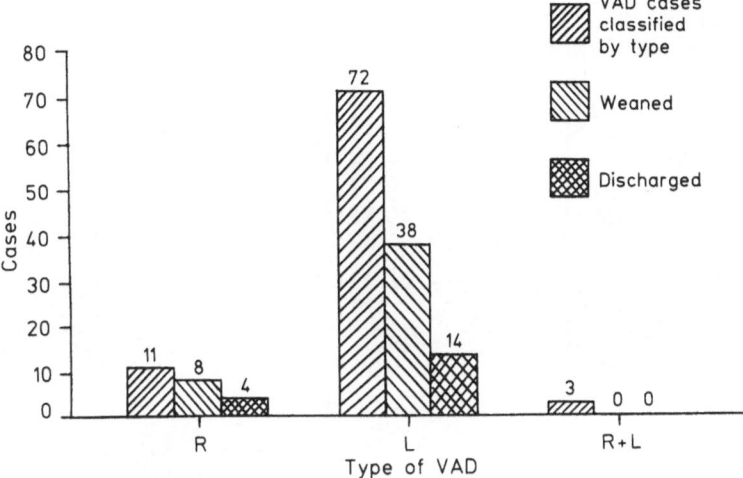

Fig. 6. Clinical results according to type of VAD. *L*, left; *R*, right

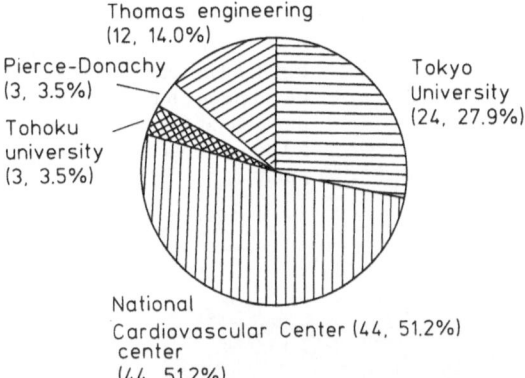

Fig. 7. Types of blood pump used in ventricular assistance

infarctions or had undergone cardiotomy. In addition, four patients (4.7%) had undergone medical therapy (Fig. 4).

Types of VAD

Left ventricular (LVAD), right ventricular (RVAD), and biventricular (BVAD) assist devices have been employed. Seventy-two patients (83%) received an LVAD, 11 (12%) an RVAD, and 3 (3%) a BVAD (Fig. 5). The clinical results according to type of VAD are shown in Fig. 6. Comparison with data from other countries shows that RVADs have been used relatively more often in Japan. The fact that the worst clinical results have been obtained with BVADs matches the experience in other countries.

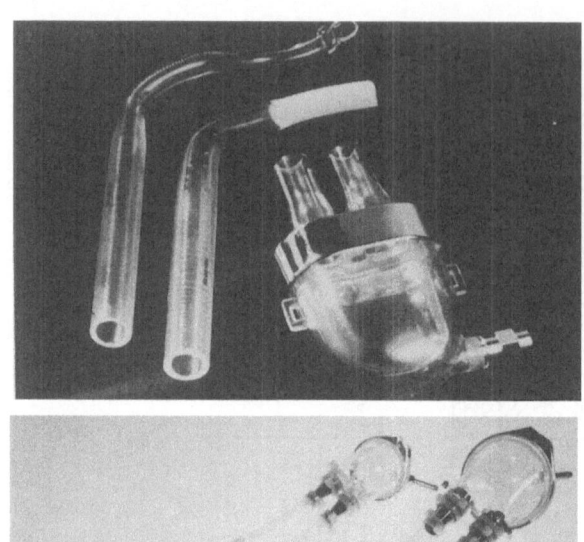

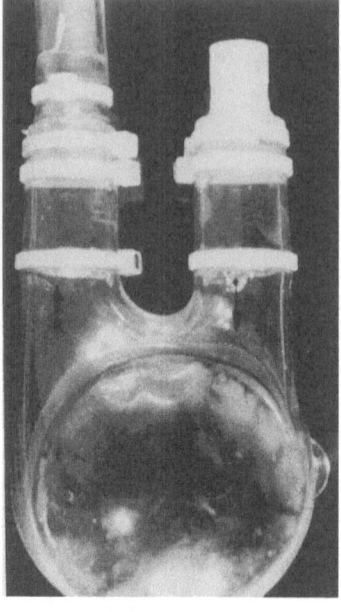

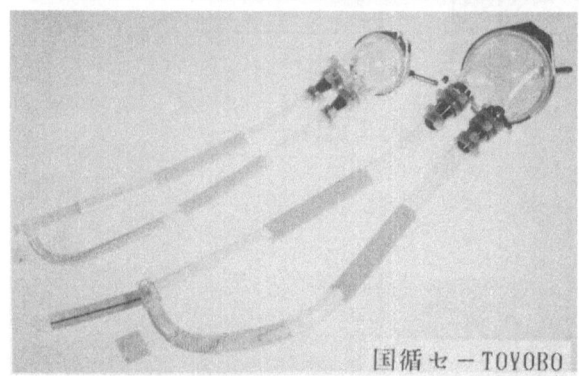

Fig. 8. a University of Tokyo
blood pump. **b** National Cardiovascular Center blood pump.
c Thomas Engineering blood
pump

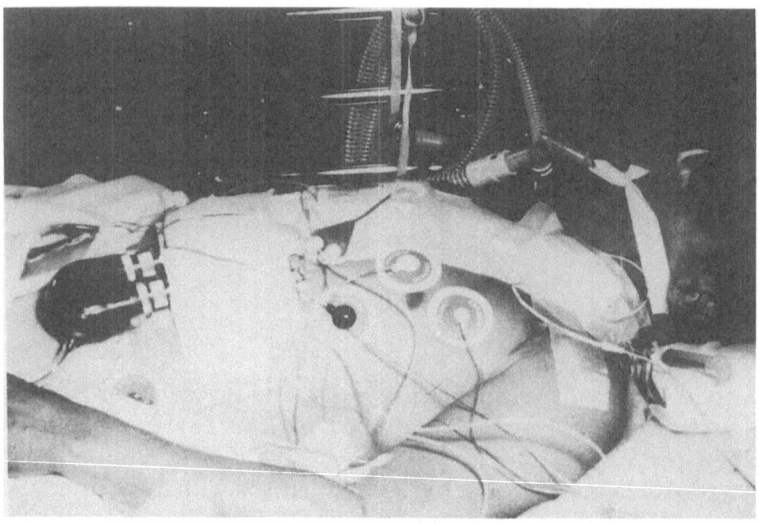

Fig. 9. Use of the University of Tokyo blood pump in left ventricular assistance

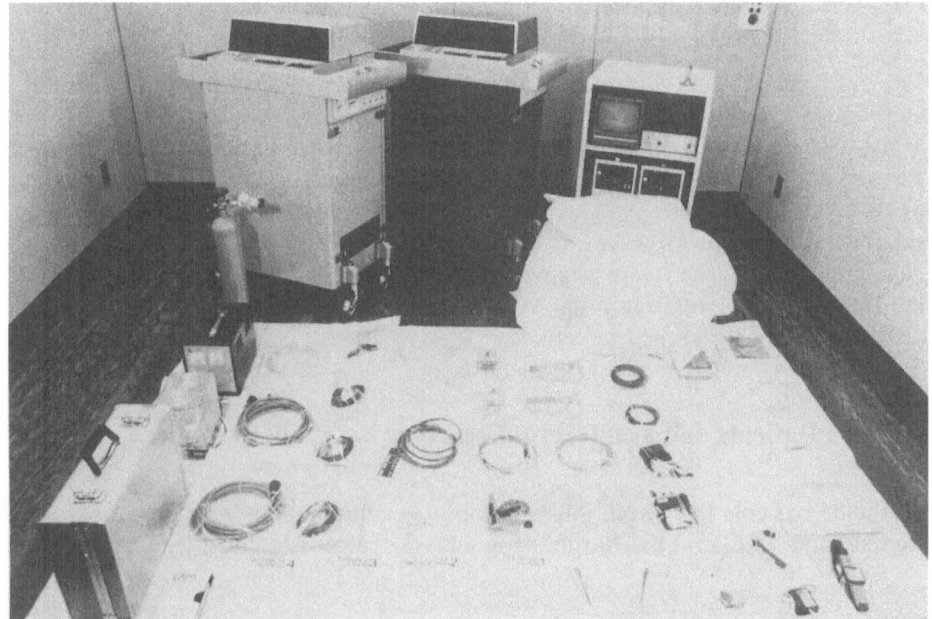

Fig. 10. Driving unit and accessories of CORAT system (Tokyo University)

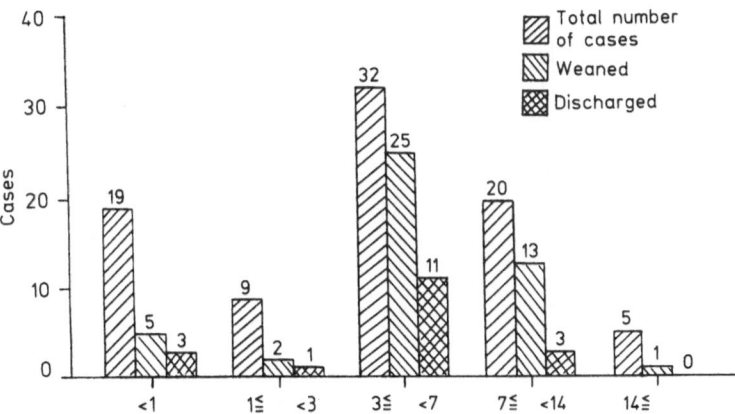

Fig. 11. Clinical results according to duration of VAD support

Blood Pumps Used in Ventricular Assistance

Five types of blood pump (pulsatile) were used: the National Cardiovascular Center pump (44 cases), the University of Tokyo pump (24 cases), the Thomas Engineering pump (12 cases), the University of Tohoku pump (3 cases), and the Pierce-Donachy pump (3 cases) (Figs. 7–9). The driving unit and accessories of CORAT (Tokyo University system) are shown in Fig. 10.

Duration of VAD Support

The duration of VAD support and the corresponding clinical results for 85 of the 86 patients are shown in Fig. 11. The duration ranged from 1 h to 70 days, and in most cases was less than 14 days. Duration of VAD support varied between weaned and nonweaned cases. Of the 52 patients receiving VAD support from 3 to 14 days, 38 (73%) were weaned and 14 (27%) discharged. These results are considered fairly good. However, in those receiving VAD support for less than 3 days, only seven (25%) were weaned and four (14%) discharged. The corresponding figures for patients receiving VAD support for more than 14 days were one (20%) and zero (0%) respectively.

Weaned Patients and Long-Term Survivors

Of the 85 patients for whom information is available 46 (54%) were successfully weaned and 18 (21%) discharged (Fig. 12); the latter are considered to be long-

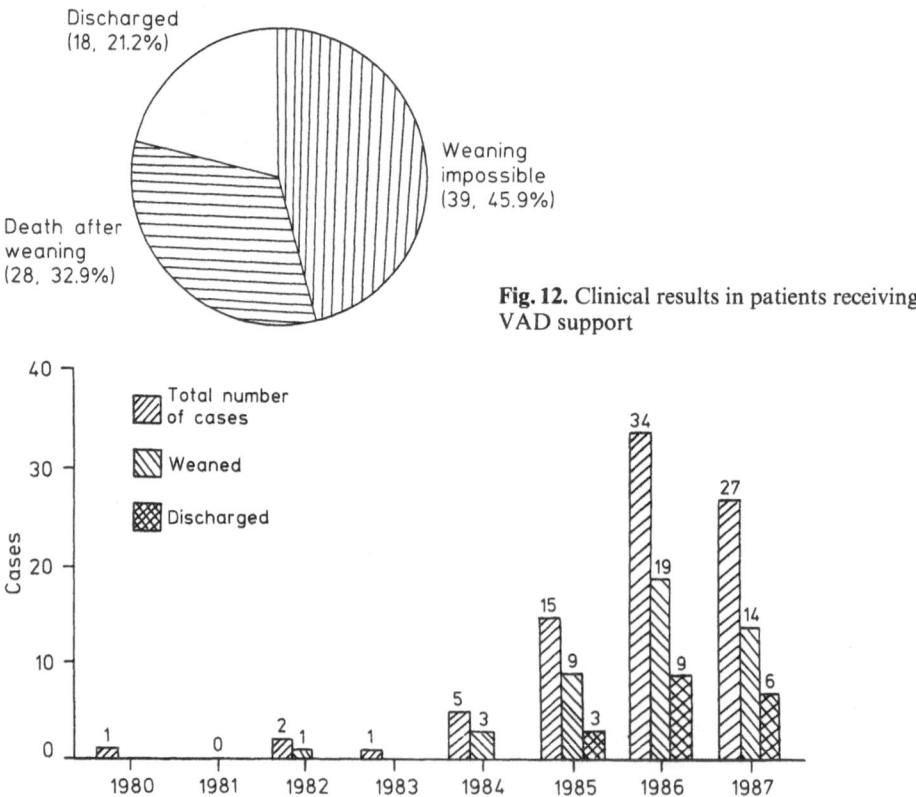

Fig. 12. Clinical results in patients receiving VAD support

Fig. 13. Numbers of weaned patients and long-term survivors (discharged patients) according to year of VAD application

Table 1. Complications/causes of death in VAD patients

Complication	No. of patients
Renal insufficiency	30
Bleeding	26
MOF	26
Infection and sepsis	22
LOS	12
Thrombus and emboli	11
Respiratory insufficiency	11
Right heart failure (LVAD)	8
Disseminated intravascular coagulopathy	4

MOF, multiple organ failure; LOS, low cardiac output syndrome

term survivors. The numbers of weaned patients and long-term survivors according to year of VAD application are shown in Fig. 13.

Complications and Causes of Death

The major complications and the causes of death are shown in Table 1. The most frequent of these were renal insufficiency, bleeding, and multiple organ failure (MOF). While in the nonweaned cases the causes of death were related to circulatory insufficiency, in the weaned cases they were bleeding and multiple organ failure.

Summary

Between May 1980 and December 1987 86 instances of VAD support were registered in Japan. In 72 patients LVADs were used, in 11, RVADs, and in 3, BVADs. The duration of VAD support ranged from 1 h to 70 days, and in most cases was 7–14 days.

The weaning rate was 54% and the discharge rate, 21%. The most frequent complications were renal insufficiency, bleeding, and MOF. The causes of death in the nonweaned cases related to circulatory insufficiency; however, in the weaned cases the causes of death were bleeding and multiple organ failure.

13. Centrifugal Pumps in Clinical Practice

L. A. R. GOLDING, R. W. STEWART, and F. D. LOOP

Nonpulsatile blood pumps are the most frequently used devices for postcardiotomy mechanical ventricular assistance and it is estimated that in the United States over 1500 patients a year now receive postoperative support. Our initial experience with mechanical ventricular assistance was with the Hemadyne (Medtronic) centrifugal pump, as an aid to weaning patients from cardiopulmonary bypass following corrective cardiac surgical procedures. This system was discontinued and we, like many other groups, now use the Biopump (Biomedicus). This latter device is also used in standard cardiopulmonary bypass and as part of an extracorporeal membrane oxygenating system.

Devices

Medtronic Blood Pump

The initial device used in this patient series was the 1861 centrifugal blood pump manufactured by the Hemadyne division of Medtronic, Inc. The blood-contacting surfaces were either composed of or covered with thromboresistant materials. Flows were measured via an ultrasonic Doppler flow probe placed externally on the outflow cannula. The system was provided with unique integral wire-reinforced cannulas coated with thromboresistant materials [1–7].

Biopump

The Biopump is a magnetically coupled commercially available device in which the acrylic pump head, composed of a single moving part, rotates. Incoming blood is accelerated over a set of parallel cones and produces a constrained vortex with flow in proportion to the revolutions per minute. Inlet and outlet ports of the pump accept standard 3/8-in (0.95-cm) tubing and flow is monitored by an inline disposable electromagnetic flow probe positioned in the outflow tubing. The drive console has an internal battery pack to allow transport and can function either in direct contact with the pump head or by connection to a remote unit distant from the drive console. In association with the Biopump, standard Tygon tubing is used to connect the ports of the acrylic pump head to the inflow and outflow cannulas. In general the cannulas used have been those that are readily available in the operating room, although on occasion we have used special cannulas.

Assisted Circulation 3
F. Unger (Ed.)
© Springer-Verlag Berlin Heidelberg 1989

Blood Access

Many cannulation techniques have been described in association with ventricular assist devices. Our preference in the postcardiotomy setting has been to position a 32-FR or 36-FR armored venous cannula into the left atrium through a buttressed-Teflon suture in the right superior pulmonary vein into the left atrium. Arterial access has, in most cases, utilized the existing arterial cannula positioned into the ascending aorta. We have generally avoided apical ventricular cannulas in an attempt to minimize any further myocardial damage. In contrast, we believe a ventricular drainage cannula to be mandatory in bridging to cardiac transplantation.

Clinical Material

Centrifugal blood pumps have mainly been used as an aid to weaning from cardiopulmonary bypass when low cardiac output state followed cardiac surgical procedures. In more recent years, these devices have also been used as a bridge to cardiac transplantation [8]. Since 1978, 61 patients have undergone attempted support with a centrifugal blood pump at The Cleveland Clinic Foundation. In ten patients adequate support was not achieved and the patients died within a brief period following the attempted support. Fifty-one patients were able to be hemodynamically supported with the centrifugal blood pump, which was used as a left ventricular assist (LVA) in 37, a right ventricular assist (RVA) in 10, and a biventricular assist (BVA) in four. The indication for use was persistent extreme low cardiac output state following cardiac surgery in 44 and as a bridge to cardiac transplantation in seven. In all cases a low cardiac output incompatible with survival was present despite maximal supportive measures including cardiotonics, vasodilators, and intra-aortic balloon pumping. Intra-aortic balloon pumping was continued and provided pulsatile perfusion in all cases except in three patients who were awaiting transplantation.

Anticoagulation was routinely instituted when bleeding had ceased; the activated clotting time was maintained at 150% of the normal value by continuous intravenous heparin. In our early experience with the Biopump, pump heads were changed routinely every 48 h, but most recently were changed only when there was evidence of malfunction. The longest use of a single pump head has been 10 days.

Case Report

A 23-year-old white man (patient 6, Table 3) had progressive onset of congestive heart failure; cardiac catheterization showed normal coronary arteries and severe cardiomyopathy. He was accepted for cardiac transplantation and during the next several weeks required increasing doses of cardiotonic agents to manage his progressive low-output state. He finally became unresponsive to all pharmacological intervention and balloon pumping and he was placed on LVA support. This was instituted without the aid of cardiopulmonary bypass by placing a drainage cannula through a pursestring suture in the right superior pulmonary vein, across the mitral valve, and into the left ventricle, with the return cannula in the ascending aorta. This technique was used because left ventricular apex was not accessible. The patient was returned to the intensive care unit; flow was maintained at 4 l/min and all pharmacological support was rapidly discontinued. He did well for the first 5 days but then showed progressive evidence of severe hemolysis despite changing the pump head at 10 days, which showed no evidence of thrombus formation. The hemolysis necessitated intermittent transfusion and we decided to replace the small-bore arterial cannula. Following this, the hemolysis rapidly abated (to 4 mg/dl) and flow was maintained at 4.5 l/min. During the 31 days of support, the pump head was changed on three occasions, the final change being after 29 days of support. During that time he was extubated and limited mobility was possible by using the remote drive unit. After 31 days an appropriate donor organ was found. He was discharged home 14 days after successful transplantation and remains in good health.

Results

From 1978 through 1987, centrifugal support with either the Medtronic or Biomedicus pump has been attempted at our institution in 61 patients, or 0.02% of the cardiac surgery patients in that time period. The patients' ages ranged from 23 to 72 years and the period of mechanical assistance ranged from 12 h to 31 days. Of the 51 patients who were stabilized hemodynamically, 25 (49%) were able to be weaned from support after regaining partial or total recovery of ventricular function. Eleven patients (21.6%) were discharged from the hospital. The longest survivor is now 98 months postoperative and he is fully active (Table 1).

The major cause of death was failure to recover adequate ventricular function. For patients who were successfully weaned, recurrence of ventricular failure remained the major cause of mortality although sepsis was a major factor in 4 of 14 and stroke in 3 of 14.

When postcardiotomy patients were subdivided on the basis of the type of mechanical assistance, almost all the survivors were patients supported with LVA

Table 1. Nonpulsatile mechanical assistance

	LVA	RVA	BVA	Total
No. of cases[a]	37	10	4	51
Weaned	19 (51%)	4 (40%)	2 (50%)	25 (49%)
Survived	10 (27%)	1 (10%)	0	11 (22%)

[a] There were also 10 additional abortive attempts,

Table 2. Postcardiotomy mechanical assistance

	LVA	RVA	BVA	Total
No. of cases	31	10	3	44
Weaned	19 (61%)	4 (40%)	2 (66%)	25 (57%)
Survived	7 (23%)	1 (10%)	0	8 (18%)

(Table 2). The sole survivor of RVA was a patient who, following transplantation, had right ventricular failure and required support for 57 h postoperatively. We have had no survivors of BVA.

Multifactorial analysis in a consecutive series of 23 patients supported with the Biopump was undertaken to determine prognostic factors for survival. While not statistically significant, female sex, early evidence of significant renal failure, and persistent right ventricular failure were features that appeared associated with a poor outcome. With the exception of the one survivor of 31 days of support, all other surviving patients have been supported for periods of less than 4 days prior to weaning or transplantation and have shown early recovery of ventricular function.

Discussion

Since the initiation of our cardiac transplantation program, there has been an increasing need for mechanical assistance due to increasing difficulty of donor procurement.

Bridging has been attempted in seven cases; in one patient the attempt was abortive, because adequate support could not be achieved and he died in the operating room. The periods of support for the other six patients ranged from 2½ to 31 days (mean 11 days) (Table 3). These patients have demonstrated several problems.

One patient was supported immediately following surgery because of inability to be weaned from cardiopulmonary bypass. The other patients had been ac-

Table 3. LVA bridge/transplant (Biomedicus pump)

Patient no.	Age (year)	Indication	Duration	Tx	Survival
1	39	Pre-Tx	5 days	No	No
2	44	Pre-Tx	9 days	No	No
3	43	Pre-Tx	15 days	No	No
4	56	Pre-Tx	2½ days	Yes	Yes
5	50	Postop.	3 days	Yes	Yes
6	23	Pre-Tx	31 days	Yes	Yes

cepted as cardiac transplant candidates and had deterioration and inadequate response to balloon pumping and cardiotonic agents. Three patients ultimately underwent cardiac transplantation and all three are presently surviving.

Our initial bridge/transplant patient was a 39-year-old man who had suffered a massive myocardial infarction. He remained in cardiogenic shock, unresponsive to the standard support with drugs and balloon pumping, and was accepted as a transplant candidate. He was well supported with good flow on the LVA device but developed evidence of sepsis. Subsequently a decision was made to attempt weaning and he rapidly died. As a result of this experience, when sepsis occurred in a second patient (patient 3, Table 3), probably associated with one of the monitoring lines, support was not discontinued but an intensive 10-day course of antibiotics appropriate to the organism was given. There was good response, and repeat blood cultures after completion of the course showed a complete absence of infection. Unfortunately, however, 24 h prior to notification of an available donor organ, evidence suddenly developed of cerebral dysfunction consistent with cerebral emboli. This occurred on the 14th day of support and by the 15th day there was evidence of irreversible and severe brain damage and support was discontinued. Autopsy confirmed massive myocardial damage, no evidence of thrombus in the pump, but evidence of mural thrombus being the source of the cerebral emboli. In this patient, the drainage cannula had been placed into the left atrial appendage with return to the ascending aorta. Hemodynamic tracings showed that although for the majority of time he was maintained in a depulsed mode, there were occasional episodes of intermittent ejection from his own ventricle. We believe that there was relative stasis in his native ventricle and that this was the exciting source of his cerebral emboli. Since then ventricular drainage only has been used in pretransplant patients. The patients supported for 2½ and 3 days had uncomplicated courses and donor hearts were rapidly found for them.

Because of the patient (No. 3) with cerebral emboli, in the 31-day case, ventricular drainage was ensured by placing a 32-FR armored venous cannula through the mitral valve into the ventricle. There was no difficulty with drainage but there were significant problems associated with hemolysis (peak serum hemoglobin level was 1500 mg/100 ml). The direct cause of this was a very small-bore long arterial return cannula, with an internal diameter of 2 mm. Change of this cannula, which resulted in a significant bleeding episode, caused a complete resolution of the hemolysis.

Three patients have been maintained in an essentially nonpulsatile mode for periods of 5, 9, and 31 days as the intra-aortic balloon pump was removed in an attempt to minimize the risk of infection (Fig. 1). In all three cases, the absence of pulsatility created no obvious systemic organ effects, and there was a complete recovery of the renal dysfunction. Flows were maintained at a minimum cardiac index level of 2.4 l/min/m^2. Another patient (patient 2, Table 3) illustrates two problems. First is the potential for bleeding associated with any invasive procedure in a patient maintained in a partially heparinized state. The introduction of the chest tube resulted in a large hemothorax and some impairment of respiratory function and difficulty in evacuating the blood. The second problem was persistent right ventricular failure that necessitated continuing use of isopro-

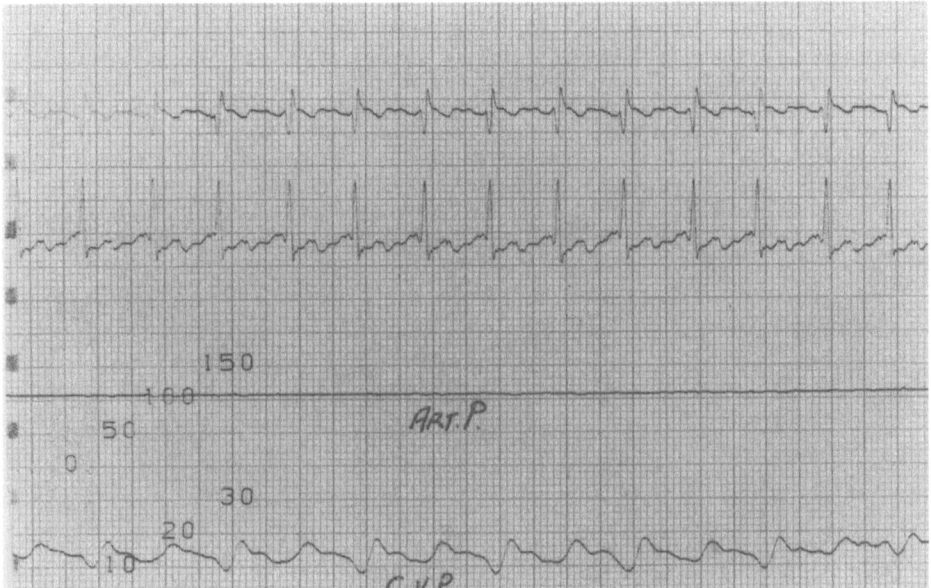

Fig. 1. Hemodynamic trace from patient on Biopump LVA at 4 l/min pretransplant

terenol. This was probably a poor prognostic sign and biventricular support should have been considered.

Conclusion

Centrifugal pumps are the simplest and most readily available devices for mechanical ventricular assistance and the relatively low cost makes them the first choice for postcardiotomy use. Their use in bridging to cardiac transplantation is uncertain due to the limited durability of the pump head but is possible with careful management. Pulsatile perfusion may be important for recovery of myocardium but does not seem necessary for pretransplant support to maintain the function of other systemic organs if adequate flow and pressure are provided.

References

1. Golding LAR (1984) Centrifugal pumps. In: Unger F (ed) Assisted circulation 2. Springer, Berlin Heidelberg New York Tokyo, pp 143–152
2. Golding L, Loop FD, Nosé Y (1985) Clinical and experimental use of the centrifugal pump. New developments in cardiac assist devices, vol 6. pp 92–102
3. Pennington DG, Golding LAR, Hill JD, Joyce L, Magovern GJ, Phillips SJ, Rose D (1986) Temporary mechanical support for cardiogenic shock. Trans Am Soc Artif Intern Organs 32:629–632

4. Golding LR, Jacobs G, Groves LK, Gill CC, Nosé Y, Loop FD (1982) Clinical results of mechanical support of the failing left ventricle. J Thorac Cardiovasc Surg 83:597–601
5. Golding LAR, Harasaki H, Gill CC, Jacobs G, Loop FD, Nosé Y (1981) Clinical mechanical ventricular support. Artif Organs 5 (Suppl):565–567
6. Golding LR, Loop FD, Sandberg GW, Jacobs G, Lewis RC (1981) Left ventricular assist device support: twenty-one month survival. Cleve Clin Q 48:373–377
7. Pennington DG, Swartz MT, McBride R (1986) Clinical experience with temporary nonpulsatile ventricular assist systems. Artif Heart 1:105–113
8. Zumbro GL, Kitchens WR, Galloway RF (1986) Mechanical assistance for bridging to heart transplantation and support of the failing transplanted heart. J Heart Transplant 5:382

14. Mechanical Support for Postcardiotomy Heart Failure

C. D. Campbell, D. J. Tolitano, K. T. Weber, H. H. Hines Jr., and R. L. Replogle

Introduction

Cardiac failure remains a life-threatening complication for certain patients undergoing intracardiac repair. Despite improvements in surgical techniques, better methods of myocardial protection, and improved postoperative care, patients are frequently at risk of developing postoperative low output syndrome. Approximately 1% of cardiac surgical patients cannot be weaned from extracorporeal circulation in spite of adequate volume loading, the use of ionotropic support, and initiation of intra-aortic balloon pumping. In such cases, the ventricular assist devices (VADs) have been recognized to mechanically aid the failing heart and reverse the low output state.

The concept of mechanical support for the failing left ventricle was first proposed by Clauss et al. [1] in 1961. By 1968, Kantrowitz and associates [2] had developed and refined the first intra-aortic balloon pump (IABP). Through the efforts of Moulopolous and others [3], this device evolved into the present-day IABP.

Clinical evidence for the efficacy of left ventricular assist devices (LVADs) remained questionable until 1980, when the National Heart, Blood and Lung Institute evaluated short-term left ventricular assistance by comparing various types of mechanical aids [1, 4–8]. This report focused attention primarily on the failing left ventricle. As the use of ionotropic support, IABPs, and LVADs improved, a small group of patients emerged who could not be separated from extracorporeal circulation due to a failing right ventricle. The failing right ventricle emerged as a unique clinical entity similar to postcardiotomy left ventricular failure, benefiting also from mechanical cardiac assistance. Current therapy at major centers incorporating mechanical assist devices is based on the premise that the low output state will allow the failing heart to recover from a reversible injury. The frequent occurrence of postcardiotomy ischemia may be due to several factors such as poor myocardial protection, overdistention of the left ventricle, emboli, coronary spasm, or technical problems. Whatever the etiology, the end product of cardiac failure is a demand for oxygen consumption which cannot be met, thus leading to cardiac demise.

Assisted Circulation 3
F. Unger (Ed.)
© Springer-Verlag Berlin Heidelberg 1989

Devices for Ventricular Assistance

The IABP has been used successfully to relieve refractory ventricular failure both intraoperatively and postoperatively. The IABP acts to reduce the afterload of the LV while increasing the blood flow to the coronary arteries. Because the effectiveness of the IABP is dependent upon a certain level of ventricular function, patients in severe ventricular failure benefit minimally. This limiting factor is absent with the use of the mechanical assist devices. A variety of mechanical circulatory support devices have been developed over the years utilizing roller pumps and the Anstadt pump as well as intraventricular balloons [9–11]. The latter two have demonstrated problems of extreme invasiveness and cranial venous congestion [12], and have been abandoned.

In 1975, Bernstein et al. [13] were the first to use the vortex pump with heparin for long-term support. The roller pump which was initially used required a reservoir and the use of anticoagulation. The occlusive nature of the roller pump can cause high afterload pressure with disruption of the lines or with low preloads can cause gaseous emboli to develop. Bass and Langmore [14] showed that the pump allowed gas to come out of solution, thus increasing the complication rate.

Mandl [15], in 1977, compared the vortex pump and roller pump and found that the incidence of emboli was significantly less with the centrifugal pump. The large pressure ranges and transient negative pressures produced by the roller style device encouraged emboli formation. The current Biomedicus centrifugal pump has excellent hematological and hydraulic characteristics [16]. This device consists of rotating cones that employ a centrifugal force to move blood through a vortex pumphead. The advantage of the Biomedicus centrifugal pump is that it is nonocclusive and the inner tubing creates a negative charge. These factors result in less trauma to blood cells, decreasing the need for heparinization and resulting in a lower incidence of gaseous emboli. If inflow (to machine) and outflow (to patient) sides of the Biomedicus centrifugal pump become occluded, there is a compensatory drop in flow which lowers the line pressure, thus reducing the incidence of formation of gaseous microemboli from the tubing.

Indications for Use

Patients can develop severe ventricular dysfunction from temporary ischemia associated with cardiopulmonary bypass. It is difficult to predict which patients will develop this "ischemic damage." At present, indications for the use of mechanical assistance have been adopted by most centers with active programs. Two general patient groups have benefited. The first group consists of those patients who undergo successful open-heart surgery but cannot be weaned from extracorporeal circulation by conventional methods. The second group contains patients who are weaned from extracorporeal circulation and later develop ventricular dysfunction with low output syndrome and do not respond to ionotropic support and intra-aortic balloon pumping. The criteria used for placement of VADs in these two groups are:

 1. Left ventricular end-diastolic pressure greater than 20 torr
 2. Systolic blood pressure less than 80 torr
 3. Cardiac index less than 2 l/m^2
 4. Left atrial pressure greater than 25 torr
 5. Central venous pressure greater than 20 torr with right ventricular failure
 6. Decreased urine output
 7. Overdistention of either right or left ventricle
 8. Failure to correct abnormality with maximum does ionotropes
 9. Failure to correct abnormality with IABP
10. Persistent right heart failure despite adequate left ventricular function

There are contraindications to the use of the Biomedicus VAD. The contraindications are: (a) advanced age associated with severe cerebral vascular disease or peripheral vascular disease and (b) malignancies or severe pulmonary hypertension.

The key to a successful outcome is the early use of ventricular assistance. Because the Biomedicus device acts on the premise that the ischemia is reversible, time must not be wasted on conventional methods to save the patient.

Technique

Once it has been determined that mechanical assistance of the heart is necessary, the Biomedicus pump console is brought into the operating room (Fig. 1). Two

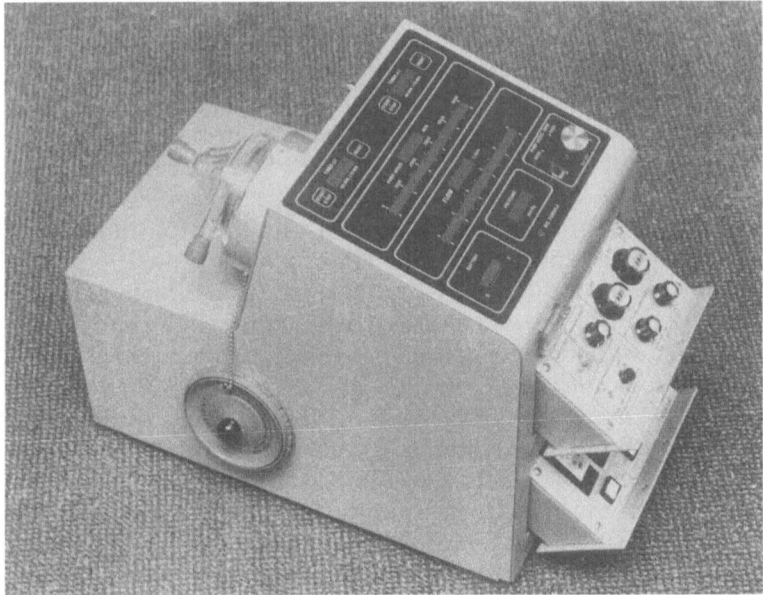

Fig. 1. Biomedicus centrifugal pump console with 80-cc pumping chamber

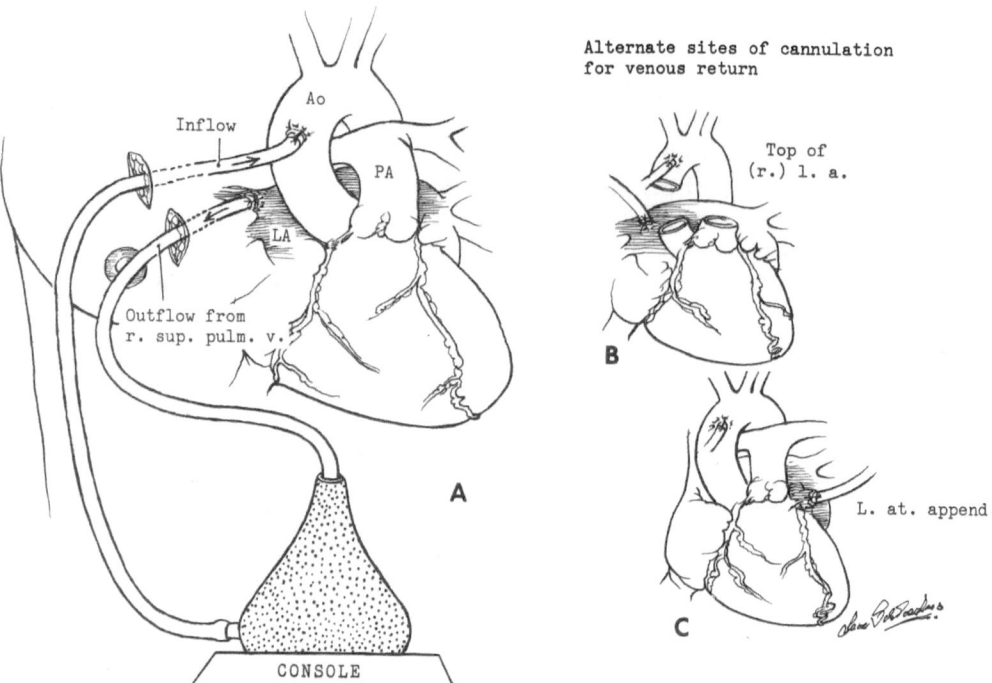

Fig. 2 A–C. Left ventricular assist device. An IABP is usually placed. The simplest placement of outflow cannulas is at the right superior pulmonary vein (**A**) or the roof of the left atrium (**B**) or the left appendage (**C**)

pumps should always be available in case biventricular failure requires pumping of both right and left hearts. If left ventricular failure is the predominant problem, left ventricular pumping is employed (Fig. 2). This is usually instituted with the patient on cardiopulmonary bypass. A Teflon buttressed pursestring suture is placed either in the roof of the left atrium between the superior cava and aorta or at the junction of the right superior pulmonary vein with the left atrium. We have not utilized the left atrial appendage although others have used this for placement of the outflow cannula. A 32- or 34-F wirewound caval catheter is then placed through the pursestring suture and inserted 5 cm into the left atrium. This outflow cannula is secured with a rubber tourniquet. The suture extending from it is secured over a plastic button, and Hemaclips are placed across the rubber tourniquet so that it can be left in the mediastinum with the cannula exiting the sternotomy wound. The outflow venous cannula is then attached to $3/8 \times 3/32$ in tubing measuring approximately $4\frac{1}{2}$–5 ft in length. We have recently obtained heparinized tubing for use in this particular instance. The tubing is attached to the disposable pumphead. By filling the patients with the heart-lung machine, we allow the left atrial pressure to rise and fill the tubing back to the pumphead. After all air has been removed, the pumphead is placed in the Biomedicus console. Using the console, the inflow portion of the tubing is filled without difficulty. At this point, cardiopulmonary bypass is decreased and with ionotropic and intra-aortic balloon support, discontinued. The tubing is then removed from the arterial infusion cannula and the inflow tubing to the Biomedicus pump attached quickly to the arterial infusion cannula, which in almost all instances is a 24-F wirewound catheter. Then, after all air is out of the system, left ventricular assistance is begun, beginning at a flow rate of about 2 l/min. In attempting to wean the patient from the heart-lung machine, it is relatively easy to determine the degree of bypass necessary to maintain a left atrial pressure of 10–50 mmHg with adequate arterial pressure. This depends on the severity of left ventricular dysfunction and in most instances is 2–3 l/min. Volume restoration during this period can be easily accomplished by attaching the arterial tubing from the heart-lung machine to the caval cannula in the right atrium. This is especially helpful during protamine infusion with its inherent vasodilatation. At the completion of the protamine infusion, the venous cannula is removed from the right atrium. A left atrial line is always utilized along with Swan-Ganz catheterization for determining cardiac outputs and right atrial pressures. After adequate hemostasis and careful treatment of the aortic infusion site to prevent unnecessary bleeding, the mediastinum is irrigated profusely with antibiotic solution. The skin is then closed with running suture to approximate the skin edges very tightly. The sternum is not closed. The inflow and outflow cannulas are brought out through the incision in the superior portion of the sternotomy incision. It is important not to have high pump flows on the left side because it is easy to overpump the right ventricle, which in almost all instances has some element of failure also. A cardiac index of 2–2.2 l/m^2 is all that is necessary at this particular time and should maintain adequate perfusion of other organ systems.

If primary right ventricular dysfunction is noted, recognized by a central venous pressure above 20 mmHg with a low left atrial pressure and low cardiac output, a right ventricular assist device (RVAD) is incorporated (Fig. 3). This right ventricular failure is usually seen in patients after mitral valve replacement or with massive right ventricular infarction. A pursestring Teflon buttressed suture is placed in the main pulmonary artery and a 22-F wirewound arterial infusion cannula is inserted during or even after cardiopulmonary bypass has been discontinued. If two right atrial cannulas are in place, one of these is disconnected from the heart-lung machine and placed in the body of the right atrium. It is usually a 32- or 34-F wirewound catheter. This is attached to the outflow tubing, and the pumphead is allowed to fill through this tubing. With complete filling, the pump is used to fill the inflow tubing and this is then attached to the arterial infusion cannula in the main pulmonary artery. Right ventricular pumping is begun at about 2 l/min. With right ventricular bypass instituted, heart-lung machine flow is gradually decreased and the patient is removed from the pump oxygenator. It is common at this time as blood is returned to the left ventricle to observe a left atrial pressure rise as there is always some degree of left ventricular failure. Therefore, it is important not to overpump the left ventricle by flowing 4 or 5 l/min with the RVAD. A flow of 2–3 l/min is frequently all that is necessary to maintain a cardiac index of 2–2.2 l/m^2. During this time, protamine is given. The second venous cannula is removed from the right atrium and the arterial infusion cannula is removed. The rubber tourniquets are secured, the tourniquet is buried in the

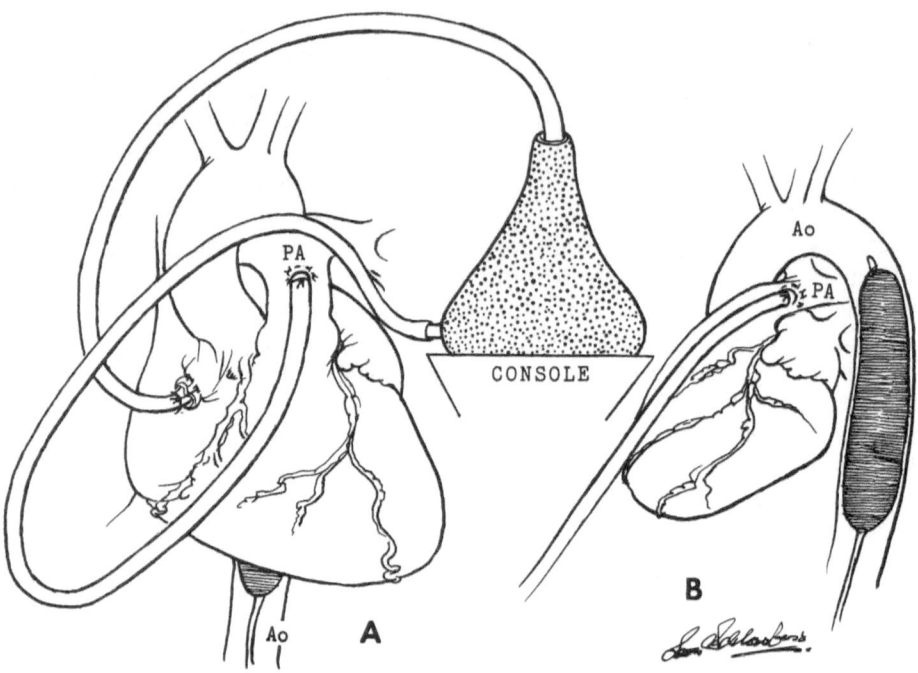

Fig. 3. Right ventricular assistance with inflow cannulas in the main pulmonary artery **A, B** IABP for the left side

mediastinum, and the cannulas are brought out through the sternotomy incision.

If biventricular failure is a problem, the patient is placed on right ventricular bypass and then left ventricular bypass with use of two Biomedicus pumps (Fig. 4). Flow with the two pumps is synchronized to maintain left and right atrial pressures of 10–15 mmHg and a cardiac index of at least 2–2.2 l/m². Literally all of these patients will have a previously placed IABP through either the femoral artery or transthoracically. This will aid even those patients with right ventricular failure. In one instance, we have used a two-stage right atrial cannula for right ventricular assistance, which we routinely do without heparinization. To our chagrin, we found upon removal that the first stage was completely thrombosed, probably secondary to stasis or low flow through the primary stage o the two-stage cannula. This did not lead to any sequelae, but because of this experience we discontinued the use of the two-stage cannula for right ventricular assistance. The cannulas are wirewound to make them more flexible so that they can be positioned and more easily moved most advantageously to the incisional site (Fig. 5). It should also be noted that the measurement of left atrial and right atrial pressure is mandatory in determining the degree of left and right ventricular failure. After closure of the skin, the patient is transferred to the intensive care unit. Volume restoration is maintained with packed red blood cells, fresh frozen plasma, and the use of platelets if hematological and coagulation profile demon-

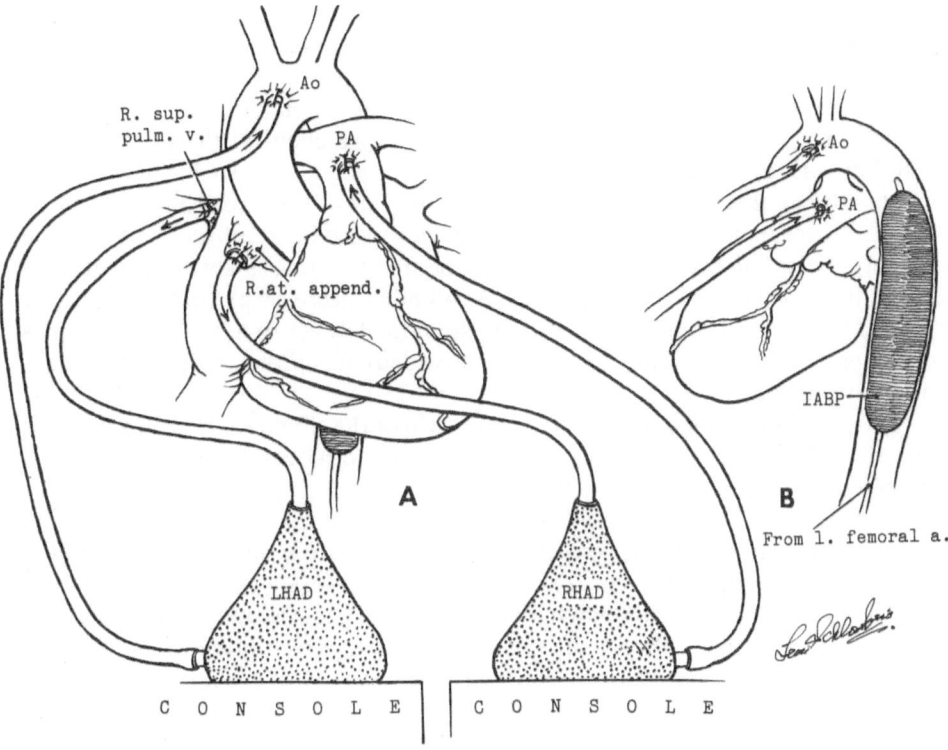

Fig. 4. Biventricular assistance requiring two pump consoles and synchrony of ventricular flows (**A**), (**B**) IABP position

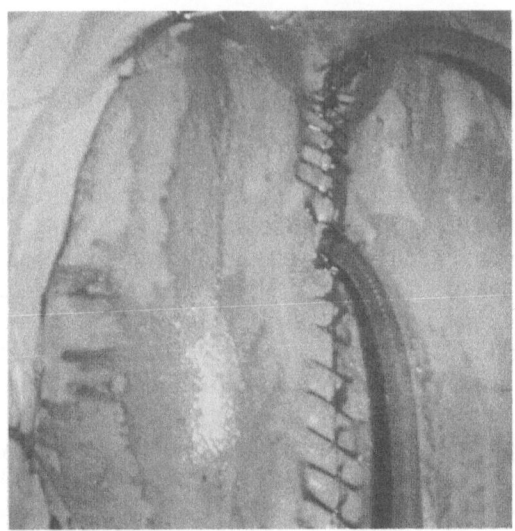

Fig. 5. Two cannulas exiting sterno-tomy wound. The arterial infusion cannulas are lying superiorly

strates the need for these blood products. Patients with RVADs are not anticoagulated whereas patients with LVADs or biventricular assistance are anticoagulated, usually beginning after 6 h or when mediastinal bleeding has slowed. We begin heparin intravenously at 100–200 units per hour, maintaining an activated clotting time of approximately 150 s. Originally, we changed the pumphead at 48 h, but with the aforementioned regime of anticoagulation we have found this unnecessary as there is usually only a small amount of thrombin on the rotor or impellers after removal of the device. The device is usually removed at 48 h at the earliest, depending on the status of the patient. Flow rate is always maintained during this period at 2 l/min or greater. At 48 h, we decrease pump flow for a few minutes to 1.5 or 1 l/min in an attempt to see good left ventricular ejection. If this is apparent and the patient can maintain an adequate cardiac index, we prepare to remove the device.

The patient is totally heparinized, after which the flow rate is reduced to 1 l/min. If cardiac output is maintained and there is no inordinate rise in the atrial pressure, the patient is prepared for surgery.

At the time of surgery, there is frequently a large amount of thrombus in the mediastinum. The thrombus is removed completely before discontinuation of the assist device. Multiple cultures are obtained.

The infusion cannula is removed and the pursestrings secured. Similar attention is directed to the outflow cannula, after which the chest tubes which had previously been placed are irrigated profusely and cleaned of old clot. During this period patients are usually stable, although frequently they require increased ionotropic support. An infusion cannula is then placed through the superior portion of the wound and brought into the mediastinum for irrigation with dilute 0.5% povidone-iodine. The sternum is then reapproximated with wire. The remaining incision is closed in anatomical fashion. The povidone-iodine irrigation is continued at 1 l/24 h for 48 h or until the mediastinal culture have proved negative. The irrigation catheter and chest tubes are then removed.

Results

In our series, six patients had placement of RVADs (Table 1). All six patients had severe myocardial dysfunction. Four of them had undergone mitral valve replacement. One underwent mitral valve replacement through the ventricle after resection of a large pseudoaneurysm and coronary bypass graft. The second patient had an acute inferior myocardial infarction with cardiogenic shock secondary to severe mitral insufficiency. The third patient developed a thrombosed mitral prosthesis while being treated for end-stage cardiomyopathy. The fourth patient had mitral valve replaement after undergoing a previous mitral commissurotomy. The left atrium was calcified and thrombosed at the time of surgery. One patient had a coronary bypass graft procedure after a recent anterior septal infarction. The sixth patient underwent closure of an acute posterior inferior ventricular septal defect. The average age of these six patients was 63 years. All patients were easily weaned from the heart-lung machine. Flow rates varied from 2 to 4.5 l/min. All patients had IABP support with two placed transthoracically. The patient with

Table 1. Right heart assistance: diagnosis and procedure

Case[a]	Age	Eject fraction	Diagnosis	Procedure	X-clamp time	Sur-vival	ECC
1	63	22	CAD, LV, aneurysm	MVR, CABG X 1, resection LV neurysmectomy	81	Yes	4'19"
2	58	25	MS	MVR, removal calcified L. atrial thrombus	89	Yes	3'22"
3	43	30	CAD	CABG X 5	68	No	3'50"
4	64	25	Thrombosed M. valve	MVR-redo	66	No	3'43"
5	72	40	Ac. VSD CAD	VSD closure	81	Yes	3'10"
6	61	35	Ac. MR/CAD	MVR	55	No	3'6"

MR, Mitral regurgitation; MVR, Mitral valve replacement; CAD, Coronery artery disease; LV, Left ventricle; VSD, Ventriculer septal defect.
[a] All patients had IABPs

coronary artery disease died 8 h after insertion of the device secondary to biventricular failure. The patient with a thrombosed mitral valve and severe cardiomyopathy died 20 days postoperatively of ventricular fibrillation. The third death occurred in the patient undergoing acute mitral valve replacement for papillary muscle rupture. She died five days postoperatively after the RVAD was removed at 48 h. The three remaining patients had the device removed at 48, 96, and 144 h and all are alive after 1 year, for a 50% salvage rate.

Twelve patients had placement of a Biomedicus LVAD (Table 2). There were four long-term survivors, for a 33% salvage rate. Five of the 12 patients had valvular replacement with or without concomitant coronary artery surgery. One patient had an acute ventricular septal defect with double coronary artery bypass operation. The remaining six patients had coronary artery bypass surgery. Two of these patients had disastrous complications. Both arrested in the catheterization laboratory and were brought to the operating room while external cardiac massage was being performed. Neither of these patients survived. Another patient with a previous history of two myocardial infarctions and associated complete heart block preoperatively had five bypass grafts. Another patient had an acute myocardial infarction with cardiogenic shock. One of four survivors in this group was a patient who had routine coronary artery bypass including bilateral mammary grafts and a saphenous vein graft. This patient, with good left ventricular function, survived after left ventricular assistance and is doing well. The second survivor with left main coronary artery disease and recent anterior myocardial infarction had placement of the LVAD for a short time intraoperatively and is currently a long-term survivor. A third survivor had a myocardial infarction 5 months preoperatively with progressive congestive heart failure and severe aortic stenosis. He underwent aortic valve replacement and double coronary artery bypass. The fourth survivor suffered completed heart block, congestive heart failure, failed balloon valvuloplasty, and an ejection fraction of 22% with a wedge

Table 2. Left heart assistance: diagnosis and procedure

Case[a]	Age	Eject fraction	Diagnosis	Procedure	X-clamp time	Sur-vival	ECC
1	53	55	CAD	CABG X 3	63	Yes	4'48"
2	59	60	MR, CAD	MVR, CABG X 1	72	No	3'56"
3	64	40	L MAIN, AC MI	CABG X 2	29	Yes	7'16"
4	59	45	AS, CAD	AVR, CABG X 2	110	Es	5'58"
5	56	30	AC MI, C shock	CABG X 2	18	No	1'30"
6	60	35	AC MI, MR S/P CABG X 3, C arrest OR	MVR-REDO CABG X 1	58	No	3'26"
7	63	35	AC MI, C shock AC VSD	VSD, CABG X 2	19	No	4'41"
8	53	32	CAD, HRT block	CABG X 5	60	No	1'51"
9	49	0	Cath. dissection L MAIN, C arrest CPR TO OR	CABG X 2	38	No	2'8"
10	50	0	Cath. dissection C arrest CPR TO OR	CABG X 1	20	No	2'34"
11	53	22	AS ht. block failed valvuloplasty	AVR	78	Yes	2'44"
12	67	50	AS AC MI arrested in OR	AVR, CABG X 2	101	No	5'11"

AC MI, Acute myocardial infarction.
[a] All patients had IABPs

Table 3. Biventricular assistance: diagnosis and procedure

Case	Age	Eject fraction	Diagnosis	Procedure	X-clamp time	Survival	ECC
1[a]	47	35	CAD	CABG X 3	40	Yes	2'25"
2	81	30	AR, TR	AVR-TVR, REDO	151	No	6'22"

AR, Aortic regurgitation; TR, Tricuspid regurgitation.
[a] IABP could not be placed

pressure of 33 torr. He underwent aortic valve replacement and is a long-term sur-vivor after left ventricular assistance. In this group of 12 patients, two were brought to the operating room dead, and two arrested during anesthestic induc-tion. Seven of the eight remaining patients had severe coronary or valvular dis-ease.

Two patients had biventricular assistance (Table 3). One had an acute inferior myocardial infarction with severe left ventricular dysfunction. She underwent triple coronary artery bypass necessitating left and right Biomedicus pump sup-port. She was discharged from the hospital doing well. The lone death from biven-tricular assistance was an 81-year-old man who had previously undergone aortic

Table 4. Results of cardiac assistance (Biomedicus pump)

No. of cases	No. removed from bypass	Survival[a]	% survival
RVAD–6	5	3	50%
LVAD–12	7	4	33%
BVAD–2	1	1	50%

[a] Survival-hospital discharge

valve replacement with complete heart block and was admitted with aortic and tricuspid insufficiency, congestive heart failure, and bacterial endocarditis. He underwent aortic and tricuspid valve replacement and insertion of a permanent pacemaker. The patient died in the early postoperative period. Therefore, one of two patients with a biventricular assist device was a long-term survivor, for a 50% salvage rate. Table 4 shows overall survival with left, right, and biventricular assistance. It may be noted that, contrary to other reports in the literature, almost all of these patients were acute or chronically ill preoperatively and considered high-risk candidates for cardiac procedures.

Discussion

Various mechanical techniques to aid and salvage the failing heart have been attempted over the years. In 1957, Stuckey and associates [17] used the heart-lung machine in selected cases of myocardial infarction. Salisbury et al. [18] in 1960, compared the effects of different types of mechanical assist device in experimental heart failure. Liotta and associates [19] reported the first clinical use of an LVAD in 1963. Litwack and associates [11] designed an LVAD consisting of a pair of cannulas, one sutured to the left atrium and another sutured to the ascending aorta, connected to a roller pump for left atrial to aortic bypass. Pennington and colleagues [20] described the utilization of a centrifugal blood pump capable of flows of 5 l/min. This, combined with intra-aortic balloon pumping, produced pulsatile perfusion. Holub et al. [21] and Norman and associates [22] described clinical work with left ventricular assistance using a pericorporeal pneumatic assist device.

In 1980, Parr and associates [23] reported the first survivor in the postcardiotomy period with right ventricular failure treated with a pneumatic assist device. This patient had a large left ventricular aneurysm extending into the right ventricle. The authors noted that this patient had an occlusion of the right coronary artery, and because of poor distal vasculature revascularization was not performed.

In 1984, Pennington and associates [24] in a review noted that 15 survivors of VAD support for postcardiotomy shock from four different centers had an excellent chance for a prolonged, high quality of life.

Kormos and associates [25] described four patients who required ventricular support with the Biomedicus centrifugal pump. One patient with right ventricular failure did well and is alive 13 months postoperatively. Three other patients had an LVAD placed. One is a long-term survivor doing well 7 months postoperatively. The other two deaths were attributed to poor left atrial drainage and/or persistent low output syndrome. Park and colleagues [26] reported their experience using the mechanical Biomedicus pump in 41 patients. The majority of these patients had coronary artery bypass alone or in combination with other procedures. Thirty-two patients were placed on LVAD, two on RVAD alone, and seven on biventricular assistance. There were ten long-term survivors in the LVAD group: a survival rate of 31%. One of two patients survived right ventricular assistance. Two of seven patients survived biventricular assistance, for a 29% salvage rate.

Dembitsky and others [16] used a centrifugal RVAD in six patients who underwent a variety of cardiac procedures. The assist period lasted from 3 to 96 h and the intra-aortic balloon was used in five of six cases. All patients initially responded to the assist device with decreased pulmonary pressures and increased contractility of the right ventricle. However, only four of the six were successfully weaned from the device, with one being a long-term survivor.

Phillips and colleagues [27] discussed the use of the Biomedicus centrifugal pump as a percutaneous device in patients suffering acute cardiac arrest who could not be resuscitated with standard methods. An oxygenator was placed in the system and bilateral femoral venous cannulation was performed along with arterial cannulation for inflow. Three of five patients survived cardiac arrest, although the authors did note that limited flow rates were obtained because of the size of the inflow and outflow cannulas.

In our series over the last 5 years, six patients had refractory right ventricular failure and were treated with right ventricular bypass utilizing the Biomedicus centrifugal pump. There were three survivors for an overall survival rate of 50%. Twelve patients had insertion of a Biomedicus LVAD. There were four long-term survivors for an overall survival of 33%. Two patients had biventricular assistance, with one long-term survivor for a survival of 50%. All of these patients were removed from the heart-lung machine with initial pump flows ranging from 2 to 4.5 l/min. In almost all instances after the institution of right or left ventricular bypass, the opposite ventricle demonstrated evidence of some ventricular impairment; thus, it is extremely important not to overpump the nonbypassed ventricle by simply maintaining a cardiac index of 2–2.2 l/m^2. Duration of bypass ranged from 8 to 192 h. The device was easily placed from the atrium to the pulmonary artery or aorta. The device is placed early before irreversible myocardial damage occurs. The sternum was not closed in any patient but in all patients the skin was reapproximated with suture to prevent infection. None of the patients with right ventricular assistance received anticoagulation, but flow rates were maintained at at least 2 l/min. Patients receiving left ventricular assistance were maintained on a heparin drip. All patients undergoing removal of the device had mediastinal irrigation with dilute povidone-iodine for 48 h. The IABP was usually removed 48 h after cardiac assistance was discontinued. The Biomedicus centrifugal blood pump is inexpensive, easy to use, and will become standard armamentarium in most hospitals dealing with critically ill patients. The Biomedicus, left, right, and biventricular assist devices may salvage 30%–50% of these previously hopeless patients.

References

1. Clauss RH, Birtwell WC, Albertal G et al. (1961) Assisted circulation 1. The arterial counterpulsation. J Thorac Surg 41:447
2. Kantrowitz A, Tjonnelarel S, Freud PS et al. (1968) Initial clinical experience with intraaortic balloon pumping in cardiogenic shock. JAMA 203:113
3. Moulopolous S, Topaz S, Kolff WJ (1962) Diastolic balloon pumping (with CO2) in the aorta: a mechanical assistance to the failing circulation. Am Heart J 63:667
4. Golding LAR (1982) Mechanical assist of the failing heart. In: Vidt DC (ed) Cardiovascular therapy. Davis, Philadelphia
5. Rose DM, Colvin SB, Culliford AT et al. (1982) Long term survivor with partial left heart bypass following perioperative myocardial infarction and shock. J Thorac Cardiovasc Surg 83:484
6. Pennington DB, Codd JE, Merjavy JP et al. (1984) The expanded use of ventricular bypass systems for severe cardiac failure as a bridge to cardiac transplantation. Heart Transplant 3:170
7. Golding LR, Jacobs G, Groves LK et al. (1982) Clinical results of mechanical support of the failing left ventricle. J Thorac Cardiovasc Surg 83:597
8. Pennock JL, Pierce WS, Wisman CB et al. (1983) Survivor and complications following ventricular assist pumping for cardiogenic shock. Ann Surg 469
9. DeBakey ME (1971) Left ventricular bypass pump for cardiac assistance. Clinical experience. Am J Cardiol 27:3
10. Spencer FR, Eiseman B, Trinkle JK, Rossi NP (1965) Assisted circulation for cardiac failure following intracardiac surgery with cardiopulmonary bypass. J Thorac Cardiovasc Surg 49:56
11. Litwak RS, Koffsky RM, Jurado RA et al. (1976) Use of a left heart assist device after intracardiac surgery. Technique and clinical experience. Ann Thorac Surg 21:191
12. Soroff HS, Birtwell WC et al. (1965) Support of systemic circulation and left ventricular assist by synchronous pulsation of extramural pressure. Surg Forum 16:184
13. Bernstein EF, Delaria GA, Johansen KH et al. (1975) Twenty four hour left ventricular bypass with centrifugal blood pump. Ann Surg 181:412
14. Bass RM, Langmore DB (1969) Cerebral damage during open heart surgery. Nature 222:30
15. Mandl JP (1977) Comparison of emboli production between a constrained vortex pump and a roller pump. Am Sect Proceedings 27
16. Dembitsky NP, Darby PO, Raney AA et al. (1986) Temporary extracorporeal support of the right ventricle. J Thorac Cardiovasc Surg 91:518
17. Stuckey JH, Vewnan MM, Dennis C et al. (1957) The use of the heart lung machine in selected cases of acute myocardial infarction. Surg Forum 8:342
18. Salisbury PE, Cross CE, Rieben PD, Lewin PJ (1960) Comparison of two types of mechanical assistance in experimental heart failure. Circ Res 8:431
19. Liotta D, Hull CW, Walter SH, Dooley DA et al. (1963) Prolonged assisted circulation during and after cardiac or aortic surgery. Prolonged partial LV bypass by means of extracorporeal circulation. Am J Cardiol 12:399
20. Pennington DG, Merjavy JP, Swartz MT, William VL (1982) Clinical experience with a centrifugal pump ventricular assist device. Trans Am Soc Artif Intern Organs 28:93
21. Holub DA, Hibbs CW, Sturm JT et al. (1979) Clinical trials of an abdominal left ventricular assist device: progress report. Trans Am Soc Artif Intern Organs 25:197
22. Norman JC (1981) The role of assist devices in managing low cardiac output. Cardiovasc Dis Bull Texas Heart Inst 8:19

23. Parr GVS, Pierce WS, Rosenberg G, Waldhause JA (1980) Survival of right ventricular fail-
    ure after repair of left ventricular aneurysm. J Thorac Cardiovasc Surg 80:79
24. Pennington DG, Swartz MT, William VL (in press) Clinical experience with temporary non-
    pulsatile ventricular assist systems. The centrifugal pump for ventricular assist. First Inter-
    national symposium current problems for further development on artificial heart and assist
    devices. Trans Am Soc Artif Intern Organs (in press)
25. Kormos RL, Scully HE, Goldman BS et al. (in press) Clinical use of a centrifugal pump for
    circulatory support following cardiac surgery (in press)
26. Park SB, Liebler SA, Magovern GJ et al. (1986) Mechanical support of the failing heart. Ann
    Thorac Surg 42:627
27. Phillips SJ, Ballantine B, Slonine D (1983) Percutaneous initiation of cardiopulmonary by-
    pass. Ann Thorac Surg 36:223

15. Technique and Results with a Roller Pump for Ventricular Assistance

D. M. ROSE, M. CONNOLLY, J. N. CUNNINGHAM JR., and F. C. SPENCER

Introduction

Although it is relatively infrequent for the utilization of ventricular assist devices (VADs) to be required for profound heart failure following cardiac surgical procedures, there have been a number of reports of increasing success with the use of these devices [1–6]. Furthermore, the role of VADs has expanded with their utilization as a bridge to transplantation [7, 8] and as a support device for patients with cardiogenic shock following myocardial infarction [9]. A variety of devices for ventricular assistance have been employed. We have used a roller pump driven device since 1978, and this system is relatively effective, easy to use, and inexpensive. This report summarizes our experience with the use of a roller pump left ventricular assist device (LVAD) and right ventricular assist device (RVAD) and also a newly developed percutaneously inserted LVAD.

Materials and Methods

Since January 1978 at New York University Medical Center, New York, NY, July 1982 at Maimonides Medical Center, Brooklyn, NY, and January 1986 at the State University Hospital, Health Science Center at Brooklyn, Brooklyn, NY, we have utilized an LVAD in 72 patients and an RVAD in seven patients following cardiac surgical procedures. In addition, a percutaneously inserted LVAD has been used in five patients with profound cardiogenic shock following acute myocardial infarction.

Technique of Insertion

Left Ventricular Assist Device
A 28- to 32-F venous cannula is inserted through a pursestring suture into the left atrium, either through the left atrial appendage or through the right superior pulmonary vein. A 5- to 6-mm arterial cannula is inserted through a pursestring suture into the ascending aorta (Fig. 1). The tip is advanced beyond the left subclavian artery in order to decrease the potential for cerebral embolization. Cannulas exit through the sternotomy or through separate parasternal incisions (Fig. 2). The cannulas are connected to 3/8 × 1/16 in. silicone tubing (Dow Corning, Midland, Michigan), which is connected to a portable roller pump (Fig. 3).

Assisted Circulation 3
F. Unger (Ed.)
© Springer-Verlag Berlin Heidelberg 1989

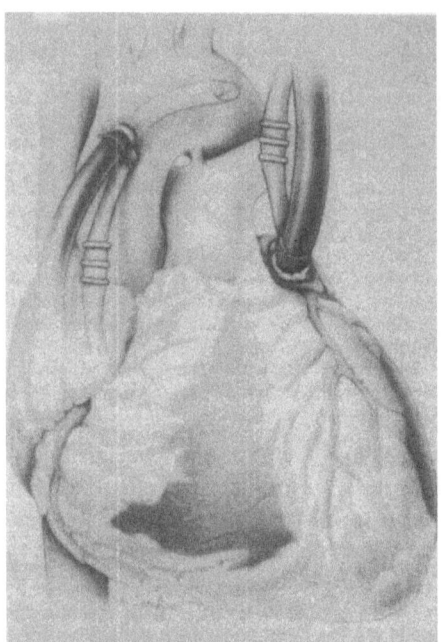

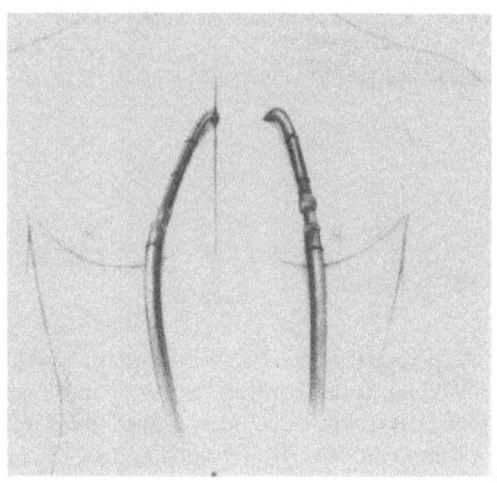

Fig. 1. Intracardiac location of aortic and left atrial cannulas

Fig. 2. Position of cannulas as they exit the sternum

With this device, maximal flow rates of 3.5–4 l/min can be attained. After insertion of the LVAD flow rates of 2–4 l/min are provided in order to maintain adequate systemic perfusion and discontinue cardiopulmonary bypass. Left atrial pressure is maintained between 5 and 12 mmHg, inotropic agents are used to augment right heart function, and an intra-aortic balloon is used to provide counterpulsation.

When closing the chest, it is critically important to avoid cardiac compression, and to open the pericardium widely. In some patients, the sternum may not be closed without compressing the heart, and in these patients it is necessary to leave the sternum open and only close the skin. In some patients it may not be possible to close the skin, and synthetic material may be used to cover the sternal defect.

The patient's heart rate, central venous pressure, pulmonary artery pressure, left atrial pressure, and systemic pressures are all continuously monitored. Cardiac output is determined with a balloon-tipped thermodilution pulmonary artery catheter.

If postoperative bleeding is not great, patients are partially heparinized (250–750 units/h), 4–6 h following surgery. The activated clotting time (ACT) is maintained between 150 and 250 s with this regimen.

Right Ventricular Assist Device
The technique for insertion of the RVAD is similar to that of the LVAD. A 28- to 32-F venous cannula is inserted into the right atrium through a pursestring suture. A small arterial cannula is inserted into the main pulmonary artery through

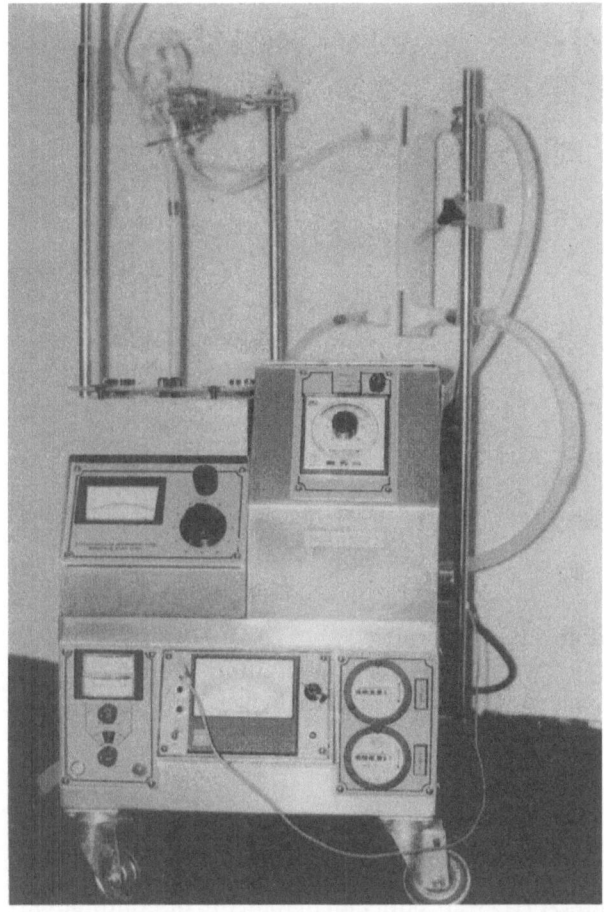

Fig. 3. Portable roller pump
that is employed for ventricular
assistance

a pursestring suture. Cannulas are connected to the Silastic tubing, which is then
connected to a portable roller pump.

Flow rates of 2.5–4 l/min are employed. Similar precautions concerning pericardial constriction and sternal compression are observed. Patients are generally
placed on pulmonary artery vasodilators and inotropic agents to enhance myocardial function. Vasoconstrictors can be infused through a left atrial line. Patients are heparinized in a fashion similar to that used with the LVAD.

Percutaneous Left Ventricular Assist Device
In five patients with profound left ventricular failure following acute myocardial
infarction, refractory to intensive medical therapy, a percutaneous LVAD has
been inserted. A specially designed venous cannula (Fig. 4) (Electrocatheter
Corp., Rahway, NJ) can be introduced through the femoral vein and passed
fluoroscopically over a guide wire into the right atrium and then via a transseptal
route, can be introduced into the left atrium. Blood can be returned to the patient

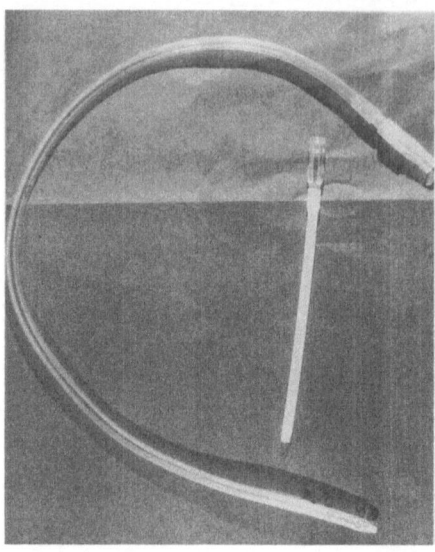

Fig. 4. Percutaneous femoral arterial and left atrial cannulas

with another cannula inserted into the femoral artery (Fig. 4). Flow rates of 1.5–3 l/min can generally be achieved with this system. In addition, inotropic agents and coronary vasodilators are given to the patient. Patients are systemically heparinized as previously described.

Indications (Table 1)

Left Ventricular Assist Device

Indications for utilization of an LVAD were either an inability to discontinue cardiopulmonary bypass (57 patients), or cardiac arrest 1–12 h postoperatively (15 patients). About one-fourth of patients (15 of 57) who could not initially be weaned from cardiopulmonary bypass sustained a pre-bypass cardiac arrest either during cardiac catheterization, attempted percutaneous transluminal coronary angioplasty (PTCA), or anesthetic induction. Standard techniques were em-

Table 1. Indications for insertion of VAD

	LVAD (open)		RVAD	Per-cutaneous
	Nonsurvivors	Survivors		
Inability to discontinue CPB	35	22	5	
Preop. cardiac arrest	11	8	1	2
Postop. cardiac arrest	7	8	1	
Cardiogenic shock following acute MI			1	5

CPB, cardiopulmonary bypass

ployed in attempting to discontinue cardiopulmonary bypass in these patients. These included volume loading, atrial-ventricular pacing infusion of inotropic agents, and insertion of an intra-aortic balloon. All patients demonstrated severe left heart failure with an elevated left atrial pressure (>25 mmHg) and systemic hypotension (mean blood pressure <50 mmHg), and cardiopulmonary bypass could not be discontinued without the use of an LVAD.

Fifteen patients sustained a postoperative cardiac arrest as a result of graft spasm (six patients), refractory arrhythmias (six patients), or acute graft thrombosis (three patients). These patients required reinstitution of cardiopulmonary bypass in order to be resuscitated and insertion of an LVAD to be weaned from cardiopulmonary bypass.

Right Ventricular Assist Device

In patients with isolated right heart failure [usually manifested by an elevated central venous pressure (>20 mmHg), a low left atrial pressure (<8 mmHg), systemic hypotension (systolic blood pressure <70 mmHg), a low cardiac index (<1.5 l/min/m^2), and an elevated pulmonary vascular resistance], a trial of inotropic agents, pulmonary vasodilators, and systemic vasoconstrictors infused directly into the left atrium was usually attempted. In most patients an intra-aortic balloon was also inserted. In five of the seven patients, cardiopulmonary bypass could not be discontinued without the use of right heart bypass. In one other patient, acute right coronary graft thrombosis occurred 6 h postoperatively, and following graft revision the patient had an RVAD inserted. One other patient with a large inferior wall myocardial infarction arrested during cardiac catheterization. This patient was placed on cardiopulmonary bypass and an RVAD was inserted.

Percutaneous Left Ventricular Assist Device

All patients in whom a percutaneous LVAD was inserted were in profound cardiogenic shock following acute myocardial infarction. They had all been given a trial of intensive medical therapy including coronary vasodilators, inotropic agents, and intra-aortic balloon counterpulsation. Three of five patients had a cardiac arrest in the cardiac cath lab and could be successfully resuscitated only after insertion of the LVAD. All patients had attempted PTCA and this was successful in four of them.

Preoperative Clinical Characteristics and Operations Performed (Table 2)

There were no major differences in the clinical characteristics of nonsurviving and surviving patients in whom an LVAD was inserted following cardiac surgery. The types of operations performed were also similar in both groups of patients, as was the period of aortic occlusion.

It has generally been our impression in the last few years that more of the patients who require a VAD postoperatively have come to the operating room in profound cardiogenic shock (failed PTCA, left main coronary artery dissection, evolving myocardial infarction, ruptured ventricular septum, ruptured papillary muscle, etc.).

Table 2. Clinical characteristics of patients with VADs

	LVAD		RVAD	Per-cutaneous LVAD
	Nonsurvivors	Survivors		
Age	60.1 ±2.0	59.8 ±2.3	63.4±3.1	69.7±4.1
Preop CI (l/min/m²)	2.17±0.1	2.34±0.10	2.2±0.1	1.3±0.1
EF (%)	40.7 ±2.5	44.4 ±2.6	38.5 ±5.2	–
Operation	31 CAB	24 CAB	3 CAB	–
	5 AVR	3 AVR+CAB	2 CAB+closure VSD +LV aneurysm	–
	3 CAB+LV aneurysm +closure of VSD	2 CAB+LV aneurysm +closure of VSD	1 MVR+CAB	
	3 MVR+CAB	1 MVR+CAB	1 acute RV infarction	–
AXC (min)	66.7± 8.1	73.6± 9.6	52.3± 9.5	–
CBP (min)	236.1±22.8	228.1±28.1	14.5±30.6	–
VAD (h)	36.4± 6.1	44.1± 4.6	68.3±10.1	24±16.5

CI, cardiac index; EF, ejection fraction; AXC, aortic cross-clamp time; CPB, cardiopulmonary bypass; VAD, ventricular assist device; CAB, coronary artery bypass; AVR, aortic valve replacement; LV, left ventricle; VSD, ventricular septal defect; MVR, mitral valve replacement; RV, right ventricle.

Table 3. Clinical experience with roller pump VADs

	Total patients	Early survivors	Late survivors
LVAD (open)	72	30 (41.7%)	21 (29.2%)
RVAD (open)	7	2 (28.6%)	0
LVAD (closed)	5	0	0

Results (Table 3)

Left Ventricular Assist Device

Thirty patients (41.7%) were weaned from the LVAD 24–96 h following insertion (Fig. 5). These patients had gradual recovery of their left heart function, allowing gradual discontinuation of the left heart bypass. Causes of death in the 42 non-

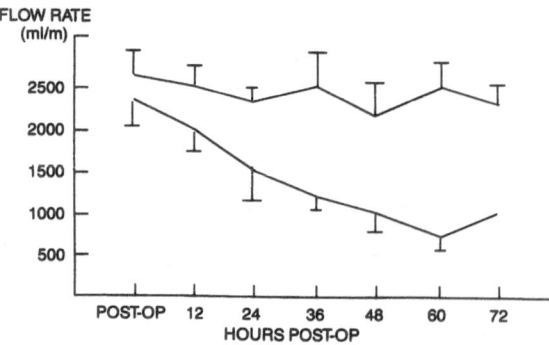

Fig. 5. Flow rates of nonsurviving (*upper line*) and surviving (*lower line*) patients. Note that there is improvement of ventricular function in many patients as early as 12 h postoperatively

Table 4. Status of patients weaned from LVAD

Early deaths (21–90 days), $n=9$	Pulmonary emboli: Sepsis (pulmonary, pancreatic, colon, renal):	2 patients 7 patients
Late deaths (4 months, 4 years), $n=2$	Sudden "cardiac" death	
Long-term survivors, $n=19$	11 patients NYHA I 7 patients NYHA II 2 patients NYHA III	

surviving patients included severe coagulopathy, refractory arrhythmias, biventricular failure, and massive neurological injury. Often a combination of these factors was present, contributing to the demise of the patients.

Nine patients died 21–90 days postoperatively: seven as a result of sepsis and multisystem failure and two from pulmonary embolism. Of the 21 long-term survivors, there were two late deaths, 4 months and 4 years postoperatively, both from cardiac causes. In the 19 long-term survivors, 11 patients are New York Heart Association class I, seven patients New York Heart Association class II, and two patients New York Heart Association class III (Table 4). No preoperative or intraoperative patient factors appear to be predictive of patient survival.

Right Ventricular Assist Device
Two patients were weaned from the RVAD 48 and 72 h following insertion. One patient expired 5 days postoperatively from multisystem failure and sepsis and one patient expired 10 days postoperatively from pneumonia. Of the five patients who could not be weaned, three had profound coagulopathy, one had severe hypoxemia and "shock lung," and one had a massive neurological injury and the RVAD was discontinued. Two of these nonsurviving patients had premature discontinuation of the RVAD: shortly following removal of the device they had a rapid return of right heart failure and the device had to be reinserted. Both of these patients developed profound coagulopathy and expired 72 and 96 h postoperatively.

Percutaneous Left Ventricular Assist Device
No patient could be weaned from the percutaneous LVAD although four patients did have successful PTCA. Two patients expired from refractory ventricular fibrillation (2 and 4 h following insertion). One patient had a massive air embolus from the pump 6 h following insertion (the only patient in the entire series in whom this occurred). Two patients expired from progressive biventricular failure at 48 and 72 h.

Discussion

Left Ventricular Assist Device
Certainly, many factors can produce profound postoperative cardiac failure, including previous myocardial infarction with depressed ventricular dysfunction,

active ongoing ischemia or infarction, inadequate myocardial protection, and incomplete myocardial revascularization [10–12]. Additionally, coronary artery vasospasm either in the native coronary artery, vein graft, or internal mammary artery can produce significant myocardial failure and arrhythmias [13, 14].

It has been suggested that during the initial reperfusion period an oxygen supply and demand imbalance exists, and despite adequate reperfusion there may be cellular and metabolic abnormalities that could impair ventricular function [15, 16]. This would cause the myocardium to act as if it had been "stunned," as has been suggested by Braunwald and Klouer [17]. As these investigators have shown, acute coronary artery occlusion for only 15 min can result in functional and metabolic abnormalities for as long as 7 days [16]. Thus, despite adequate revascularization, some patients may have persistent cardiac failure as a result of the myocardium being stunned.

Previous experimental studies indicate that left ventricular bypass and left atrial bypass can both effectively unload the left ventricle and can arrest infarct expansion [9, 18, 19]. Thus, marginally perfused ischemic tissue with could ultimately infarct may be salvaged with the utilization of left heart bypass. Obviously, a critical determinant of ultimate survival is the extent of irreversibly infarcted tissue as compared to the amount of reversibly injured ischemic tissue, and this ratio may be favorably affected with the use of left heart bypass.

It is not clear what is the optimal or necessary period of time left heart support should be provided. The device we have employed is not capable of providing flow rates as high as the device employed by Pierce and associates [2]. With the device we have utilized, surviving patients will demonstrate evidence of left ventricular recovery as early as 12 h postoperatively, and most surviving patients will show improvement in left ventricular function within 48 h postoperatively [1, 9] (Fig. 5).

We have been reluctant to maintain flow rates in excess of 3 l/min for prolonged periods in our patients, since we felt that this could produce significant hemolysis and destruction of blood elements. However, if larger arterial and venous cannulas were inserted, this most likely would not occur. The Hershey group [2] has supported patients with their LVAD for as long as 25 days (mean 6.8 days). Thus, the optimal period of left heart support varies considerably with the type of assist device employed. The device that Pierce and co-workers have utilized is capable of providing flow rates of up to 6.5 l/min. Therefore, it seems that with more complete left heart bypass, patients can be successfully supported for longer periods.

Right Ventricular Assist Device

The causes of right heart failure can be similar to those of left heart failure (active ongoing ischemia or infarction, inadequate myocardial protection, incomplete revascularization, vasospasm, etc.) [20–22]. In addition, right heart failure can be exacerbated or caused by increased pulmonary vascular resistance [23]. Often a combination of these factors (right heart ischemia and elevated pulmonary vascular resistance) will be present. While we personally have not had any experience with pulmonary artery balloon counterpulsation, there have been some encouraging results with this modality [24, 25].

The effects of right heart bypass on pulmonary microcirculation and lung water formation have not been clearly elucidated experimentally. There are some recent experimental data which suggest that right heart bypass may have a deleterious effect on pulmonary function [26]. Thus, this support device may, in some instances, create further pulmonary injury and elevate pulmonary vascular resistance, further impairing right heart function.

It is evident from experimental and clinical data that the right heart can often recover sufficiently to permit removal of the support device [2, 20, 21]. However, we have observed, quite dramatically, an insidious return of profound right heart failure and cardiac arrest, in two patients in whom there was premature discontinuation of the RVAD. The recurrence of right heart failure may be a result of an increase in pulmonary vascular resistance that has gone undetected.

Clearly, in many patients there is evidence of biventricular failure [5]; however, there is often a predominance of one chamber failure and thus either an RVAD or an LVAD can be successfully employed. Our experience with biventricular assistance is minimal, although it does seem from the experience of others that patients with severe biventricular failure will generally go on to cardiac transplantation if they are suitable candidates [2, 8].

Percutaneous Left Ventricular Assist Device
Finally, although the results with the percutaneous LVAD have been poor, we feel that such devices are still in the early phases of development. All of the patients in whom the device was employed were extremely ill, either in profound cardiogenic shock or having an active cardiac arrest. Hopefully, as we gain further experience and expertise, this modality will become a useful adjunct in patients with acute evolving myocardial infarction and potentially reversible left ventricular dysfunction.

Conclusion

In summary, reasonably good results can be achieved with a roller pump type of VAD. Further experience obviously needs to be obtained in treating patients with acute evolving myocardial infarction. For the VADs to gain widespread use, refinement of all existing devices will be necessary, making them less complicated and more economical, and enhancing patient survival.

References

1. Rose DM, Laschinger J, Grossi E et al. (1985) Experimental and clinical results with a simplified left heart assist device for treatment of profound left ventricular dysfunction. World J Surg 9:11
2. Pae WE, Pierce WS, Pennock JL et al. (1987) Long-term results of ventricular assist pumping in postcardiotomy cardiogenic shock. J Thorac Cardiovasc Surg 93:434
3. Pennington DG, Bernhard WF, Golding LR et al. (1985) Long-term follow-up of postcardiotomy patients with profound cardiogenic shock treated with ventricular assist device. Circulation 72:206

 4. Park SB, Liebler GA, Burkholder JA et al. (1986) Mechanical support of the failing heart. Ann Thorac Surg 42:627
 5. Pennington DG, Merjavy JP, Swartz MT et al. (1985) The importance of biventricular failure in patients with postoperative cardiogenic shock. Ann Thorac Surg 39:16
 6. Zumbro GL, Kitchens WR, Shearer G et al. (1987) Mechanical assistance for cardiogenic shock following cardiac surgery, myocardial infarction, and cardiac transplantation. Ann Thorac Surg 44:11
 7. Hill JD, Farrar DJ, Hershon JJ et al. (1986) Use of a prosthetic ventricle as a bridge to cardiac transplantation for postinfarction cardiogenic shock. N Engl J Med 314:626
 8. Pennock JL, Pierce WS, Campbell DB et al. (1986) Mechanical support of the circulation followed by cardiac transplantation. J Thorac Cardiovasc Surg 92:994
 9. Rose DM, Grossi E, Laschinger J et al. (1986) Strategy for treatment of acute evolving myocardial infarction with pulsatile left heart assist device. Can this modality increase survival and enhance myocardial salvage? In: Bregman D (ed) Critical care clinics, new techniques in mechanical support, vol 2. Saunders, Philadelphia, p 251
10. Buda AJ, MacDonald IL, Anderson MJ et al. (1981) Long-term results following coronary bypass operation. Importance of preoperative factors and complete revascularization. J Thorac Cardiovasc Surg 82:383
11. Hilton CJ, Beubl W, Acker M, Levinson HJ, Millard RW, Riddle R, McEnany MT (1979) Inadequate cardioplegic protection with obstructed coronary arteries. Ann Thorac Surg 28:323
12. Kennedy JW, Kaiser GL, Fisher LD et al. (1981) Clinical and angiographic predictors of operative mortality from the collaborative study in coronary artery surgery (CASS). Circulation 63:793
13. Buxton AE, Goldberg S, Harken A et al. (1981) Coronary artery spasm immediately after myocardial revascularization. Recognition and management. N Engl J Med 304:1249
14. Lockerman ZS, Rose DM, Cunningham JN et al. (1987) Reperfusion ventricular fibrillation during coronary artery bypass surgery and its association with postoperative enzyme release. J Thorac Cardiovasc Surg 93:247
15. Kloner RA, Ellis ST, Lange R et al. (1983) Studies of experimental coronary artery reperfusion: effects on infarct size, myocardial function, biochemistry, ultrastructure and microvasculature damage. Circulation 68 [Suppl I]:I-8
16. Ellis SB, Henschke CI, Sandor T et al. (1983) Time course of functional and biochemical recovery of myocardium salvaged by reperfusion. J Am Coll Cardiol 11:1047
17. Braunwald E, Klouer RA (1982) The stunned myocardium – prolonged, postischemic ventricular dysfunction (Editorial). Circulation 66:1146
18. Pennock JL, Pae WE, Pierce WS et al. (1979) Reduction of myocardial infarct size. Comparison between left atrial and left ventricular bypass. Circulation 59:275
19. Grossi EA, Laschinger JC, Cunningham JN et al. (1984) Time course in myocardial salvage with left heart assist in evolving myocardial infarction. Surg Forum 35:322
20. Dembitsky WP, Daily PO, Raney AA et al. (1986) Temporary extracorporeal support of the right ventricle. J Thorac Cardiovasc Surg 91:518
21. O'Neill MJ, Pierce WS, Wisman CB et al. (1984) Successful management of right ventricular failure with the ventricular assist pump following aortic valve replacement and coronary bypass grafting. J Thorac Cardiovasc Surg 87:106
22. Cohn JN (1979) Right ventricular infarction revisited. Am J Cardiol 43:666
23. Vlahades GJ, Turley K, Hoffman JIE (1981) The pathophysiology of failure in acute right ventricular hypertension. Hemodynamic and biochemical correlations. Circulation 63:87
24. Spence PA, Weisel RD, Easdown J et al. (1985) The hemodynamic effects and mechanism of action of pulmonary artery balloon counterpulsation in the treatment of right ventricular failure during left heart bypass. Ann Thorac Surg 39:329
25. Symbas PN, McKeown PP, Santora AH et al. (1985) Pulmonary artery balloon counterpulsation for treatment of intraoperative right ventricular failure. Ann Thorac Surg 39:437
26. Toporoff B, Marini C, Grubbs PE et al. Improvement of left ventricular compliance utilizing a right ventricular assist device in sepsis induced acute respiratory distress syndrome (ARDS). Surg Forum

16. Clinical Experience
with the Thoratec Ventricular Assist Device

J. H. Lawson and G. Cederwall

Clinical experience with the Thoratec ventricular assist device has been wide-spread, with cases in 38 hospitals in nine countries in Europe, Asia, and North America. A summary of that clinical experience in the last 7 years, March 1981 through February 1988, is presented below.

The Thoratec System

The Thoratec ventricular assist system consists of the Pierce/Donachy prosthetic ventricle and the Thoratec dual drive console. The Pierce/Donachy prosthetic ventricle was developed at the Hershey Medical Center of Pennsylvania State University and was first used clinically by Dr. Pierce during the late 1970s [1, 2]. The prosthetic ventricle is a sac-type pneumatically actuated blood pump made from either a segmented polyurethane (Biomer, Ethicon, Somerville, N.J.) in the P/D 1 model or from a copolymer blend (BPS-215M, Thoratec, Berkeley, California) in the P/D 2 model [3]. The paracorporeal prosthetic ventricle receives blood from the patient's left or right atrium via a 51-F cannula and returns the blood to the ascending aorta or pulmonary artery through a low porosity woven polyester graft. Direct cannulation of the left ventricular apex can be used in place of left atrial cannulation when the intention is to proceed to cardiac transplantation. The blood pump has been described in several articles [1–5].

The Thoratec dual driver provides pneumatic actuation for either one or two prosthetic ventricles in several modes of operation. There is an asynchronous mode which pumps at a predetermined fixed rate with a variable stroke volume and an EKG synchronous mode which allows counterpulsation. But the most frequently employed mode of operation is referred to as the volume or full-to-empty mode, which provides a fixed stroke volume with a variable rate that responds to the patients' physiological condition on a beat-to-beat basis [6].

Patients

The Thoratec system is used for temporary circulatory support of patients in acute cardiac failure pending recovery of the natural heart or as a bridge to cardiac transplantation. These two categories will be referred to as "recovery" and "bridge" patients respectively.

Assisted Circulation 3
F. Unger (Ed.)
© Springer-Verlag Berlin Heidelberg 1989

Table 1. Patient profile

	Average	Maximum	Minimum
Age (years)	49	77	13
Body surface area (m^2)	1.87	2.75	1.25
Weight (kg)	76	144	36
Period of support (days)	5.5	74.0	0.1

Table 2. Average values by patient group

	Combined	Recovery	Bridge
Age (years)	49	54	42
Body surface area (m^2)	1.87	1.90	1.84
Weight (kg)	76	79	72
Period of support (days)	5.5	3.5	8.4

The system is generally used when acute cardiac failure, defined as a cardiac index of less than 1.8 l/min/m^2 with a systolic pressure of less than 90 mmHg and an atrial pressure of more than 20 mmHg, cannot be corrected with appropriate drugs or an intra-aortic balloon.

Different clinical investigators have developed variations in the operative and postoperative procedures to treat specific anatomical and pathological conditions. These procedures have been described in the literature [2, 7–10].

The Thoratec system has been used to treat left ventricular failure, right ventricular failure, and biventricular failure. In a few cases, the system has been used in combination with other circulatory support devices, such as centrifugal pumps or intra-aortic balloon.

A total of 164 patients have been treated with the Thoratec system in the last 7 years. There have been 123 males and 41 females. Characteristics of this group of patients are listed in Tables 1 and 2.

Results

Of the 164 patients, 59, or 36%, are either convalescing in hospital or have been discharged alive. This figure can be somewhat misleading because it includes two distinctly different groups of patients with two different results. In the bridge group of patients, the long-term results are much more favorable than in the recovery group.

The Thoratec system has supported 96 recovery patients, of whom 77 (80%) have been patients who could not otherwise be weaned from cardipulmonary bypass after an open-heart operation. The remaining patients were treated for acute cardiac failure due to cardiomyopathies, myocardial infarctions, or posttrans-

Table 3. Mortality results, recovery group

	Alive	Dead	Total	% alive
Wean from CPB	14	63	77	18%
Cardiomyopathy	1	5	6	17%
Postinfarction	1	5	6	17%
Posttransplant	0	7	7	0%
Total	16	80	96	17%

Table 4. Mortality by age in the recovery group

Age in years	Survivors	Total patients	% survivors
Less than 30	2	5	40%
30–50	8	26	31%
More than 50	6	62	10%

Table 5. Type of ventricular functional replacement

	Left	Right	Both	Mixed	Total
Recovery patients	48 (50%)	15 (16%)	25 (26%)	8 (8%)	96
Survivors	8	4	4	0	16
Bridge patients	12 (18%)	0	49 (72%)	7 (10%)	68
Survivors	9	0	33	1	43
Total patients	60 (37%)	15 (9%)	74 (45%)	15 (9%)	164

plant failure. Mortality results for each indication are presented in Table 3. Table 4 shows mortality by age in the recovery group.

The causes of death have not been reported or reliably determined in all cases in this patient group but most frequently cited have been multiorgan failure (57%), bleeding, both surgical and coagulopathies (22%), sepsis (8%), thrombosis and thromboembolus (3%), and other miscellaneous causes (11%). There have been no deaths reported as a result of device failure.

The Thoratec system can replace the function of the left, right, or both ventricles of patients in acute heart failure. In addition, some patients have had the Thoratec system for one ventricle while the other ventricle has been supported with another device (a mixed system). The type of support for each patient category is shown in Table 5.

In an attempt to save the lives of potential cardiac transplant recipients who suffer cardiac failure before a suitable donor heart can be found, the Thoratec system has been used to support or bridge the patients until they can be transplanted. The results in this group of patients are presented in Table 6.

The proliferation of cardiac transplant programs in the United States and the rapid growth of transplant cases has made it very difficult to find sufficient heart

Table 6. Results of bridge to cardiac transplantation

Patients implanted as a bridge	68
Patients who died without transplantation	15 (22%)
Patients currently awaiting transplantation	3
Transplanted patients	50
Patients who died after transplantation	10 (20%)
Patients convalescing or discharged alive	40 (80%)

Table 7. Bridge patients by diagnostic group

Diagnosis	Implanted	Awaiting donor	Transplanted	Alive
Post-MI shock	23	0	17	17
Ischemic CM	14	1	11	8
Viral CM	3	0	3	2
Postpartum CM	3	1	1	1
Idiopathic CM	23	1	16	13
Posttransplant	2	0	2	2
Total	68	3	50	43

MI, myocardial infarction; CM, cardiomyopathy.

donors. One result of this problem is that the period of circulatory support for bridge to transplant patients has been lengthening. The Thoratec system was meant to support patients for about 2 weeks, but many cases have gone much longer, with one patient successfully transplanted after 74 days of biventricular support. There have been seven cases with more than 3 weeks of circulatory support.

The bridge group is almost evenly divided between ischemic and nonischemic heart disease patients. The diagnostic groups for these patients are shown in Table 7.

Discussion

The Thoratec system using the Pierce/Donachy blood pump has been widely employed for short-term circulatory support in patients with acute heart failure during the last 7 years. That experience has shown that the system is capable of restoring nearly normal hemodynamic conditions in patients in cardiogenic shock [4, 5, 7–10]. However, restoration of normal hemodynamics does not insure a successful outcome. While the long-term results in the bridge group of patients have been excellent, the results in the recovery group have been less satisfactory.

If we look at the patient profile for each of these groups, we see that there are two areas of significant difference between the two groups of patients, age and period of support (Table 2). Age is a factor in selecting potential transplant candidates and it is assumed that younger age should be associated with increased survival. The recommended age limit for recovery patients is 65 years. If we look at the mortality rates for various age groups (Table 4), we can see that this recommendation is valid. There have been 16 patients 65 years of age or older in this group, with no long-term survivors, though Dr. Pae and his colleagues have reported the long-term survival of a 69-year-old patient after 6.4 days circulatory support with a Pierce/Donachy pump [11].

In examining the data on mortality in the recovery group, there is one factor which stands out above all others. Of the 16 long-term survivors in this group, 14 of them were patients in three hospitals. At those three hospitals, there were 14 survivors out of 42 patients (33%), figures which are quite similar to the results achieved by Dr. Pierce and his colleagues in Hershey [11], while at the 15 other hospitals, there were only 2 survivors out of 54 patients (3.5%). It would be difficult to justify the use of such devices in the recovery group based on a 3.5% long-term survival rate, but the results in Hershey and the first group of hospitals show that there is a role for devices in the treatment of postcardiotomy cardiogenic shock.

A possible answer for the excellent results at the first three hospitals is experience, perhaps coupled with confidence in the system, which leads the surgeons to earlier and more efficacious use of it. The system is used as a last resort in every case, but the decision to use the system must be made as early as possible in the patient's course. The most often mentioned cause of death among patients in the recovery category was multiorgan failure. We believe that multiorgan failure is often a sign that intervention with a circulatory support device was instituted too late in the patient's course, when cardiogenic shock had become irreversible.

The experience of the clinical investigator does not appear to play such an important role in the bridge group. Nineteen hospitals have had at least one patient in the bridge category and there is at least one survivor in all but two of those hospitals. In 12 hospitals, the first bridge to transplant patient was a long-term survivor. In contrast, the first recovery patient has died at every one of the 18 hospitals where that procedure has been attempted.

Since the implantation procedure is the same for recovery and bridge patients, as is postoperative care, and since the two groups of patients are often treated by the same team at the same institution, it seems that patient selection is the critical element in determining a successful outcome in the recovery group.

There have been only five patients in the recovery group treated for postinfarction cardiogenic shock, with one survivor – too few to draw any conclusions about the efficacy of this treatment, but because of the large numbers of postinfarction cardiogenic shock patients this remains an important area for investigation.

Long-term survival in the bridge group of patients (Table 6) is equivalent to long-term survival in patients who have received a cardiac transplant without having undergone periods of support with a device [10], a strong indication that functional replacement of one or two ventricles as a bridge to cardiac transplantation is a viable alternative for patients in acute cardiac failure who qualify for cardiac transplantation.

In summary, there is now a significant body of clinical experience with the Thoratec ventricular assist system. This experience has shown that the system can replace the function of either or both ventricles of the heart for periods of up to 2 months. There are questions remaining in the use of such a system when the intention is to salvage the natural heart. There is some evidence that the system is useful for this purpose but patient selection and the timing of intervention must be carefully evaluated. Results of bridge to cardiac transplantation have been outstanding and there is clearly a role for such a device in any cardiac transplantation program.

References

1. Olsen EK, Pierce WS, Donachy JH et al. (1979) A two and one half year clinical experience with a mechanical left ventricular assist pump in the treatment of profound postoperative heart failure. Int J Artif Organs 2:197–206
2. Pierce WS, Parr GVS, Myers JL et al. (1981) Ventricular-assist pumping in patients with cardiogenic shock after cardiac operations. N Engl J Med 305:1606–1610
3. Farrar DJ, Litwak P, Lawson JH et al. (1988) Invivo evaluations of a new thromboresistant polyurethane for artificial heart blood pumps. J Thorac Cardiovasc Surg 95:191–200
4. Pennington DG, Samuels LD, Williams G et al. (1985) Experience with the Pierce-Donachy ventricular assist device in postcardiotomy patients with cardiogenic shock. World J Surg 9:37–46
5. Pennington DG, Merjavy JP, Swartz MT et al. (1985) The importance of biventricular failure in patients with postoperative cardiogenic shock. Ann Thorac Surg 39:17–24
6. Farrar DJ, Compton PG, Lawson JH et al. (1986) Control modes of a clinical ventricular assist device. IEEE Eng Med Biol
7. Hill JD, Farrar DJ, Hershon JJ et al. (1986) Use of a prosthetic ventricle as a bridge to cardiac transplantation for postinfarction cardiogenic shock. N Engl J Med 314:626–628
8. Carpentier A, Brugger JP, Berthier B et al. (1986) Heterotopic artificial heart as bridge to cardiac transplantation. Lancet 2:97–98
9. Farrar DJ, Hill JD, Gray LA et al. (1988) Heterotopic prosthetic ventricles as a bridge to cardiac transplantation. N Engl J Med 318:333–340
10. Hill JD, Farrar DJ, Hershon JJ et al. (1986) Bridge to cardiac transplantation: successful use of prosthetic biventricular support in a patient awaiting a donor heart. Trans Am Soc Artif Organs 32:233–237
11. Pae WE, Pierce WS, Pennock JL et al. (1987) Long-term results of ventricular assist pumping in postcardiotomy cardiogenic shock. J Thorac Cardiovasc Surg 93:434–441

17. Progress in Impeller Pumps in China *

K. X. QIAN

Introduction

Definition

The term "impeller pump", as distinct from both the vaneless Biomedicus pump and the inductive coupling powered Medtronic pump, refers to the motor-driven impeller-type centrifugal pump.

Advantages

The advantages of the impeller pump derive from its mechanism. In the impeller pump there are only two periods of energy transformation, one from electric to mechanical through the motor, another from mechanical to fluidic through the pump. Every additional energy transformation which is necessary in other types of pump needs an additional mechanism and causes energy loss and mechanical unreliability. Therefore, the impeller pump can be produced at a minimum size and weight, but with maximum efficiency and reliability. Furthermore, the impeller pump imitates the natural heart in function rather than mechanism. There are thus no inflow and outflow valves, no flexible diaphragm, and no compliance chamber.

Problems

Applications of the impeller pump have been limited mainly to assistance of the heart because of certain outstanding problems. Above all, the reduction of hemolysis is significant for long-term performance. The generation of a pulsatile flow with low hemolysis has long been within sight but beyond reach. The bearings and sealing of the rotor are also a difficult problem.

Progress

Much progress has been achieved in Shanghai toward solving the current problems of the impeller pump. An analytical method with three-dimensional dy-

* Project Supported by Chinese Academy of Sciences.

Assisted Circulation 3
F. Unger (Ed.)
© Springer-Verlag Berlin Heidelberg 1989

namics for impeller design and an experimental method for investigating the hemolysis factors were established. The main factors causing excessive hemolysis
were subsequently ascertained. Both the impeller assist heart, including the nonpulsatile and the pulsatile impeller pump, and the impeller total heart were developed. Their size and weight have been minimized and their index of hemolysis has
been reduced to an acceptable range. A friction-free magnet-ferrofluid sealing
construction was also introduced. This paper presents a general outline of all
these advances.

Analytical Method of Impeller Design

Design Conceptions

The new analytical method of impeller design with three-dimensional dynamics
focused on blood damage, hemolysis, shear stress, Renold shear, and velocity
variations: Blood damage is the most important problem of the impeller pump,
and hemolysis is the most serious form of blood damage. Shear stress is the mechanical force with the greatest effect on hemolysis and turbulent shear (i.e.,
Renolds shear) carries more danger to erythrocytes than does laminar shear (i.e.,
Newton shear). The product of velocity variations measured in two directions
perpendicular to each other determines the Renolds shear. The velocity variation
in a peripheral direction is largest as the impeller changes its rotating speed
periodically in the process of generating a physiological pulsatile flow. Therefore,
the impeller design should ensure no velocity variation, no turbulence.

Fundamental Equations

The current empirical method of impeller design with two-dimensional dynamics
cannot be qualified to meet the requirements of a blood pump. In particular, the
velocity distribution in the impeller designed according to the current method is
analytically unknown. Therefore, it is scarcely possible to discuss the question of
how to reduce the velocity variation in the impeller, and even more impossible to
deal with the question of how to reduce the velocity variation in a peripheral direction.

From the rotation-free equation

$$\text{rot } \vec{C} = 0 \tag{1}$$

and the equation when there is no dead-water area in impeller,

$$\vec{W} \neq 0, \tag{2}$$

where $\vec{C}$ and $\vec{W}$ are the absolute and relative velocities of blood cells, a simplified,
analytical method of impeller design has been derived [1, 2].

Equation 1 could also be deduced from the continuity equation, the motion
equation, and the energy equation of relative velocity [1, 2]:

$$\text{div } \vec{W} = 0 \tag{3}$$

$$\frac{D\vec{W}}{Dt} - \omega^2\vec{r} + 2\vec{\omega}\times\vec{W} = -\nabla P \tag{4}$$

$$P + \frac{W^2}{2} - \frac{u^2}{2} = Po \tag{5}$$

in which $\vec{W}$ is the relative velocity of blood cells in the impeller, as mentioned above, ω is the rotating speed of the impeller, $\vec{r}$ is the radial vector in cylindric ordinate (r, φ, z), $u = \omega r$, P is the pressure of blood flow, and Po is the atrial pressure.

There is a relation between $\vec{C}$ and $\vec{W}$

$$\vec{C} = \vec{W} + \vec{\omega} \times \vec{r}. \tag{6}$$

Thus Eq. (1) can be expressed as

$$\text{rot}\,\vec{W} = -2\vec{\omega}. \tag{7}$$

Velocity Distributions

The partial differential equation (Eq. 7) is solvable in some special examples [1, 2]:

In an axial impeller $(W_r = 0)$, $\vec{W} = (0, -\omega r + c/r, c_1)$ (8)

In a radial impeller $(W_z = 0)$, $\vec{W} = (c_1/r, -\omega r + c/r, 0)$ (9)

In a mixed-flow impeller, $\vec{W} = (c_1/r, -\omega r + c/r, c_2)$.   (10)

Equations (8)–(10) express the analytical velocity distribution in axial, radial, and mixed-flow impellers respectively.

Stream Surfaces

According to the relation between the stream surfaces ψ_1, ψ_2 and the relative velocity $\vec{W}$:

$$\vec{W} = \nabla\psi_1 \times \nabla\psi_2, \tag{11}$$

together with Eqs. 8–10, ψ_1, ψ_2 could be obtained by solving some other partial differential equations [1, 2]:

For an axial impeller: $\begin{cases} \psi_1 = c_1(-\omega r^2/2 + c\ln r) \\ \psi_2 = r\varphi/(-\omega r + c/r) - z/c \end{cases}$ (12)

For a radial impeller: $\begin{cases} \psi_1 = -c_1 z \\ \psi_2 = \varphi - \omega r^2/2c_1 - c\ln r/c_1 \end{cases}$ (13)

For a mixed-flow impeller: $\begin{cases} \psi_1 = -c_1 z + c_2 r^2/2 \\ \psi_2 = \varphi + \omega r^2/2c_1 - c\ln r/c_1 \end{cases}$ (14)

Equations (12)–(14) represent the stream surface forms in the impellers of different types. Equation (11) can also be certified from continuity equation (3).

Shroud and Vane

In an impeller with reasonable design the shroud and vane should be the stream surfaces, because neither flow departure nor impact between the impeller surface and the stream surface is desirable or permissible. Thus Eqs. 12–14 can be taken as the shroud (ψ_1) and vane (ψ_2) of impellers of different types.

Figure 1 shows the shroud forms of different impellers: cylindrical (axial impeller), disk shaped (radial impeller), and parabolic. The parabolic stream surface has a simple geometrical and physical significance [3]. As a cup with water rotates, the contacting surface of the water and air is a parabola. But in impeller design, the gravity of blood is neglected; a Coriolis force which is produced by relative motion and rotation plays the same role as gravity.

The vane forms of different impellers are: axial helical spiral $\varphi = cz$ for axial impellers [let $c = 0$ in ψ_2 in Eq. 12], and a form overlapped by parabola $\varphi = C_1 r^2$ and logarithmic spiral $\varphi = C_2 \ln r$ for radial and mixed-flow impellers [Eqs. 13 and 14]. The axial helical spiral vane and the radial logarithmic spiral vane which were applied in blood pumps are shown in Fig. 2. The logarithmic spiral vane also has a dynamic and physical significance [3]. With this vane the ratio of the peripheral velocity component and the radial velocity component (i.e., W_φ / W_r) remains constant from the root to the top of vane.

The dimensions of the impeller were determined by current design methods.

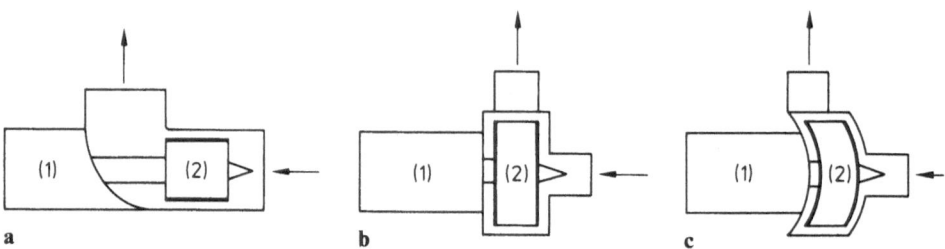

a   b   c

Fig. 1 a–c. The shroud forms of different impellers. (*1*) motor; (*2*) impeller. **a** Cylinder (axial impeller); **b** disc (radial impeller); **c** parabola (mixed-flow impeller)

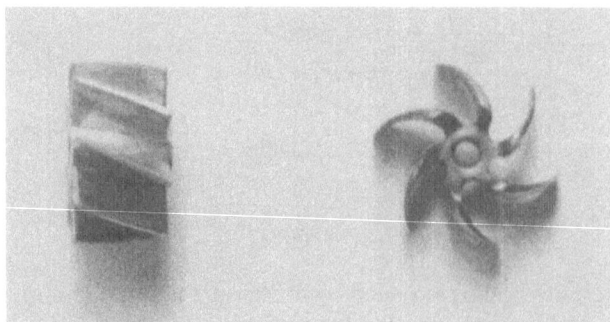

Fig. 2. Impellers with an axial helical spiral vane (*left*) and a radial logarithmic spiral vane (*right*)

Impeller Assist Heart

Nonpulsatile Pump

The nonpulsatile impeller pump is of the mixed-flow type according to pump theory [4] (Fig. 3). It consists of an impeller, a motor with a housing, a sealing box and pump housing. The impeller has the parabolic form of shroud and six logarithmic spiral vanes:

$$\begin{cases} \psi_1 = z - c_1 r^2 \\ \psi_2 = \varphi - c_2 lnr \end{cases}.$$ (15)

The total weight of the pump is 240 g, including the 190-g motor.

The nonpulsatile pump was first tested with saline. Against 100 mmHg pressure the pump output reached as high as 8 l/min. At the design point of 4 l/min volume and 100 mmHg pressure, the consumed power was 2.7 W (15 V × 0.18 A). That means, the total efficiency of the motor and the pump reached 33%, and the pump efficiency reached about 60% [5].

For hemolysis testing the nonpulsatile impeller pump was compared with the roller pump made in Shanghai and SARNS 7000 roller pump (Figs. 4, 5). In each case fresh citrated porcine blood was used. The results revealed that the hemolysis with the nonpulsatile impeller pump was about one-fifth of that with the Shanghai roller pump and 1/3.5 of that with the SARNS 7000 roller pump [6].

In animal experiments the nonpulsatile pump was used as an extracorporeal left ventricular assist device in dogs and goats (Fig. 6). The bypass ratio was adjusted to 40%–50% of the total flow (Fig. 7). The plasma hemoglobin of experimental goats was mostly lower than that of calve with a pneumatic diaphragm pump in identical experiments.

Pulsatile Pump

The pulsatile impeller pump involved changing the RPM of the impeller periodically through inputting voltage of a square wave form. Reduction of hemolysis

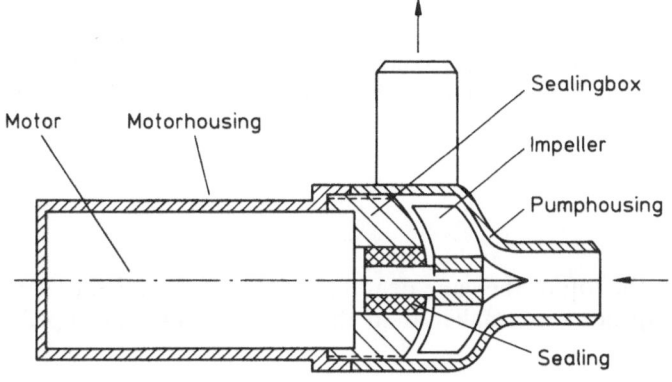

Fig. 3. Schematic drawing of a nonpulsatile impeller pump

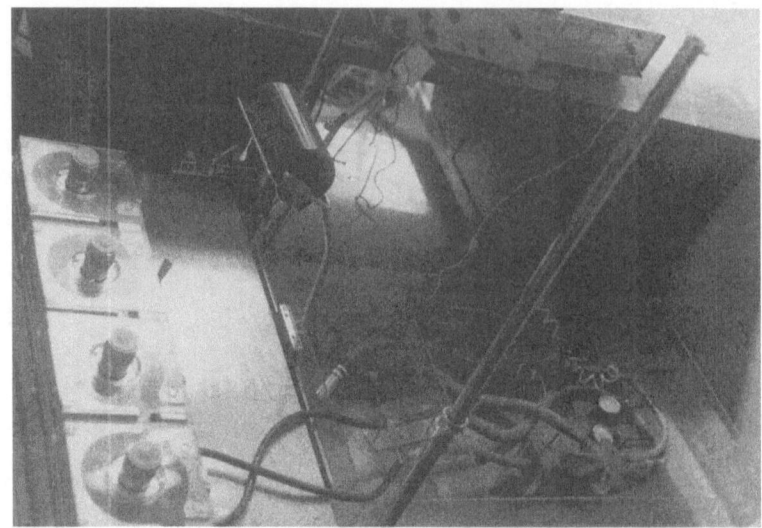

a

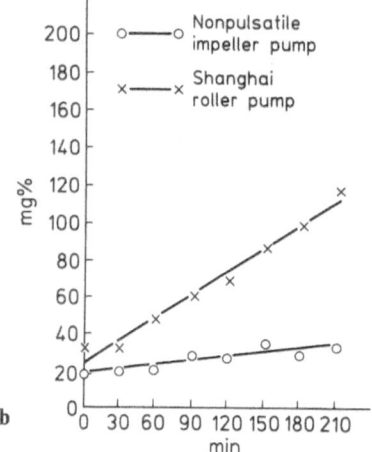

b

Fig. 4 a, b. Hemolysis testing of the nonpulsatile impeller pump compared with the roller pump made in Shanghai. a The pumps in testing. b The hemoglobin in plasma. The slope of the oblique lines indicates the index of hemolysis of the two pumps

with the pulsatile blood flow was achieved according to Eqs. 12–14 by use of a twisted vane ($\varphi = c\,zlnr$), compacted by an axial helical spiral ($\varphi = cz$) and a radial logarithmic spiral ($\varphi = clnr$) [7], in which the velocity variation in a peripheral direction was minimized:

$$\begin{cases} \psi_1 = z - c_1 r^2 \\ \psi_2 = \varphi - c_2 zlnr \end{cases} . \tag{16}$$

The velocity triangle at the top of the vane demonstrated that the velocity variation in the twisted impeller was smaller than that in the untwisted impeller (Fig. 8).

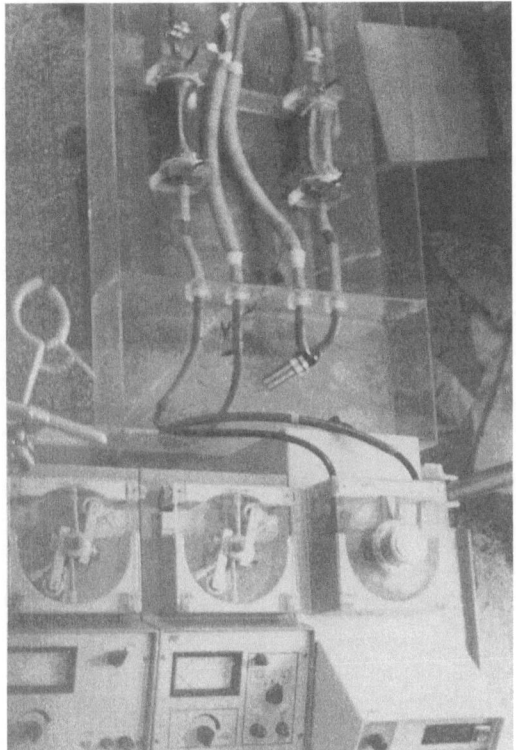

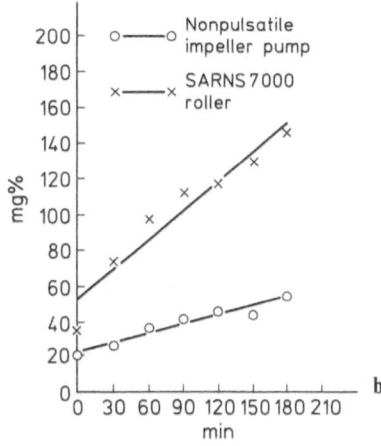

Fig. 5 a, b. Hemolysis testing of the nonpulsatile impeller pump compared with the SARNS 7000 roller pump. a The pumps in testing. b The experimental results

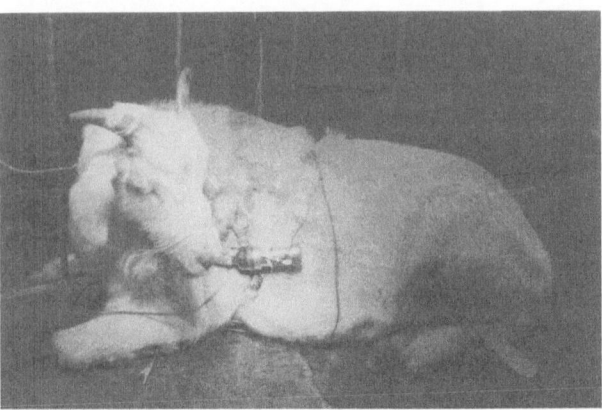

Fig. 6. Left ventricular assistance in a goat, using the nonpulsatile impeller pump

Except for the vane form there is no difference between the nonpulsatile and the pulsatile pump in construction (Fig. 9). Both are of the mixed-flow type, and both impellers have a parabolic shroud.

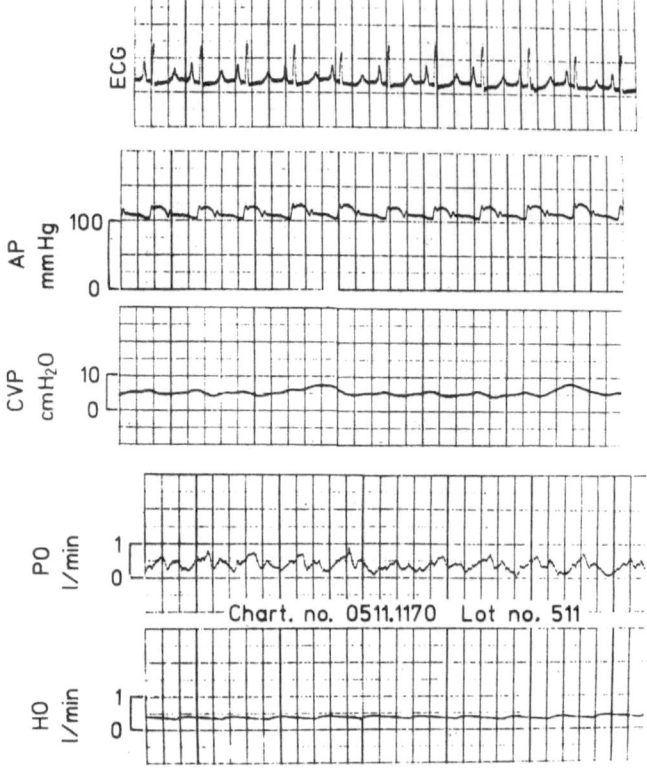

Fig. 7. The hemodynamics of the nonpulsatile impeller pump in an animal experiment. *ECG,* electrocardiogram; *AP,* aortic pressure; *CVP,* central venous pressure; *PO,* pump output; *HO,* heart output

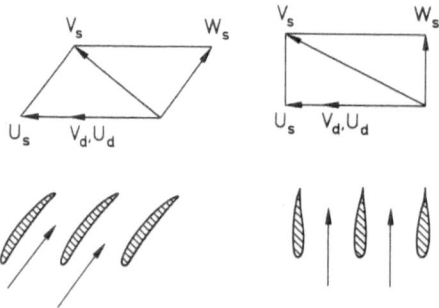

Fig. 8. The velocity triangle at the top of the vane demonstrated that the velocity variation ($V_s - V_d$) in the twisted impeller (*left*) is smaller than that in the untwisted impeller (*right*), V_s, systolic absolute velocity; W_s, systolic relative velocity; U_s, systolic peripheral velocity; V_d, diastolic absolute velocity

In contrast to the diaphragm pump, the pulsatile impeller pump fills and ejects simultaneously as the impeller rotates at high speed; its mean output is varied with systolic and diastolic voltages, with systolic period, and with the afterload. The pulsatile frequency has no effect on pump output; the pressure pulsatility is determined by voltage pulsatility.

The pulsatile impeller pump was tested repeatedly together with the nonpulsatile impeller pump to determine the index of hemolysis. Results showed the index of hemolysis of the pulsatile impeller pump to be about 0.020, slightly more than that of the nonpulsatile impeller pump (0.015). The pulsatile impeller pump

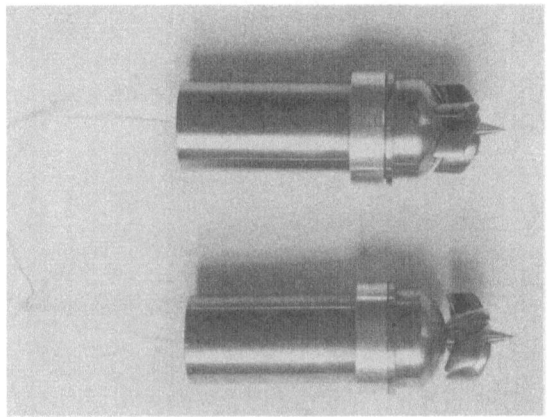

Fig. 9. Except for the impeller vane form there is no difference between the nonpulsatile pump (*above*) and the pulsatile pump (*below*)

was then compared with a self-made diaphragm pump and the Danish Polystan pulsatile pump (Figs. 10, 11). The results revealed that the hemolysis with the pulsatile impeller pump was about one-sixth of that with the self-made diaphragm pump and 1/13 of that with the Danish Polystan pulsatile pump [6].

The pulsatile impeller pump was employed as a left ventricular assist device in dogs and goats. The bypass flow was adjusted to 40%–50% of total flow (Fig. 12). The blood counts, the hemoglobin, and the hematocrit remained fairly constant, and the free hemoglobin remained below 50 mg% in first 20 h postoperatively [8].

Impeller Total Heart

Based on the analytical method of impeller design and the development of the impeller assist heart, a prototype total impeller heart was designed [9, 11].

The device possesses a DC motor with double output shafts, onto which the left and right impellers are directly fixed (Fig. 13). Each of two sealing boxes between the motor housing and the pump housing has a magnet-ferrofluid construction, providing frictionless sealing of the rotor. Because of the different pressure–volume ratios, there are some differences between the left and the right impellers. The left impeller is of mixed-flow type and has an outside diameter of 30 mm, while the right impeller is of axial type and has an outside diameter of 25 mm. The vanes of both impellers are twisted, compacted by a radial logarithmic spiral and an axial helical spiral. Both have a logarithmic spiral angle of 30°, but the axial helical angle of the left impeller is 30°, while that of the right impeller is 45°.

As the motor changes its RPM periodically, the left and right pumps eject simultaneously, producing a physiological pulsatile flow (Fig. 14). The volume is adjusted by changing the motor voltage and the systolic period, and equilibrium of both pumps is achieved by the self-modulating property of the impeller pump.

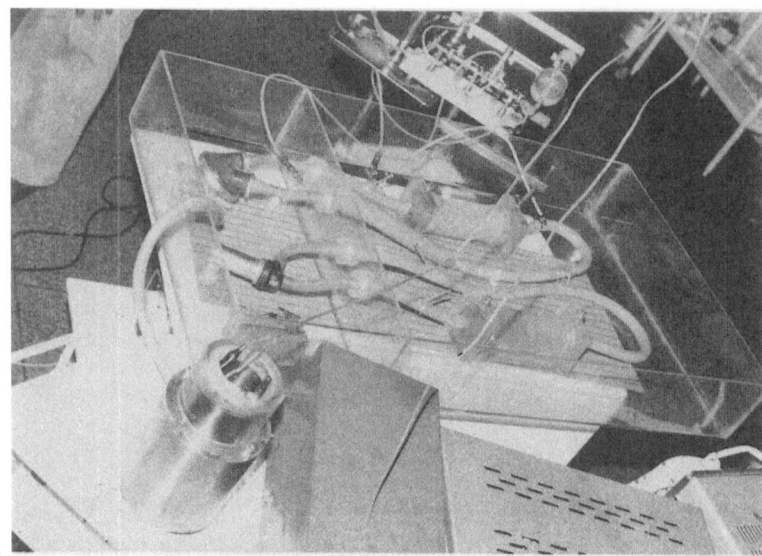

a

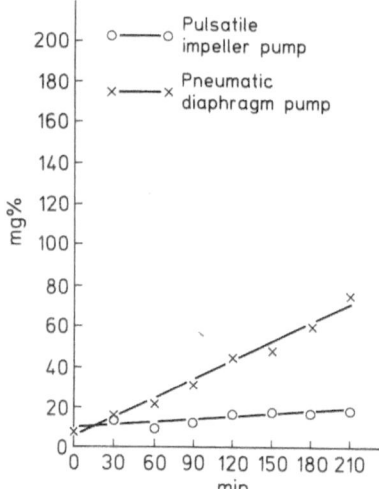

Fig. 10 a, b. Hemolysis testing of the pulsatile impeller pump compared with a self-made diaphragm pump. **a** The pumps in testing. **b** The experimental results

The device weighs 365 g. For anatomical suitability, the development of a disk form motor is now under consideration.

Hemolysis Reduction

Experimental Method for Investigating the Hemolysis Factors

The idea of hemolysis reduction was important through out the development of the impeller pump, not only in its design, as described above, but also in its manu-

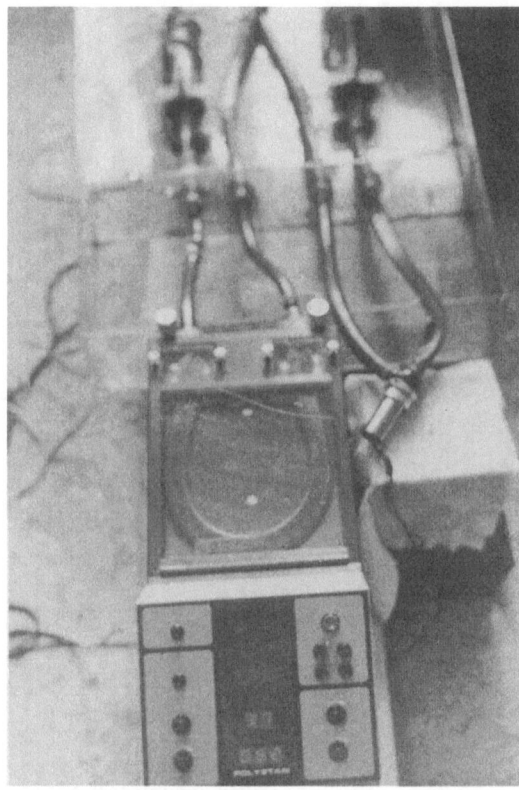

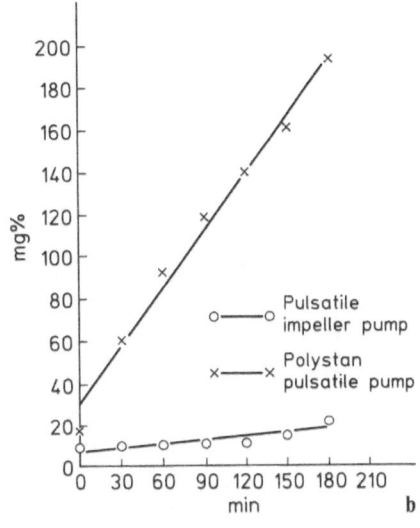

mg%

Pulsatile impeller pump

Polystan pulsatile pump

min b

Fig. 11 a, b. Hemolysis testing of the pulsatile impeller pump compared with the Polystan pulsatile pump (Denmark). **a** The pumps in testing. **b** The experimental results

facture. There are many difficulties in achieving a low hemolysis impeller pump. First, the factors causing excessive hemolysis in impeller pumps are unknown, and there is no effective method, either theoretical or empirical, for identifying these factors. Second, there are many factors which might bring about excessive hemolysis, and all these factors always act together, so it is difficult to distinguish them. Third, errors could take place at many points during hemolysis testing making it difficult to reproduce the results.

As is well-known, shear stress is the main mechanical force causing hemolysis, but what causes shear? According to up-to-date fluid mechanics both Newton shear τ_N and Renolds shear τ_R are involved:

$$\tau_N = \eta \frac{\partial V}{\partial y}, \qquad \tau_R = \varrho \overline{u'v'} \tag{17}$$

where η is viscosity of blood, V is the absolute velocity of blood cells at the top of the impeller vane, y is the gap between the pump housing and the vane top, ϱ is the density of blood, and u', v' are velocity variations measured in two perpendicular directions. By current method the shear stress is calculated by Eq. 17, and the hemolysis S could be estimated accordingly:

$$S = K \cdot t \cdot \tau^2 \tag{18}$$

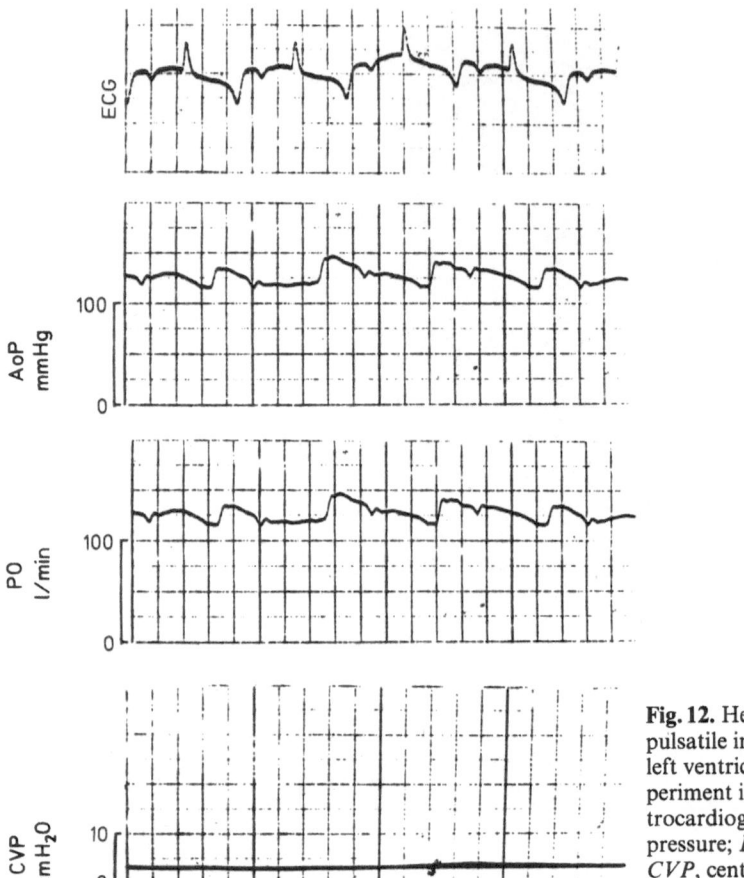

Fig. 12. Hemodynamics of the pulsatile impeller pump in a left ventricular assistance experiment in a dog. *ECG*, electrocardiogram; *AoP*, aortic pressure; *PO*, pump output; *CVP*, central venous pressure

with S = hemolysis rate, t = exposed time, τ = shear, and K = constant, determined by blood viscosity η and the ratio of blood surface A over blood volume V:

$$K = f\left(\frac{1}{n} \cdot \frac{A}{V}\right). \tag{19}$$

The velocity of the flow could be also calculated by means of Eq. 11, in which ψ_1, ψ_2 should be taken as the impeller shroud and vane.

Both the measurement and the calculation of the velocity are complicated and inaccurate. Experience has shown that the results are generally unacceptable.

An experimental method for searching for individual factors influencing hemolysis has been developed by using a two-canal circulatory model [10]. Each canal consists of atrium, aorta, peripheral resistance modulator, and pressure- and volume-measuring devices. Two identical impeller pumps with only one factor different were connected to two identical canals and tested under completely identical conditions for hemolysis comparison. Alternatively an impeller pump changed only one factor in the middle of the hemolysis testing period. The free hemoglobin in systems was taken to evaluate the hemolysis of the pump. In these

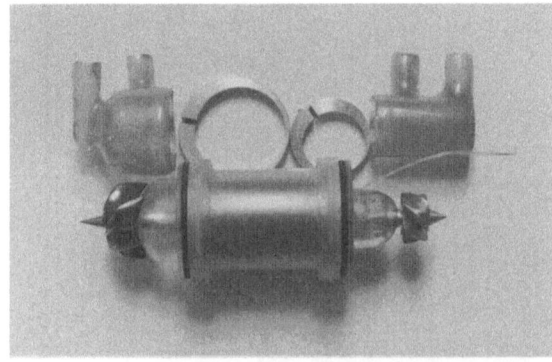

Fig. 13. The prototype design of an impeller total heart

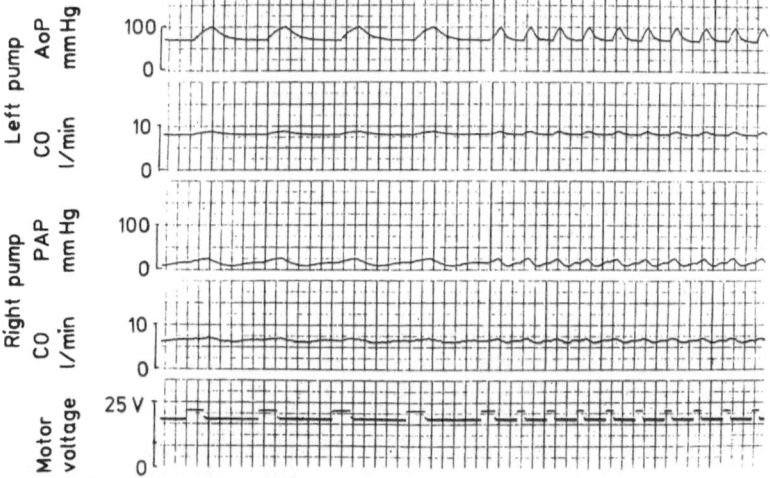

Fig. 14. The left pump and the right pump eject simultaneously as the impeller rotates at high speed. The frequency has almost no effect on pump output

ways the effect of each factor on the hemolysis of the impeller pump could be clarified. By use of this method, some factors were certified to have a great effect on pump hemolysis.

Efficiency

Two identical impeller pumps in a two-canal circulatory model were tested simultaneously (Fig. 15). One delivered the blood flow with a constant volume and pressure changed hourly in a stepwise fashion. Another delivered the blood flow with a constant pressure and volume changed hourly in a stepwise fashion. The index of hemolysis of the pump did not change with changing pressure, but the volume did have an obvious effect on the hemolysis (Fig. 16). The index of hemolysis seems to increase with decreasing efficiency η of the pump, and to decrease

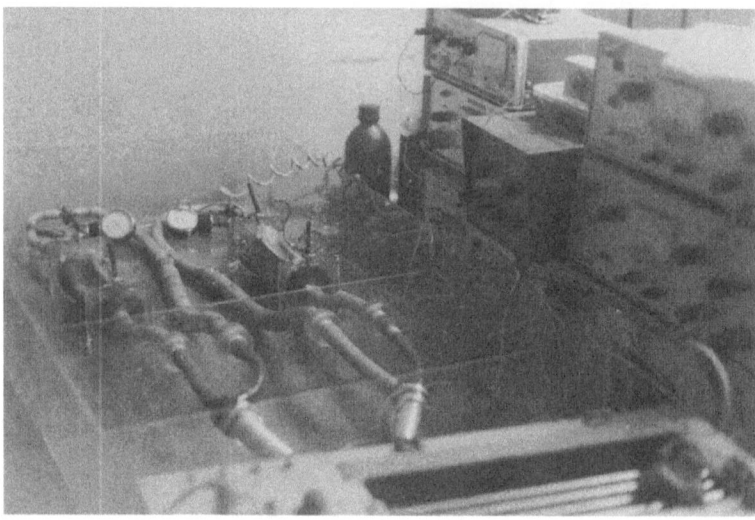

Fig. 15. Two identical impeller pumps with only one different factor were tested in completely identical conditions

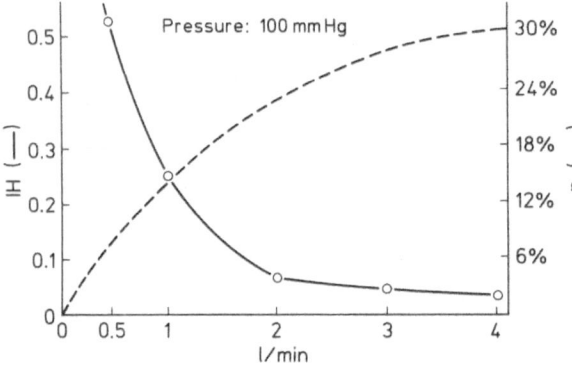

Fig. 16. The index of hemolysis (*IH*) of the impeller pump decreases with increasing η

with increasing η. The low efficiency of pumping indicates heavy dynamic loss and bad hydraulic property, and results in intensive turbulence and huge Renolds shear. The impeller assist heart is designed to generate 4 l/min blood flow against 100 mmHg mean pressure; at this design point the pump achieves highest efficiency. Figure 16 suggests that if the drift of volume from the design point is not too large, smaller than 2 l/min for example, the index of hemolysis of the pump is acceptable. Therefore, there is promise that reduction of hemolysis can be realized by improving the efficiency of the pump.

Impeller Vane Angle

Five impellers with different vane angles (Fig. 17) were tested. Two identical pumps with two different impellers were compared in a two-canal circulatory

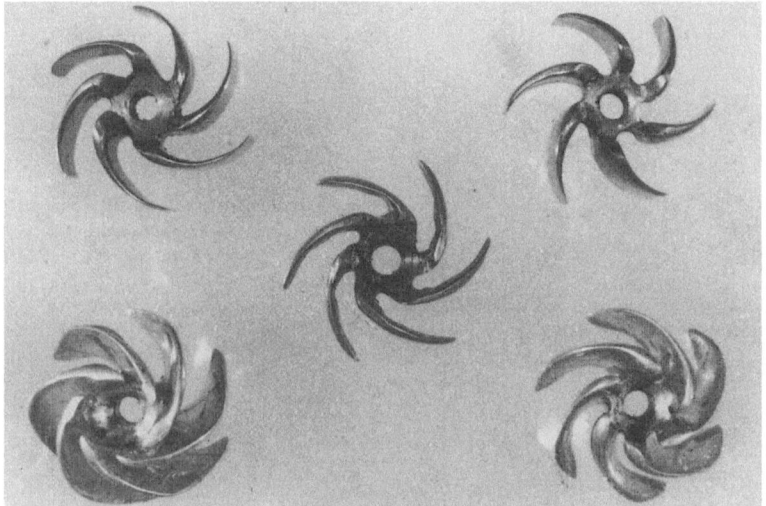

Fig. 17. Five impellers with different axial helical spiral angles and radial logarithmic spiral angles were tested to assess the optimal vane angles of both the nonpulsatile impeller pump and the pulsatile impeller pump

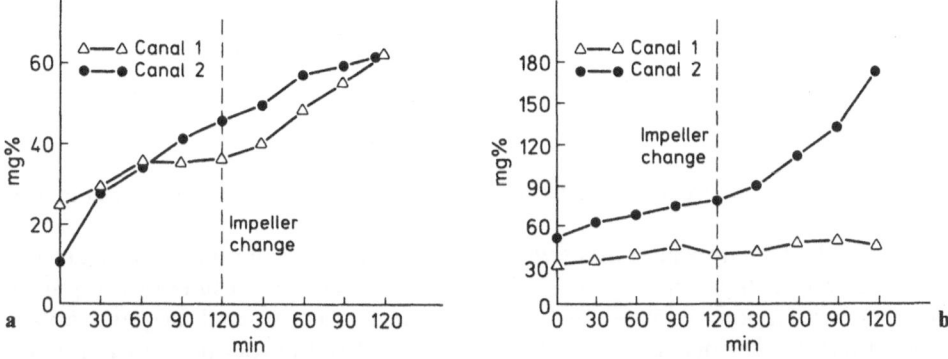

Fig. 18. The effect of the vane angle on the hemolysis of the impeller pump in **a** nonpulsatile and **b** pulsatile pumping

model. After 2 h the pumps were dismantled and the impellers were exchanged for another two different impellers. The testing then continued for a further 2 h. In this way the optimal vane angle for both the nonpulsatile and the pulsatile pump could be determined. According to the experimental results the effects of the vane angle is greater on hemolysis of the pulsatile pump than on hemolysis of the nonpulsatile pump (Fig. 18).

Roughness of the Blood-Contacting Surfaces

Blood-contacting surfaces in the impeller pump include the impeller vane surface, the sealing box surface, and the pump housing inner surface; of these the last-

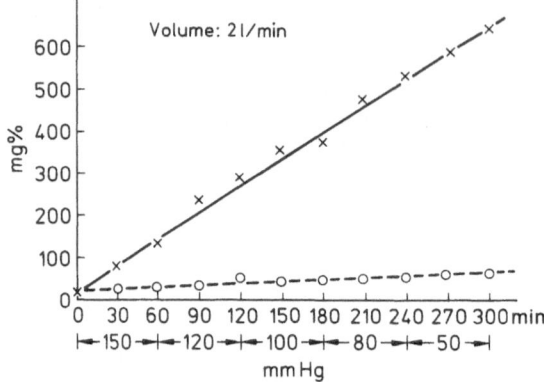

Fig. 19. The effect of the roughness of blood-contacting surfaces on hemolysis. × — × Rough housing, o—o Polish housing

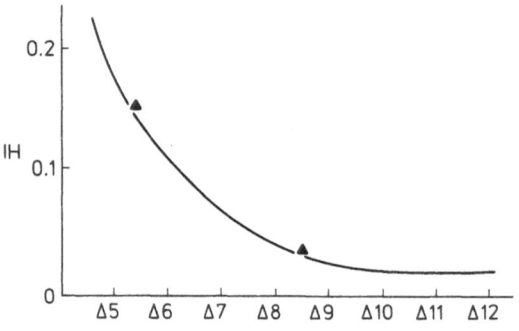

Fig. 20. The experimental results suggest that the polish degree of the blood-contacting surfaces should not be lower than Δ9 anywhere in the impeller pump. *IH*, index of hemolysis

mentioned has the greatest effect on pump hemolysis according to experimental experience.

Two identical impeller pumps with different roughness of pump housing inner surface were compared. Figure 19 shows the comparative results of the pump housing with a polished inner surface (polish degree Δ8–Δ9) and the pump housing with a rough inner surface (polish degree Δ5–Δ6). In order to confirm the relation between the pressure pumped and hemolysis, the afterload of both pumps was changed every hour.

Figure 20 is the relation between the index of hemolysis of the impeller pump and the polish degree of the blood-contacting surfaces. It suggests that the polish degree of the blood-contacting surface should not be lower than Δ9 anywhere in the impeller pump.

Other Factors

Other factors were also confirmed to have a significant effect on pump hemolysis [10], e.g., the prerotational swirl of blood flow at the inlet of the pump, the poor concentricity and the dynamic disequilibrium of, in particular, the rotor of the impeller due to inaccurate manufacture. By eliminating all these factors one by one, hemolysis could be reduced to an acceptable range.

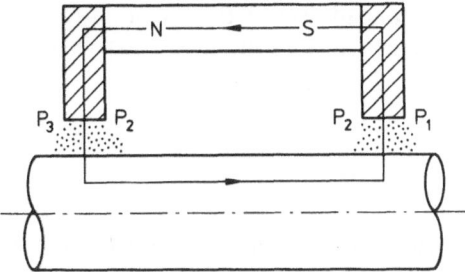

Fig. 21. The frictionless magnet–ferrofluid sealing construction

Bearing and Sealing

From the schematic drawing of the impeller pump (Fig. 3) it is clear that the motor shaft extends into the pump housing directly, without any additional bearing. The sealing of the motor shaft is a serious problem of such motor-driven type impeller pumps. With the usual sealing method there is friction which results in heating. Lubrication and cooling are necessary, otherwise the heat generation would bring about thrombosis.

A new sealing method has been successfully applied in the impeller pump. It is based on the reciprocal action of a magnet and ferrofluid. Between the magnet (stator) and the motor shaft (rotor), a few drops of ferrofluid fill the gap and prevent penetration of blood into the motor housing (Fig. 21). Ferrofluid is a suspension with numerous fine ferromagnetic particles suspending in water or oil. The size of these particles is about 80 Å. To keep the magnetic particles from sticking together, every particle is coated with nonferrous material. The intensity of the magnet and the saturation of the ferrofluid must be appropriate to the pressure of sealed blood. There is a relation between them:

$$P = P_2 - P_1 = \mu \int_{H_1}^{H_2} M dH . \tag{20}$$

Here P is the pressure to be sealed (see Fig. 21), μ is magnetic conductivity, H is magnetic density, and M is magnetic intensity of ferrofluid.

Because the ferrofluid could be dissolved in the blood, it is necessary to separate them. The construction "air–ferrofluid–blood" is unsafe, and should be replaced by "air–ferrofluid–air–blood."

Discussion

The progress in the development of impeller pumps has been achieved by solving certain problems. However, other problems remain to be solved. One such problem is thrombus formation along the inlet edge of the vane, which is sometimes observed after animal experiments with a low dosage of anticoagulant (ACT 150–200 s). As survival is prolonged, new problems will surely be discovered. Much further development of the impeller pump lies ahead. But by the use of up-to-date science and technology, all the problems promise to be soluble, avoidable, or at least reducible.

References

1. Qian KX (1987) The applications of 3-dimensional theory in designing impeller of the blood pumps. Chin J Eng Maths 4 (2)
2. Qian KX (1987) An analytical method of impeller design and its applications in blood pumps. Chin J Biomech 2 (2)
3. Qian KX (1989) A new total heart design via implantable impeller pumps. J Biomaterial Applications 4 (1)
4. Qian KX et al. (1983) Prototype design of an implantable nonpulsatile diagonal pump. Proceedings ISAO
5. Qian KX et al. (1985) A fully implantable nonpulsatile impeller pump assists the circulation of the free-walking goat. Proceedings, ISAO
6. Qian KX et al. (1988) Hemolysis test of nonpulsatile and pulsatile impeller blood pumps. Clin Phys Physiol Meas 9 (2)
7. Qian KX et al. (1989) The realization of a pulsatile implantable impeller pump with low hemolysis. Artif Organs 13 (2)
8. Qian KX et al. (1988) A new impeller blood pump design: in vitro and in vivo studies. Perfusion 3 (3)
9. Qian KX et al. (1987) Toward an implantable impeller total heart. Trans ASAIO
10. Qian KX (1989) Experience in reducing the hemolysis of impeller assist heart. Trans ASAIO 35 (1)
11. Unger F, Genelin A, Hager J, Kemkes BM, Koller I, Schistek R (1984) Functional heart replacement with nonpulsatile assist devices. In: Unger F (ed) Assisted Circulation 2. Springer, Berlin Heidelberg New York Tokyo

18. The Sealless and Bearingless Rotor Blood Pump System: Adaptation to the Circulatory System and In Vitro Advantages in Efficiency, Flow Characteristics, and Boundary Conditions of Thermal Heat Up

G. Bramm and D. B. Olsen

The long-term application of blood pump systems on the basis of conventional displacement concepts involves many insufficiencies due to unavoidable characteristics of the mechanical function which provoke inevitable material wear and embrittlement. The consequent desire to avoid all sorts of material loading has led to the new concept of the free-floating, magnetically suspended rotor blood pump [1–3]. This concept has found application in some laboratory models of blood pump, and in vitro results with these pumps have been published [4, 5]. In the following, we discuss the characteristics of these types of pump operating on a circulatory system and the advantages displayed in vitro.

Characteristics When Operating on a Circulatory System

In a theoretical study some of the most important hydraulic blood flow parameters have been isolated in order to predict the operating characteristics when the pump is connected to a natural circulatory system.

The pressure-flow characteristics of the heart and circulatory system can be clearly represented by transformation of the hydraulic into electrical parameters. The Frank-Starling effect in the heart and circulatory system can be described by means of an idealized model with concentrated elements. The model is based upon a circulatory system which is reduced in complexity but which does take into account the arterial compliance, peripheral resistance, and venous compliance, as shown in Fig. 1.

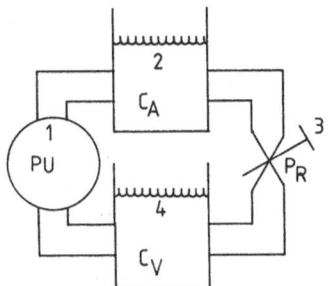

Fig. 1. Schematic idealized fluid model of heart and circulatory system, with concentrated properties (compliance, resistance etc.). *1*, pump (*PU*); *2* arterial pressure reservoir (C_A); *3*, peripheral resistance (P_R) (λ = variable); *4*, venous volume reservoir (C_V)

Assisted Circulation 3
F. Unger (Ed.)
© Springer-Verlag Berlin Heidelberg 1989

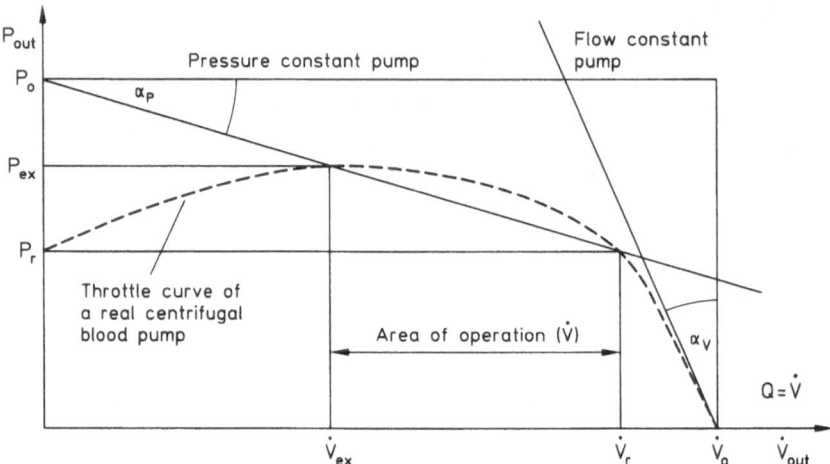

Fig. 2. Flow–pressure pattern of volume- and pressure-constant pumps and the real throttle curve of centrifugal blood pump models. P_{ex}, pressure under exercise; P_{out}, pressure at pump output; P_0, pressure of idealized pressure-constant pump; P_{ex}, pressure under exercise of a real centrifugal pump; P_r, pressure in rest of a real centrifugal pump; $\dot{V}_r$, flow in rest of a real centrifugal pump; $\dot{V}_0$, flow of idealized pressure-constant pump; $\dot{V}_{out}$, flow at pump output; α, tangent angle

The pressure-flow correlation of the flow source (heart or pump) is characterized as pressure "constant" or flow "constant," whereby these properties are idealized and concentrated in reservoirs and throttle elements. The realistic flow-pressure pattern in the operation area of centrifugal blood pumps is denoted in Fig. 2 by the dotted line, while the tangent angle represents the degree of idealization (throttle curve of a centrifugal pump).

The transformation of the fluid dynamic parameters into electrical values reduces the fluid system's complexity and allows an equational treatment in the electronic/electrical discipline, where such networks are commonly used. Pressure P^1 is thereby transformed into voltage U, flow $\dot{V}$ is equivalent to current I, and volume V is transformed into charge Q. Such transformation results in an electric diagram in which elements typically form a "floating potential" circuit (Figs. 3, 4). Equational representation of the circuit (Table 1) demonstrates that the venous pressure (potential U_P) is under a constant peripheral resistance dependent on the circulatory filling volume (charge Q). This makes possible effective control of the validity of this model: The resulting venous pressure/filling volume correlation is well-known and of great benefit in the operation of heart-lung machines. In cases of reduced cardiac output the operator makes use of the correlation by filling up the incorporated volume in order to achieve a rise in venous return pressure, which in turn leads to an increasing cardiac output due to the Frank-Starling effect.

---

[1] To avoid confounding factors, the pressure P does not identify the filling but rather the output pressure of the heart or blood pump, as determined by the peripheral resistance and the output flow or the cardiac output.

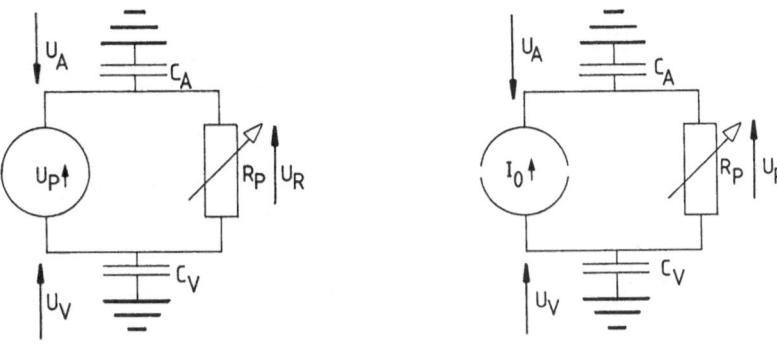

Fig. 3   Fig. 4

Fig. 3. Floating potential circuit of flow-constant pump type. C_A, arterial compliance; U_A, arterial potential; U_P, pump pressure potential; U_V, venous potential; C_V, venous compliance; R_P, peripheral resistance; U_R, peripheral resistance; cross potential

Fig. 4. Floating potential circuit of pressure-constant pump type. C_A, arterial compliance; U_A, arterial potential; I_0, pump flow potential; C_V, venous compliance; R_P, peripheral resistance; U_R, peripheral resistance cross potential; U_V, venous potential equivalent

Table 1. Equational representation of a "floating potential" circuit

---

Arterial pressure reservoir:

$\Delta V_A = C_A \cdot \Delta P_A \cong$ El. capacitance: $\Delta Q_A = C_A \cdot U_A$

Venous pressure reservoir:

$\Delta V_v = C_v \cdot \Delta P_v \cong$ El. capacitance: $\Delta Q_v = C_v \cdot \Delta U_v$ whereas, because of the compliance
relationship $C_v = C_A$

Peripheral resistance:

$R_P = \dfrac{\Delta P}{\dot{V}} \cong R = \dfrac{UR}{I}$

This coincidence of model and reality demonstrates that the reduction of the model's complexity is a valid and legitimate measure which does not render invalid conclusions drawn (e.g., predictions of the system response) when an operative parameter is varied.

The more interesting question and the subject of this investigation is the influence of the Frank-Starling effect upon the operational pressure-flow pattern. Numerical investigation shows that the Frank-Starling effect is a sort of forward closed loop controller which influences the cardiac output in such a way that increasing venous return elevates the cardiac output (current I_0).

The Frank-Starling correlation is approximated as a linear function between venous return pressure (U_V) and cardiac output flow (I_0). Analysis of the influence of the Frank-Starling effect on the system yields the following results: as the peripheral resistance R_P decreases, the pressure gradient between venous and arterial pressure decreases related to the absolute values of the venous and arterial

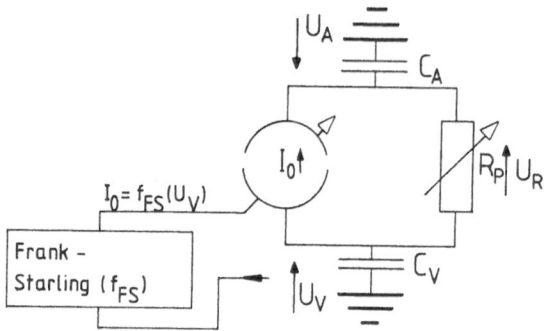

Fig. 5. Electrical analogue to the natural heart, including the Frank-Starling effect with the linear approximation: $I_0 = f_{FS}(U_V)$. C_A, arterial compliance; U_A, arterial potential; I_0, pump flow potential, varied by Frank-Starling effect; C_V, venous compliance; U_R, peripheral resistance, cross potential; R_P, peripheral resistance; U_V, venous potential

compliance (preconditions: $C_A > 0$, $C_V > 0$, $C_V > C_A$), so that in addition a certain blood volume

$$V \cong Q = \Delta U_R \frac{1}{\dfrac{1}{C_P} + \dfrac{1}{C_V}} \tag{1}$$

is transported from the arterial to the venous reservoir.

The generated venous pressure inflow increases according to the Frank-Starling effect (f_{FS}). The cardiac output in turn transports part of the venous volume back to the arterial side and mainly increases the peripheral cross-flow, which results in an elevated peripheral perfusion pressure.

$$U_{v_0} + U_{R_0} = U_{A_0}, \qquad U_{v_1} + U_{R_1} = U_{A_1} \quad \text{with} \quad U_{R_0} > U_{R_1}$$

$$U_{v_1} > U_{v_0}, \qquad U_{A_1} < U_{A_0}. \tag{2}$$

In consequence an elevated venous pressure $P_V(U_V)$ and a reduced arterial pressure are established. Reaction of the heart to a pressure rise caused by the Frank-Starling effect results in an elevated flow $\dot{V} (\cong I_0)$. This must be interpreted; the reduction in peripheral perfusion pressure, caused by variation in peripheral resistance, is largely compensated by the Frank-Starling effect. This can be proved in the model when the peripheral resistance increases, with corresponding consequences for the perfusion pressure. The Frank-Starling effect on this case decreases the perfusion pressure on behalf of the reduced cardiac output.

The conclusion can be drawn that the natural evolution process has by way of the Frank-Starling effect, given rise to a sort of feedback system to overcome the disadvantages in basic circulatory stability of the nearly volume-constant pumping characteristic of the natural "displacement muscle" heart. In fact the theoretical model developed demonstrates that the Frank-Starling effect changes at least in the tendency of the nearly volume-constant pumping characteristic towards a nearly pressure-constant characteristic, which implies that stable organ perfusion pressures are achievable.

Proceeding from this idealized investigation to the actual P-V operation characteristic of artificial displacement blood pump types (angle α_P and α_V, Fig. 2) does not lead to new findings but to a reduction in the mentioned effects. As a consequence of the developed dependencies it is in principle possible to dispense with the Frank-Starling effect in the electronic control, if centrifugal blood pumps are applied in an operative area of nearly constant pressure. Moreover the circulatory stability is achievable even with avoidance or failure of all controller functions. So in principle it is possible to dispense with all control of the venous return pressure of centrifugal blood pump types. It is, however, advisable to control the venous inflow pressure in order to achieve a pressure niveau which is superior to that of the tissue, otherwise venous collapse can be induced; this must be avoided under all circumstances.

Conclusions

Depending upon the actual point of operation the P-V characteristic of a centrifugal blood pump comes very close to that of a pressure-constant pump type. Numerical studies of fluid-electric modeling show that this type of pump can dispense with the Frank-Starling effect without a significant reduction in circulatory stability. This indicates that, due to the fail save operation requirements (MTBF = mean time between failure), centrifugel pumps are extremely suitable for life-support systems because of a possible save operation even in the event of controller failure or defect.

Advantages of the Laboratory Model and Ongoing Developments

The circulatory stability achieved with centrifugal pumps, together with the advantages which can be expected to accrue from their sealless and nontouching mode of operation, indicates that the projected pump type is one of the most promising avenues for the long-term application of cardiac assist devices and artificial hearts. The proven advantages in terms of blood treatment and operational characteristics are, however, achieved at the expense of simplicity in blood pump model design: it is a fact that the valveless, bearingless, and nontouching mode of operation of the magnetically suspended rotor blood pump model generates a very complex structure and an even more complex module physical law network. Optimization of the function requires the participation of a large number of disciplines, as illustrated by Fig. 6.

As an example one of the most important passways of optimization is shown in Fig. 7. The electromagnetic conversion efficiency of the driving system (right side) presupposes the temporary and spatial field distribution and amplitude of the magnetic suspension and driving field in order to generate driving and suspension forces. The conversion efficiency itself is, however, correlated with the torque speed, which influences (over the outer passway; Fig. 7) the field distribution. But the conversion efficiency is also responsible for the heat dissipation of the suspension and driving system, so that the blood-contacting surface temperature is in turn mainly influenced by the torque speed. On the other hand the torque-speed correlation is responsible for the circumferential velocity of the rotor, which in

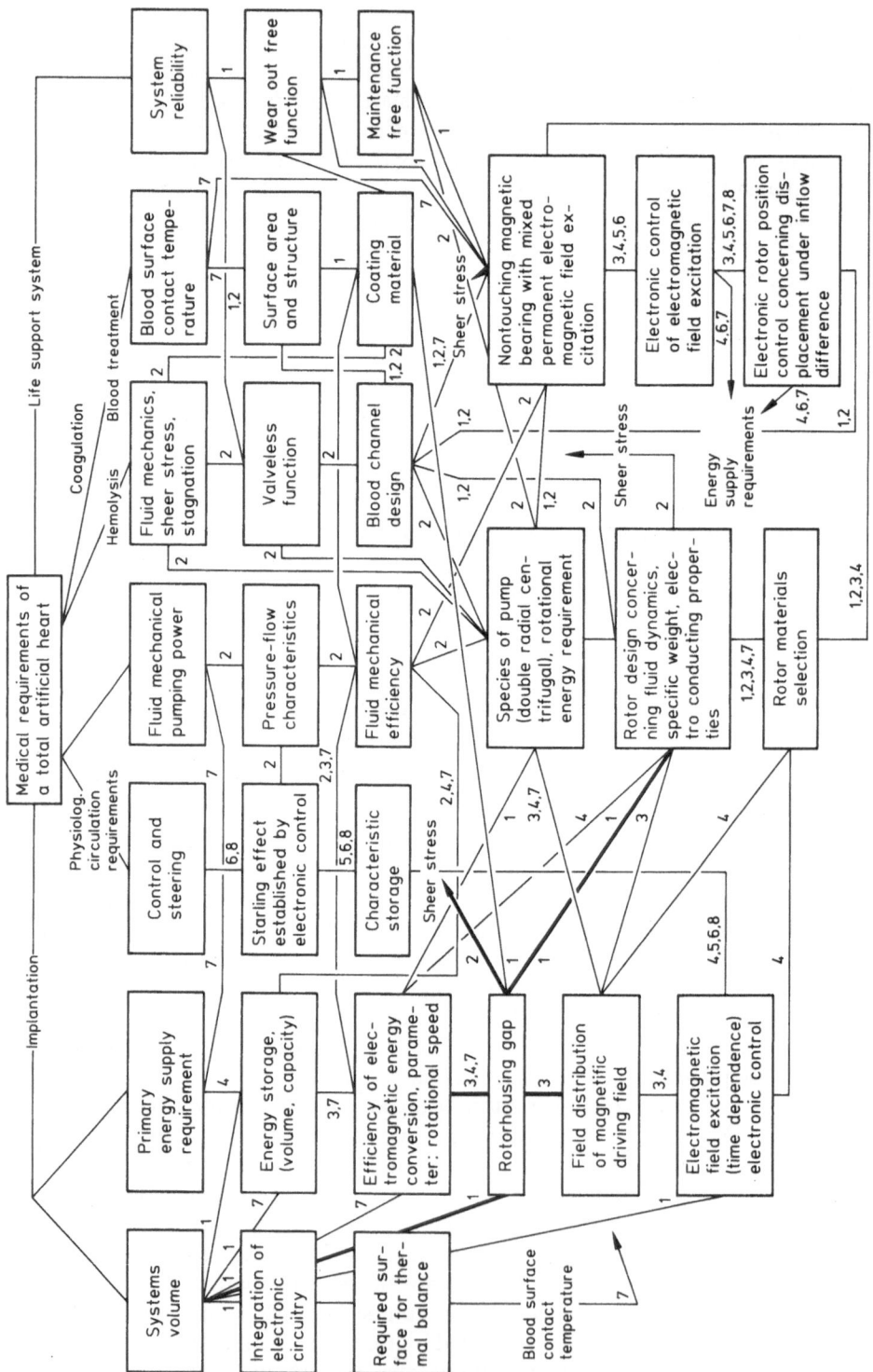

Fig. 6. Research and development interdependencies and interdisciplinary inter relationships in functional optimization. *1*, mechanical (degree of motion freedom, etc.); *2*, fluid dynamics; *3*, magnetic field physics; *4*, electro physics; *5*, electronics; *6*, electronic control; *7*, Physics; *8*, electronic measurement

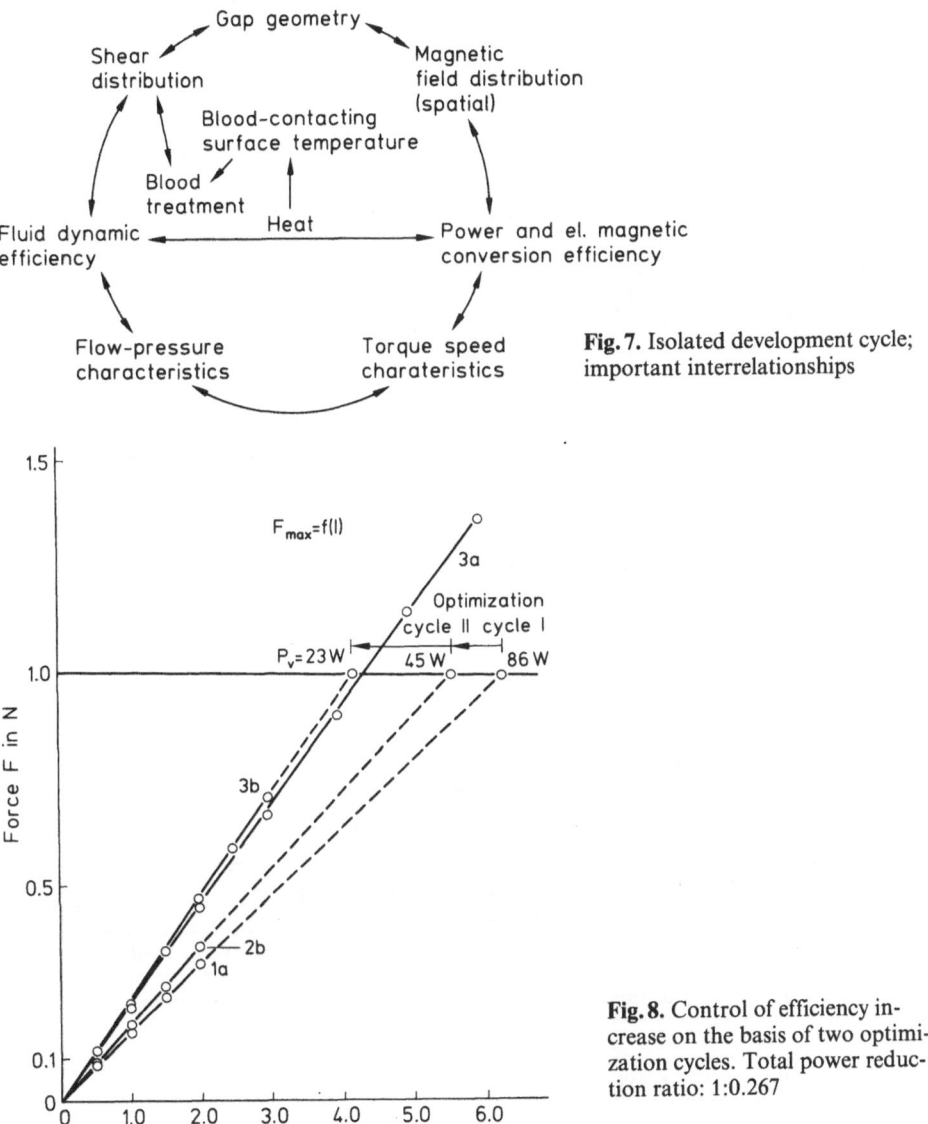

Fig. 7. Isolated development cycle; important interrelationships

Fig. 8. Control of efficiency increase on the basis of two optimization cycles. Total power reduction ratio: 1:0.267

turn induces a certain shear stress in the blood at a certain rotor housing gap geometry. However, the rotor housing gap is one very important parameter in connection with conversion efficiency optimization. This indicates the high degree of interdisciplinary dependence, which in practice means that almost no operational or design parameter can be varied without severe consequences for all other parameters and corresponding consequences for the blood treatment.

Optimization is hence only possible by stepwise progress in numerical modeling and quantitative analysis. Figure 8 shows an example for the progress in reducing the supply power of the magnetic suspension system under the influence of two serial numerical optimization cycles in magnetic field distribution.

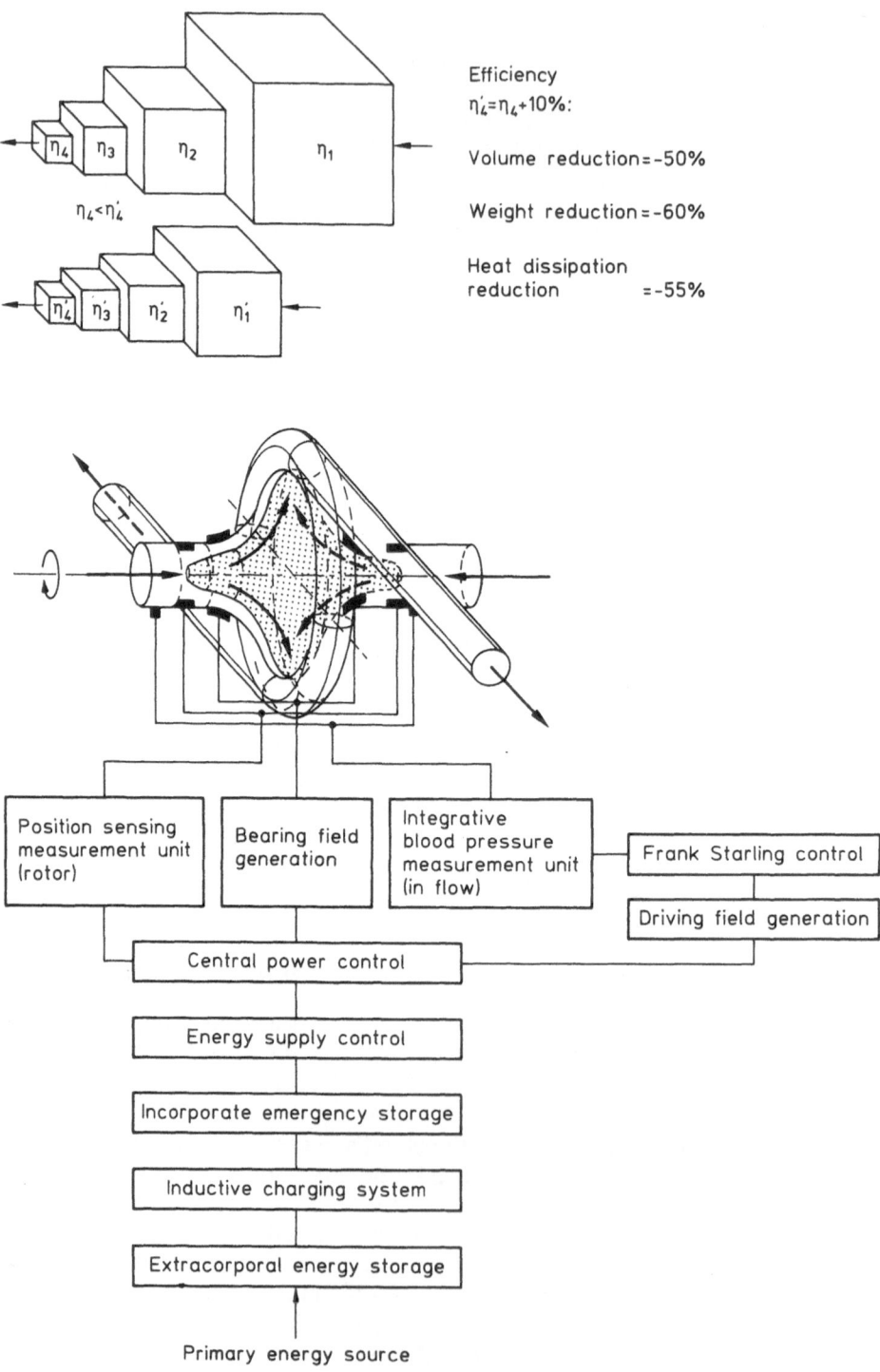

Efficiency
$\eta'_4 = \eta_4 + 10\%$:

Volume reduction $= -50\%$

Weight reduction $= -60\%$

Heat dissipation
reduction $= -55\%$

Fig. 9. Module structure and influence of efficiency of the different modules

Table 2

Cause of power dissipation	Output power (W)	Efficiency η	Power dissipation (W)
Inductive energy transmission (implanted module)	10.5	0.6	4.1
Electrochemical energy storage	9.56	0.9	0.96
Power electronic rotational field	7.56	0.75	1.92
Electromagnetic rotational field generation	5.46	0.6	2.18
Power loss in the rotor	4.2	0.7	1.26
Power: magn. bearing (no acceleration)	0.2		0,2
Hydromechanic losses in the pump	1.2	0.4	3
Sum of power dissipation (implanted device)			13.72

From the point of view of implantation, one of the most critical data is the total power consumption of pump, because all of the supply energy which is not converted into hydraulic power heats up the system. The absolute thermal tolerance, as examined by several authors in animal implantation, was shown to be 0.95–1.1 W/kg body weight [7–10]. At this tolerance the power balance shown in Table 2 must be established. The sum of 13.72 W under rest conditions corresponds to a total efficiency of 8.7%. A body weight of 60 kg would thus result in a total power to heat conversion of 62.8 W under maximum exercise. The hydraulic energy then exceeds 5 W.

Figure 9 shows the module structure of an incorporated blood pump with inductive storage battery charge. The significance of the module efficiency in the balancing is very different. The last modules close to the blood transport source (η_4) influence the total volume, total weight, and power dissipation to a much greater extent, than do the first energy conversion modules close to the input energy source (h_1). A relatively minor increase in efficiency, e.g., 10%, in module

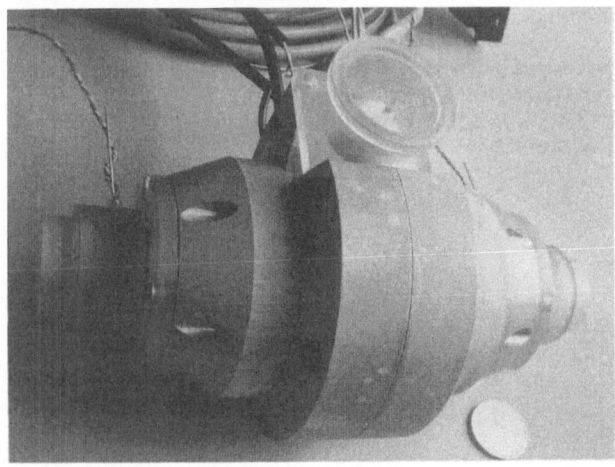

Fig. 10. Last laboratory model of a nontouching, magnetically suspended rotor blood pump

η_4 reducs volume, size, weight, and heat dissipation by more than 50%. This underlines the importance of fluid dynamic pump optimization and optimization of driving energy conversion.

At the current state of development and optimization, a third improved model, which is advanced in some important modules, has been assembled and will be examined in in vitro tests in the future (Fig. 10).

References

1. Bramm G, Novak P, Olsen DB (1981) A free-floating body as the rotor of a centrifugal blood pump for LVAD or TAH. Eur Soc Artif Organs Proc (Copenh) 8:41–45
2. Bramm G, Novak P, Olsen DB, Ruge I (1982) Axial centrifugal blood pump with magnetically suspended rotor life support systems. Proceedings, IX annual meeting of the ESAO, 1982. p 215–219
3. Bramm G, Novak P, Olsen DB, Ruge I (1982) A radial centrifugal blood pump with magnetically suspended rotor. 2nd int workshop. J Artif Organs 5(3):161–163
4. Bramm G, Olsen DB, Novak P, Ruge I (1982) Seal- and bearingless blood pump conception for long term application to avoid coagulation and to reduce hemolysis. Proceedings, World congress on medical physics and biomedical engineering, pp 5, 25
5. Bramm G, Olsen DB, Novak P, Ruge I (1983) Ventil- und lagerfreie Blutpumpen zur Reduzierung von Blutschäden im Langzeiteinsatz. 17th Annual meeting at the German society of biomedical technology, Suppl 28:3
6. Bramm G, Olsen DB (1984) Reduction of coagulation and hemolysis by sealless and bearingless blood pump systems for long-term application. In: Unger F (ed) Assisted circulation 2. Springer, Berlin Heidelberg New York Tokyo
7. Gillis MF, Walkup PC (1969) Studies on the effect of added andogenous heat and on heat exchanger designs. Report, Battelle memorial institute, Pacific Northwest Lab, Richland, Wash
8. Pegg C, Sandberg G, Lee R, Huffman P, Normann J (1969) Effects of intracorporeal Sr 90–Am 241/Be sources (RES) simulating radiation fields from Pu-238-fueled artificial heart (Abstract). Fed Proc 28(2):789
9. Norman JC, Harvex RJ, Covelli VH, Mc Candlers W, Bernhard WF (1967) Implantable power sources: continuing studies. Proceedings of 20th Annual Conference on Engineering in Medicine and Biology, Boston, vol 9, no 3/4
10. Natl Heart Lung and Blood Inst (1980) Performance definitions for energy systems. Report, contractors meeting of the device and technology branch. National Heart Lung and Blood Institute, Bethesda
11. Bramm G, Ruge I (1981) New control and system – conception of a heart-lung-machine. Proceedings IIIrd meeting of the ISAO, Paris 1981, suppl vol 5, pp 372–375
12. Bramm G, Koschke P, Gaab M (1982) Cavity resonator sensing system. In: Proceedings World Congress on Medical Engineering. MPBE, Hamburg

19. The Spindle Pump – A Nonpulsatile Blood Pump for Assisted Circulation *

J. HAGER, F. BRANDSTAETTER, O. DIETZE, I. KOLLER, and F. UNGER

During the past few years the development of nonpulsatile blood pumps has been encouraged as an alternative to membrane pumps. Most of these pumps were planned for left ventricular or biventricular assistance and only some for cardiac replacement [1, 3, 6, 8, 10, 12–14]. While all were very durable and reliable, it quickly became apparent that they were plagued with various problems, such as traumatic hemolysis, thromboembolic complications, and sealing difficulties [1, 3, 7, 14]. Despite these problems several short-term clinical applications were risked [2, 9, 11, 15]. To deal with these limiting factors we chose the spindle pump concept, the essential aim being to achieve, by proper design, sufficient volume output at low rpm rates so as to minimize blood trauma [4, 5].

Development of the Spindle Pump

The form of the spindle pump is very simple; it consists of a U-shaped Plexiglas housing, with two connectors for inflow and outflow ports, and a spindle (initially made of polyvinylchloride and later of Teflon because of its low surface tension), with three windings, an axle bearing, and an electric motor (Fig. 1). The function-

* With support of the Austrian Research Council, project no. P 5186 and the National Jubiläumsfond, project no. 2341.

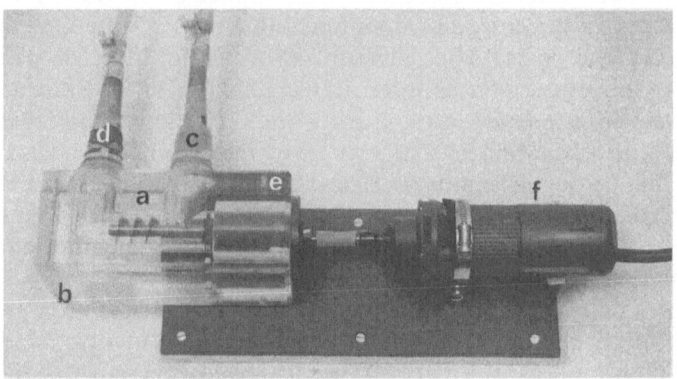

Fig. 1. View of the spindle pump (third prototype). *a*, spindle; *b*, housing; *c*, inflow tract; *d*, outflow tract; *e*, sealing and ball bearing; *f*, electric motor (of Bosch Comp., 220 V, 500 W)

ing of this blood pump is based on two components: by rotation of the spindle, the fluid, due to its viscosity, begins to rotate in the screw windings and is forced against the cylinder walls by centrifugal force; simultaneously it is pushed forward by the screw blades.

The main problem in developing this pump was calculation of the spindle's dimension, the base for this calculation being a quadratic equation:

$$(d_a^2 - d_k^2) \cdot \frac{\pi}{4} \cdot a \cdot n - \frac{d_a - d_k}{2} \cdot (a - f) \cdot v = V^*$$

d_a = external diameter of the spindle screw (cm)
d_k = internal diameter of the spindle screw (cm)
a = screw pitch (cm)
n = revolutions per second (in hertz, since measured inductively with a frequency meter)
f = thickness of screw blades (cm)
v = back-flow speed of the fluid that is a result of the induced pressure differential (cm/s)
V^* = fluid volume pumped per second (cm^3/s)

On the basis of given values (first the goal of 4 l moved per minute in mock circulation by a pressure difference of 130 torr between inflow- and outflow-tract at 3500 rpm was established), the following figures were determined: 4 cm as the smallest external diameter and different values for the internal diameter between 1.38 and 2.43 cm. It should be noted that the presence of three screw windings has no bearing on the equation.

Tests of the diverse prototypes as left ventricular assist devices (LVAD) were performed in mock circulation and in animal experiments with calves (weighing 74–106 kg).

The operation technique was as follows: after left-side thoracotomy with resection of the fifth rib, double purse-string sutures were applied on the descending aorta immediately after the aortic arch and, after opening the pericardium, on the left atrial appendage of the heart. After heparinization with 330 IE/kg body weight the outflow cannula of the device (aortic arch cannula A211-95, Stöckert-Shiley, diameter 8.7 mm) was inserted into the aorta and the inflow cannula (venous catheter V121-50, Stöckert-Shiley, diameter 50 F) into the left ventricular cavity via the left atrium through the mitral valve. The cannulas were connected to the spindle pump and after air removal of the system left ventricular assistance began. In all experiments the animals were kept heparinized according to the results of active clotting time tests.

The first prototypes had a good pumping capacity in mock circulation and showed a favorable hemodynamic effect in animal experiments but involved a still unacceptable traumatic hemolysis. Even at low speeds (3600–4800 rpm, depending on the arterial pressure of the experimental calf) to achieve nonpulsatility (Fig. 2) it was not possible to restrict blood trauma to a level within acceptable limits; the rate of hemolysis after 10 h of pumping was nearly or over 50 mg% free hemoglobin.

ECG

AP
(mm Hg)   150
            0

CVP
(mm Hg)   40
            0
LAP
(mm Hg)   30
            0

LVP   150

(mmHg)   0

RPM   4200

            0

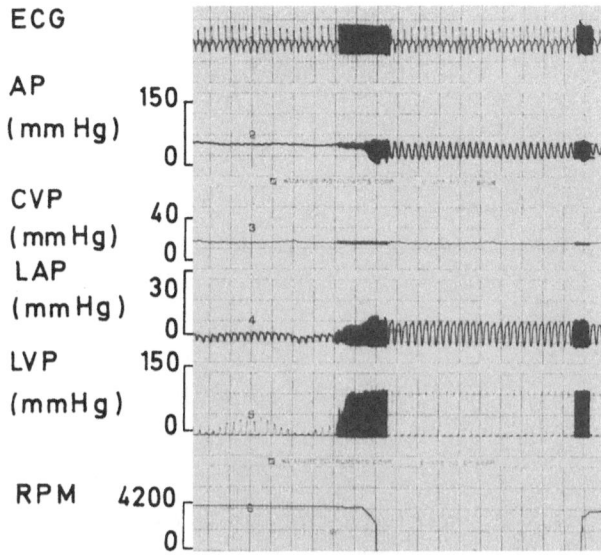

Fig. 2. Hemodynamics of the spindle pump (sixth prototype) in LVAD position in a calf experiment. *AP*, arterial pressure; *LAP*, left atrial pressure; *LVP*, left ventricular pressure; *CVP*, central venous pressure

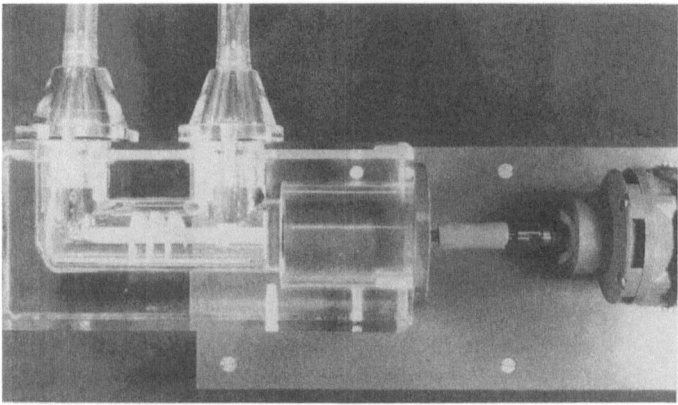

Fig. 3. Tenth prototype of the spindle pump. The inner diameter of the spindle is 1.38 cm; the outer diameter, 4 cm; the thickness of the screw blades, 1.8 mm

Various modifications were therefore made in the internal diameter and in the pitch (Fig. 3). Also, the initial 4 l moved per minute were corrected upwards, since the pump in animal experiments was not "elastic" enough, to 6 l/min (by a pressure difference between inflow- and outflow-port of 130 torr at 3500 rpm). The external diameter of the spindle screw was consequently enlarged to 4.5 cm and for the internal diameter two alternative values were determined: 2 and 3.5 cm. In the interest of a light spindle with a small practical design, the first alternative was initially put into practice. However, the next pumps were despite a decreasing of the revolution number to 3000 rpm not successful in controlling traumatic hemolysis because of the excessive vacuum effect (Figs. 4, 5).

ECG

AP
(mmHg)

LAP
(mmHg)

LVP
(mmHg)

RPM

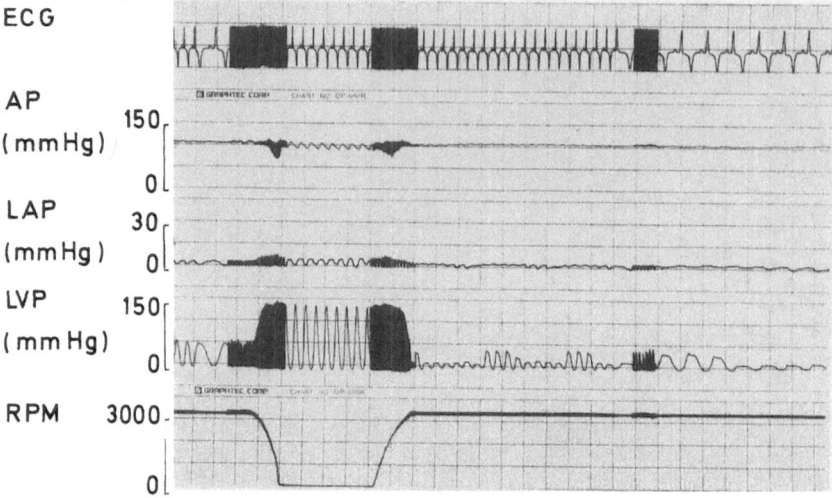

Fig. 4. Hemodynamic changes with the spindle pump (11th prototype) in a calf with normal heart functions

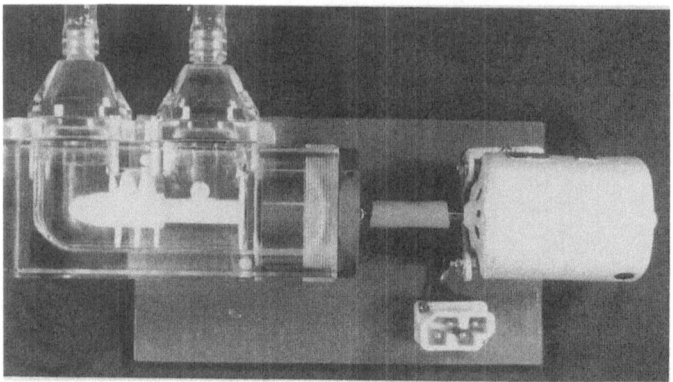

Fig. 5. Twelfth prototype of the spindle pump. The housing is newly designed; the inner diameter of the spindle is 2 cm in the area of the screw blades (to the rear, 1.4 cm); the outer diameter is 4.5 cm

As a consequence, the second alternative solution of the quadratic equation for the inner diameter was considered, e.g. 3.5 cm. The now enlarged spindle had a detrimental effect on the axle bearing because of it's weightiness resulting that is was made of Teflon which has a high density ($\varrho = 2.5$ g/cm^3). Moreover the spindle screw was subject to additional vibrations through which damage to the cylinder walls became a possibility.

Therefore, a modification of the spindle was undertaken in which the gap between the cylinder walls and the outer edge of the screw blade was enlarged from a tolerance minimum to 0.06 cm (Fig. 6). A further effect of this was a reduction

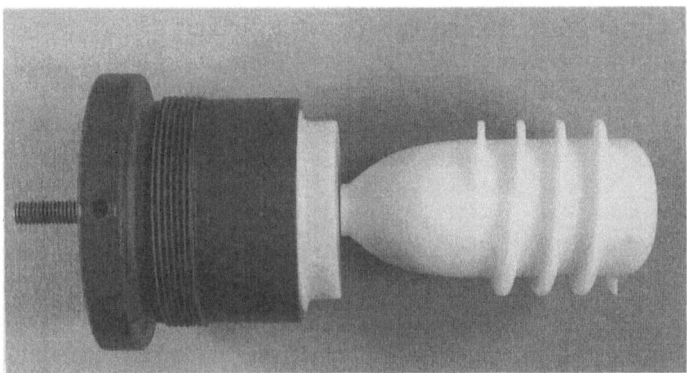

Fig. 6. Completely redesigned spindle (15th prototype). Enlarged (inner diameter, 3.5 cm) and in typical streamline form

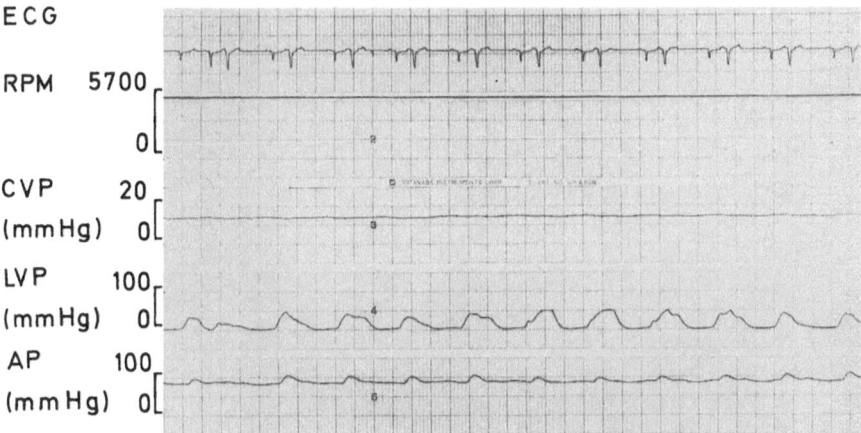

Fig. 7. Hemodynamic study in a calf experiment with the 15th prototype of the spindle pump as LVAD. A speed of 5700 rpm is necessary to achieve a nonpulsatile blood flow, given an arterial pressure of the animal of 100 mmHg

in the velocity gradient of the blood in the gap, which had an ameliorating influence on the blood trauma. However, the pump thereby sacrificed efficiency. Although designed for an output of 6 l/min against a pressure differential of 130 torr at 3300 rpm, in the mock circulation it only achieved 6 l/min against 100 torr at 6000 rpm. Depending on the arterial pressure of the experimental animal, in the calves experiments a speed up to 6000 rpm was necessary to achieve a nonpulsatile flow (Fig. 7). These high speeds led to critical values in the design construction.

For this reason a further change was made in the internal diameter of the spindle. While keeping the external diameter and the pitch constant, the internal diameter was adjusted to 2.75 cm, i.e., an average of the values in the two solutions (Figs. 8, 9). With these dimensions the pump moves in mock circulation 4 l

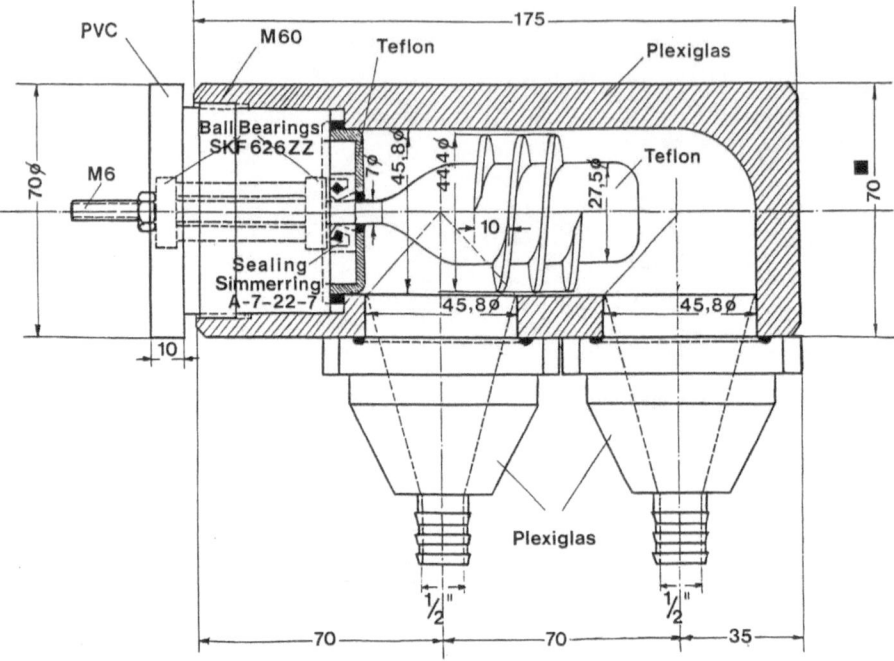

Fig. 8. Cross-sectional view of the spindle pump

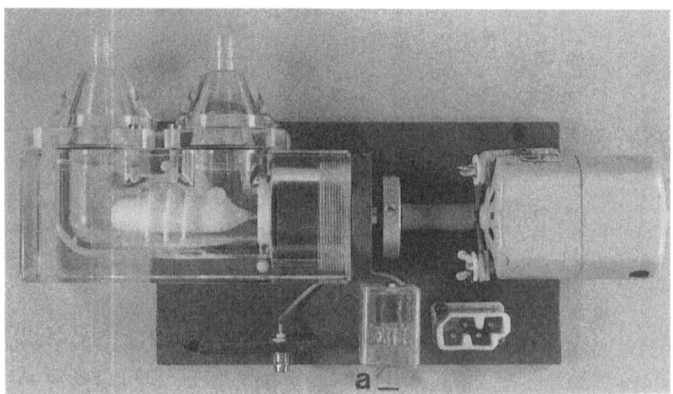

Fig. 9. Sixteenth prototype of the spindle pump. *a*, Measuring instrument for speed

water per minute against 130 torr at 4740 rpm and 6 l/min against 130 torr at 4980 rpm at a stroke volume of 9.5 cm³ and a cross-sectional loss of 1.68 cm².

These figures were confirmed in animal experiments (Fig. 10); depending on arterial blood pressure (the hearts were not damaged), a speed of up to 4800 rpm was necessary to attain a nonpulsatile flow (Fig. 11). Measurements with an electromagnetic flow meter recorded flow rates between 6 and 9 l/min depending,

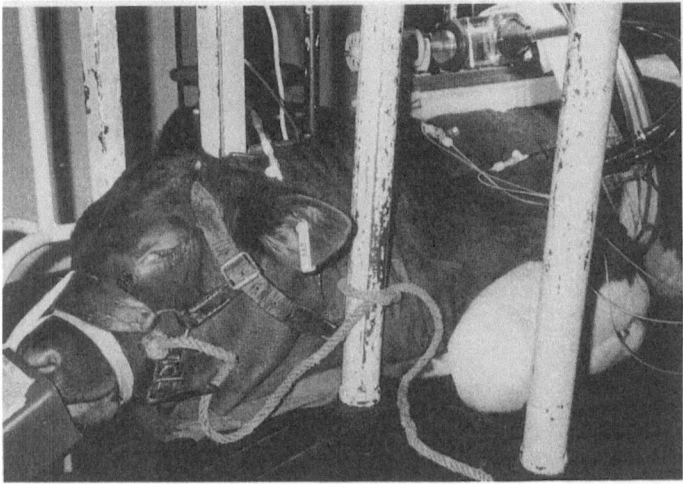

Fig. 10. Left ventricular assist experiment with calf

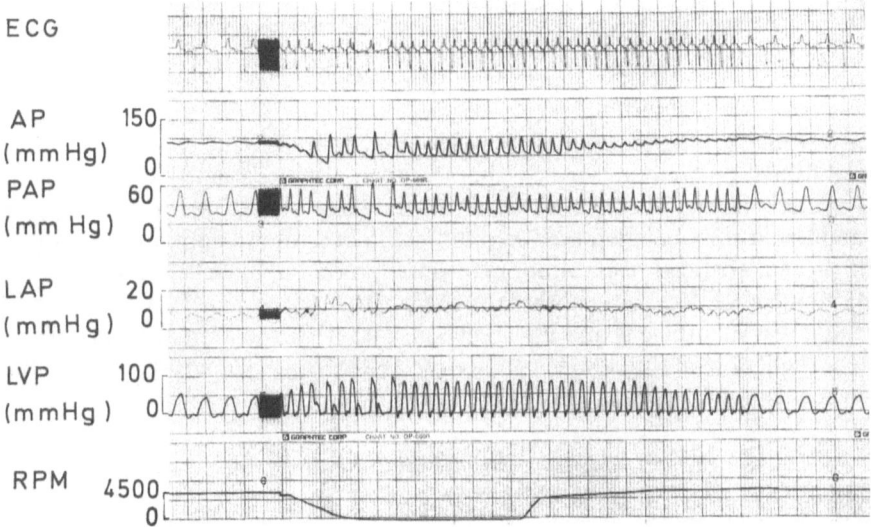

Fig. 11. Hemodynamics in a calf experiment with the 16th prototype in LVAD position (*PAP*, pulmonary artery pressure)

again, on the arterial blood pressure of the experimental animal. Traumatic hemolysis remained within acceptable limits and also stayed within the norm, or slightly above, during longer experiments (up to 63 h of pumping).

To investigate the effects of nonpulsatile blood flow on body tissues, numerous specimens of various organs were collected from the experimental animals and examined histologically and by electron microscopy. Figure 12 shows a light-microscopic section of a lung specimen (the lungs of calves are known to be par-

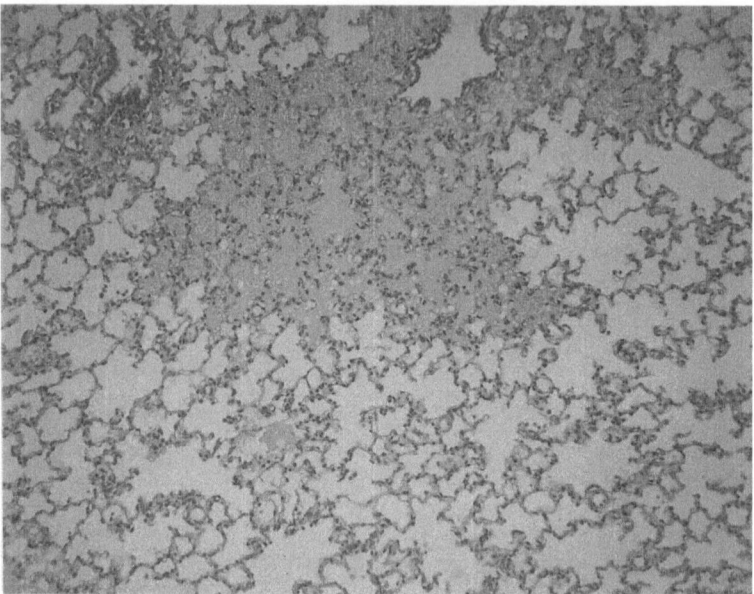

Fig. 12. Circumscribed dystelectatic area in a otherwise inconspicuous lung parenchyma (CAB, 30 ×)

ticularly vulnerable) after 30 h of pumping. Substantial tissue changes could not be established; only circumscribed alterations were to be found. Most of the lesions existed – as histological investigations showed – already before pumping began and could thus be attributed mainly to the operation (right lateral position of the thorax, artificial respiration, manipulation on the lungs, etc.). An increase in the number of lesions was seen in the postoperative phase, if the animal's breathing was insufficient and assistance necessary. If the animal remained respirated, the lesions in the lungs were barely progressive. Therefore, only a minimal influence can be assumed from pumping conditions.

Discussion

Assisted circulation or replacement of the human heart can be performed with pulsatile or nonpulsatile blood pumps. Up to now it has not been quite clear whether a pulsatile flow is necessary for perfusion of the body. It can therefore be seen as a great challenge to nature to assist or to replace a failing heart with nonpulsatile blood pumps [3, 6, 14, 15]. This possibility has been known for 25 years; Saxton and Andrew in 1960 were among the first to report the observation that in animal experiments the circulation adjusts to a pulseless flow [12].

Our experiments with the spindle pump used as LVAD have clearly demonstrated that this device completely relieves the left ventricle and effects partial functional heart replacement [4, 5]. This could be observed in long-term experiments within the first 24 h where the heart was impaired in its function due to the operation.

As a result of their simple design centrifugal pumps are very durable. Nevertheless, their two major disadvantages cannot be denied: thrombus formation and traumatic hemolysis. Unlike impeller and toroidal blood pumps, in which the formation of thrombi within the pump is a limiting factor, the spindle pump has the advantage that the axle entrance is continuously rinsed, and areas of stagnation do not develop [1, 3, 4, 6, 8, 14]. At the same time, rinsing the axis of the spindle helps to avoid overheating. The second major problem of many pulseless blood pumps, traumatic hemolysis, has presented the general problem in the development of the spindle pump [4, 5]. Several modifications of the spindle have been necessary to arrive at an adequate prototype with which the level of traumatic hemolysis remains within acceptable limits.

It became apparent in animal experiments that the main reason for blood stress was not the speed but the suction effect of the spindle pump. Although it was possible to reduce the speed to 3000 rpm, the hemolysis rate could not be lowered to a tolerable level. With our newest prototype it has become possible to obtain a nonpulsatile blood flow with a speed of 4200–4800 rpm, depending on the arterial blood pressure of the experimental animal. Survival tests (involving up to 63 h of pumping) showed that with this number of revolutions and with this design of the spindle (using a greater gap between housing and rotor), the rate of traumatic hemolysis remained within acceptable limits.

Our three acute and five survival experiments with this newest prototype have demonstrated that both problems – stress on blood cells and stress on body tissues caused by the spindle pump and its special characteristics – have largely been solved.

References

1. Affeld K, Schichl K, Yoganathan A (1986) Nonpulsatile blood pumps – summary of the ESAO workshop 1985. Herrmann Föttinger Institut, TU, Berlin
2. Belcher P, Glenville B, Cooper L (1987) Successful use of a right ventricular assist device. Br Heart J 58:162–165
3. Golding LAR (1984) Centrifugal pumps. In: Unger F (ed) Assisted circulation 2. Springer, Berlin Heidelberg New York Tokyo, pp 142–152
4. Hager J, Brandstaetter F, Koller I, Unger F (1986) The spindle pump – a new concept for a nonpulsatile blood pump. In: Nosé Y, Kjellstrand C, Ivanovich P (eds) Progress in artificial organs – 1985. ISAO Press, Cleveland, pp 354–358
5. Hager J, Brandstaetter F, Koller I, Unger F (1988) Left heart assistance with the spindle pump. Int J Artif Organs 11:465–468
6. Lefemine AA, Dunbar J, DeLucia A (1986) Concepts in assisted circulation. Texas Heart Inst J 13:23–37
7. Magovern GJ, Park SB, Maher TD (1985) Use of a centrifugal pump without anticoagulants for postoperative left ventricular assist. World J Surg 9:25–36
8. Olsen DB, Bramm G (1985) Blood pump with a magnetically suspended impeller. Trans Am Soc Artif Intern Organs 31:395–399
9. Pennington DG, Merjavy JP, Swartz MT, Willman VL (1982) Clinical experience with a centrifugal pump ventricular assist device. Trans Am Soc Artif Intern Organs 28:93–99

10. Qian KX, Wang HS (1986) A fully implantable nonpulsatile impeller pump assists the circulation of the free-walking goat. In: Nosé Y, Kjellstrand C, Ivanovich P (eds) Progress in artificial organs – 1985. ISAO Press, Cleveland, pp 464–467
11. Rose DM, Laschinger J, Grossi E, Krieger KH, Cunningham JN, Spencer FC (1985) Experimental and clinial results with a simplified left heart assist device for treatment of profound left ventricular dysfunction. World J Surg 9:11–17
12. Saxton GA, Andrew CB (1960) An ideal heart pump with hydrodynamic characteristics analogous to the mammalian heart. Trans Am Soc Artif Intern Organs 6:288–291
13. Thoma H, Losert U, Schwanda G, Stöhr H, Wolner E (1984) Development of implantable centrifugal pumps. In: Atsumi K, Maekawa M, Ota K (eds) Progress in artificial organs – 1983. ISAO Press, Cleveland, pp 152–157
14. Unger F, Genelin A, Hager J, Kemkes BM, Koller I, Schistek R (1984) Functional heart replacement with nonpulsatile assist devices. In: Unger F (ed) Assisted circulation 2. Springer, Berlin Heidelberg New York Tokyo, pp 163–174
15. Yozu R, Golding LAR, Jacobs G, Harasaki H, Nosé Y (1985) Experimental results and future prospects for a nonpulsatile cardiac prosthesis. World J Surg 9:116–127

20. Various Designs of Nonpulsatile Blood Pumps

R. Schistek

Hydrodynamic Pumps

A subset of rotary pumps are the hydrodynamic pumps. The basic parts of a hydrodynamic pump are the housing and a set of rotating blades mounted on a wheel. The energy is transmitted from the pumping wheel to the pumped fluid by hydrodynamic forces, similar to the lift of an airfoil in an airplane. For increased efficiency there can be a stator, which consists of nonmobile blades that direct the flow going into or coming out of the pumping wheel.

The pumps are classified according to the direction of the flow inside the pump: axial, radial, and diagonal. The blades of the pumping wheel can be replaced by a large surface, which moves the fluid by friction forces. Pumps are characterized by their throttle curves (Fig. 1), which show the relationship between the pump flow and the pressure at the pump outlet at increasing outflow resistance at a certain speed of rotation.

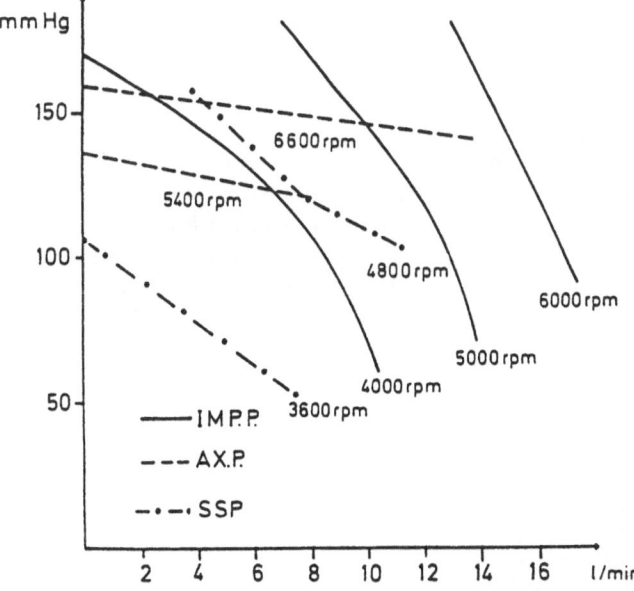

Fig. 1. Comparison of throttle curves of a radial (IMP.P.), an axial pump (AX.P.), and a spindle pump (SSP)

Assisted Circulation 3
F. Unger (Ed.)
© Springer-Verlag Berlin Heidelberg 1989

Compared with the axial pumps, the radial pumps react to increasing resistance with a greater increase in pressure. Axial pumps perform better in high-flow and low-pressure ranges. Pumping wheels can be calculated for certain flow conditions. The flow conditions are characterized by pressure difference across the pump, the flow, and the speed of rotation. The relationship between these parameters is given by Euler's equation. Jarvik et al. [1] described the calculation for an axial pump used in an implantable pulsatile heart driver. Under such conditions the efficiency is optimal; under other, less optimal conditions, the efficiency of performance drops. Therefore, the expedient layout of the pump in vivo will always compromise these optimal conditions. Radial pumps and bladeless pumps allow a larger range of reasonable pumping conditions. Axial pumps are the smallest of the hydrodynamic pumps in relation to the pump flow.

Hydrodynamic Blood Pumps

As the hydrodynamic pumps are simple in construction, with only one moving part, they have been proposed as blood pumps since the report of Saxton and Andrews in 1960 [2]. Though centrifugal pumps have been used clinically for temporary support, long-term application and intracorporeal implantation have not been successful, for several reasons: namely sealing and heat at the axle of the pumping wheel and dead-water spaces [2]. In order to make the pump smaller, suitable for total implantation, and to avoid dead-water spaces we constructed an axial blood pump for total implantation.

The Axial Blood Pump

Various axial pumps were tested in mock circulation. In order not to be limited in high-flow regions, we chose pumps larger than necessary. Our axial blood pump for animal experiments consists of a copper U-shaped housing in which a pumping wheel (impeller) is mounted. For its use as a TAH, the outflow part of the U-housing of the right pump was twisted at the level of the impeller, so that

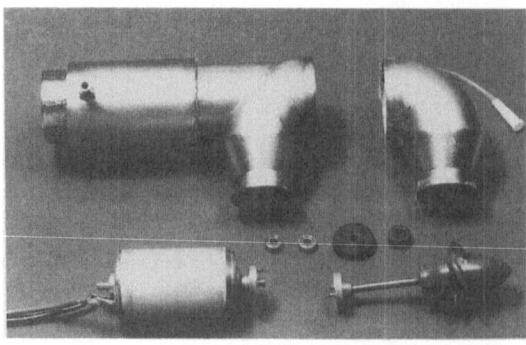

Fig. 2. Axial blood pump

the ouflow was pointed to the left when implanted, for better access to the pulmonary artery. The housing of the DC motor is flanged, as is the pump housing, for better heat conduction. The dimensions are $180 \times 40 \times 70$ mm; the weight is 850 g. The inner and outer surfaces are covered with polyurethane. For total implantation, a water-cooling system had to be employed (Fig. 2). In mock circulation a flow of 17 l/min at 6000 rpm and an arterial pressure of 100 mmHg were achieved. With low outflow resistance even a flow of up to 40 l/min was possible. The overall efficiency was between 12% and 20%.

Animal Experiments

Two types of animal experiments were performed. In the first group the pump was applied as a paracorporeal assist device, for either left or biventricular assist. In the second group two pumps were implanted to function as a total artificial heart.

Ventricular Assistance

In six acute experiments the pump was used as a left ventricular assist device (LVAD), in four cases with a beating heart and in two as a biventricular assist device (BVAD) for ventricular fibrillation (functional heart replacement). The experimental animals were calves, ranging in weight between 80 and 110 kg. A left thoracotomy was performed. The left ventricle was cannulated through the left auricle across the mitral valve. The blood was returned via a Dacron graft anastomosed end-to-side to the descending aorta. For biventricular assistance the right ventricular cannula was inserted in the right ventricle through the right

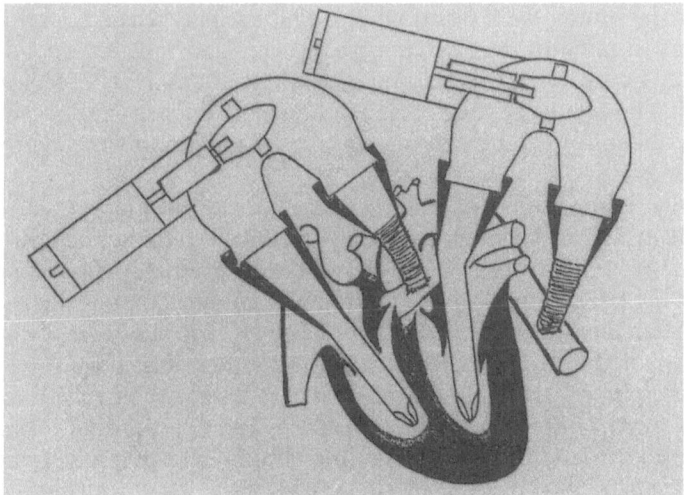

Fig. 3. BVAD with axial pumps

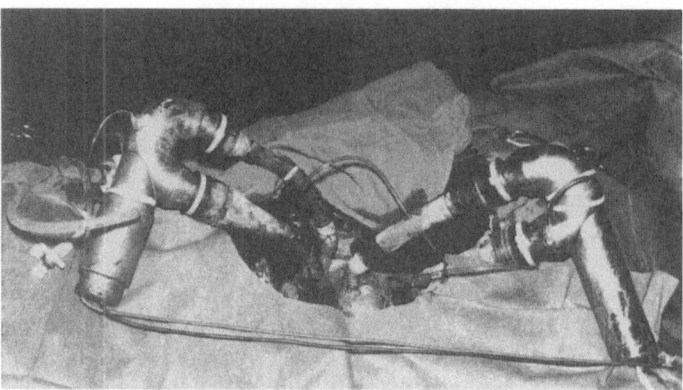

Fig. 4. BVAD with axial pumps

auricle. The return cannula was connected to a Dacron graft and this was sewn to the pulmonary artery (Figs. 3, 4). Anesthesia was continued until the experiment was terminated.

Hemolysis was measured by free plasma hemoglobin. Urine excretion was taken as a parameter of adequate cardiac output. Aortic pressure, pulmonary artery pressure, left and right atrial pressure, and voltage and current of the electric motors were documented.

Total Heart Replacement

Total cardiopulmonary bypass was initiated according to the technique described by Olsen and Murray [4]. The natural heart was excised at the level of the atrioventricular and arterial valves. Cuffs, similar to those used for the implantation of a pneumatic heart, were sewen to the left and right atria, aorta, and pulmonary artery. The axial pumps were positioned so that the part which contains the electric motor was situated in the ventral costophrenic gap. The closed side of the U of the housing pointed toward the inner side of the sternum. The electric motors were parallel. The planes of the U-shaped housings opened in an angle of 45°–90°, where by the inflow and outflow openings of the pump were nearly in the same line (Fig. 5).

Compression of the right atrium was observed in all cases, but it never led to a significant inflow obstruction. Through a venting line the air in the pump housing could be removed. Weaning from bypass was started by gradually increasing the rotation speed of the left pump. The right pump was connected after the left pump was started. After this the right pump was started. Then the flow of the heart-lung machine was reduced gradually. When the total cardiac output had been taken over by the pumps, the cannulas of the heart-lung machine were removed. The rotation speed of the pump was adjusted by hand, according to the atrial pressures. On the one hand, the atrial pressures should be kept low. On the other hand, inflow occlusion of the pump by sucking in of the atrial wall should be avoided by not emptying the atrium completely. It is typical of the hydrody-

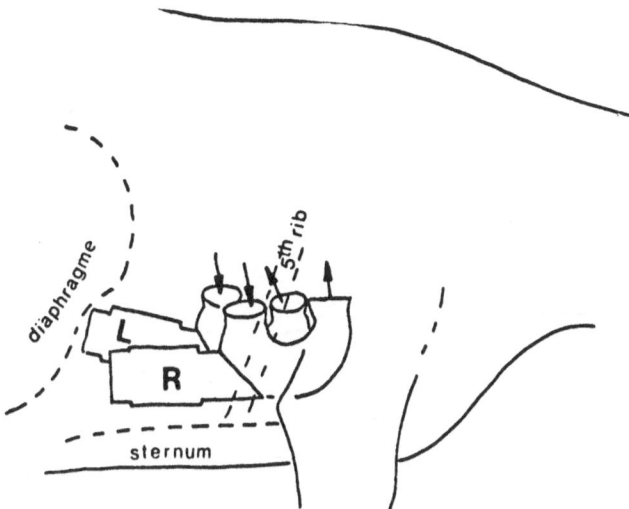

Fig. 5. TAH with axial pumps

namic pumps that the inflow pressure drops very low when the inflow is occluded. In contrast, in pulsatile membrane pumps, where the pump acts as fluid amplifier, such negative pressures are never reached. We tried to keep the aortic pressure above 60 mmHg. In all experiments, heparin administered for CPB was not reversed with protamine.

Results

Ventricular Assist

These experiments were performed mainly to show the effect of the pump on the circulation and blood damage. With the LVAD, a nonpulsatile flow in the aorta could be created. Though the natural heart was still beating, the total flow was taken over by the pump. With the BVAD it was shown that the whole circulation could be maintained by the pumps.

Total Heart Replacement

The pumps were placed in the thoracic cavity so that the thorax could be closed. In two cases it was necessary to mobilize the inferior vena cava and the right atrium to allow unimpeded flow into the pump. The maximum time of artificial circulation was 8.5 h. Reflexes and spontaneous breathing were demonstrated. Reasons for terminating the experiments were bleeding in two animals and technical defects in other two. After 2 h of pumping, the level of free plasma hemoglobin reached a mean of 92 mg% and did not rise higher. The concentration of fibrinogen and platelet count were reduced to half of the baseline value. In two cases, the blood gases were normal at the end of the experiment.

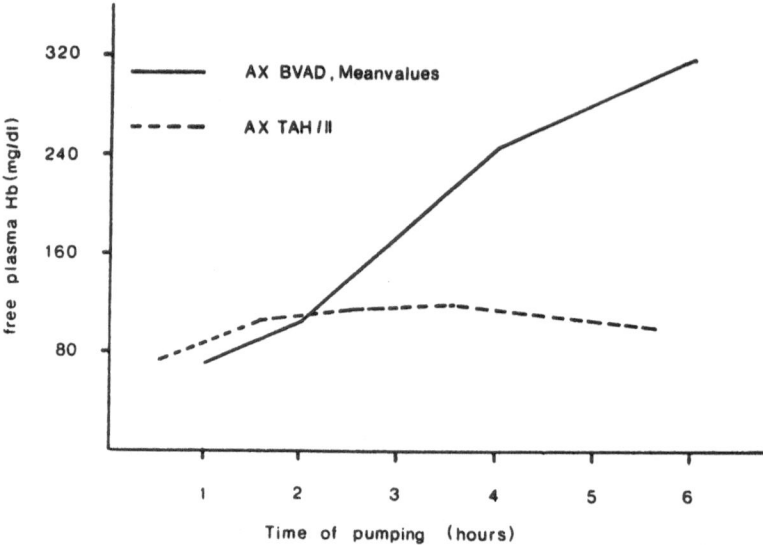

Fig. 6. Comparison of mean free plasma hemoglobin in ax-TAH and ax-BVAD experiments

Hemolysis was significantly different in the LVAD, BVAD, and TAH groups: free plasma hemoglobin ranged between 250 mg% and 500 mg% in the LVAD group with the beating natural heart, and it was 220 mg% in the BVAD group and 80 mg% in the TAH group at the end of the experiment (Fig. 6). Technical problems with the pumps (e.g., loose electric wire, incompetent sealing of the motor housing) occurred in all groups. Thrombotic depositions were found in the gap between hub and sealing of the axle. There was no sign of gross emboli at necropsy.

Discussion

It was shown that it is possible to built axial blood pumps that meet the hemodynamic requirements for total heart replacement. Circulation could be maintained for up to 8.5 h by two axial pumps; urine excretion manifested adequate cardiac output. Thrombotic deposits were found, as in our previous study with another type of centrifugal pump [5]: despite the facts that the longest pumping time was 8.5 h and that systemic heparinization was maintained throughout, thrombi were found in the gap between the impeller and the sealing. Therefore, it has to be assumed that thromboembolism can occur when using this pump as well. Hemolysis was the highest in the LVAD experiments. In BVAD it was much lower, but still higher than that in TAH experiments. This difference can be explained partly by the different pumping conditions. In left ventricular assistance the pump had to overcome the pressure built up by the natural heart and the resistance of the cannulas. Moreover, the pump flow is only a part of the systemic output. For these pumping conditions, a radial or a piston-type pump would meet the requirements much better. In our BVAD experiments the natural heart was excluded from circulation by setting it in fibrillation. The total cardiac output was produced by two pumps, and there was no pressure produced by the heart that had to be overcome. Even better conditions could be achieved by using the pumps as an orthotopic artificial heart. Here, the long cannulas used in the paracorporeal position could be avoided. Though free plasma hemoglobin was comparatively low in the TAH group, it is still too high, even for the chronic animal experiments. It is likely that the plateau in the TAH free hemoglobin curve is due to hemodilution by blood loss and nonhemic volume substitution. Renal excretion of hemoglobin also has to be considered.

The poor hydraulic efficiency, caused by our overestimation of the pump size and omission of a stator, could be an additional a reason for the high traumatization of the blood. To overcome this inefficiency and its attendant hazards we constructed a pump according to Euler's equation for the following conditions:

Mean pressure	80 mm Hg
Rotation speed	10 000 rpm
Flow	8 l/min
Thickness of blades	1 mm
Efficiency assumed	0.7

The result was a pumping propeller with an outer diameter of 1.5 cm and a hub diameter of 1 cm. The maximum relative fluid speed inside the pump was calculated to be 9 m/s (32 km/h!).

Another important aspect was to avoid the weak points of nonpulsatile pumps by avoiding the blood contact with sealing and axle. An ideal, but a technically sophisticated, solution is the magnetically suspended rotor pump, as proposed by Olsen and Bramm [7]. Another solution would be a rotary pump in which inlet and outlet are peripheral and the centrifugal forces allow the air to float in the center of the pump. It is possible to modify it so that an air bubble is stabilized in the center of the pump, which separates the blood from the axle and the sealing. We have constructed such a system with a side-channel pump (Fig. 7). In our initial experiments with the side-channel pump (R. Schistek, unpublished data) the

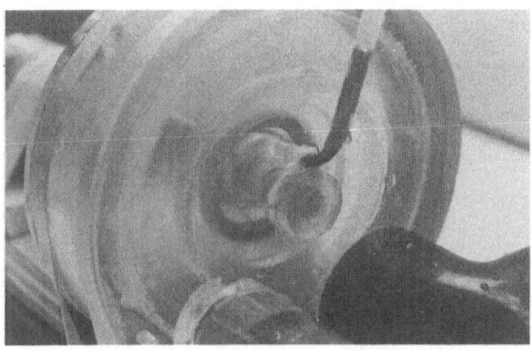

Fig. 7. Side-channel pump: the air bubble can be seen in the center of the pump. Inlet and outflow tubes are seen at the bottom

central air bubble was created. However, we have not yet solved the problem of keeping the axle actually dry.

References

1. Jarvik RK, Nielsen SD, Orth J, Summers RL, Isaacson MS, Kolff WD (1978) Development of a reversing electrohydraulic energy converter for left ventricular assist devices. Annual report, Devices and Technology Branch, Division of Heart and Vascular Diseases, National Heart and Lung Institute, Washington DC
2. Saxton GA, Andrews CB (1960) An ideal heart pump with hydrodynamic characteristics analogous to the mammalian heart. Trans Am Soc Artif Intern Organs 6:288–291
3. Golding LR, Murakami G, Harasaki H et al. (1982) Chronic nonpulsatile blood flow. Trans Am Soc Artif Intern Organs 28:81–85
4. Olsen DB, Murray KD (1984) The total artificial heart. In: Unger F (ed) Assisted circulation, 2nd edn. Springer, Berlin Heidelberg New York Tokyo, pp 197–228
5. Hager J, Schistek R, Stoss FF, Unger F, Kemkes BM (1983) Biventricular assisted circulation with the impeller pump. Acta Chir Austr 15:121–128
6. Kolff WJ (1988) The tenth Hastings lecture: experience and practical considerations for the future of artificial hearts and of mankind. Artif Organs 12(1):89–106

Part III
Bridging to Transplantation

21. The Use of Artificial Hearts for Bridging to Transplantation

F. UNGER

The idea of using an artificial heart as a bridge to a consecutive transplantation dates back to 1969, when Cooley performed the first bridge in a patient with postoperative cardiac failure. To date, and especially in the past 9 years, 111 artificial hearts have been used and 74 pulsatile ventricular assist devices.

The main indications for using a TAH or an LVAD are: (a) a patient awaiting transplantation whose condition is deteriorating, (b) acute cardiogenic shock, (c) postoperative cardiac failure syndrome, and (d) graft rejection. The patients have to meet all requirements for a consecutive transplantation so that the donor organ is not spoiled. There are hearts available (Jarvik 7-70, Berlin, Ellipsoid, Penn-State) which are driven pneumatically. In 72 of the patients who received a TAH (64%) a consecutive transplantation has been performed, and 29 of these are alive (40% of the transplant-group population, 26% of the total; Fig. 1).

A positive outcome can be expected in people under 40 years of age and who are on the device for a week, to avoid organ malfunction, but are weaned off as soon as the whole organism has recovered.

This chapter presents the latest results from eight of the 29 groups dealing with TAH implantation. Dr. Frazier and Dr. Cooley report on their experience since 1982. They have used 30 IABPs, three LVADs, three VADs, and two TAHs in 26 patients. They discuss the selection criteria in detail in respect to the individual outcome.

Drs. Icenogle and Copeland, from Arizona, also report their experience. They used seven TAHs in six patients for bridging, and two of them survived (33%). They report on the severe complications, especially embolism, which is created in the Jarvik heart within the DH-junction inside the blood chamber, and severe infection.

Dr. Griffith, from Pittsburgh, used the Jarvik heart in 26 cases as a bridge; nine patients survived the transplantation. In his paper the contraindications are

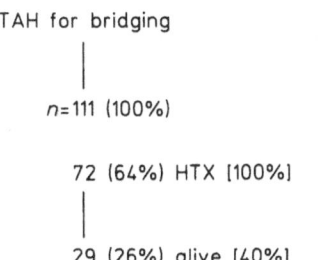

TAH for bridging

$n=111$ (100%)

72 (64%) HTX [100%]

29 (26%) alive [40%]

Fig. 1. Results of TAH used for bridging to transplantation (*HTX*) in 111 patients

Assisted Circulation 3
F. Unger (Ed.)
© Springer-Verlag Berlin Heidelberg 1989

exactly defined. He points out the incidence of severe infections and the source of thromboembolization.

In 1986 the editor performed the first European bridge-to-heart transplantation with the Ellipsoid heart. The Ellipsoid heart was evaluated in long experimental series in calves and has been used since 1977 clinically as an LVAD. The main goal of its design was to eliminate all stagnation areas within the blood chamber to avoid thrombus formation. This goal was achieved in 20 cases with an LVAD and with four TAH implantations; in three cases Dr. Wolner form Vienna used the Ellipsoid heart. Dr. Trubel from the Vienna group reports on five cases, three using the Unger design and two the Berlin design.

In Philadelphia, Dr. Kolff and his father, the great pioneer Dr. W.J. Kolff, developed the "Philadelphia heart system." The lens-shaped ventricle consists of three pieces which are vacuum molded. This technique allows great reproducibility and is inexpensive in production. Dr. Kolff performed feasibility studies in seven cadavers. The design criteria are very clear. This heart is now being reproduced by the groups in Berlin and Vienna.

Dr. Loisance thinks that mechanical support for bridging is not necessary. He shows the superior effectiveness of the modern catecholamines, such as enoximone, and he thinks that with proper administration, bridging with artificial ventricles can be avoided.

The Salt Lake City group, with Dr. Paulis and Dr. Olsen, addresses the problems of designing artificial ventricles. In general, bridging is still a therapeutic concept which will be realized clinically step by step.

Most survivers are patients who received a chance to live literally at the last possible moment. Despite the generally good first results, patients must be selected more carefully so that bridging does not spoil the valuable donor heart. Claims have been made that bridging can make transplantation unnecessary. This is wishful thinking, because in bridging the overall survival is only 26%. The TAH as a bridging device is to be considered only in combination with a transplant program. The indication for bridging is also given in a highly selected group of patients with postoperative cardiac failure. Paulis and Olsen describe the critical parts of the Jarvik TAH and its sites for thrombus formation [1]. The Jarvik TAH has been successful as a bridge in 55% of cases.

Reference

1. Olsen DB, Unger F (1975) Thrombi formation within the artificial heart. J Thorac Cardiovasc Surg 82:157–168

22. Use of Cardiac Assist Devices as Bridges to Cardiac Transplantation: Review of Current Status and Report of the Texas Heart Institute's Experience

O. H. FRAZIER and D. A. COOLEY

With the introduction of the potent and more selective immunosuppressant cyclosporin A (CsA) in the early 1980s [1–3], cardiac transplantation changed from an experimental procedure into an accepted therapeutic modality. Since that time, transplantation has offered the only hope for numerous patients with end-stage heart disease. Donor availability has not kept pace with the growing number of patients awaiting cardiac transplantation, however, and approximately 20% of potential transplant recipients die before a suitable donor can be found [4]. This dilemma has led to a renewed interest in "staged" cardiac replacement, using mechanical circulatory support to sustain these patients during the critical waiting period.

At the Texas Heart Institute, hemodynamically unstable heart transplant patients are immediately considered for a cardiac assist device. Indications for mechanical support are progressive heart failure unresponsive to medical therapy, signs of low perfusion (increased BUN and creatinine, increased total bilirubin, increased A-VO$_2$ differences), refractory angina, and uncontrolled arrhythmias.

Our first choice for mechanical assist is the intra-aortic balloon pump (IABP), which is easy to insert, simple to operate, and can effectively augment the cardiac output. When the IABP proves ineffective, more escalated forms of support – a left ventricular assist device (LVAD), a biventricular bypass pump, or a total artificial heart (TAH) – are considered.

This chapter reviews the background, comparative features, and current status of these cardiac assist devices and presents an overview of our experience with staged cardiac transplantation since July 1982, when the Texas Heart Institute reestablished its program in cardiac transplantation, using CsA for immunosuppression.

Types of Cardiac Assist Devices

Intra-aortic Balloon Pump

The IABP is a means of partial circulatory support that has been used extensively and successfully at our institution (Fig. 1). Developed by Moulopoulos and colleagues [5] in 1962 and first used clinically by Kantrowitz [6] in 1968, this device gained widespread acceptance in the management of high-risk operative patients with low cardiac output owing to reversible ventricular dysfunction [7–9]. The IABP was the first assist device to be successfully used for staged cardiac trans-

Assisted Circulation 3
F. Unger (Ed.)
© Springer-Verlag Berlin Heidelberg 1989

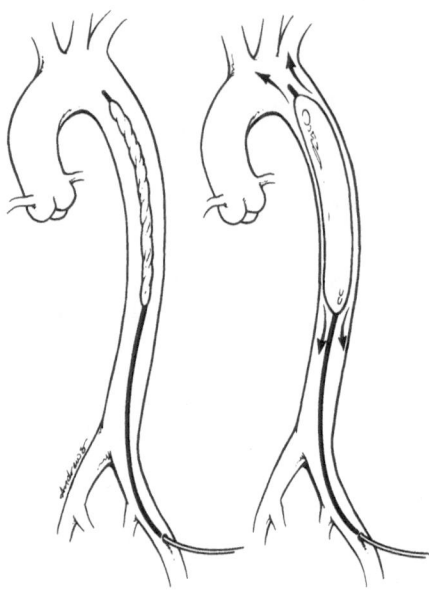

Fig. 1. Schematic representations (deflation/inflation) of the IABP

plantation: this breakthrough was reported in 1978, by Reemtsma and associates [10], who used the device to support three patients with hemodynamic deterioration until heart transplantation could be performed; all three survived and were able to leave the hospital.

The IABP's effectiveness is based on improving the circulation [11]: balloon deflation reduces the impedance to systolic ejection and thereby decreases the cardiac wall tension or afterload (-10%) and decreases oxygen consumption (-10%); phased inflation of the balloon during diastole then results in augmentation of the coronary circulation. Thus, coronary diastolic blood flow and myocardial oxygen delivery are both enhanced. The cardiac output may rise by as much as 30% – an increase from 550 to 800 ml/min is typical (Table 1) – and renal function is improved (Table 2). Complications of IABP use are generally minimal, although lower limb ischemia can occur and dissection has been reported [12]. The IABP should not be implanted when peripheral vascular occlusive disease is present. In our series, infection occurred in three patients and femoral artery thrombosis in one patient.

Because the IABP can only assist the function of the failing left ventricle, the technique's usefulness is limited in circumstances requiring an actual substitute

Table 1. Effects of IABP on hemodynamic status ($n = 16$ patients)

	Cardiac index (l/min/m²)	Systemic vascular resistance (dynes s cm⁻⁵)
Minimum change	↑ 0.7	↓ 462
Maximum change	↑ 2.07	↓ 2392
Mean change (of all pts)	↑ 1.39	↓ 1203

Table 2. Effects of IABP on renal function ($n = 16$ patients)

	BUN (mmol/l)	Creatinine (mg/dl)
Minimum change	↓ 16	↓ 0.3
Maximum change	↓ 43	↓ 3.4
Mean change (of all pts)	↓ 31	↓ 2.1

for left ventricular function. Moreover, the IABP provides very little assistance to the failing right ventricle. When the patient does not remain stable on IABP and when mechanical assistance is needed, an LVAD is often the alternative of choice.

Left Ventricular Assist Device

In the early 1970s, the Cullen Cardiovascular Research Laboratories of the Texas Heart Institute became heavily involved in the investigation of LVADs. Extensive implantations and operative tests in calves were conducted to determine both the effectiveness and the limitations of these devices. This experience led to the first clinical implantation of the LVAD as a bridge to transplantation, in 1978, when Norman and colleagues [13] used an abdominal left ventricular assist device (ALVAD) to support the circulation of a patient with "stone heart" for 5 days until orthotopic transplantation could be performed. Although the patient died 14 days after receiving the donor heart, the ALVAD's ability to provide complete circulatory support, even in the face of absent right ventricular function, was demonstrated.

The first LVAD-assisted staged cardiac transplantation to result in long-term survival was performed in September 1984, by Oyer and associates, at Stanford University. The patient, a 51-year-old man with ischemic cardiomyopathy, was sustained by an LVAD for 9 days before undergoing an orthotopic cardiac transplant. The patient remains alive and well.

Unlike the IABP, which is a volume-displacement pump that augments the existing circulation and depends on a regular electrocardiographic signal, the LVAD is a true blood pump that can capture the entire cardiac output while the biological heart remains in place and that can improve hemodynamic parameters (Table 3). Because the LVAD can be activated either synchronously or asynchronously, it is not dependent upon the natural heart's function. Potential complications associated with LVAD use include bleeding, thromboembolism, hemolysis, renal failure, and infection related to the necessity for percutaneous cannulas.

Our institution now uses, under FDA protocol, the Thermedics Model 14 LVAD (Thermedics Corporation, Waltham, Massachusetts), a pusher-plate blood pump that is pneumatically powered by an external control system (Figs. 2, 3). The inflow and outflow conduits, which consist of 20-mm-diameter woven Dacron grafts, are attached to the left ventricular apex and the ascending aorta, respectively. Each conduit contains a glutaraldehyde-preserved porcine xenograft

Table 3. Clinical LVAD: percent change in hemodynamics from pre- to postimplantation

	Study 1	Study 2	Study 3
HR (bpm)	↓ 2%	↑ 5%	↑ 17%
RAP (mm Hg)	NC	↑ 22%	↓ 21%
PAP (mm Hg)	↑ 6%	NC	↓ 9%
PCWP (mm Hg)	↓ 54%	↓ 28%	↓ 50%
AoP (mm Hg)	↑ 3%	↑ 13%	↑ 9%
CI (l/min/m^2)	↑ 4%	↑ 63%	↑ 84%
SVR (dynes)	↓ 4%	↓ 34%	↓ 35%
PVR (Wood units)	↑ 203%	↑ 25%	↑ 6%
Urine (ml/h)	↑ 237%	↓ 39%	↑ 259%

HR, heart rate; RAP, right atrial pressure; NC, no change; PAP, pulmonary arterial pressure; PCWP, pulmonary capillary wedge pressure; AoP, aortic pressure; CI, cardiac index; SVR, systemic vascular resistance; PVR, pulmonary vascular resistance

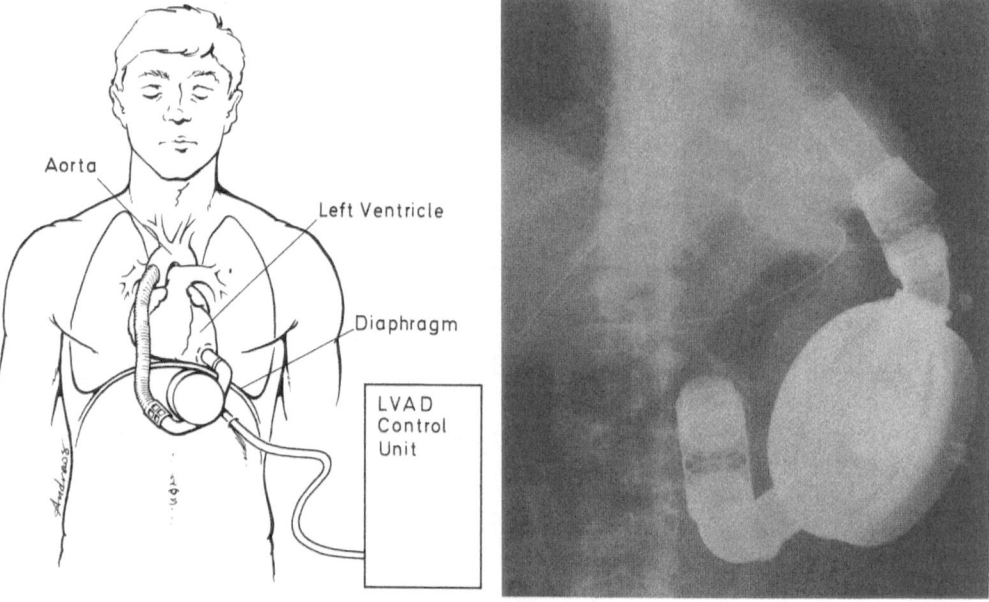

Fig. 2   **Fig. 3**

Fig. 2. Schematic representation of the implanted LVAD

Fig. 3. Roentgenogram showing the position of the implanted device

valve. The flexible pump bladder and metal components are covered with a prosthetic interface consisting of randomly distributed, flocked polyester fibrils; these provide a uniform blood/material surface that promotes the development of a thin fibrin-cellular coagulum (Fig. 4). The device has a maximum stroke volume of 85 ml and provides either synchronized counterpulsation or fixed-rate pumping.

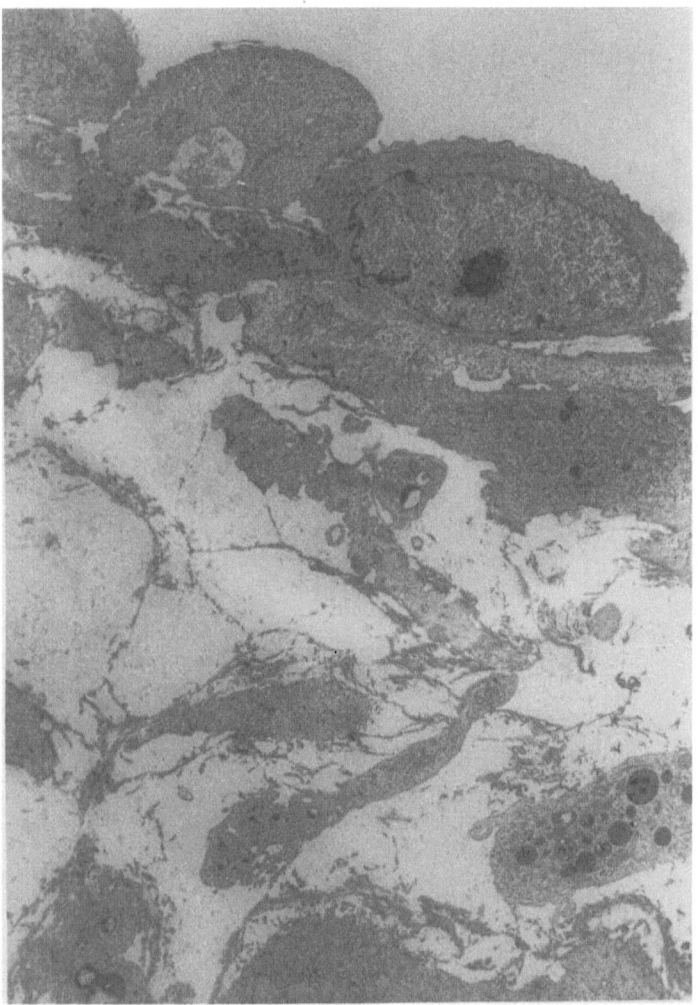

Fig. 4. Scanning electron micrograph showing formation of a pump lining composed of cellular elements from a patient's bloodstream

Whereas patients with isolated left ventricular failure and in some instances of associated right ventricular failure can usually be sustained with LVAD pumping alone, patients with biventricular failure who do not respond to inotropic drugs may need biventricular support to survive. In both instances, support is continued until the patient's renal and hepatic functions improve sufficiently to attempt transplantation.

Ventricular Bypass Pump

The Biomedicus Biopump (Biomedicus, Eden Prairie, Minnesota) extracorporeal centrifugal system was initially developed by Kletschka and Rafferty [14] for use

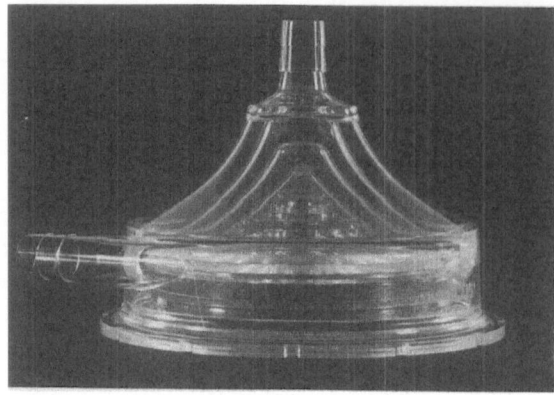

Fig. 5. The Biomedicus Biopump

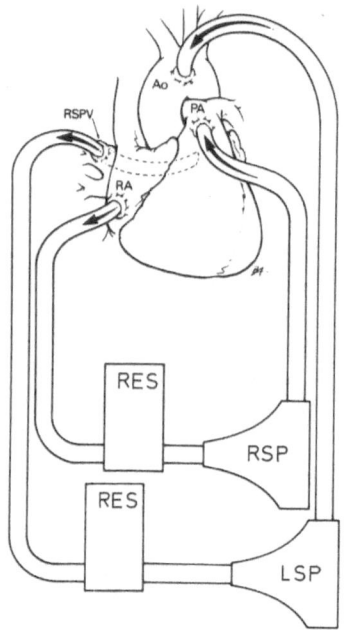

Fig. 6. Schematic representation of the ventricular bypass circuit. *Ao*, aorta; *PA*, pulmonary artery; *RSPV*, right superior pulmonary vein; *RA*, right atrium; *RES*, reservoir; *RSP*, right side pump; *LSP*, left side pump

as an artificial heart. Since its introduction in 1976, however, it has mainly been used to provide cardiopulmonary perfusion for open-heart surgery and to furnish temporary mechanical support for the failing heart [15–17].

The Biopump system consists of a portable console and a disposable pump head. The pump (Fig. 5) operates according to the same principle as a cyclone, moving the fluid gently by means of smooth rotator cones and providing flows that range from less than 100 ml to over 10 l/min. The hydrodynamically designed rotator cones are fabricated from nonthrombogenic acrylics. The basic flow is nonpulsatile and demand-responsive – that is, the rate and pressure are adjusted automatically, depending on the degree of resistance encountered and the amount of fluid returned (Fig. 6). The pulsatile controls allow nonsynchronous pulsatile operation, with variations in both rate and pressure. However, clinical experience to date does not indicate that pulsatile flow is necessary for survival.

In comparison to traditional roller-type pumps, centrifugal blood pumps offer several advantages: they reduce trauma to blood elements, thus decreasing the risk of hemolysis; they necessitate little or no heparinization; they do not need either compliance chambers or valves; they will not pump or suck air around the atrial cannulation site; and they will not pump against resistance. The Biomedicus Biopump can provide a cardiac output in excess of basic metabolic requirements. It is easy and safe to operate. In our hospital, no additional technicians are required. Because it involves the use of percutaneous cannulas, however, the risk of infection is increased.

Total Artificial Heart

The world's first staged cardiac transplantation took place at our institution in April 1969 [18]. The patient, a 47-year-old man with terminal cardiac disease who could not be weaned from cardiopulmonary bypass, was supported with a Liotta pneumatic double-ventricle prosthesis for 64 h until a donor heart could be found. Although he succumbed to pneumonia 32 h after transplantation, this case demonstrated the feasibility of staged cardiac replacement and encouraged further development of cardiac prostheses. In July 1981, we implanted an Akutsu Model III, Series 3 TAH in a 36-year-old man who could not be weaned from cardiopulmonary bypass despite IABP support. The TAH sustained the patient for 54 h until cardiac allografting could be performed, but he died approximately 1 week later of multiple organ failure [19]. The first TAH-assisted staged cardiac transplantation to result in long-term survival was performed in a 25-year-old man by Copeland and associates of the University of Arizona [20].

Total artificial heart research has been the focus of worldwide efforts, and several hearts are available, all of which have separate left and right ventricles; highly smooth, seam-free polyurethane blood-contacting sacs; tilting disk valves; vessel-to-prosthetic ventricle quick connectors; and an ejection fraction of 70% or greater [21]. One of the most successful models has been the Jarvik-7 TAH (Symbion, Inc., Salt Lake City, Utah), which captured public attention in December 1982 when it was implanted in Barney Clark in Salt Lake City; Clark was subsequently sustained by the device for 112 days. The Jarvik-7 TAH was later used as a permanent system in four other patients. Numerous transplant centers have been authorized – including the Texas Heart Institute – to use the Jarvik-7 TAH for staged cardiac transplantation. Only one center (Humana Heart Institute, Louisville, Kentucky) has been authorized to implant the device on a permanent basis [22].

The Jarvik-7 TAH (Figs. 7, 8) closely resembles the Akutsu III model developed in our laboratory (Fig. 9). Its two spherical polyurethane ventricles can be "quick-connected" to the natural atria (by means of Dacron felt cuffs) and to the great vessels (by means of Dacron grafts). Each blood chamber contains two Medtronic tilting disk valves of pyrolytic carbon. The diaphragm consists of three layers of Avcothane, with graphite between the blood-contacting layer and the

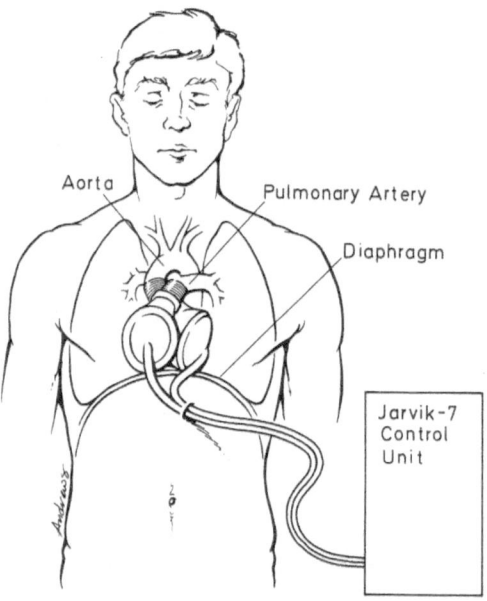

Aorta

Pulmonary Artery

Diaphragm

Jarvik-7
Control
Unit

Fig. 7. Schematic representation of the Jarvik-7 TAH implanted for use as a bridge for staged cardiac transplantation

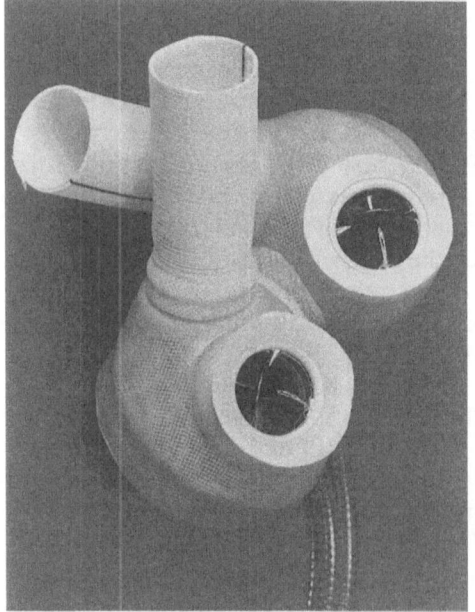

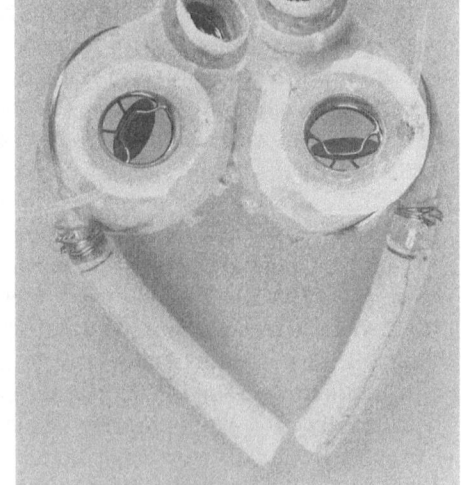

Fig. 8. The Jarvik-7 TAH

Fig. 9. The Akutsu III TAH

air-contacting layer. Each ventricle offers a maximum end-diastolic volume of 150 ml and a maximum stroke volume of 100 ml, for an ejection fraction of 67%. Unfortunately, the Jarvik-7 TAH will not fit easily in all normal-sized adult patients, and external power is required.

The TAH's advantages include the fact that it is available and is relatively simple to operate. Disadvantages include the necessity of removing the natural heart, the geometric limitations of the device, the obligatory nature of the device, the external location of the power source, and the risk of inadvertent interruption [23]. Thrombosis, infection, and multisystem organ failure have been the most troublesome complications associated with TAH implantation.

Clinical Experience

From July 1982 through June 1987, we performed staged cardiac transplantation in 38 CsA-treated patients, or 19.7% of our total patient population (Table 4). Thirty patients were supported by an IABP, three were sustained by an LVAD, three others were kept alive with a ventricular bypass pump, and two were supported by a Jarvik-7 TAH.

Intra-aortic Balloon Pump

The 30 IABP-supported patients included 29 men and 1 woman, ranging in age from 39 to 66 years (mean, 48 years). The preoperative diagnosis was ischemic cardiomyopathy in 17 cases (56%) and idiopathic cardiomyopathy in 13 cases (44%). In all but one case, the intra-aortic balloon was inserted percutaneously, in the intensive care unit, with the use of local anesthesia; the exception involved a patient who was admitted to our institution with the balloon already in place. While on IABP support, each patient had an increase in cardiac index, ranging from 0.7 to 2.07 l/min/m^2 (mean, 1.39 l/min/m^2), and a concomitant decrease in systemic vascular resistance, ranging from 462 to 2392 dynes s cm^{-5} (mean, 1203 dynes s cm^{-5}). The duration of IABP support ranged from 1 to 37 days (mean, 8.25 days). Twenty-one patients (70%) underwent successful transplantation, but nine (30%) died before a suitable donor could be found.

Left Ventricular Assist Device

Three patients were sustained by a Thermedics LVAD for 19 to 41 days. The first patient, a 47-year-old man with end-stage cardiac disease secondary to ischemic cardiomyopathy, was supported by the LVAD for 41 days. A heterotopic cardiac

Table 4. Staged cardiac replacement, July 1982 through June 1987 ($n = 38$ patients)

Device	No. of patients	No. of patients who underwent transplantation
Intra-aortic balloon pump	30	21
Left ventricular assist device	3	3
Ventricular bypass pump	3	2
Jarvik-7 total artificial heart	2	1

transplant was then performed, and the LVAD was removed uneventfully. Myocardial recovery was evidenced by the pretransplant right and left ventricular ejection fractions, which were 17% and 26%, respectively. Although the patient survived cardiac transplantation, he died of liver failure 49 days later.

The second patient, a 53-year-old man with idiopathic cardiomyopathy, received an LVAD after suffering a cardiac arrest secondary to ventricular arrhythmias. His condition stabilized, and the LVAD supported him for 19 days until transplantation could be performed. Unfortunately, his condition deteriorated, and he died of multiple organ failure and infection.

The third patient to undergo LVAD-assisted staged transplantation was a 37-year-old man with end-stage idiopathic cardiomyopathy and severe perfusion-related organ dysfunction, whose condition deteriorated rapidly after hospital admission. After LVAD implantation, the patient's hemodynamic and peripheral organ function stabilized. At heterotopic heart transplantation 25 days later, the patient's heart was 30%–50% smaller than it had been before LVAD implantation. Improved myocardial contractility suggested that the heart had recovered during the period of mechanical support. The donor heart failed, however, and the patient could not be weaned from cardiopulmonary bypass.

Ventricular Bypass Pump

Three patients have been supported with the Biomedicus centrifugal pump. The first case involved a 57-year-old man who had sustained an acute myocardial infarction (ejection fraction, 13%) and was transferred to our institution for possible heart transplantation. Several hours after admission, he suffered a cardiac arrest. An intra-aortic balloon was inserted, and the patient was immediately transferred to the operating room, where a right aortocoronary artery bypass and a left ventricular aneurysmectomy were performed. Because the IABP could not support the patient, biventricular bypass was necessary to wean him from cardiopulmonary bypass. The Biomedicus pump maintained excellent circulation, with flows ranging from 4.5 to 6.0 l/min. When a donor heart became available 9 h later, orthotopic heart transplantation was performed. On the 26th postoperative day, the patient had to be reintubated because of bilateral lung infiltrates, pleural effusion, and hypoxemia. Despite maximal support, he died 30 days after transplant, of *Pseudomonas* pneumonia, respiratory failure, and sepsis.

The second patient to undergo staged transplant with a Biomedicus centrifugal pump was a 50-year-old man with ischemic cardiomyopathy who was also transferred to our institution as a transplant candidate. Left heart bypass was instituted, and although an improvement in hemodynamic function was seen, the patient needed increasing inotropic support. He ultimately succumbed to multisystem failure before a transplant could be performed.

A third patient, a 9-year-old boy who weighed 35 kg, became the first child to undergo staged cardiac transplantation. This patient was admitted for treatment of idiopathic cardiomyopathy, but had suffered a cardiac arrest preoperatively. A Biomedicus pump was used to sustain him for 12 h until orthotopic transplantation could be performed. Although the patient had previously been oliguric, his kidney function was restored during the period of pump support. Three months after transplantation, he continues to do well. This pump is uniquely satisfactory for pediatric patients.

Total Artificial Heart

The Jarvik-7 TAH has been used in two patients as a bridge to transplantation. The first case involved a 41-year-old man with a 5-year history of idiopathic cardiomyopathy, who was already being supported by an IABP when he was admitted to the Texas Heart Institute. The patient's mentation and urine output continued to deteriorate, and his cardiac output decreased. After 10 days on the IABP, his heart continued to fail and was replaced with a Jarvik-7 TAH. Because his spine-to-sternum diameter was 11.9 cm, implantation of the artificial heart required several surgical maneuvers to prevent obstruction of the venous return and allow approximation of the sternal edges. During the patient's 31 days of TAH support, his cardiac output was maintained between 4.5 and 7.5 l/min. Reoperation was required 5 days after implantation, to control bleeding attributed to heparinization. The patient's pulmonary and renal function subsequently normalized, and 31 days after implantation, the Jarvik-7 TAH was replaced with an orthotopic cardiac allograft. This patient suffered numerous complications, including a *Candida albicans* infection of the Dacron graft, and required eight additional major operations. Despite these setbacks, he has recovered completely and has returned to his home.

The second patient to receive a TAH as a possible bridge to transplantation was a 42-year-old man who was referred for treatment of end-stage idiopathic cardiomyopathy after his condition underwent rapid deterioration. Because the IABP proved insufficient for his needs, a Jarvik-7 TAH was implanted. Nevertheless, his condition continued to deteriorate, and he died 4 days later, of multisystem organ failure.

Comments

Selection criteria for mechanical devices have not yet been firmly established. Infection and multiple organ failure still pose the greatest threats to survival for these patients. At our institution, the devices are chosen on a case-by-case basis, depending on anatomical fit, cardiac function, pulmonary vascular resistance, and other factors. According to Pennock and associates [23], if a single LVAD can provide hemodynamic stability, this device is preferable to a TAH. If the choice lies between a TAH and a biventricular pump, however, the TAH is preferable if the patient's chest is large enough to accommodate it. Whereas paracorporeal ventricular assist devices are associated with overall survival rates that approach 90%, TAH usage results in reported survival rates of approximately 50% [4]. These data lack meaning since there is no current agreement for implementation of these devices. We feel that the bulk of patients can be supported by the IABP.

Once an appropriate device has been selected, a high degree of skill is required in order to provide optimal conditions for implantation and postoperative care. Collaboration with various related departments (hematology, infectious diseases, renal services, physical therapy, etc.) is crucial. Proper selection of the patient for implantation is also of major importance, as well as deciding to perform the procedure before profound dysfunction of the vital organs supervenes, which may result in failure of the procedure itself.

With respect to the 38 cases in which we have used cardiac assist devices as bridges to cardiac transplantation, 21 (70%) of the 30 IABP patients underwent successful transplantation, but nine (30%) died before a suitable donor became available. The eight patients who required escalated mechanical assistance all recovered sufficiently to become better candidates for transplantation, but two deteriorated and died before donors could be found. Of the six who underwent transplantation, two have survived and are doing well. One of these patients, who was sustained for 30 days on a Jarvik-7 TAH, has recovered and has returned to his home, where he remains well 15 months after transplantation. The other, a 9-year-old boy who was supported with left heart bypass, is doing well and has returned home to normal activity.

The largest crisis today in the field of heart transplantation is the inadequate availability of heart donors. Estimates of the need for cardiac replacement vary from 15000 to 30000 per year, depending on selection criteria. The shortage of donors may make staged cardiac transplantation an important part of therapy for end-stage heart disease patients. At the Texas Heart Institute alone through May 1987, 564 patients had been referred for transplantation; 355 were accepted by the Medical Review Board, and 187 were transplanted. Those who die are generally young individuals primarily with single organ disease who could have the opportunity for active lives with a donor heart. The use of assist devices as bridges to transplantation also eliminates some of the urgency associated with transplantation, allowing physicians to keep their patients in better health prior to transplant. The ideal device is one that does not require the patients placed on the transplant list to supersede other equally moribund patients.

The performance of the various cardiac assist devices with respect to antithrombogenicity, compression of other organs, influence on blood components, etc. is still being evaluated. Thus, although hemodynamic stabilization has occurred with each of the devices described above, further experience is needed to determine the optimal therapeutic system for mechanical circulatory support in staged cardiac transplantation.

References

1. Kahan BD (1982) Cyclosporin A: a new advance in transplantation. Texas Heart Inst J 9:253–266
2. Cooley DA, Frazier OH, Kahan BD (1982) Cardiac transplantation with the use of cyclosporin A for immunologic suppression. Texas Heart Inst J 9:247–251
3. Cooley DA, Frazier OH, Painvin GA et al. (1983) Cardiac and cardiopulmonary transplantation using cyclosporine for immunosuppression: recent Texas Heart Institute experience. Transplant Proc 15(4) (Suppl 1):2567–2572

4. Pae WE, Pierce WS (1986) Combined registry for the clinical use of mechanical ventricular assist pumps and the total artificial heart. J Heart Transplant 5:6–7
5. Moulopoulos SD, Topaz S, Kolff WJ (1962) Extracorporeal assistance to the circulation and intraaortic balloon pumping. Trans Am Soc Artif Intern Organs 8:85–89
6. Kantrowitz A, Tjonneland S, Freed PS et al. (1968) Initial clinical experience with intraaortic balloon pumping in cardiogenic shock. JAMA 203(2):135–140
7. Bolooki H (ed) (1977) Clinical application of intra-aortic balloon pump. Futura, Mount Kisco, NY
8. Johnson MD, Holub DA, Winston DS et al. (1977) Retrospective analysis of 286 patients requiring circulatory support with the intraaortic balloon pump. Cardiovasc Dis Bull Texas Heart Inst 4:428–440
9. Igo SR, Hibbs CW, Trono R et al. (1978) Intra-aortic balloon pumping: theory and practice. Experience with 325 patients. Artif Organs 2:249–256
10. Reemtsma K, Krusin R, Edie R et al. (1978) Cardiac transplantation for patients requiring mechanical circulatory support. N Engl J Med 298:670–671
11. Urschel CW, Eber L, Forrester J (1970) Alterations of mechanical performance of the ventricle by intraaortic balloon counterpulsation. Am J Cardiol 25:546–551
12. Isner JM, Cohen SR, Virmani R et al. (1980) Complications of the intraaortic balloon counterpulsation device: clinical and morphologic observations in 45 necropsy patients. Am J Cardiol 45:260–268
13. Norman JC, Cooley DA, Kahan BD et al. (1978) Total support of the circulation of a patient with postcardiotomy stone-heart syndrome by a partial artificial heart (ALVAD) for 5 days followed by heart and kidney transplantation. Lancet 1:1125–1127
14. Kletschka HD, Rafferty EH, Olsen DA et al. (1975) Artificial heart. III. Development of efficient atraumatic blood pump. A review of the literature concerning in vitro testing of blood pumps for hemolysis. Minn Med 58:757–781
15. Dixon CM, Magovern GJ (1982) Evaluation of the Bio-pump for long-term cardiac support without heparinization. J Extracorporeal Tech 14:331–336
16. Lynch MF, Peterson D, Baker V (1978) Centrifugal blood pumping for open heart surgery. Minn Med 26:72–76
17. Beckman D, Siderys H (1986) Prolonged left heart bypass with the BioMedicus vortex centrifugal pump. Contemp Surg 29:69–73
18. Cooley DA, Liotta D, Hallman GL et al. (1969) Orthotopic cardiac prosthesis for two-staged cardiac replacement. Am J Cardiol 24:723–730
19. Cooley DA, Akutsu T, Norman JC et al. (1981) Total artificial heart in two-staged cardiac transplantation. Cardiovasc Dis Bull Texas Heart Inst 8:305–319
20. Copeland JG, Levinson MM, Vaughn C et al. (1986) The total artificial heart as a bridge to transplantation. JAMA 256:2991–2995
21. Pennock JL, Wisman CB, Pierce WS (1982) Mechanical support of the circulation prior to cardiac transplantation. Heart Transplant 1:299–305
22. DeVries WC (1985) Replacement of the failing heart: role of mechanical support in cardiac transplants. Presented at the American Society for Artificial Internal Organs Meeting, Atlanta, May 1985
23. Pennock JL, Pierce WS, Campbell DB et al. (1986) Mechanical support of the circulation followed by cardiac transplantation. J Thorac Cardiovasc Surg 92:994–1004

23. Experience with the Total Artificial Heart as a Bridge to Transplantation

T. ICENOGLE and J. G. COPELAND

Introduction

The artificial heart has stirred considerable interest and controversy in the lay and medical press. The controversy arising from stroke complications and quality of life issues has stalled efforts to implant the device permanently. The clinical indications for the artificial heart are now largely limited to "bridge to transplantation."

The artificial heart as a bridge to transplantation is not a new idea. Dr. Cooley and colleagues first implanted an artificial heart for this indication in 1969 [1, 2] and again in 1981 [3]. Unfortunately both of these patients died. Dr. Copeland, at the University of Arizona, used the "Phoenix Heart" in an attempt to save a young transplant recipient with acute failure of his donor heart [4]. The Phoenix Heart was an experimental design for use in calves but it sustained the patient for 11 h until another donor was found. The patient died following retransplantation but this event stimulated several transplant centers to consider the artificial heart as a reasonable tool in the transplant surgeon's armamentarium. The first clinical success of the artificial heart as a bridge to transplantation was in a 25-year-old male at the University of Arizona in September of 1985. This patient remains alive and well and has returned to work as an assistant manager in a grocery store. Since then several transplant centers have successfully used the artificial heart as a bridge to transplantation. This chapter will explore data from the world experience and at the University of Arizona in the use of the artificial heart as a bridge to transplantation.

The current status and history of cardiac transplantation must be understood to comprehend the proper role of the artificial heart as a bridge to transplantation. Following Dr. Christian Barnard's first transplant in 1968, there was a flurry of activity around the world. Initial mortality rates were high and so most centers ceased efforts in clinical heart transplantation. Stanford University continued its program and, through intensive research, several developments contributed to improved survival. Better immunosuppression and the development of the endocardial biopsy to monitor for acute rejection were major achievements. The introduction of cyclosporin led to increased survivals, and now triple drug therapy (cyclosporin, azathioprine, and prednisone) has improved the outcome further by decreasing severe rejections and infections [5]. The survival for heart transplantation is now between 70% and 90%, with many experienced centers boasting rates in the low 90s. Heart transplantation is no longer considered experimental and most patients can look forward to a quality life-style with few limitations. Many of the clinical problems in heart transplantation have been solved but the dilemma concerning the patient with severe cardiac failure without an immediate donor remains. Clinicians are now "pushing the envelope," using the artificial heart as an attempt to save these desperately ill patients.

The World Experience

There have been 69 implants in 67 patients from April 1969 to 1 June 1987 [6], as a bridge to transplantation. The device most commonly used has been the Jarvik-7-70 (40), which has a theoretical filling volume of 70 cc. The Jarvik-7 with a 100 cc filling volume was second, with 21 implants. Other heart types have included the Penn State Heart (2), the Ellipsoid heart (4), Berlin (1), Liotta (1), Akutsu III, Series 3 (1), and the Phoenix Heart (1). Data on all implants is not available, yet trends have appeared. The implant time for most bridged patients has been less than 2 weeks (range 0.5–244 days). The mean age has been 40 years, with a range of 17 to 58 years. Indications for implantation have included ischemic heart disease (42%), cardiomyopathy (39%), viral myocarditis (7%), congenital defects (3.6%), postpartum (3.6%), and valvular heart disease (3.6%) [7]. Most patients have been anticoagulated with heparin and dipyridamole, with some centers using aspirin as well. Postoperative bleeding requiring reoperation has been common in the early experience [8] but hemolysis has not [9]. Data on 45 bridged patients reveal a 13% incidence of proven stroke but only one patient died as a result [6]. The single death was attributed to multiple emboli secondary to stasis in the left atrium resulting from inflow occlusion from poor fit [7]. Device infections have occurred in 17 patients, with some infections involving just the drive lines and others the entire prosthesis. The overall survival following transplantation with a donor heart has been from 50% to 70% [6, 10, 11]. When one considers the number of transplant centers involved in artificial heart research, and the reality that these patients would have certainly died without support, then these preliminary data are indeed impressive. Unfortunately, progress in medicine is often made after repeated failures in the early stages of investigation. By sharing clinical experience, physicians can learn and improve the clinical outcome. Brief review of the experience at the University of Arizona illustrates the successes and pitfalls involved in the use of the artificial heart as a bridge to transplantation.

The University of Arizona Experience

At the University of Arizona in Tucson there have been seven implants in six patients (Table 1). Relevant points in each case are discussed with an attempt to illustrate lessons learned.

Case 1. A 33-year-old man with ischemic cardiomyopathy received a heart transplant in March 1985. Initial graft function was sluggish and required excessive inotropic support. Subsequently, the donor was found to have suffered *Pseudomonas* sepsis documented by positive blood cultures not apparent at the time of

Table 1. Case details

Patient	Age	Sex	Weight	Heart disease	Device	Outcome
1. T.C.	33	M	65.5	Ischemic	Phoenix	Died
2. M.D.	25	M	103	Myopathy	Jarvik-7	Alive
3. B.C.	40	F	65	Viral	Jarvik-7-70	Died
4. B.S.	43	F	84	Congenital	Jarvik-7-70	Died
5. J.S.	39	M	79.5	Myopathy	Jarvik-7-70	Alive
6. S.G.	39	M	43	Myopathy	Jarvik-7-70	Died

surgery. The patient suffered a cardiac arrest 24 h after transplantation and was resuscitated with open chest massage (1 ½ h) then placed on cardiopulmonary bypass (7½ h). The Phoenix Heart, designed for use in calves, was the only heart available and was implanted as an emergency measure. The device adequately supported the patient's blood pressure (110–120 mmHg systolic), and a urine output of greater than 100 cc per hour resulted. The sternum could not be closed and the chest had to be reopened once for bleeding. Another donor heart was located and transplanted after 11 h of support. The new donor had poor graft function and the patient died 33 h later of pulmonary edema, *Pseudomonas* pneumonia, and low cardiac output.

This case illustrates several points in the management of artificial heart patients. A well planned and conceived artificial heart program is necessary for a success. The device and its management are sufficiently complicated that "emergency" implantation is an invitation to disaster. In retrospect, implantation of the heart should be for sufficient duration to allow for recovery from physiological and surgical insults. The time for recovery should allow the patient to become a better transplant candidate and improve his chances for survival.

Case 2. A 25-year-old 103-kg man with chronic cardiomyopathy, presumed to be viral, was admitted in a critical condition. He had an ejection fraction of 10%, acidosis, hypotension, and delirium. A donor was unavailable and a Jarvik-7 was implanted. The technique of implantation has been described [12]. There were no problems with fit or postoperative bleeding. Initial cardiac output was in the 5–6 l/min range and urine output was excellent. Peripheral pulses were poor and the patient had a high core temperature (38–38.5 °C), suggesting an inadequate cardiac output for this patient's size. The cardiac output was increased to 7–8 l/min by using diastolic vacuum and raising the drive pressures. The pulses became bounding, the core temperature dropped, and the peripheral skin temperature rose. This series of events illustrated the control of cardiac output available with the artificial heart and the fact that some patients may require higher outputs than what is thought to be adequate.

This patient had pulmonary edema at the time of implantation and over the next 4 days was diuresed 18 l. The patient's lungs cleared but there were two adverse effects. First, the drop in preload forced a decrease in cardiac output. Second, there was a concentration of clotting factors and the platelet count also rose during this time. These effects were probably contributory to platelet and thrombin deposition at the inflow and outflow valve mounts [13]. The patient suffered a stroke on the 7th day, evidenced by right hemiparesis and expressive aphagia. The CAT scan of the brain was normal and his neurological deficit eventually resolved completely.

A different approach to prevention of thromboembolism is now followed. An attempt is made to keep the heart rate and cardiac output high to wash the valve surfaces and valve mount crevices. Aggressive diuresis is tempered by decreasing fill volumes and signs of hemoconcentration. The patient's condition is also closely monitored for changes in coagulation studies. The liver may recover dramatically following implantation and coagulation factor levels may become elevated. The coagulation studies are followed every 6 h and the partial thromboplastin time is maintained at 1½-2 times normal with heparin. The platelet count is also closely monitored and persantine 75–100 mg p.o. every 6 h is given to blunt platelet function. These maneuvers will hopefully reduce the formation of thrombus in the device.

The patient received a donor heart 9 days after implantation. He suffered from toxoplasmosis transferred in the donor heart but overcame this complication. The patient recovered completely and returned to work.

Case 3. A 40-year-old 65-kg woman presented after a 1-week history of influenza-like symptoms and severe vomiting. She was hypotensive (BP 83/63) upon admission to the emergency room of the referring hospital and an echocardiogram showed global hypokinesis. She was transported to the University of Arizona where a heart biopsy showed myocardial necrosis. Influenza A antigen was demonstrated in both nasopharyngeal secretions and in the heart biopsy. Treatment with steroids, azathioprine, amantadine, and inotropic support was undertaken. The patient's condition deteriorated, as evidenced by pulmonary edema requiring 100% FIO_2, mild hepatic insufficiency, and rapidly progressing renal insufficiency. The Jarvik 7-70 was implanted without significant problems.

Mediastinal bleeding occurred on the 2nd and 4th postoperative days and each episode followed attempts to achieve adequate heparinization. Vigorous chest tube stripping resolved one episode of tamponade. Mediastinal reexploration was considered but an excellent donor was identified. The cytotoxic antibody screen was twice negative prior to cardiac transplantation.

The patient was transplanted successfully on the 4th postoperative day but required reexploration for mediastinal bleeding. A retrospective cross-match with the donor was positive for cytotoxic antibodies and the patient suffered a cardiac arrest on the 2nd day following transplantation. Cardiopulmonary resuscitation was administered and she was transferred to the operating room and placed upon cardiopulmonary bypass. The family was consulted and they strongly desired a second implantation of the Jarvik 7-70. This was accomplished successfully but the patient suffered a series of serious complications.

Several complications related to the artificial heart were demonstrated. A paucity of atrial tissue precluded positioning of the heart to the left and the patient developed inflow occlusion of the right heart. The inferior vena cava was compressed and ascites developed. Catheterization showed a 10-mm gradient at the inferior vena cava – atrial junction. At reoperation this problem was solved by first, placing traction on the right heart using an umbilical tape sling from the

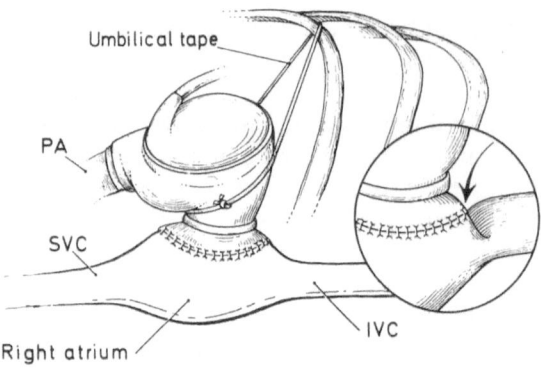

Fig. 1. Method used to correct obstruction of inferior vena cava (*IVC*) in patient B.C. Umbilical tape passed around a rib pulls device anteriorly. *PA*, pulmonary artery; *SVC*, superior vena cava

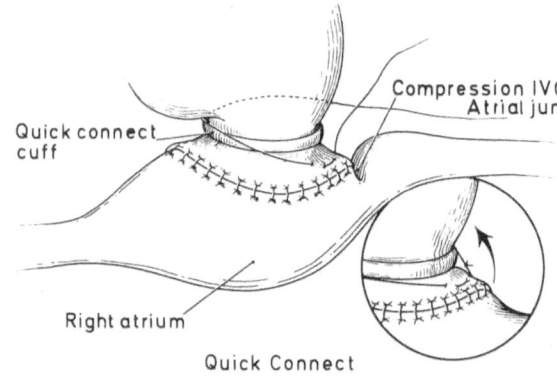

Fig. 2. Method used to correct obstruction of inferior vena cava (*IVC*) patient B.C. Horizontal mattress suture pulls cuff anteriorly

left lateral rib to the right ventricle (Fig. 1), and second, turning up the inferior edge of the right atrial quick connect, which was compressing the inferior vena cava. This was accomplished using horizontal mattress sutures from the cuff of the tricuspid valve mount to the inferior edge of the atrial quick connect (Fig. 2).

This patient recovered from a series of complications (Table 2) and eventually became ambulatory. Cytotoxic antibodies prevented her from receiving a cross-matched negative donor despite her excellent physical condition.

This case illustrates the dangers of implantation in patients with acute viral myocarditis. The physiology of this disease is poorly understood and the patients should be considered immunologically unstable. This patient never successfully cleared her viral infection until given an experimental antiviral agent, yet she seemed to have a hyperactive immune system in that she made cytotoxic alloantibodies to 70%–100% of a random panel of donors and had high titers of a number of autoantibodies.

This patient eventually developed a drive line infection which ascended to involve the entire prosthesis. The device was extensively debrided and the chest irrigated with betadine and antibiotic solutions. An attempt was made to suppress her hyperactive immune system using total nodal irradiation (2000 rads) and plasmapheresis. Her autoantibody levels fell and the patient was transplanted but the heart failed from hyperacute rejection.

Table 2. Complications in patient B. C.

	Days after 2nd implant	Treatment
Infections		
Influenza A sepsis	0– 12	Intravenous ribavirin
Candida sepsis	12– 21	Intravenous amphotericin B
Enterobacter sepsis	18– 31	Intravenous imipenum
Herpes simplex sepsis; intermittent urinary tract infections	43– 52	Intravenous acyclovir
Drive line infection	30–244	Local treatment
Mediastinal infection	220–244	Debridement drainage
Surgical complications		
Inferior vena cava compression	0– 9	Decompression
Delayed splenic rupture	23	Splenectomy
Other complications		
Renal failure	0– 78	Dialysis and continuous hemofiltration
Prolonged intubation	0– 41	Extubation
Pancreatitis	0– 8	Nasogastric drainage
Ileus	0– 60	Intravenous alimentation
Persistent cytotoxic antibodies; autoantibodies	0–244	Plasmapheresis, total nodal irradiation (2000 rads)
Transient ischemia attack	212	

This patient was supported for 245 days and was free of embolism for 212 days. Her embolic event presented with left facial palsy and upper extremity weakness and the symptoms eventually resolved. This event occurred during a time when she was septic with infection of her prosthesis and the embolism may have been related to infected graft material. Other complications prevented heparin anticoagulation for more than 80 days during this implant period, but at explantation the ventricles and atrial quick connect areas were free of thrombus. This patient maintained a 6–7 l/min cardiac output and heart rate of 125 bpm throughout her implant and the vigorous washing of valve surfaces may have contributed to the rarity of embolization.

Case 4. A 43-year-old female with Epstein's anomaly decompensated after implantation of an automatic defibrillator. A Jarvik 7-70 was implanted and although the fit seemed adequate, the ventricular filling curves dampened when the chest was closed. Severe pulmonary edema developed and after 72 h the chest was reopened and the filling curves improved. Metallic supports were placed across the sternum to hold it open and just the skin was closed. The patient's course was continued downhill and the device was turned off on the 9th postoperative day. The patient was brain dead and a postmortem examination showed severe compression of both atria, with flattening of pulmonary veins and intra-atrial thrombus and numerous cerebral infarcts.

This patient illustrates the dangers of poor fit. She was moderately obese (weight 84 kg) but had a small skeleton. She had a large pericardium as a result of her cardiac disease and there was little initial concern about the adequacy of her chest to accept the device. The chest, however, was too small, which led to compression of the atrium with the resultant thrombus formation and embolization.

A variety of techniques can allow a small chest to accept an artificial heart. The pericardium can be incised above and below the left phrenic nerve to allow the heart to move to the left. The atrial connects can cut to allow the ventricles to rotate into the left chest. The drive lines must be brought out such that the ventricles will not compress the pulmonary veins or vena cava. It is sometimes helpful to use artificial heart dummies or sizers at the time of implantation to determine the best exit sites for the drive lines. It is of critical importance to assure that the fit is adequate at the time of the implantation. Filling curves will often indicate if there is a problem. When doubt exists concerning right atrial compression, a venous catheterization should be performed before transferring from the operating room. A central venous pressure can be obtained from an internal jugular catheter and the inferior vena cava can be catheterized to determine whether there is a gradient at the atrial-caval junction. It is important to determine whether there is any evidence of compression before leaving the operating room.

Case 5. A 39-year-old male transplant recipient mistakenly received an ABO incompatible heart. This error was discovered shortly after completion of the procedure and the Jarvik-7-70 was implanted soon thereafter. The transplanted heart was having atrial dysrhythmias and poor ventricular function within only a few hours of the transplant. This patient was supported for 12 days and then retransplanted. He recovered completely.

This case illustrates aspects of the artificial heart candidate selection. The decision to implant the device is often difficult. The device must be implanted before the patient suffers irreversible end-organ failure. Once irreversible end-organ failure is established then the patient is no longer a heart transplant recipient. Procrastination may lead to end-organ failure or a severely debilitated state such that recovery will be prolonged, if obtainable at all.

Case 6. A 39-year-old 43-kg white male was transferred in agonal condition from a distant hospital. The patient was in severe cardiogenic shock despite multiple inotropic agents at pharmacological doses. He was obtunded, emaciated, and after a rapid pretransplant workup, represented a high-risk candidate. The Jarvik-7-70 heart was implanted and his chest was the smallest we had ever encountered. Using the techniques documented above there were no problems with inflow occlusion following implantation. The left lower lobe was compressed by the device and became completely atelectatic. He remained somnolent for 6 days but eventually awoke and was neurologically intact. He was extubated and given rigorous nutritional and physical therapy. The patient made a remarkable but slow recovery from his preoperative status. Neurological, hepatic, and renal function became normal. After 28 days of support the patient received a heart transplant.

At the time of operation the adhesions were dense and dissection difficult. A hole in the pulmonary artery was made in an attempt to surround the aorta. Once the transplanted heart was in place, an attempt was made to decorticate the entrapped left lower lobe. Dense adhesions in the left chest bled profusely. In spite of all efforts the patient's bleeding could not be controlled and he died in the operating room.

This unfortunate case illustrates two pitfalls in artificial heart management:

1. Patients who are in severely debilitated states are poor candidates for the artificial heart. While they may have reversible end-organ failure, the time required for recovery is so long that adhesions have time to become firmly established. The device is then explanted at a time of worst adhesion formation (3–8 weeks), making the operation most difficult. Placing artificial heart recipients at the top of the transplant list is appropriate because the ideal time to transplant them seems to be less than 2 weeks.

2. While fit problems can be solved with a variety of techniques, the problem of pulmonary compression and atelectasis remains. Attempting to decorticate a lung soon after bypass can lead to profuse bleeding. A decortication with resultant air leaks is to be avoided in the new transplant because the steroid immunosuppression may lead to prolonged air leak. The problem with pulmonary compression remains as a difficult roadblock in using the artificial heart in patients with small chest cavities.

Summary

The total artificial heart has demonstrated clinical success when used as a bridge to transplant. The current success rate of 50%–70% compares with a success rate of heart transplantation of about 90% at the first year. While this success rate is an admirable achievement for the early experience, much can be learned and achieved so that the success rate will be commensurate with that of cardiac transplantation.

Problems with bleeding and hemolysis have largely been solved with the experience to date. Fit problems with the resultant inflow occlusion have been successfully managed up to a point. Problems with pulmonary compression and adhesions remain technical challenges for the future.

Artificial heart candidate selection remains a difficult problem. A candidate must be viewed first as a heart transplant candidate. The goal of successful heart transplantation must not be lost in the clamor and rush to stabilize the dying cardiac patient. End-organ failure must be reversible and the patient's condition sufficiently amenable to allow a rapid recovery once the device is implanted. Patient selection is a matter of judgment but the severely debilitated, patients with acute viral myocarditis, and transplant patients with acute rejection are in a higher risk group. The problem with adhesions is sufficient reason for artificial heart recipients to be placed high on the transplant list.

The experience to date has revealed a number of limitations of the currently used devices. Time, experience, and better technologies will provide devices and techniques to improve upon the current results. Progress in medicine is often slow, but patient and diligent effort should improve the clinical outcome for the critically ill cardiac patients who require the use of the artificial heart as a bridge to transplantation.

References

1. Cooley DA, Liotta D, Hallman GL et al. (1969) Orthotopic cardiac prosthesis for two staged cardiac replacement. Am J Cardiol 24:723–730
2. Cooley DA, Liotta D, Hallman GL et al. (1969) First human implantation of cardiac prosthesis for staged total replacement of the heart. Trans Am Soc Artif Intern Organs 15:252–23
3. Cooley DA (1982) Staged cardiac transplantation: report of three cases. Heart Transplant 1:145–163
4. Copeland JG, Levinson MM, Smith R et al. (1986) The total artificial heart as a bridge to transplantation: a report of two cases. JAMA 256:2991–2995
5. Andreone PA, Olivani MT, Elick B et al. (1986) Reduction of infectious complications following heart transplantation with triple drug immunotherapy. J Heart Transplant 5:13–19
6. Artificial Heart Registry. Department of Artificial Heart, University Medical Center, Tucson
7. Copeland JG, Smith RG, Icenogle TB, Ott RA (in press) Early experience with the total artificial heart as a bridge to cardiac transplantation. Surg Clin North Am
8. Joyce LD, Johnson KE, Pierce WS et al. (1986) Summary of the world experience with clinical use of total artificial hearts as heart support devices. J Heart Transplant 5:229–235
9. Levinson MM, Copeland JG, Smith RG et al. (1986) Indexes with hemolysis in human recipients of the Jarvik-7 total artificial heart: a cooperative report of fifteen patients. Heart Transplant 5:236–248
10. Cabrol C, Gandjbakhch CI, Pavie A et al. (1986) Use of a total artificial heart as a bridge to transplantation. J Heart Transplant 5:390
11. Griffith BP, Hardesty RL, Kormos RY (1987) Temporary use of the Jarvik-7 total artificial heart before transplantation. N Engl J Med 316:130–134
12. Levinson MM, Copeland JG (1987) Technical aspects of total artificial heart implantation for temporary applications. J Cardiac Surg 2:3–19
13. Levinson MM, Smith RG, Cork RC et al. (1986) Thromboembolic complications of the Jarvik-7 total artificial heart: case report. Artif Organs 10:236–244

24. Temporary Use of the Jarvik-7 Artificial Heart – The Pittsburgh Experience

B. P. Griffith

Nearly concurrently with the development of the pneumatic artificial heart [1, 2], cardiac transplantation emerged from an experimental to a therapeutic procedure [3]. By 1987, the International Cardiac Transplant Registry had 4600 entries, and current 1-year expectation for survival exceeds 80% [4]. The increased use of cardiac transplantation has prolonged the waiting period even for those patients who are most critically ill – from less than 5 days in 1980, when cardiac transplantation was performed in five centers in the United States, to more than 42 days in 1986, when the procedure was performed in more than 60 centers [3]. Our group has previously shown that there is a group of mortally ill patients who might survive if their circulation could be temporarily and safely supported by an intravenous, inotropic system and the intra-aortic balloon pump (IABP) [5].

This chapter describes the experience at Presbyterian-University Hospital, where 16 patients have received the Jarvik-7 artificial heart in an attempt to bridge them to cardiac transplantation. In all instances the patients who were candidates for cardiac transplantation were not expected to live for more than a few hours.

Selection of Patients

All 16 patients who received the total artificial heart (TAH) were candidates for cardiac transplantation; ten suffered with cardiomyopathy, and six had end-stage ischemic disease. All but one were men, and the average age was 47 years (range: 27–59). Thirteen patients became candidates for the TAH when they developed cardiogenic shock in spite of the use of intravenous inotropes and the IABP (Table 1). The average duration of support with inotropes was 23 days (range: 2–83 days), while with the IABP it was 13 days (range: 2–65 days). These patients

Table 1. Indications for implantation of the Jarvik-7 artificial heart

	No. of patients	No. transplanted	No. alive
Cardiogenic shock while waiting for donor heart	13	11	7
Acute rejection of donor organ (within 24 h of transplant	1	1	1
Primary failure of donor heart	2	2	0

Assisted Circulation 3
F. Unger (Ed.)
© Springer-Verlag Berlin Heidelberg 1989

Table 2. Clinical characteristics of 13 patients given the Jarvik-7 artificial heart

Characteristics[a]	Patient no. and indication						
	1 Cardio-myo-pathy	2 Acute infarction	3 Cardio-myo-pathy	4 Cardio-myo-pathy	5 Ischemic heart disease	6 Acute intra-operative rejection	7 Unex-pectedly injured donor heart
Intravenous inotropic drugs (days)	33	7	10	54	11	–	12
Intra-aortic balloon pump (days)	22	3/2[b]	5	15	1	–	1
Preimplantation cardiac index (l/min/m²)	1.1	<1.0	1.3	1.4	–	1.1	–
Serum creatinine (mg/dl)	1.6	1.1	4.1	1.3	1.8	2.0	0.7
8-h urine output (ml)	275	300	100	250	0	–	700
Bilirubin (mg/dl)	1.1	1.3	8.0	2.1	6.4	1.5	1.0
Radiographic pulmonary edema	Yes	Yes	Yes	Yes	Yes	–	No
Mental obtundation	Mild	Moderate	Severe	Mild	Moderate	–	None
Days with implant	4	13	18	2	6	9	2
Outcome	Home for 10 mo	Home for 6 mo	Dead[c]	Dead[d]	Home for 3 mo	Home for 3 mo	Dead Unknown

[a] To convert values for creatinine and bilirubin to micromoles per liter, multiply by 88.4 and 17.1, respectively

[b] A biventricular assistance was used for 2 days

[c] Died of candidal sepsis and multiorgan failure

[d] Died with rejection 60 days after transplantation

were judged unlikely to survive a few hours, and once the decision to implant the device was made, the procedure was conducted as an emergency (Table 2). The cardiac index in the recipients ranged from less than 1.0 to 1.4 l/min/m². All had some degree of mental obtundation, which was severe in three. Prior to selection, high doses of diuretics were required to maintain hourly urinary outputs of 10–50 ml/h; one patient was anuric. The serum creatinine concentration averaged 2.0 mg/dl (180 μmol/l) and ranged from 1.1 to 4.1 mg/dl (97–360 μmol/l). Acute pulmonary edema was noted radiographically in the 13 patients awaiting their first cardiac transplant, and four of these required urgent preoperative tracheal intubation and mechanical ventilation. When it appeared that medical treatment and intra-aortic counterpulsation were failing, an attempt was made to discuss the possible need for the TAH before the clinical condition deteriorated. Informed consent for the use of the TAH was obtained in advance and at the time of implantation from four recipients and from all the families.

The decision to implant the TAH was prompted by a progressive decline in cardiac function, which was associated with cardiopulmonary resuscitation in four patients. One of the cardiac arrests occurred in another hospital, where a biventricular support system (Biomedicus) was implanted in order to maintain

Patient no. and indication								
8 Cardio-myo-pathy	9 Cardio-myo-pathy	10 Cardio-myo-pathy	11 Ischemic heart disease	12 Cardio-myo-pathy	13 Ischemic heart disease	14 Cardio-myo-pathy	15 Failure of donor heart	16 Ischemic heart disease
11	2	3	18	28	41	13	13	83
2	1	2	8	16	41	1	–	65
1.6	1.7	1.2	1.2	1.5	1.7	1.76	3.6	1.8
1.6	2.6	2.2	1.3	2.5	2.5	1.5	1.2	2.5
180	0	300	620	300	500	30	450	500
7.3	4.3	1.3	5.4	4.1	0.6	1.1	1.0	1.9
Yes	Yes	No	Yes	Yes	Yes	Yes	Yes	Yes
Mild	Mild	Severe	Moderate	Moderate	Mild	None	Severe	Mild
8	4	4	5	35	13	6	7	1
Home for 16 mo	Home for 16 mo	Dead Unknown	Dead Infection	Dead Infection	Dead Infection	Home for 10 mo	Dead Infection	Dead Hemorrhage

the patient's life (Fig. 1). Later, the patient was transferred to our hospital for substitution of the Jarvik-7 (Fig. 2) and subsequent transplantation.

Three patients became candidates as a consequence of failed transplantation (Table 1). In one recipient the need to bridge was due to an inexplicable failure of the donor heart to function 12 h after transplantation. In another patient, a donor's heart was belatedly found to have extensive myocardial contusion with atrial septal rupture not diagnosed by echocardiographic examination of the donor. Lastly, one patient developed hyperacute rejection of the heart within an hour of transplantation, presumably due to rare preformed antiendothelial antibodies to the donor that were found to be present retrospectively [6].

In Pittsburgh contraindications to implantation have grown from notions to absolutes based on our experience (Table 3). Patients were not included if at the moment of implantation they would not have been considered candidates for cardiac transplantation had a donor heart been available. Although subsequently proven wrong in at least two cases, we attempted to exclude candidates with active infection. While anuria was present in two recipients, it was of short duration (<2 h), and those with established acute tubular necrosis were not chosen. No patient was considered (a) who had had a previous sternotomy (for fear of post-

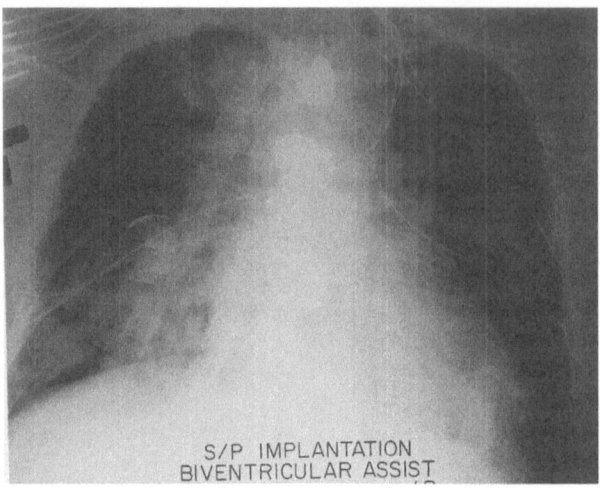

Fig. 1. Radiograph from patient #2, who required biventricular assistance with Biomedicus pumps prior to transfer to Presbyterian-University Hospital

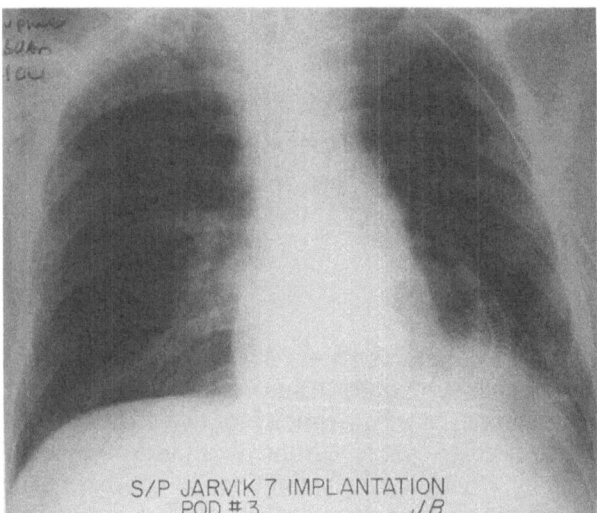

Fig. 2. Radiograph from patient #2 after implantation of the Jarvik-7 artificial heart. Marked clearing of pulmonary edema in Fig. 1 is evident

operative hemorrhage in the anticoagulated patient from lysed adhesions), (b) who weighed less than 115 lb with an anterior vertebral (T10) to sternal distance of less than 8 cm, or (c) who had elevation of preformed antibodies (percent reactive antibodies > 20%). Lastly, we have learned in two instances that unresponsive or comatose patients are poor candidates because of an uncertain prospect for neurological recovery. It is especially important to assess the latter after cardiopulmonary resuscitation.

Table 3. Contraindications to bridge to transplantation with the Jarvik-7 artificial heart

Contraindication	Explanation
1. Presence of active infection	Postimplant infection
2. Previous sternotomy	Hermorrhage from lysed adhesions in anticoagulated recipient
3. Age > 60 years	Reasonable expectation of survival and limited other secernment systemic illnesses
4. Evidence of preformed antibodies to HLA antigens (percent reactive antibodies > 20)	Increased likelihood of not finding compatible donor postimplantation
5. Established acute tubular necrosis	High risk of postimplant and transplant difficulties
6. Unresponsiveness or coma	Risk of implanting device in patient with poor prospect of neurological recovery
7. Small size, weight < 115 lb, vertebral-sternal dimension < 8 cm	Poor fit of device with high likelihood of pulmonary and/or systemic venous obstruction

Operative Procedure – Postimplant Care

The operation is performed through a median sternotomy in a fashion similar to that described by DeVries et al. [2]. One-third of our patients required a return to the operating room because of excessive mediastinal hemorrhage and/or atrial tamponade (Fig. 3). The latter was easily diagnosed from drive line air wave forms (Fig. 4). The pericardium is not removed in the patient. The pneumatic drive lines exit through skin incisions below the left lateral costal arch at the anterior axillary line. The aim is to position the TAH so that the left ventricle is drawn inferiorly and laterally and the right ventricle is pulled to the left of the sternum anteriorly.

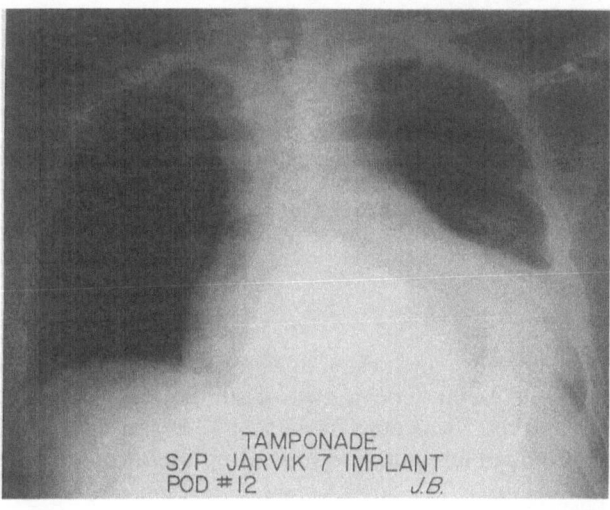

TAMPONADE
S/P JARVIK 7 IMPLANT
POD #12   J.B.

Fig. 3. Radiograph from patient #2 on the 12th postimplant day showing enlargement of the pericardial shadow

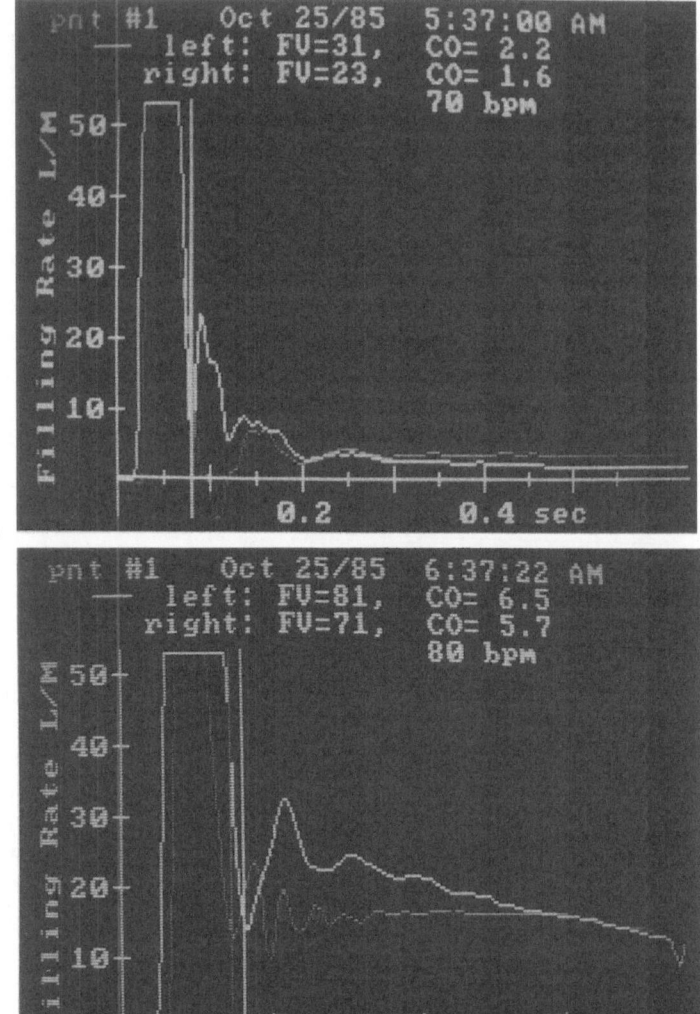

Fig. 4. a Graph of diastolic filling phase from analysis of drive line air wave form showing severe impediment of filling and low left and right stroke volumes. **b** Graph of diastolic filling from analysis of drive line air wave form after operative removal of pericardial blood and release of atrial tamponade

This prevents obstruction of pulmonary and systemic venous return and permits closure of the sternum. The 100-ml Jarvik-7 device was used in our first three patients, while the 70-ml "mini" Jarvik-7 was used in the last 13 because we found it was easier to implant and provided adequate outputs of up to 7 l/min at heart rates of 118–120/min.

All patients remained in the surgical intensive care unit, and the function of the artificial ventricles was monitored by the cardiac diagnostic unit that is integral to the Utah heart-drive console. For the first 12–24 h, a physician, usually a surgical resident from the surgical research laboratory, remained at the bedside; thereafter, the physician was immediately available by page from within the hospital. Information from the cardiac monitor was telephoned to the homes of the investigators. Anticoagulation with heparin and dipyridamole was started as soon as the mediastinal drainage slowed, usually within 8 h of the operative procedure. Intravenous heparin was initially given at a dose of 500 units per hour, and the dose was increased hourly until a partial thromboplastin time between 2 and 2.5 times the control value was reached. Dipyridamole, 75 mg, was given by nasogastric tube or by mouth every 8 h.

Our inclination was to substitute a donor heart for the TAH as soon as circumstances became reasonable. On occasion, patients were not listed as priority candidates for cardiac transplantation for a few days so that pulmonary edema, renal insufficiency, and/or mental obtundation could resolve or stabilize. While we considered renal insufficiency or failure undesirable prior to transplantation, we believed that, in view of other problems previously shown to be associated with long-term use of the TAH, it should not be considered a contraindication. The only absolute contraindication to transplantation was uncontrolled infection.

The immunosuppressive regimen followed after transplantation was similar to that used in routine cases except that azathioprine was avoided. All patients received 500 mg methylprednisolone when the transplanted organ was reperfused and 125 mg every 8 h for three doses. Thereafter, except for treatment of acute rejection, steroids were limited to 20 mg prednisone daily. Cyclosporine was withheld preoperatively and begun at a dose of 2.5 mg/kg every 12 h in the first few postoperative hours when the patient was stable and exhibited adequate cardiac and renal functions. The dose was usually adjusted upward to a targeted whole blood level (RIA Sandoz) of 700 ng/ml. Some consideration of a lowered dose was made for those individuals with abnormal renal function. Rabbit antithymocyte globulin was given intramuscularly for 5 days.

Results

Function of the Jarvik-7 Device

The drive functions of the Jarvik-7, including pressure and percentage of systole, were adjusted to ensure complete ejection of blood from the ventricles. Physiological cardiac outputs were maintained between 5 and 7.5 l/min. Transient rises in central venous pressure and left atrial pressure occurred during coughing, during endotracheal suctioning, and when patients became animated because of visitors. None of these episodes required a change of the drive functions. After the first 24 h of support, heart rate and left and right drive-pressure settings required little or no adjustment, even when the patient changed from a supine to an erect position. Serious hemolysis did not occur, and plasma hemoglobin concentrations

Table 4. Causes of death with the temporary artificial heart (16 patients)

Cause	During implant	After transplant
Infection	1	4
Bleeding	1	0
Medical noncompliance	–	1
Failure of donor heart	–	1
Rejection of donor heart	–	1 [a]
	2/16	7/14

[a] In setting of reduced immunosuppression with mediastinitis

never rose above 20 mg/dl. Thrombocytopenia occurred in two patients, one with candidal sepsis and the other after 24-h biventricular support with the Biomedicus pumps.

Survival

The actuarial survival of all patients who received the TAH was 50%. Two of 16 patients died prior to transplantation, one with sepsis from fungus and the other with hemorrhage from a torn pulmonary arterial anastomosis (Table 4). Fourteen patients received cardiac allografts, and seven continue to survive without restrictions. Infection within the mediastinum caused the death of four patients after transplantation. In three of these patients, mediastinitis was not recognized prior to transplantation but occurred within the first 2 post-transplant weeks. Of the remaining three deaths, one was due to sudden and still unexplained failure of the donor heart 8 h postoperatively, one to acute rejection of the donor heart on the 60st postoperative day in the setting of reduced immunosuppression and treated mediastinitis, and one to medical noncompliance (thus death occurred late, during the 9th postoperative month).

Infection

Six of nine deaths were related to infection [7]. One patient died of bacterial and fungal sepsis prior to transplantation, and five others succumbed with mediastinitis. In only one of these patients was mediastinitis diagnosed prior to transplantation. This patient was transplanted on the 36th postoperative implant day with evidence of persisting localized mediastinitis and died promptly with sepsis. The diagnosis was made early after transplantation by culture of pericardial and pleural fluid, except in the only successfully treated case, in which a localized infection was detected 3 weeks after transplantation.

Infected sputum or frank pneumonia occurred in all six patients who died from infection. In three of these patients, the same organism appeared to be related to the subsequent mediastinitis (*Serratia marcescens*, 2; *Pseudomonas*, 1), and in one patient the organisms (*Enterobacter aerogenes* and *Candida albicans*) caused sepsis which resulted in death prior to transplantation. The two additional cases were due to *Mycoplasma hominis*, a bacterium difficult to isolate from the sputum but one known to reside within the respiratory system. The culture of the mediastinum obtained during the transplant procedure was sterile in all patients except in the one with mediastinitis and pneumonia from *Pseudomonas*. Between 2nd and the 22nd post-transplant day, intrathoracic cultures became positive. An ascending infection from the pneumatic drive lines was not detected in any of the patients. The inside of the TAH was infected by *Candida albicans* in the patient who died with bacterial and fungal sepsis prior to transplantation. In this case, endocarditis-like lesions were found adjacent to the outflow valves and within the aortic and pulmonary conduits.

Factors, including age, number of sternotomies, duration of TAH implant, days of support on the mechanical ventilator prior to infection, and duration of preoperative inotropes and IABP, were assessed to determine their possible influence on subsequent lethal infections [7]. While those patients with infection were older and required longer preoperative periods of support, the differences did not reach statistical significance. Interestingly, the number of days of mechanical ventilation and requirement for a repeat sternotomy due to bleeding were essentially the same in both groups. Acute renal failure frequently accompanied septic complications and was believed to be a result of the infection, not the cause.

Thrombosis and Thromboembolism

Cerebral embolism occurred in one patient who was receiving a large dose of heparin (1200 units/h) but whose partial thromboplastin time was only 37 s (control 30 s), and most explanted devices showed some deposition of small thrombi (1–3 min) in the inner and outer crevices formed between the polished valve rings and their isoplast housings (Fig. 5). These findings occurred variably in the major and minor orifices of the atrioventricular, aortic, and pulmonary valves. In two Jarvik-7 100-ml hearts, large red thrombi were found; one was loosely adherent to the suture line connecting the left atrium to the polyurethane-covered inlet cuff, and the other adhered to the polyurethane diaphragm at its point of connection to the rigid left ventricular housing (Fig. 5). There was no evidence of wear to the valves, housings, or blood and air diaphragms.

Discussion

The use of the TAH as a bridge device has brought criticism because this application increases the number of mortally ill candidates waiting for donor hearts, and the poorer results after transplantation in these TAH bridge patients suggest some wastage of donor organs [8]. The actuarial survival of all recipients of the TAH in Pittsburgh has been 50% (Fig. 6), a result significantly below the 85% national average 1st-year survival after heart transplantation alone. Advocates of the experiment counter that temporary use of the device is ideal as valuable information can be learned that ultimately might benefit a large number of patients

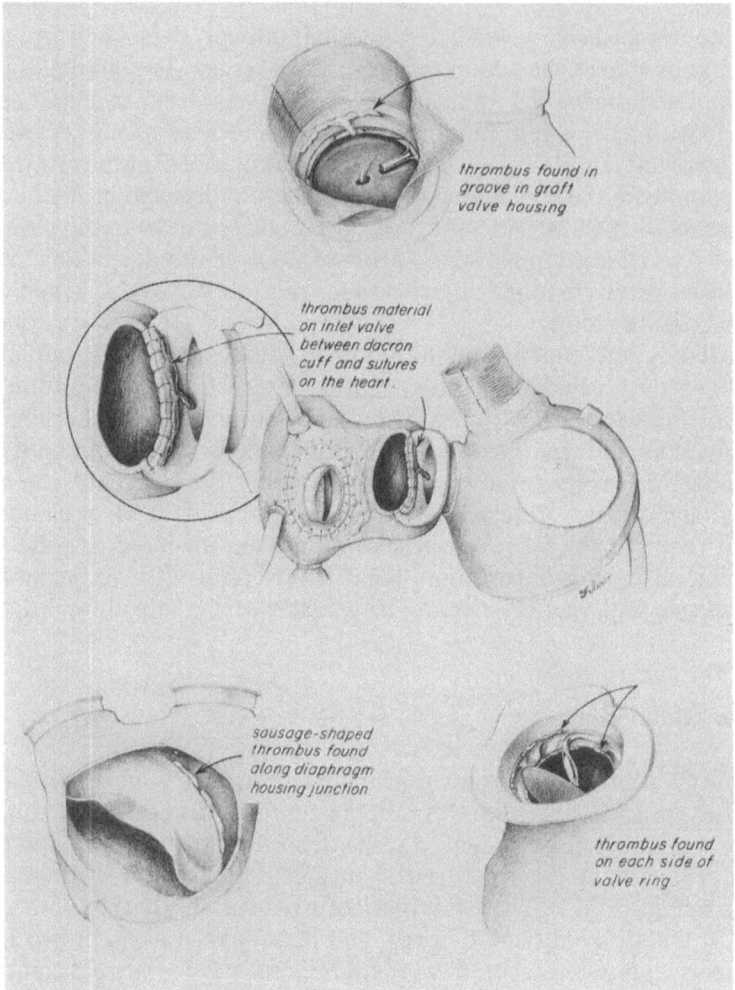

thrombus found in groove in graft valve housing

thrombus material on inlet valve between dacron cuff and sutures on the heart.

sausage-shaped thrombus found along diaphragm housing junction

thrombus found on each side of valve ring

Fig. 5. Site of thrombus found in explanted artificial heart

when clinical strategies and technology progress to produce a more therapeutic permanent device [9, 10]. We have chosen to be conservative in selection; currently we select as candidates those with reasonably recoverable situations and prefer not to use the heart as a triage for large numbers of patients who may or may not recover enough to become transplant candidates. Experts agree that the key to the selection of candidates likely to ultimately benefit from the bridge is an understanding that the TAH should not be used to resurrect patients dying from prolonged cardiopulmonary arrest or advanced degrees of renal and hepatic failure, and should not be used in those with any evidence of coexisting sepsis or pneumonia [11]. The rates of survival after transplantation reflect our perhaps ill-

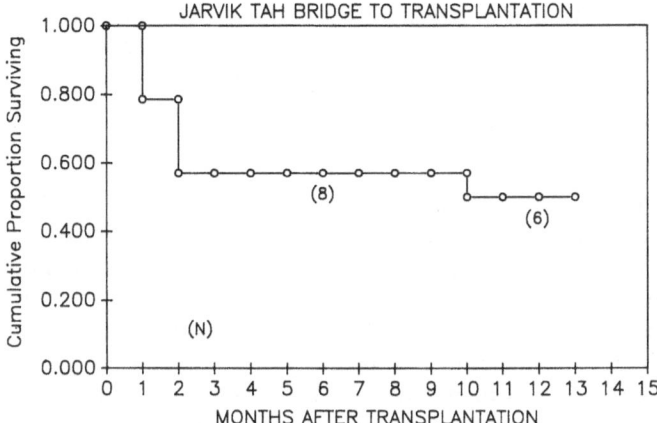

Fig. 6. TAH bridge-to-transplantation survival – Pittsburgh

advised preference to be more aggressive with transplantation in those with implantation-related complications, including pneumonia, mediastinitis, and renal failure. This preference suggests our unwillingness to become involved in a complicated, chronic implant with minimal hope for a therapeutic result.

There have been four major complications subsequent to the implantation of the TAH as a bridge, and these include perioperative hemorrhage, thromboembolism, infection, and multiorgan failure [6, 12]. Up to one-third of the patients have required a return to the operating room to address excessive perioperative bleeding. The problem is due to multiple suture lines and the requirement for aggressive use of early therapeutic anticoagulation out of fear for thromboemboli from the Jarvik-7 device. The relatively low (1/16) but still unacceptable rate of thromboembolic phenomena in this application of the device compared to that occurring with its permanent use is due to good fortune, its short-term application (which has averaged 13 days), and an aggressive protocol of anticoagulation based on the lessons learned from DeVries et al. [13]. It is likely that pumps of better design will lessen the risk of stroke, but based on experience from the permanent implants of DeVries, the threat from the embolism from pseudo-endocarditis will continue [14, 15]. Most investigators were aware of a significant risk of infection with the interim use of the TAH as lethal infection had been the cause of death in every long-term survivor of the permanently implanted TAH. Because clinical and animal infections generally were diagnosed after 4 weeks, it was hoped they could be minimized by restricting the time of implantation to 14–21 days. While all investigators have noted significant infectious mortality, the Pittsburgh series is most remarkable for a staggering 32% (5/16) incidence of mediastinitis, which was diagnosed in all but one patient early after transplantation [6]. Deep infection of the skin buttons with spread to the periprosthetic space has not been noted in the bridged patients who have received donor hearts within 2–4 weeks of implantation, probably due to the relatively short duration of implantation. Our series suggests no difference in rates of survival or infection between the routine transplant population who were admitted for their operative procedure and those with prolonged hospitalizations supported on inotropes and the IABP. It was noted that recipients of the TAH who developed lethal infections tended toward longer periods of preoperative support with inotropes (12 vs. 30 days) and the IABP (3.4 vs. 17 days) but as with age (45 vs. 47.5 years), these differences were not found to be significant [6]. We have found that patients have been able to mount a response against their transplanted organ but believe that this response is not directly related to similar inclinations against infection.

It is most likely that the pericardial space which contains clotted blood and serum plus the prosthetic ventricle and vascular conduits represents a major problem for local host defense against infection. Realistically, almost every potential factor known to contribute to surgical infection is present in the TAH bridge-to-transplant patient, and perhaps one might question why the incidence of lethal infection is not higher. It would seem, based on the successful use of paracorporeal ventricular assist devices [16], that maintenance of a beating heart and epicardial-to-pericardial apposition is a major benefit.

In the future, we plan (a) to exclude from candidacy for the TAH all patients who are being treated for infection, (b) to reduce the level of anticoagulation early postoperatively in order to lessen the risk of bleeding and resternotomy, (c) to experiment with the use of selective antibiotic decontamination of the gastrointestinal track to reduce the likelihood of bacterial translocation and enteric pneumonias, (d) to eliminate as much as possible the pericardial space, and (e) to consider the use of omental wraps and perhaps sustained release antibiotics around the TAH. Continued work with the temporary orthotopic replacement of the heart with a mechanical one is necessary to provide insight into problems and solutions critical to expansion of this important technology.

References

1. Working Group on Mechanical Circulatory Support of the National Heart, Lung, and Blood Institute (1985) Artificial heart and assist devices: directions, needs, costs, societal, and ethical issues. National Heart, Lung, and Blood Institute, Bethesda, May 1985
2. DeVries WC, Anderson JL, Joyce LD et al. (1984) Clinical use of the total artificial heart. N Engl J Med 310:273–278
3. Griffith BP, Hardestry RL, Trento A et al. (1986) Cardiac transplantation: emerging from an experiment to a service. Ann Surg 204:308–314
4. Kaye MP (1987) The registry of the International Society for Heart Transplantation: fourth official report – 1987. Heart Transplant 6:63–67
5. Hardesty RL, Griffith BP, Trento A et al. (1986) Mortally ill patients and excellent survival following cardiac transplantation. Ann Thorac Surg 41:126–129
6. Trento A, Hardesty RL, Griffith BP et al. (1988) Role of the antibidoy to vascular endothelial cells in hyperacute rejection in patients undergoing cardiac transplantation. J Thorac Cardiovasc Surg 95:37–41
7. Griffith BP, Kormos RL, Hardesty RL et al. (1988) The artificial heart: infection-related morbidity and its effect on transplantation. Ann Thorac Surg 45(4):409–415
8. Annas GJ (1985) No cheers for temporary artificial hearts. Hastings Cent Rep 15:27–28
9. Griffith BP, Bahnson HT, Roth LH (1987) Rebuttal to George J. Annas' letter to the editor. N Engl J Med 317:315

10. Relman AS (1986) Artificial hearts – permanent and temporary. N Engl J Med 314:644–645
11. Griffith BP, Hardesty RL, Kormos RL et al. (1987) Temporary use of the Jarvik-7 total artificial heart prior to transplantation. N Engl J Med 316:130–134
12. Cabrol CE, Gandjbakhch I, Pavie A et al. (1988) Orthotopic heart transplantation survival after total artificial heart implantation. Presented at the annual meeting, Am Assn Thorac Surg, Los Angeles
13. DeVries WC (1988) The permanent artificial heart, four case reports. JAMA 259:849–859
14. Kunin CM, Dobbins JJ, Melo LG et al. (1988) Infectious complications in four long-term recipients of the Jarvik-7 artificial heart. JAMA 259:860–869
15. Gristina AG, Dobbins JJ, Grammara B et al. (1988) Biomaterial-centered sepsis and the total artificial heart, microbial adhesions vs tissue integration. JAMA 259:870–874
16. Farrar DJ, Hill D, Gray LA et al. (1988) Heterotopic prosthetic ventricles as a bridge to cardiac transplantation. N Engl J Med 318:333–340

25. First European Bridge to Heart Transplantation with the Ellipsoid-Heart

F. UNGER

The artificial heart has become a clinical reality since its first elective clinical implantation in 1982 [1]. The total artificial heart was designed and developed as a permanent substitute for a failing heart, and, as such, artificial hearts have been implanted in six patients for up to 600 days. The main limiting factor is generation of thrombi, due to the design [2], and the resulting cerebral embolism [3]. The first clinical experience with temporary use of an artificial heart was in 1969 [4] in combination with transplantation. Experience now covers five cases of cardiac failure after cardiac operation [5] and ten cases of patients with failing hearts awaiting transplantation.

The first European operation was performed with the ellipsoid heart on 6 March 1986 in Salzburg. The heart of a 26-year-old female patient failed irreversibly after an aortic valve replacement. The case of this patient is described in detail below.

Case Report

A 26-year-old female patient was admitted with an aortic restenosis. An aortic isthmus stenosis had been corrected in 1968, and an aortic valve was replaced in 1980 with a Carpentier-Edwards bioprosthesis. The bioprosthesis calcified, so reoperation was indicated this was done on 6 March 1986. The valve reconstruction was performed in extracorporal circulation, the biological valve being replaced by a Sorin valve. In the intensive care unit 2 h after the (uneventful) cardiac operation the heart started to fibrillate. Despite several attempts at defibrillating, the heart was not able to maintain sufficient circulation, so reoperation was indicated. Extracorporeal circulation could not help recovery and it was not possible after prolonged emergency cardiac care to take the patient off cardiopulmonary bypass. Total heart replacement was indicated because the patient met the normal criteria for receiving a transplant.

In mild hypothermia the heart was removed in the atrioventricular area. The pulmonary artery and the aorta were dissected. The quick connectors for the artificial heart were anastomosed by running suture on to the remaining atria and the great arteries. The artificial heart used was the ellipsoid heart (Fig. 1) [5], driven pneumatically. First, the left ventricle was connected to the left atrium, the air was removed, and it began to pump. The right ventricle was then connected, the air removed, and in it pumping then began. The airlines were led out of the chest on the left side. The artificial heart gradually assumed the entire blood vol-

Assisted Circulation 3
F. Unger (Ed.)
© Springer-Verlag Berlin Heidelberg 1989

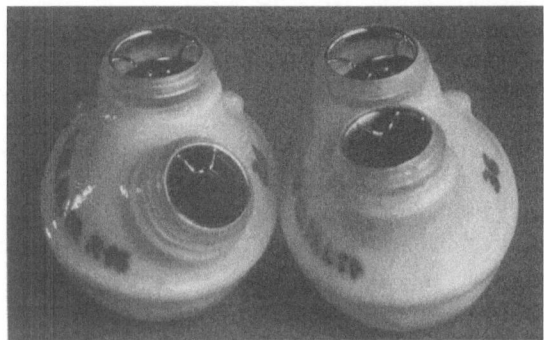

Fig. 1. The ellipsoid heart

ume, and the patient could be taken off cardiopulmonary bypass. The heparin was neutralized with protamine. The chest was drained and closed.

The patient's arterial pressure, central venous pressure, blood gases, electrolytes, creatinine, UN, leucocytes, erythrocytes, clotting, fibrinogen, lactate, and urinary output were monitored. The patient remained intubated. The artificial heart was driven by a driving console constructed by Thoma [6] and was monitored via gas pressures and gas flows. The frequency was 80 bpm, the left driving pressure 70 mmHg, and the right driving pressure 70 mmHg. During pumping the patient received heparin according the ACT. The transplantation was performed 24 h later by E. Wolner (Vienna). The artificial heart was removed. The remaining atria and vessels were trimmed, and the donor organ sewn in place. The patient died 10 days later, however, due to rejection.

The Ellipsoid Heart

The ellipsoid heart was designed to prevent areas of stagnation in the blood chamber and thereby the formation of thrombi [7]. The membrane is constructed with the end-diastolic position as its memory position (Fig. 2). The dome of the

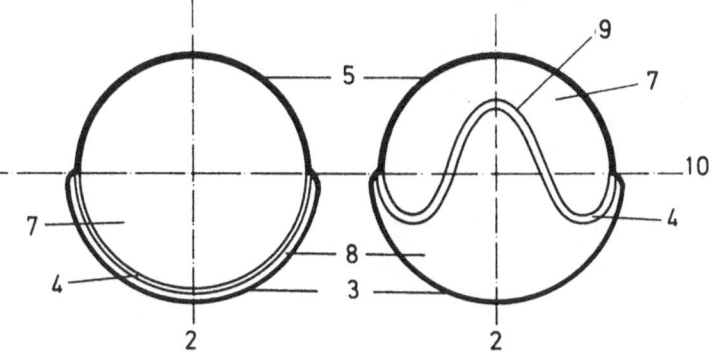

Fig. 2. Cross-section of the ellipsoid heart. *Left*, end-diastolic position (memory position). *Right*, end-systolic position

membrane increases to the maximum of the ejection beneath the valves. With this design the overall dimensions can be kept smaller than in other artificial ventricles [8]. The stroke volume is 100 ml, and the maximal output is 16 l/min. The ellipsoid heart is driven pneumatically; the driving console was developed by Thoma. To ensure adequate monitoring of the membrane, gas flow is monitored beat-by-beat [9]. The ellipsoid heart is constructed of polyurethane (Biomer), the valve-supporting structures of Teflon, and the heart base of vacuum-formed polycarbonate. The blood flow is directed by sorin valves, the inflow valves being size 29 and the outflow valves size 27.

Results

The ellipsoid heart fitted very well in the chest of the patient (Fig. 3) and could maintain a physiological perfusion of the body (Fig. 4). The patient was able to recover on the artificial heart. Adequate perfusion was demonstrated by spontaneous urinary output and especially by a decrease in lactate excess from 14 to 3.75 mmg. The platelet count declined, and total blood loss was 600 ml. Levels of C3 and C4 of the complement system declined to 0. The time spent on the total artificial heart was completely uneventful. The membrane was free of any deposits of thrombi or fibrin.

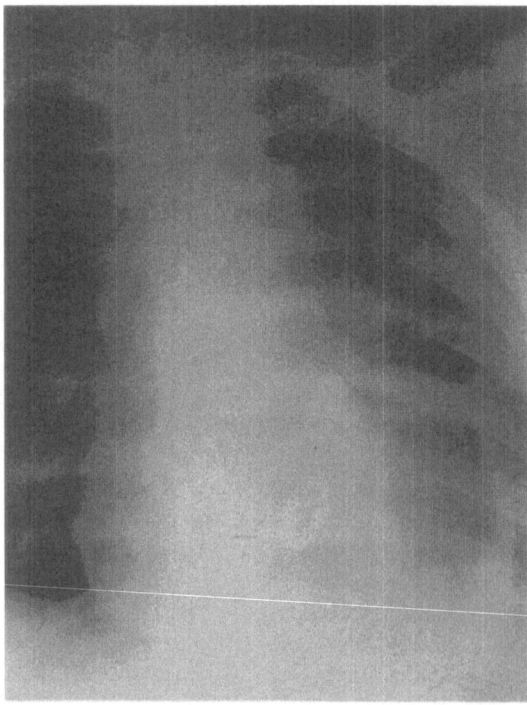

Fig. 3. X-ray with ellipsoid heart at 16 h after implantation

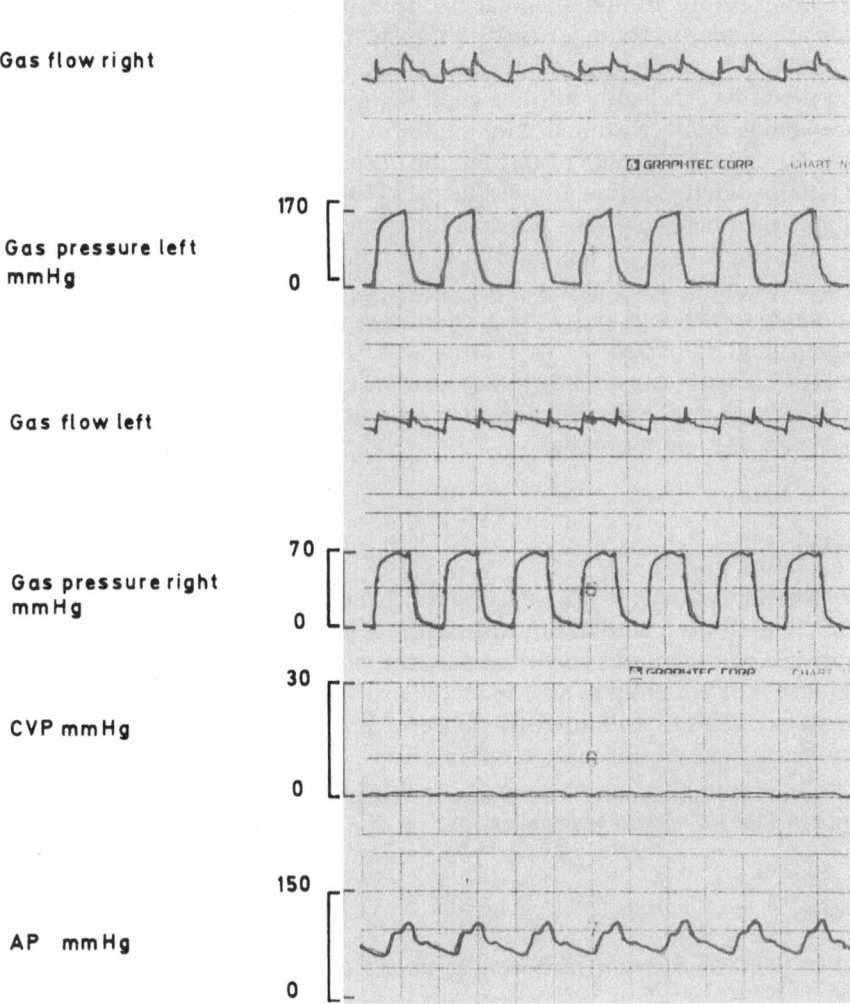

Fig. 4. Hemodynamic parameters with ellipsoid heart

Discussion

The total artificial heart has become a clinical reality for temporary use in combination with transplantation. Permanent implantation is contraindicated due to the thrombogenicity of artificial hearts [3]. To date there have been 15 clinical experiences with its temporary use: five patients have received a total artificial heart after cardiac operations and ten patients with failing heart who are awaiting cardiac transplantation have had one temporarily. It seems that those with a failing heart after a cardiac operation have less chance of survival than patients whose heart is failing before an imminent cardiac transplantation. Indications for the operation are similar to those for cardiac transplantation.

The artificial heart guaranteed adequate hemodynamic performance. The ellipsoid heart fitted excellently into the chest without compromising surrounding structures and without twisting or kinking the atrium. The inside of the artificial heart was free of any deposits of thrombi or fibrin such as were found in earlier clinical studies of left ventricular assist devices [10]. In retrospect, in the case described here the time chosen for transplantation was too early. Based to this experience, the ellipsoid heart was used in May 1986 by E. Wolner in Vienna in a patient with a failing heart and waiting for transplantation. The ellipsoid heart was implanted for 10 days and performed uneventfully, so that the patient could be extubated and mobilized.

The artificial heart can already be used without hesitation as a bridge to transplantation. Based on the first 30 clinical investigations, designs must be reevaluated to ensure safe temporary use.

Summary

In a 26-year-old patient it was necessary to implant an artificial heart and thereafter to perform a cardiac transplantation. The ellipsoid heart fitted excellently into the chest without compromising the surrounding structure. With the artificial heart the patient was able to recover sufficiently to allow the following transplantation. This first clinical experience inspires confidence in using artificial hearts more often as a bridge to transplantation.

Acknowledgements. With support of the Austrian Research Council, the Austrian Research Foundation and the Kurt Polzer Foundation.

References

1. Kolff WJ (1984) Questions and prediction. In: Unger F (ed) Assisted circulation 2. Springer, Berlin Heidelberg New York Tokyo, pp 8–10
2. Levinson MM, SMith RG, Cark RC, Gallo J, Emery RW, Icenogle TB, Ott RA, Burns GL, Copeland IG (1986) Thromboembolic complications of the Jarvik-7 total artificial heart: case report. Artif Organs 10:236–244
3. Unger F, Olsen DB, Oster H, Kolff WJ (1976) Material and design factors in thromboembolisation in total artificial heart recipients living 100–2000 hours. Eur Surg Res 8:105–116
6. Thoma H (1984) Drive and management of circulation support systems. In: Unger F (ed) Assisted circulation 2. Springer, Berlin Heidelberg New York Tokyo, pp 339–366
7. Unger F (1977) Konstruktion und tierexperimentelle Befunde mit einer neuen Form eines künstlichen Herzens: das Ellipsoidherz. Wien Klin Wochenschr 89 (Suppl):65
8. Henning E, Mohnhaupt A, Bücherl ES (1976) Effect of filling pressure on the performance of pneumatically driven blood pumps. Eur Soc Artif Organs 3:27
9. Unger F, Deutsch M, Faschin W, Horcher E, Losert U, Mohl W, Stellwag F, Thoma H, Weißkirchner R, Wolner E, Navratil J (1977) Automatic driving systems for artificial hearts. Med Instrum 11:208
10. Wolner E, Deutsch M, Losert U, Stellwag F, Thoma H, Unger F, Polzer K, Navratil J (1978) Clinical application of the ellipsoid left ventricular assist device (E-LVAD). Artif Organs 2:268–274
11. Unger F (1986) Artificial heart – assisted circulation. Curr Opinion Cardiol 2:66

26. The Total Artificial Heart in Clinical Practice – The Vienna Experience and Point of View

W. Trubel and E. Wolner

Introduction

More than 30 years have passed since Kolff and his co-workers performed their first successful implantation of a total artificial heart (TAH) in a dog [1]. Survival times of more than 6 months were later achieved by different groups in experiments [2], and the first clinical implantation of a TAH was performed by Cooley and his team in 1969 [3].

In contrast to ventricular assist devices (VADs), which are used to provide temporary mechanical support to a failing heart and are removed after cardiac recovery, clinical TAH implantation is an irreversible step leading either to subsequent heart transplantation (HTx) or to permanent TAH replacement. There is an ongoing discussion as to whether, in a bridging procedure, preference should be given to a TAH or a VAD.

At present bridging to HTx is the main indication for clinical TAH implantation, which is usually performed in patients with biventricular failure. Up to the end of June 1987, 77 TAH implantations had been performed as a bridge to transplantation; 62 patients were transplanted successfully, and 35 (56%) of them survived [4].

A TAH bridging procedure should only be performed if the recipient shows no contraindications to HTx, such as infection, systemic diseases (malignancies or neurological or endocrinological diseases), vital organ dysfunctions, recurrent embolization and pulmonary infarction, fixed pulmonary hypertension, psychological disorders, or an age of more than 60 years [5, 6]. Patients in whom later HTx is contraindicated can still be candidates for permanent VAD or TAH replacement, as has already been performed in some cases [4]. The lack of natural donor organs could become another indication for such a procedure. At present the prognosis of permanent VAD or TAH replacement is poor, and long-term complications like recurrent embolizations, infections, and technical dysfunctions have to be solved. VAD and TAH systems with an implantable driving unit and a transcutaneous energy supply are under construction and some are in experimental use, but it will take years before an artificial circulation support will be an adequate substitute or source of relief for a natural heart.

Clinical TAH bridging has been performed by 19 teams in seven countries; eight different devices have been implanted [7]. At the IInd Department of Surgery, University of Vienna, where artificial hearts have been constructed and in experimental use since 1975, five clinical TAH implantations for bridging to HTx have been performed [8]. On three occasions the "ellipsoid heart" was used, and

Assisted Circulation 3
F. Unger (Ed.)
© Springer-Verlag Berlin Heidelberg 1989

on two, the "Berlin TAH." Both systems work with membrane pumps and an external driving unit and have been described previously [9, 10].

Clinical Use of the TAH for Bridging to HTx

At our clinic two groups of patients are potential candidates for a temporary TAH: deteriorating HTx candidates who cannot receive a donor heart in time [12] and patients who cannot be weaned off mechanical circulatory support after open-heart surgery. Up to now all bridging patients have belonged to the first group (four patients had dilated cardiomyopathy and one a large anterior wall infarction).

The goal of temporary TAH implantation is to take over the function of the failing heart and to maintain circulation. After restoration of circulation by the TAH, the patient has to be brought into a condition which allows HTx; that means none of the contraindications mentioned above may exist.

Owing to the poor preoperative hemodynamics and/or increased extracorporeal circulation (ECC) time, dysfunctions of other vital organs have to be expected. Therefore the decision on TAH implantation should be taken promptly.

Surgical Procedure

Under total ECC the patient's own heart is removed along the atrioventricular border and the origin of the great arteries. Then the connectors for the TAH ventricles are anastomosed to the residual atria, pulmonary artery, and aorta. The tubes for moving the driving membranes of the artificial ventricles are led to the mediastinum through the abdominal cavity as an additional barrier against infection. First the left and then the right TAH ventricle is connected to the atrium, great vessel, and driving tube, and after careful and complete evacuation pumping can be started. After decannulation of the heart-lung machine, thoracotomy is closed, including sternal cerclage.

Medical and Technical Procedure

The patients are kept separately in the postoperative ICU as they are at additional risk of infection from the driving tubes and all invasive catheters.

The medical treatment is similar to that in other patients after open-heart surgery [13]; only the driving of the TAH and pharmacological regulation of blood pressure need close medicotechnical cooperation [14].

Driving Mode

According to the Frank-Starling mechanism the TAH ventricles are driven in a partial filling – full ejection driving mode. As the vasomotoricity is unstable, especially during the early postoperative period, pressure-related driving of the TAH alone does not guarantee adequate perfusion of the patient's body. Measurement of arterial and central venous oxygen saturation and calculation of the percentage of tissue oxygen utilization provide information on the cardiac output actually needed, to which the left TAH ventricle is adapted. The pumping of the right TAH ventricle is adjusted to an optimal filling pressure for the left pump, avoiding an overload of the lung circulation. The arterial pressure, which is based on the cardiac output of the TAH and the systemic vascular resistance of the patient, is kept within the physiological range by administration of vasoactive medication [15].

Only if the patient is free of infection and all vital organs function sufficiently is a suitable donor heart accepted and HTx performed.

A lot of risks and medical and technical problems accompany TAH bridging; these have to be recognized and avoided to improve results and the number of long-term survivors.

Complications Related to TAH Implantation

Preoperative Status of the Patient

Depending on the duration and severity of the basic cardiac disease, the general condition of the patient and the vital organ functions may be more or less impaired due to chronic and/or acute heart failure. The preoperative status is an important factor determining the postoperative recovery of the patient and the prognosis for the whole procedure. An overlooked infection, for instance, is usually aggravated by TAH implantation, and it is hardly possible to bring the patient into a transplantable condition. The decision to implant a mechanical cardiac support should be made as soon as possible after failure of medical intervention, and the duration of severe circulatory insufficiency should be kept as short as possible.

Surgical Problems

In contrast to the excision of the patient's heart for one-stage HTx [16], the fibrous ring of the atrioventricular valves should be saved for fixation of the connectors for the TAH ventricles. Maximum atrial retention facilitates "physiological" pumping (see above). The fixation of the connectors in a fibrous tissue provides greater security than fixation to the rather thin atrial walls, which is important for the tension movements related to the valve and membrane movements of the nonelastic TAH system. After explantation of the device the affected tissue close to the former atrial anastomosis can also be excised before HTx.

In patients with a small thorax and/or no pathological heart enlargement, there might not be enough space for standard size TAH ventricles. Excision of the remaining pericardium to place parts of the system in the left pleural cavity is a solution, but may cause atelectasis of the inferior lobe of the left lung, with danger of infection and delayed recovery. Therefore nowadays smaller TAH ventricles are also available and in use [11, 17]. Another advantage of a smaller ventricle is the higher blood flow through the system, which may lead to a reduction in the incidence of thrombosis [18].

Cardiopulmonary bypass (CPB) is always necessary in a TAH implantation, in contrast to the situation when a VAD is used. The use of membrane oxygenator and intraoperative hemofiltration are state of the art for such a procedure.

Complications During TAH Bridging

Postoperative Bleeding and Anticoagulation

Hemorrhage in the early postoperative period can be evoked by the reduced number and activity of blood platelets [19] and as a hangover of heparin effects. Mass transfusion of stored blood may initiate specific and nonspecific immunoreactions, which can cause rejection problems after HTx. Resubstitution of the patient's own blood, which is led through a cell saver system [20], is one solution to this problem during the first few postoperative days.

In contrast to experimental experiences, thromboembolic events have been observed only seldom in the clinical use of TAH when anticoagulation therapy has been performed consistently during the bridging period [18]. This may be because the bridging period usually does not last long enough for pannus formations to overgrow the atrial connectors and to induce recurrent thrombus formation in the valve apparatus with subsequent multiple embolizations [21]. Other sources of thrombus formation are microlesions in the driving membranes and areas of blood stasis in the TAH ventricles. Modern technology avoids such areas by specific membrane and ventricle constructions. Covering of the inner surface of the whole system with an autologous endothelial cell layer and the use of bioprosthetic valves may also help to solve the problem of thromboembolism in the future, with a view to the permanent implantation of artificial circulatory devices.

Infection

The risk of infection during TAH pumping is high, owing to three main factors.

1. Transcutaneous driving tubes
2. Invasive catheters
3. Limited mobilization of the patient

In most systems in clinical use the driving tubes have to be led transcutaneously from the external driving unit to the mediastinum. Even though various kinds of skin button have been developed, infections along the driving tubes, even causing mediastinitis, have been reported [22, 23]. At least in the early postoperative period the patients have to be monitored by invasive catheters, which may be another source of infection. Inside the TAH an endocarditis-like infection appears mainly at sites of predilection like valve rings, suture lines, and connectors [21]. After recovery from TAH implantation, mobilization of the patient is limited depending on the system in use, and immobilization becomes another risk factor for local and general infection. Most of the patients on TAH who could not be transplanted suffered from incurable infection [4, 7].

Dysfunction of Vital Organs

Depending on the preoperative status of the patient and the duration of the circulatory insufficiency, dysfunctions of vital organs may appear after TAH implantation. Renal function, for instance, is often impaired after TAH implantation [24, 27]; even acute renal failure with oligoanuria has been observed and had to be treated by hemofiltration or hemodialysis. It could be demonstrated experimentally that a TAH circulation itself does not disturb renal function [25]. Postoperative renal function in patients who have undergone open-heart surgery significantly depends on preoperative circulation, preoperative renal function, and duration of CPB [26]. We were able to observe a complete recovery of renal function under TAH circulation, a recovery which was not influenced by the subsequent HTx and immunosuppression [27].

Due to the poor preoperative hemodynamics all grades of diffuse or focal cerebral dysfunction can appear. Recovery to a transplantable condition can only seldom be expected, the likelihood depending on the severity of the dysfunction. We observed such a complication in one of our patients; in his autopsy typical neuropathological findings due to low cardiac output [28] were detected.

Device Dysfunction
Device dysfunctions in TAH patients, such as breakdown of a valve [29], temporary disconnection, or kinking of drive lines, were observed. Fortunately up to now no TAH patient has died of such an event.

Before a TAH system comes into clinical use, it has to go through a number of in vitro tests and experimental long-term runs. All the technology is based on a maximum of security, since dysfunctions in any part of the system may have fatal consequences.

Future TAH systems, especially the fully implantable ones, should be equipped with control and alarm mechanisms [30] which enable transcutaneous check-up by a wireless reception. "Physiological" driving algorithms and control mechanisms in fully implantable devices for permanent use will have to be developed and optimized within the next few years.

Psychological Aspects
Having no own heart and being completely dependent on a machine can be a big psychological problem for a TAH recipient. After postoperative return of consciousness it can take hours, even days, until the patient recognizes his temporary state, even though he had agreed to this procedure preoperatively. Besides psychological care, frequent visits by close relatives and friends should help to overcome anxious hyperreactions and stress.

Duration of Bridging
The ideal duration of TAH bridging is a topic of global discussion, and bridging periods have lasted from a few hours up to 8 months [4, 7]. Long-term survival rates of patients undergoing HTx after TAH bridging do not correlate with the duration of TAH pumping. Following the latest discussions at international meetings the most opportune time for transplantation (taking into consideration all the above-mentioned possible complications during TAH bridging) seems to be between 10 and 20 days after TAH implantation.

If a bridging patient cannot achieve a transplantable condition, the temporary TAH implantation may become a permanent one. The man factors precluding

HTx are recurrent rejection, persisting organ failure, and incurable infection [4, 7, 8]. The patient then has to be kept on the TAH. Complications of long-term pumping like recurrent thromboembolism, persisting organ failure, and infection are still the main reasons for the bad prognosis in these patients [7].

Complications After HTx That Are Related to Bridging

Surgical Problems
In contrast to the situation when a one-stage HTx is performed, the tissue of the remaining atria and those parts of the great arteries close to the former anastomoses may be affected by the TAH system. Necrotic tissue should be excised before the donor heart is implanted to avoid bleeding, delayed healing, and infection. The tunnels of the former driving tubes need extra surgical treatment such as drainage and suturing to avoid fistula formation.

Infection
Naturally the risk of infection is always higher after a two-stage HTx due to multiple factors such as the duration of immobilization and monitoring by invasive catheters, the short time lapse before reoperation, and initiation of immunosuppressive therapy; post-transplantation care has to pay special attention to this.

Hypersensitization and Rejection
Different TAH bridging centers have reported on therapy-resistant transplant rejections in bridging patients, leading to reimplantation of a TAH or the patient's death [8, 31]. Humoral rejection mechanisms may be stimulated by multiple blood transfusions and/or other antigen contacts during the bridging period, leading to a higher titer of circulating cytotoxic antibodies. Alterations of immunological parameters such as increased complement activation and marked lymphopenia after TAH implantation have been observed [32]. Therefore the necessity of cytotoxic antibody screening and/or lymphocyte cross-matching in bridging patients before HTx is being discussed at present [31].

Future Developments

Though a number of ethical, medical, and technical problems remain to be solved, it is obvious that the human heart can be replaced by an artificial one at least for some time. Even if the availability of donor hearts could be increased by liberalization of the law and improved organization, the demand for heart replacements will still exceed the supply of natural donor organs. The artificial heart does not yet seem ready to serve as a permanent replacement; fully implantable systems with only an external energy supply are under development, and the problems of the inner surfaces of the devices may also be solved in the future. The goal is to create an artificial heart that works like the natural heart – or even better. The coming years will reveal the possibilities and limitations of such a development.

References

1. Akutsu T, Kolff WJ (1958) Permanent substitutes for valves and hearts. Trans Am Soc Artif Intern Organs 4:230–235
2. Jarvik RK, Olson DB, Kessler TR, Lawson J, English J, Kolff WJ (1977) Criteria for human artificial heart implantation based on steady state animal data. Trans Am Soc Artif Intern Organs 23:535–536
3. Cooley DA, Liotta D, Hallmann GL, Bloodwell RD, Leachmann RD, Hilan JD (1969) First clinical implantation of a total artificial heart. Trans Am Soc Artif Intern Organs 15:68–69
4. Olson DB (1987) ISAO International registry, TAH-bridge to transplant experience, patient status as of June 30, 1987. Latest data periodically published in Artif. Organs or directly available via the Institute of Biomedical Engeneering, University of Utah
5. English TA, Spratt P, Wallwork J, Cory-Pearce R (1984) Selection and procurement of hearts for a transplantation. Br Med J [Clin Res] 288:1889–1891
6. Jamieson SW, Oyer PE, Reitz BA, Baumgartner WA, Bieber CB, Stinson EB, Shumway NE (1981) Cardiac transplantation at Stanford. Heart Transplant 1(1):86–91
7. Joyce LD, Johnson KE, Pierce WS, DeVries WC, Semb BK, Copeland JG, Griffith BP, Cooley DA, Frazier OH, Cabrol C, Keon WJ, Unger F, Buecherl ES, Wolner E (1986) Summary of the world experience with clinical use of total artificial hearts as heart support devices. J Heart Transplant 5(3):229–230
8. Trubel W, Losert U, Schima H, Rokitansky A, Spiss CK, Coraim F, Laczkowics A, Wolner E (1987) Total artificial heart bridging: a temporary support for deteriorating HTX-candidates. Thorac Cardiovasc Surg 35(5):277–283
9. Unger F (1977) Konstruktion und tierexperimentelle Befunde mit einer neuen Form des künstlichen Herzens: das Ellipsoidherz. Wien Klin Wochenschr 89(3) [Suppl]:65
10. Akutsu T, Jarvik RK, Zartnack S (1986) Blood pumps. In: Buecherl E (ed) Proc Sec World Symp Artif Heart, vol 1. Vieweg, Braunschweig, pp 59–112 (Adv System Analysis)
11. Jarvik RK, DeVries WC, Semb BK, Koul B, Copeland JG, Levinson MM, Griffith BP, Joyce LD, Cooley DA, Frazier OH, Cabrol C, Keon WJ (1986) Surgical positioning of the Jarvik-7 artificial heart. J Heart Transplant 5(3):184–195
12. Pierce WS (1983) Artificial heart and blood pumps in the treatment of profound heart failure. Circulation 68(4):883–884
13. Haider W (1980) Intensivbehandlung nach herzchirurgischen Eingriffen. In: Steinbereithner K, Bergmann H (eds) Intensivstation, -pflege und -therapie. Thieme, Stuttgart
14. Schima H, Trubel W, Coraim F, Huber L, Müller MR, Redl G, Losert U, Thoma H, Wolner E (1987) Control of the total artificial heart: new aspects in human versus animal experience. Artif Organs (manuscript submitted)
15. Rokitansky A, Trubel W, Coraim F, Schima H, Laczkovics A, Müller MR, Buxbaum P, Schreiner W, Losert U, Haider W, Wolner E (1987) Clinical TAH-bridging in Vienna: hemodynamics and regulation. Artif Organs (in print)
16. Lower RR, Shumway NE (1960) Studies on orthotopic transplantation of the canine heart. Surg Forum 11:18–19
17. Joyce LD, Pritzker MR, Kiser JC, Nicoloff DM, Kersten TE, Von Rueden TJ, Eales F, Johnson KE, Jorgensen ChR, Gobel FL, Van Tassel RA (1986) Use of the mini Jarvik-7. Total artificial heart as a bridge to transplantation. J Heart Transplant 5(3):203–204
18. Lewinson MM, Smith RG, Cork RC, Gallo J, Emery RW, Icenoglet B, Ott RA, Burns GL, Copeland JG (1986) Thromboembolic complications of the Jarvik-7 total artificial heart: case report. Artif Organs 10(3):236–244
19. Müller MR, Wohlfahrt A, Lee A, Trubel W, Zilla P, Fasol R, Wolner E (1987) Observations on human thrombocytes during TAH replacement. Artif Organs (in print)
20. Saggau W, Späth J, Tanzeem A, Storch HH, Schmitz W (1982) Erfahrungen mit dem Haemonetics-Cell-Saver in der offenen Herzchirurgie. Anästh Intensivther Notfallmed 17:51–57
21. Weidemann H (1985) Künstlicher Totalherzersatz – Korrelation klinischer, hämodynamischer und morphologischer Befunde in 4 Entwicklungsphasen 1972–1984, chap 3. Klinikum Charlottenburg der Freien Universität Berlin, pp 91–92

22. Murray KD, Hughes S, Bearnson D, Olsen DB (1983) Infection in total artificial heart recipients. Trans Am Soc Artif Intern Organs 24:539–540
23. Murray-Leishure KA, Aber RC, Rowley LJ, Applebaum PC, Wisman CB, Pennock JL, Pierce WS (1986) Disseminated *Trichosporon beigelii* (cutaneum) infection in an artificial heart recipient. JAMA 256(21):2995–2996
24. Westenfelder C, Haus RM, Border WA, Muniz H, Duffy D, Menlove RL, Bananovsky RL (1983) Renal function in the first artificial heart patient. Am Soc Nephrol 16:42–43
25. Westenfelder C, Haus RM, Border WA, Muniz H, Duffy D, Menlove RL, Bananovsky RL (1985) Renal function in calves with TAH. Trans Am Soc Artif Intern Organs 31:383–387
26. Hilberman M, Myers BD, Carvie BJ, Derby G, Jamison RL, Stinson EB (1979) Acute renal failure following cardiac surgery. J Thorac Cardiovasc Surg 77(6):880–888
27. Trubel W, Losert U, Rokitansky A, Coraim F, Schreiner W, Kovarik J, Buxbaum P, Müller MR, Wolner E (1987) Acute renal dysfunction and TAH bridging. Artif Organs (in print)
28. Peters G (1979) Spezielle Pathologie der Krankheiten des zentralen und peripheren Nervensystems, Kreislaufstörungen, 2nd edn. Thieme, Stuttgart, pp 150–151
29. DeVries WC, Anderson JL, Joce LD et al. (1984) Clinical use of the total artificial heart. N Engl J Med 310(5):273–278
30. Mays JB, Hastings WL, Williams MA, Barker LE, DeVries WC (1986) Drive system management of emergency conditions in three permanent total artificial heart patients. Trans Am Soc Artif Intern Organs 32:221–225
31. Levinson MM, Smith RG, Cork R, Gallo J, Icenogle T, Emery R, Ott R, Copeland J (1986) Three recent cases of total artificial heart before transplantation. J Heart Transplant 5(3):215–216
32. Stelzer GT, Ward RA, Wellhausen SR, Mcleish KR, Johnson GS, DeVries WC (1987) Alterations in select immunologic parameters following total artificial heart implantation. Artif Organs 11(1):52

27. The Philadelphia Heart System – An Implantable Artificial Heart for a Transplant Center

J. KOLFF, P. WURZEL, and J. B. RIEBMAN

Introduction

The human implantation of the first total artificial heart (TAH) in 1969 by Cooley [1, 2] represented the efforts of many investigators and many years of research. During this and other implants to follow, the TAH clearly demonstrated its capacity to anatomically and functionally replace the diseased natural heart, relieving heart failure and restoring cardiac hemodynamics to normal. Further laboratory investigation was stimulated by these results and has since led to the development of more advanced device designs which incorporate advances in biocompatibility and mechanical reliability of the components and driving systems. Select clinical applications of the currently available devices have shown promising results, generating an increasing interest in more widespread clinical application of TAH devices [3–8].

As of 1 April 1987, a total of 68 TAH implantations had been performed in 17 centers throughout the world [9]. This figure includes 5 patients who received the TAH as a permanent implant and 63 who were treated with the TAH as a temporary "mechanical bridge" while awaiting cardiac transplantation. Mechanical circulatory support for limited periods with the TAH allowed hemodynamic stabilization of these patients, for whom death seemed imminent, thus providing time for an acceptable donor heart to be located. Successful transplantation was carried out in 78% of these patients. Analysis of the experience with clinical applications of the TAH has allowed researchers to evaluate the usefulness of these devices in different groups of patients, forming the basis for establishing guidelines on patient selection and ultimately on the indications for clinical use [10].

Evaluation of these patients has also revealed the range of complications and probable limitations of this therapy [11, 12]. The problems associated with the TAH include unacceptable anatomic fit, generation of thromboemboli, bleeding, stroke, hemolysis, thrombocytopenia, immunomodulation, and infections, as well as mechanical malfunction of the heart, its valves, or the driving system, and limited mobility of the implanted patient.

However, if use of the TAH is less hazardous to the patient than the disease that afflicts him, the physician and the patient should consider the use of this device. Practically speaking, use of the TAH requires both knowledge of the hazards of the device and the ability to assess the patient's illness. Most importantly, the use of a particular device needs to be personalized to the individual patient, considering his size, disease, and ability to comprehend the risks and limitations of the device as well as the risks of his disease. Our design of a new artificial heart

Assisted Circulation 3
F. Unger (Ed.)
© Springer-Verlag Berlin Heidelberg 1989

is based on our understanding of the hazards of the TAH and our experience with evaluating the critically ill cardiac patient for whom such a device may need to be used.

The Philadelphia Total Artificial Heart System

System Overview

The design features and fabrication techniques of the Philadelphia heart system (PHS) are derived from years of laboratory bench and animal studies and from the clinical experience to date with other device models. The PHS consists of two internal, pneumatically actuated blood pumps (Fig. 1) connected via 6-ft tubular air conduits (air drive lines) to an external driving console which provides pneumatic energy and computer monitoring of system performance. Within each pump is a multilayered, thin, flexible diaphragm which divides the intraventricular volume into chambers for blood and air. Pressurized air is introduced into the air chamber from the driving console which moves the diaphragm and causes the ejection of blood from the ventricle. When this air is allowed to exhaust, blood can fill the ventricle. The pneumatic controllers within the driving console alternate continuously between pressure (ventricular systole) and exhaust (ventricular systole) to create the cardiac cycle. Although other pneumatic TAH systems share these functional features, the PHS incorporates several novel features which are described below.

Ventricles

The specific geometry and size of the ventricular pumping chambers allow orthotopic implantation of the ventricles with all atrial and arterial anastomoses con-

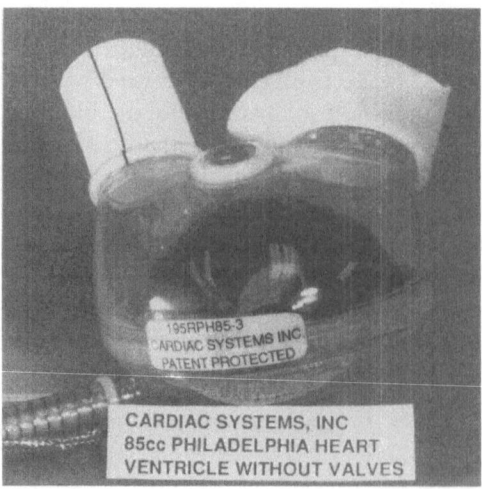

Fig. 1. Philadelphia heart system ventricles

tained within the pericardial sac. The quick connectors found on other TAH systems have been eliminated. The atrial cuffs and arterial grafts are permanently attached to the blood pump. This design of the PHS ventricles allows more efficient use of available pericardial space than does that in other TAH models; this reduces the risks of undesirable compression of adjacent pulmonary and vascular structures. It also allows the prosthetic valves to be sewn into the cuffs and grafts. This technique provides two advantages over other systems: first, the valves retain the compliant mounting arrangement for which they were designed and, second, this method eliminates the micro crevices found in other TAH valve mounts, which are believed to be a site of thrombosis.

Performance of the PHS ventricles has been engineered so that they follow a performance curve similar to the Starling curve for a natural heart beating at a fixed rate. A pumping rate and percent systole are selected for the ventricles which allow them to fill approximately 60% of their maximum stroke volume during each beat. A driving pressure is then selected for each ventricle which generates full ejection of the blood chamber. As atrial pressure increases, the ventricular filling rate (dQ/dt) increases during diastole, which creates an increase in stroke volume and subsequent cardiac output. This type of intrinsic regulation allows the PHS to respond to limited transient variations in atrial pressures without driving system adjustments. If the atrial pressure rises sufficiently to completely fill the blood chamber, the cardiac output becomes constant unless the pumping rate is increased.

The ventricular housing, intermediate and air diaphragms, and the base are all constructed from vacuum-formed polyurethane (Pellathane 2363-80AE, Dow Chemical, North Haven, Connecticut) with no metallic or hard plastic rings to hold the various components or the valves in place. The housing and base are so designed that they snap together and are sealed with only a bead of solvent glue. In order to create a seamless intima, the endocardial surface (including the pressure transducer), blood diaphragm, and valve annuli are casted from a polyurethane in dimethylacetamide solution. Ultrafine graphite is applied as a lubricant between diaphragm layers. Each ventricle has a 2-in. long Dacron outflow graft glued to the outflow port and a 1.0- to 1.5-in. diameter velour-covered cuff glued to the inflow port. Commercially available prosthetic valves are sutured into the grafts and onto the cuffs at their junctions with the ventricular housing. (For additional details on the construction of the ventricles see [13].) The volume displacement of each ventricle is approximately 200 cm^3 with an effective stroke volume of 85 cm^3.

The design of PHS ventricles was determined in part by the desire to use low-thrombogenic tissue valves which need to be sewn into an annulus. This is true whether the valves are free homografts or are premounted on stents with sewing rings. A valve annulus was incorporated into the artificial ventricles into which both tissue and mechanical valves could be sutured. The original experiments with these ventricles utilized commercially available valves of the surgeon's choice, which were sewn into the valve openings on a side table at the time of implantation. However, in order to standardize our valve usage as suggested by the United States Food and Drug Administration, we elected to utilize the St. Jude mechanical bileaflet valve. These valves were chosen because of their excellent

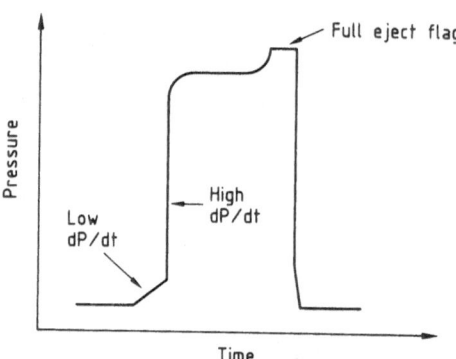

Fig. 2. Idealized air driveline waveform from Philadrive model IP pneumatic controller

flow characteristics and low-profile design. Because of the expense of these, and in fact all, commercially available valves, the next generation of Philadelphia hearts will use polyurethane trileaflet valves manufactured by methods similar to those used in ventricle construction.

Drive System

The external drive console contains an air compressor, two high-pressure back-up tanks, and two Philadrive pneumatic controls. The systolic pressure pulse supplied to the left ventricle consists of two phases. During the first phase the air has a very slow rate of pressure rise (dP/dt) (1400–3000 mmHg/s) to reduce the closing velocity of the mitral valve (see Fig. 2). This initial pressure wave lasts approximately 35 ms. The second phase is a much stronger air jet with a dP/dt of between 7000 and 12000 mmHg/s. This wave generates the ejection phase in the blood chamber and lasts until all the blood is ejected, and the diaphragm is in its full systolic position. The Philadrives then release this pressurized air, and ventricular diastole begins.

Timing and cycling of air pressure by the Philadrives is controlled by a group of industrially available pneumatic logic elements that do not require electrical energy to function but utilize instead the same air source that drives the ventricles [16]. Heart rate and percent systole are adjusted by turning knobs that affect air flow in the pneumatic logic elements. A digital display on the front panel indicates heart rate, percent systole, and duration of the low dP/dt interval period, in addition to being the visual indicator of any alarm conditions. Solid-state pressure transducers interface between the pneumatic system and a single chip microcomputer which operates the display and monitors the various system parameters. If a parameter falls outside its normal range, the microcomputer triggers an audible alarm and outputs an alarm code on the display. The required pneumatic source for the Philadrive is 25 psi at 1.8 scfm.

Results of Animal and Human Studies

The anatomic fit of PHS ventricles into the human pericardial space was a prime concern during the design and development of this heart system. Implantation of

Table 1. Seven long-term calf survivors with 85-cc artificial hearts, containing four St. Jude valves anticoagulated with coumadin

Animal (calves)	Survival (days)	Cause of Death	Weight (kg)	Renal infarcts (old/new)	Thrombus (macroscopic) Valve	Thrombus (macroscopic) Ventricle
Val	128	Terminated secondary to diaphragm system failure	154	None/one	Clear with pseudoneointima	Thrombus left
Ch	104	Elective termination	202	Few/none	Pannus	Clear
Wa	64	Cerebral hemorrhage	95	None/several	Paravalvular	One small right side
Ph	61	Cervical hemorrhage	95	None/one	Clear	Recent blood clots in left atrium and ventricle
Tor	39	Bacterial endocarditis	112	Several/several	Infected thrombus	None
We	32	Cerebral hemorrhage	95	None/one	Small at subannular hinge	None
Jed	31	Retroperitoneal hemorrhage	82	None/none	Clear	None

the ventricles into human cadavers has shown that these ventricles can fit in an orthotopic position as a TAH in a variety of patients with different chest sizes.

Acute and chronic animal implant studies have been performed both at Temple University (Philadelphia, Pennsylvania) and the University of Utah (Salt Lake City, Utah). The acute experiments focused on evaluation of new design and construction features as well as providing training for the surgical team in implantation techniques. These studies were followed by chronic animal studies for longer term device evaluation. A number of studies were performed with various valves, including tissue valves, polyurethane trileaflet valves, and various mechanical valves. In the interest of developing a device for clinical application, the St. Jude valve was selected for the later implants.

Table 1 summarizes the pertinent survival and pathology data of the six longest living chronic animal implants to date with the PHS with St. Jude valves. The longest surviving animal was electively terminated when its condition clinically deteriorated, with the diagnosis of malfunctioning left-sided diaphragm at 130 days. Each of these animals was maintained with the Philadrive control console and underwent routine interval hematologic, coagulation, and hemolysis studies. The device fit well into calves weighing as little as 78 kg without compromise of TAH function or impingement on surrounding thoracic structures. Organ function and growth curves of the implanted animals were normal, and hemodynamic studies indicated that the PHS provided adequate cardiac output at rest and during exercise. Hematologic and biochemical profiles could usually be maintained within the normal range except for the anticoagulant-effected protime [13].

Role of PHS in the Treatment of Circulatory Failure

Patient Selection: Identification of Candidates for Transplantation

At Temple University Hospital, the longitudinal care of patients with progressive heart failure is coordinated by a specially organized Heart Failure Center, dedicated to the interdisciplinary management of this disease. The Cardiothoracic Surgery Division provides an integral component of heart failure therapy, offering cardiac transplantation and temporary mechanical circulatory assistance. With centralized patient management by the heart failure center, medical therapy for the diseased heart can be continually maximized. The constant monitoring for end organ failure and progressive disability allows potential candidates for transplant to be identified early, permitting performance of surgery at the optimal time to offer the best result.

Since the inception of our transplant center in January 1984, over 420 patients have been referred for evaluation for heart and heart-lung transplantation. Thirty percent of patients could not meet the medical criteria for transplantation while 114 patients have been transplanted. In March 1988, 13 patients were on the waiting list for heart-lung transplantation and 30 patients for heart transplantation. From our own experience and that of others, we can expect 20%–26% of cardiac transplant candidates to die before a natural heart can be found for them [17, 18].

Patient Selection: Candidates for Temporary Mechanical Support

Criteria are currently evolving for identifying those transplant candidates who will benefit from temporary mechanical circulatory support with a TAH as a bridge to transplantation [10]. To demonstrate the potential for application of the TAH in heart failure seen at transplant centers such as our own, in August 1987 we profiled the 59 patients who had died after referral to our Heart Failure Center [17]. To summarize the findings, we found that survival time varied greatly. Some patients died from shock or arrhythmias within four hours from the time of consultation, before a hospital transfer could be arranged. One patient died at home 16 months postreferral after waiting 9 months for a suitable donor heart. Between these two extremes, the clinical courses of 35 deceased patients were reexamined. Five of these patients were thought to have been ideal candidates for the use of a temporary TAH. Their common clinic characteristics were as follows:

- All patients died in our own intensive care unit under closenursing surveillance.
- All patients were alert and oriented until minutes before their death.
- All patients were in cardiogenic shock from ischemic cardiomyopathy.
- All patients were good transplant candidates.
- None of the patients had evidence of sepsis.
- Three of the five patients were on partial mechanical circulatory support prior to death (two were on intra-aorta balloon pump, one was on femoral vein to femoral artery bypass).

   The unpredictable availability of a donor heart for transplantation forces critically ill patients to remain on intravenous vasopressor and/or vasodilators as well as inotropic agents for prolonged periods of time, making them prone to progressive renal failure and peripheral tissue ischemia. The diuretics become ineffective. They are dependent on intravascular monitoring lines and intra-aorta balloon pumps, with their inherent infectious complications. Pulmonary congestion and mental status wax and wane with fluctuations in blood pressure and cardiac output. This continual progressive deterioration may rapidly lead to death or impaired organ function, reducing the chances to achieve successful transplantation even after implantation of an artificial heart. Patient selection and late institution of circulatory support were sited as the major causes of death in four out of eight patients in a multicenter study with heterotopic prosthetic ventricles [18].

   Waiting periods to locate a heart for transplantation not only vary with the age, size, and blood type of the recipient but also depend on the donor criteria that are adhered to. We have now taken hearts from donors in their 50s for patients in critical need and would prefer to have a coronary angiogram on such hearts. Our current average waiting period is 4 months. The primary determinant of the length of the waiting period is the clinical status under which the recipient is listed with the donor procurement agency. Our current clinical grading system divides patients into the following four status levels:

Status 3 refers to a patient who can be maintained outside the hosital
Status 2 refers to a patient who needs hospitalization
Status 1 refers to a patient requiring intensive care unit treatment
Status 9 refers to a gravely ill patient in the intensive care unit on multiple intravenous drugs or on intra-aorta balloon pump or intubated or all of the above.

Our status 9 patients who survived to have a transplant waited an average of 4.7 days (ranging from 12 h to 14 days) for a donor to become available. The five previously described TAH candidates who died had been status 9 for several hours to as long as 10 days. We estimate that one out of seven patients who are clinically classified as status 9 in our intensive care unit, as well as occasional other patients from within our hospital or transported from other hospitals, will become candidates for TAH as a bridge to transplantation.

   Selecting between status 9 patients who can wait the average of 4.7 days for a heart transplant and those who cannot is a clinical decision that can usually be documented by a worsening hemodynamic, respiratory, and metabolic course on the records of the intensive care unit. The hemodynamic guidelines frequently used to guide the need for circulatory support are described elsewhere [10, 19]. Although vascular resistance is frequently calculated to be high (>2100 dyn s^{-1} cm^{-5}), when the patient is first seen, in this era of vasodilators, the vascular resistance may be normal or low, without cultural evidence that the patient is septic. Our goal is to support the patient in status 9 as long as possible but, when clinical deterioration jeopardizes peripheral organ function, to proceed with implantation of the TAH and reverse peripheral organ malfunction before subsequent elective transplantation.

   For some patients with secondary refractory pulmonary edema or with severe prerenal failure, a period of circulatory support with the TAH may improve respiratory and renal function, so that candidacy for heart transplantation becomes possible. The secondary organ failure that occurs with cardiogenic shock may require several weeks to several months to recover. A totally implantable artificial heart optimally designed should give adequate time for the recipient to recover secondary organ function and allow for longer intervals of support in which to find a heart for transplantation.

As we reach the numerical limits of organ donation, and as long as we have not solved the secret to successful xenografting, we are challenged to design artificial hearts that last for years and are less subject to the risks and restraints of currently available devices. The Philadelphia heart design is hoped to be a stepping stone in that direction.

The PHS was designed on the experience of previous artificial hearts and has been shown capable of pumping effectively for 4 months. Bleeding episodes were common in animal studies and were due to the requirement to anticoagulate the blood in the presence of four mechanical valves. These results suggest the increased usage of tissue valves in the TAH, which the PHS was indeed designed to allow.

References

1. Cooley DA, Liotta D, Hallman GL (1969) Orthotopic cardiac prosthesis for two-staged cardiac replacement. Am J Cardiol 24:723–730
2. Cooley DA, Liotta D, Hallman GL, Bloodwell RD, Leachman RD, Milan JD (1969) First human implantation of cardiac prosthesis for staged total replacement of the heart. Trans Am Soc Artif Intern Organs 15:252–263
3. DeVries WC, Anderson JL, Joyce LD, Anderson FL, Hammond E, Jarvik RK, Kolff WJ (1984) Clinical use of the total artificial heart. N Engl J Med 310(5):273–278
4. Copeland JG, Emery RW, Levinson NM, Copeland J, McAleer MJ, Riley JE (1985) The role of mechanical support and transplantation in treatment of patients with end-stage cardiomyopathy. Circulation 70(2):7–12
5. Levinson M, Smith R, Cole R, Gallo J, Icenogle TB, Emery R, Ott R, Copeland J (1986) Three recent cases of the total artificial heart before transplantation. J Heart Transplant 5:215–228
6. Copeland JG, Levinson NM, Vaughn C, Cheng K, Icenagle TB, Austen J, Riley JE (1986) The total artificial heart as a bridge to transplantation. JAMA 256(21):2991–2995
7. Griffith BP, Kormos R, Wei LM, Borovetz HS, Trento A, Hardesty RL (1986) Use of the total artificial heart as an interim device: initial experience in Pittsburgh with four patients. J Heart Transplant 5(3):210–214
8. Griffith BP, Hardesty RL, Kormos R, Trento A, Borovetz HS, Thompson M, Bahnsen H (1987) Temporary use of the Jarvik-7 total artificial heart before transplantation. N Engl J Med 316:130–134
9. Olsen DB, Riebman JB, DePaulis R, Durrant G, Nielsen SD (1987) Registry and tabulations of orthotopic total artificial hearts in man. Trans Am Soc Artif Intern Organs 33(3):182–191
10. DePaulis R, Riebman JB, Deleuze P, Olsen DB (1987) The total artificial heart: indications and preliminary results. J Cardiac Surg 1987 (in press)
11. Joyce LD, Johnson KE, Pierce WS et al. (1986) Summary of the world experience with clinical use of total artificial hearts as heart support devices. J Heart Transplant 5:229–235
12. Levinson MM, Smith RG, Cork RC, Gallo J, Emery RW, Icenagle TB, Ott RA, Burns GL, Copeland JG (1986) Thromboembolic complications of the Jarvik-7 total artificial heart: case report. Artif Organs 10(3):236–244

13. Wurzel D, Kolff J, Missfeldt W, Wildevuur W, Hansen G, Brownstein L, Riebman J, De-Paulis R, Kolff WJ (1987) Development of the Philadelphia heart system. ESAO 14: (in press)

14. Wurzel D, Wildevur W, Kolff J (1986) Instrumentation for deriving pneumatic TAH control signals from the drivelines pressure and flow. Trans Am Soc Artif Intern Organs 32:258–262

15. Wurzel D (1986) Cardiac prosthesis having integral blood pressure sensor. US Patent Application no 857896

16. Missfeldt W, Wurzel D, Kolff J (1986) An air powered artificial heart all pneumatic Driver. ABST internal symposium on artificial organs. Biomed Eng Transplant

17. Kolff J, Cavarocchi NC, Riebman JB, Jessup M (1988) The artificial heart; design capabilities and indications in the treatment of heart failure. Heart Failure (in press)

18. Farrar DJ, Hill JD, Gray LA, Pennington DG, McBride LR, Pierce WS, Pae WE, Glenville B, Ross D, Galbraith TA, Zambro GL (1988) Heterotopic prosthetic ventricles as a bridge to cardiac transplantation, a multicenter study in 29 patients. N Engl J Med 318:335–340

19. Inou N (1984) Quantitative approach to determine the application time of the left ventricular assist device. Artif Organ 8:458

28. Enoximone Therapy: An Alternative Strategy to Temporary Mechanical Support

D. Loisance, J. L. Dubois Rande, Ph. Deleuze, A. Tarral, M. L. Hillion, D. Lellouche, A. Castaigne, and J. P. Cachera

Urgent heart transplantation in patients in irreversible cardiogenic shock or with low cardiac output unresponsive to sympathomimetic drugs has recently been shown to be possible [1]. This life-saving procedure may be performed either immediately, if a suitable donor is available, or later following a period of mechanical support [2, 3]. Various techniques have been evaluated during the past 2 years: prolonged extracorporeal circulation with membrane oxygenation [4, 5], paracorporeal or internal ventricular assist devices (VADs) [2, 6, 7], and the implantable total artificial heart (TAH) [3, 8–12].

Initial reports on this new strategy of using a "mechanical bridge" to transplantation in urgent cases have revealed various problems [3, 9, 13–15]. Firstly, the risk of thromboembolism and cardiac sepsis as a result of insertion of such devices is substantial. Secondly, the cost of both the devices and the procedure must not be neglected at a time of rising health care expenditure. Thirdly, there is an ethical issue since the strategy leads cardiac transplantation to be performed urgently, with a higher risk of postoperative death as compared with mortality in routine waiting list candidates.

Consequently, any alternative approach to this strategy which would permit a reduced need or the temporary implantation of mechanical devices has to be evaluated. The purpose of this study is to evaluate prospectively the use of Enoximone as an alternative to the mechanical bridge to transplantation.

Protocol

The study was carried out between September 1985 and July 1987. Patients were referred to our institution from various intensive care units (ICUs) throughout Paris for immediate cardiac transplantation, or, in the case of no cardiac graft being available, for implantation of a mechanical circulatory assist device – the Jarvik-7 TAH (Symbion Inc.) or a VAD (Symbion Inc.).

At the time of admission into the ICU, a Swan-Ganz catheter was inserted at the bedside. Systemic arterial pressure was monitored via a radial artery catheter. The routine indices, such as pulmonary capillary wedge pressure (PCWP), cardiac index (CI), and pulmonary (PVR) and systemic vascular resistance (SVR), were calculated using standard formulae. Urine output was measured hourly.

The patients entering the protocol were unresponsive to optimal conventional therapy, including oxygen, fluid balance, and maximum doses of sympathomi-

Assisted Circulation 3
F. Unger (Ed.)
© Springer-Verlag Berlin Heidelberg 1989

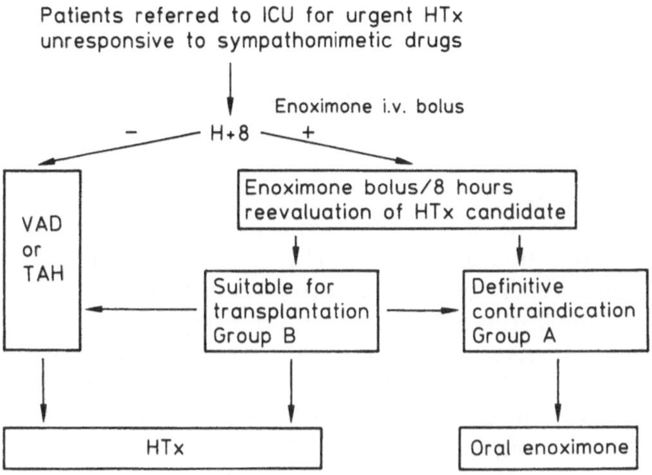

Fig. 1. Study design in patients unresponsive to sympathomimetic drugs

metics, including dopamine and dobutamine. The study plan (Fig. 1) required intravenous administration of Enoximone, in addition to existing therapy, as a 10-min bolus, at a dose of 0.5–2 mg/kg body weight. After 30 min, the clinical and hemodynamic condition was evaluated. Lack of any significant improvement or further deterioration indicated urgent cardiac replacement provided there was no evidence of sepsis. If no compatible donor organ was available, a TAH was implanted. In the case of a significant improvement, the decison concerning cardiac replacement was postponed and reconsidered after 2, 5, and 8 h; any evidence of deterioration prompted the decision for immediate surgery. Eight hours after the Enoximone dose a repeat intravenous bolus was given and the effects were carefully and continuously monitored. This period, during which the patient's condition was stabilized, allowed a more detailed consideration of the indications for urgent transplant. In particular, an active search for definitive or temporary contraindications could focus upon problems such as patient compliance and occult pathology, which had previously been neglected (Table 2). In this way patients were divided into two groups. *Group A* included those with some form of contraindication to transplantation. In these patients Enoximone therapy was continued with 8-hourly bolus doses. If continued benefit was observed, the patient was weaned off intravenous sympathomimetic drugs and oral Enoximone was introduced. *Group B* included patients with no contraindication to transplantation. They were immediately placed on the computerized national waiting list, France Transplant, for an optimized search for a compatible donor. Selection required only ABO matching; although preoperative sera were cross-matched against donor lymphocytes, the result was not known until after the operation.

Obviously if there was any clinical or hemodynamic deterioration and if no compatible donor was available, immediate TAH implantation was mandatory.

Clinical Experience

Twenty-four patients, 22 males and 2 females, entered the study. The mean age was 47 ± 11 years (19–62 years). The etiology of their heart failure was dilated cardiomyopathy in 14 patients, end-stage valvulopathy with previous valve replacement in three and ischemic heart disease in five, of whom two had undergone previous conservative surgery. One patient was admitted for retransplantation because of uncontrolled acute rejection of an allograft performed 3 months previously. He was in cardiogenic shock, unresponsive to both immunological and sympathomimetic therapy. The last patient was in profound cardiogenic shock developing within 48 h of an extensive acute myocardial infarction. The mean duration of treatment in the referring ICU was 7 days, with a range of 2–17 days. At the time of admission 17 patients were in cardiogenic shock ($CI < 2.00$ l/min/ m^2, $PCWP > 15$ mmHg, urinary output < 25 ml/h). Nine patients were in profound low cardiac output states. Individual values of hemodynamic parameters, their mean values, and standard deviation in the whole group are listed in Table 2.

Results

Immediate Results

The efficacy of Enoximone was obvious in all but two patients. This was reflected by an improvement clinically, by beneficial hemodynamic changes, and by an increase in the urinary output (Fig. 2). The increase in urinary output was even observed in patients previously anuric. After 30 min the CI had increased from baseline values by 33% and the PCWP had decreased by 46% (Fig. 3). The individual data are listed in Table 1. The heart rate did not change significantly (94 ± 16 to 95 ± 17.6 per minute), nor did the systolic blood pressure (107 ± 15 to 104 ± 7 mmHg). In two patients there was a deterioration in the initial clinical condition despite Enoximone; one was the case with acute rejection (pat. #10) and the other the case with an extensive myocardial infarction (pat. #12). They were immediately implanted with a Jarvik-7 device. One died 3 days later; following an initial dramatic improvement there was a profound peripheral vasodilatation requiring increasing adjustments of the Jarvik output. On the 3rd day the cardiac output of 12 l/min could no longer maintain an adequate systemic arterial pressure and additional pharmacological support could no longer prevent progressive neurological and renal deterioration. At autopsy, diffuse hepatic necrosis was found. Blood and tissue cultures remained negative. In the second case TAH was successful as a "bridge." Retransplantation was carried out in a routine fashion on day 6 and the patient was extubated after a further 6 days. On the 37th postoperative day the patient died from a *Candida albicans* septicemia which had been initially identified on day 22.

Table 1. Overall hemodynamic results in patients treated by intravenous Enoximone

Patients	Age	Sex	CI baseline	CI 30 min	PCWP Baseline	PCWP 30 min	SVR Baseline	SVR 30 min	PVR Baseline	PVR 30 min	Syst. BP Baseline	Syst. BP 30 min
Group A												
Pat. 1	58	M	2.18	2.10	17.00	15.00	2444.00	2400	9.16	8.82	110.00	100.00
Pat. 2	58	M	1.90	3.00	16.00	8.00	1897.00	1120	5.14	4.00	108.00	99.00
Pat. 3	63	M	1.54	2.80	34.00	14.00	2340.00	1224	6.67	6.53	103.00	96.00
Pat. 4	48	M	2.40	2.53	23.00	22.00	1770.00	1699	4.42	5.18	110.00	110.00
Pat. 5	60	F	1.80	2.02	27.00	14.00	3128.00	2410	7.30	7.28	123.00	118.00
Pat. 6	60	M	1.45	2.00	27.00	7.00	1500.00	1664	5.14	9.18	103.00	104.00
Pat. 7	33	M	2.10	4.15	37.00	15.00	1711.00	866.00	0.83	2.63	101.00	94.00
Pat. 8	31	M	2.12	3.20	32.00	23.00	2184.00	1933	5.64	5.10	157.00	139.00
Pat. 9	62	M	1.70	2.10	33.00	31.00	2830.00	1942	7.61	7.50	110.00	126.00
Pat. 10	41	M	2.00	2.00	30.00	28.00	1888.00	1320	5.27	3.63	73.00	69.00
Pat. 11	62	M	2.00	2.25	26.00	20.00	2275.00	1620	2.70	2.41	109.00	90.00
Pat. 12	59	M	1.65	2.20	32.00	17.00	2414.00	1724	5.26	4.55	110.00	108.00
Group B												
Pat. 1	29	M	1.50	3.50	40.00	11.00	2157.00	905.00	3.57	3.38	90.00	88.00
Pat. 2	38	F	1.90	3.00	24.00	9.00	2395.00	1525	4.29	3.92	110.00	100.00
Pat. 3	54	M	1.70	3.00	25.00	16.00	2080.00	1323	12.00	5.96	100.00	100.00
Pat. 4	36	M	2.00	2.70	20.00	12.00	1640.00	1407	6.86	3.41	90.00	95.00
Pat. 5	45	M	2.00	2.90	28.00	16.00	1802.00	1174	7.67	2.41	95.00	85.00
Pat. 6	61	M	2.12	3.20	30.00	23.00	2909.00	1834	8.68	4.55	110.00	125.00
Pat. 7	37	M	1.50	2.10	22.00	7.00	3081.00	2288	5.18	5.00	120.00	122.00
Pat. 8	19	M	1.54	2.70	34.00	14.00	2074.00	1300	7.03	6.04	99.00	96.00
Pat. 9	44	M	1.50	3.40	40.00	11.00	2371.00	950.00	8.21	3.59	107.00	84.00
Pat. 10	36	M	2.00	3.00	36.00	27.00	1969.00	1186	3.07	3.33	125.00	130.00
Pat. 11	52	M	1.75	1.80	29.00	17.00	1691.00	1338	3.42	2.44	95.00	90.00
Pat. 12	40	M	2.20		35.00						90.00	
Mean	47		1.85	2.67	29.04	16.54	2174.87	1523	5.76	4.73	106.17	102.21
SD	13		0.27	0.59	6.64	6.61	463.70	442.44	2.48	1.99	15.86	17.07
N. obs	24		24.00	24.00	24.00	24.00	24.00	24.00	24.00	24.00	24.00	24.00
Mean+SD	60		2.13	3.26	35.68	23.16	2638.58	1966	8.24	6.72	122.02	119.27
Mean−SD	34		1.58	2.08	22.40	9.93	1711.17	1081	3.28	2.74	90.31	85.14

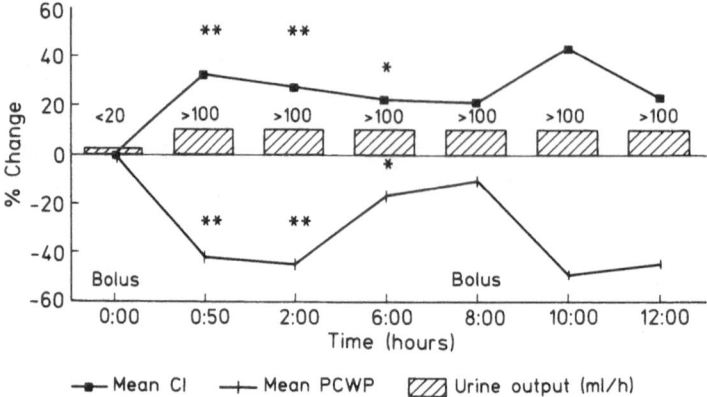

Fig. 2. Percentage changes in CI, PCWP, and urinary output in the first 12 h on intravenous Enoximone therapy. **$p < 0.001$; *$p < 0.05$

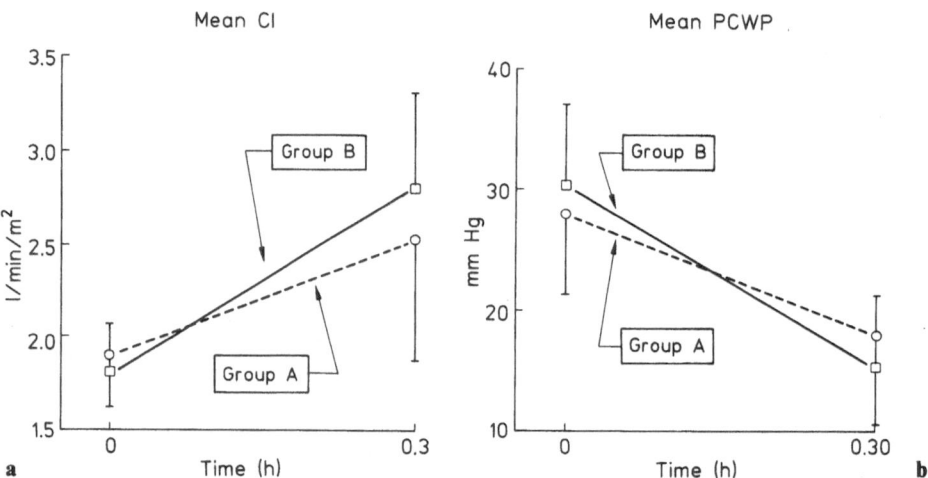

Fig. 3. Changes from control to 30-min values in **a** mean CI and **b** mean PCWP in all patients

Reevaluation of Transplant Candidates and Outcome

In the 22 patients responsive to initial intravenous Enoximone bolus there was sufficient improvement in clinical status to allow a reevaluation of the indications for cardiac transplantation. In 12 cases a contraindication was discovered (group A). The individual causes are listed in Table 2. In most cases, the contraindication was not cardiac related, but a previously underestimated problem or occult pathology. The most striking was a colonic carcinoma discovered during a colonoscopy indicated for symptoms of subacute obstruction. Commonly the contraindication related either to a potential lack of recipient compliance or to a previous history of alcohol abuse.

Table 2. Contraindications to heart transplantation in patients ($n = 12$) improved by intravenous Enoximone therapy

Diabetes	1
Neoplasia	1
Age (borderline)	3
Pulm. insufficiency	1
Proteinuria	2
Raised PVR	4
Alcohol addition	3
No psychological compliance	3

Four patients died while in the ICU despite prolonged intravenous administration of Enoximone in combination with optimal sympathomimetic drugs. The remaining eight patients were successfully weaned off intravenous therapy and oral Enoximone was introduced. Four ultimately died but survived for a mean duration of 10 months (6–17 months). Four are still alive, in NYHA class III heart failure, with a mean follow-up duration of 15 months (10–19 months). None required readmission during this time.

Ten patients were considered suitable for transplantation (group B) and were classified as high priority candidates. In all, a suitable donor was found in good time, in six cases within 48 h. In three cases the indication for implantation of a TAH was considered on two occasions, on consecutive days, but a suitable graft was found at the last minute. Three were placed on extracorporeal circulation just prior to graft harvesting. The graft organ was obtained locally in four cases and from a remote hospital in six. The mean ischemic time was 156 min, ranging from 92 to 195 min. All patients were successfully weaned off cardiopulmonary bypass.

Immunosuppression included immediate intravenous low dose cyclosporin, daily methylprednisolone, rabbit antithymocyte globulin, and azathioprine. Four patients died within the first 3 weeks: one died of septic shock related to a previous uncontrolled stomal infection, another, with previously raised pulmonary resistance, died of primary graft rejection, and two patients died of cachexia and multiple organ failure. The six surviving patients were discharged in routine time. One discontinued immunosuppression voluntarily after 5 months and died. The five surviving patients are still well in NYHA class I with a follow-up duration between 10 months and 2.5 years.

In summary, from an initial group of 24 patients referred to our hospital for immediate cardiac transplantation, unresponsive to sympathomimetic inotropes, intravenous Enoximone appeared effective in 22 cases and helped delay surgery. This prolongation of the immediate survival allowed reevaluation of the transplant candidate and ultimately reduced the indication for both temporary circulatory support and transplantation.

Discussion

In recent years cardiac transplantation has been shown to be a life-saving procedure in extremely unstable patients [1]. Various systems for temporary mechanical support of the circulation have been used to maintain the patient when no immediate cardiac graft is available [2, 3, 9, 11, 12, 14, 15]. Initially the results of these procedures appeared promising until the results of routine priority transplantation were also considered. At a time when there is a marked discrepancy between the number of suitable donor organs and potential candidates, the acceptability of such a strategy in urgent cases must be questioned. One cannot consider that a patient kept alive with a TAH or a VAD, with all of the incipient risks such as cardiac sepsis and thromboembolism, should have a regular priority for transplantation, as has been recently proposed [3]. The implantation of a mechanical device on an emergency basis may lead to the underestimation of factors that might be important determinants of the final outcome. The use of such a device in a febrile patient, or in patients with refractory cardiogenic shock following a large acute myocardial infarction, might be reasonable; however, should the ferver be in fact due to sepsis, the introduction of such a foreign body might result in irreversible problems. Equally one has to weigh up the effects that a delay in evaluating the cause of the fever before implantation might have on rapidly deteriorating cerebral or renal function. Finally the financial and human cost of the mechanical bridge to transplantation strategy is another issue presently being discussed. For these various reasons any alternative to an invasive approach in these unstable, urgent cardiac transplant candidates has to be evaluated.

Optimal control of fluid balance, load reduction, and adequate inotropic support using sympathomimetic agents have been shown to be most beneficial, and such regimens can decrease the need for urgent transplantation. Stevenson [16] has recently shown that 32 of 40 patients transferred for urgent transplantation could be discharged from the ICU and the hospital by the use of such optimal mediacl therapy, despite an initial CI of 1.9 ± 0.6 l/min/m^2. Nevertheless, among this group of patients there are some who cannot be stabilized for a significant period. For these the mechanical bridge technique remains the only alternative.

The efficacy of pretransplant medical management in urgent candidates may be improved by intravenous Enoximone therapy [17]. No adverse effects have been observed in the present study. The most striking beneficial effects have been on CI, PCWP, and urinary output. The immediate effects are similar to those observed by Farrar in left VAD bridged patients [2]. This effect was spectacular in the 17 patients who were in cardiogenic shock, since only two deteriorated clinically despite significant hemodynamic improvement. In all of these 17 patients the general criteria required for VAD or TAH implantation were present at the time of admission. Consequently a reduction from 17 to 2 in the actual number of TAH candidates implanted was obtained.

Patient survival for hours and days in combination with a clinical and hemodynamic improvement resulted from Enoximone therapy in 92% of our patients and allowed a further evaluation of the indications for immediate transplantation. The most surprising result of this procedure has been that 12 patients initially considered as good candidates for transplantation, by the referring cardiology departments, were finally refused. In each of these cases the definitive contraindication discovered during this reevaluation was not cardiac but was associated with an occult or underestimated problem such as borderline age, lack of potential compliance, or long-standing alcoholism. The prognostic significance of such associated problems has been the subject of careful analysis by other [2, 18, 19], authors and is most often underestimated when an urgent decision is necessary. Just such a situation is created by an acute uncontrolled low cardiac output state, and the benefit of prolonging survival, even for only a few hours, before an irreversible decision to operate is made, is obvious in terms of both cost and the optimal use of a scarce cardiac graft.

A comment should be made concerning the 8 of the 12 patients refused for transplantation who ultimately survived. The favorable outcome following their successful weaning off intravenous Enoximone emphasizes the benefit that may be derived from any therapy which allows the original heart to recover [4]. The actual potential for an individual heart to recover may be difficult to assess, for, despite the severity of the initial clinical and hemodynamic state, survival of a reasonable duration and quality is attainable.

The final comment relates to the risk involved in maintaining a patient, using intravenous Enoximone, while reviewing that patient daily for TAH implantation until a donor organ is available. The major theoretical issue relates to the risk of progressive organ deterioration compared to patients who have been implanted with a TAH. In all ten patients in this study who were ultimately transplanted there was no significant increase in serum creatinine and no deterioration of cerebral function. The only potential risk was sepsis. Two patients developed localized pulmonary infections and three required prolonged postoperative ventilation. This risk was nevertheless acceptable provided that the delay before transplantation was not excessive.

References

1. Editorial (1986) Transplantation around the world. J Heart Transplant 5:46–87 (abstracts)
2. Farrar DJ, Hill JD, Gray LA, Pennington DJ, McBrid LR, Pierce WS, Pae WE, Glenville D, Ross D, Galbraith TA, Zumbro GL (1988) Heterotopic prosthetic ventricles as a bridge to cardiac transplantation. N Engl J Med 318:333–340
3. Joyce LD, Johnson KE, Pierce WS, DeVries WC, Semb BKH, Copeland JG, Griffith BP, Cooley DA, Frazier OH, Cabrol C, Keon WJ, Unger F, Bucherl ES, Wolner E (1986) Summary of the world experience with clinical use of total artificial hearts as heart support devices. J Heart Transplant 5:229–235
4. Pennington DG, Codd JE, Merjavy JP et al. (1984) The expanded use of ventricular bypass systems for severe cardiac failure and as a bridge to cardiac transplantation. Heart Transplant 3:170–175
5. Loisance DY, Hillion ML, Deleuze PH et al. (1987) ECCMO as a bridge to transplantation on cardiac surgical patients. Transplant Proc 19:3786–3788
6. Hill JD, Farrar DJ, Hershon JJ, Compton PG, Avery GJ, Levin BS, Brent BN (1986) Use of a prosthetic ventricle as a bridge to cardiac transplantation for post infarction cardiogenic shock. N Engl J Med 314:626–628

7. Magovern JA, Pennock JL, Campbell DB, Pae WE, Pierce WS, Waldhausen JA (1986) Bridge to heart transplantation: the Pennstate experience. J Heart Transplant 5:196–202
8. Solis E, Leger PH, Muneretto C, Gandjbakhch I, Pavie A, Bors V, Piazza C, Szefner J, Cabrol A, Cabrol C (1988) Clinical application and patient selection in the use of a total artificial heart as a bridge for transplantation. Eur J Cardiothorac Surg 2:65–71
9. Griffith BP, Kormos RL, Wei LM, Borovetz HS, Tento A, Hardesty RL (1986) Use of the total artificial heart as an interim device: initial experience in Pittsburgh with four patients. J Heart Transplant 5:210–214
10. Griffith BP, Hardesty RL, Kormos RL, Trento A, Borovetz HS, Thompson ME, Bahnson HT (1987) Temporary use of the Jarvik 7 total artificial heart before transplantation. N Engl J Med 316:130–134
11. Unger F, Chmelizek F, Jungwirth W, Koller I et al. (1988) Artificial heart and cardiac transplantation: report on the first European combined procedure. Artif Organs 12:51–55
12. Levinson MM, Smith RG, Cork R, Gallo J, Icenogle T, Emery R, Ott R, Copeland JG (1986) Three recent cases of the total artificial heart before transplantation. J Heart Transplant 5:215–228
13. Levinson MM, Copeland JG, Smith RG, Cork RC, DeVries WC, Mays JB, Griffith BP, Kormos R, Joyce LD, Pritzker MR, Semb BKH, Koul B, Kenkis AH, Keon WJ (1986) Indexes of haemolysis in human recipients of the Jarvik-7 total artificial heart: a cooperative report of fifteen patients. J Heart Transplant 5:236–248
14. Joyce LD, Kiser JC, Nicoloff DM, Kersten TE, von Rueden TJ, Eales F, Johnson KE, Jorgensen CR, Gobel FL, ven Tassel RA (1986) Use of the mini Jarvik 7 total artificial heart as a bridge to transplantation. J Heart Transplant 5:203–209
15. Loisance DY, Deleuze P, Kawasaki et al. (1987) Total artificial heart as a bridge to retransplantation in acute cardiac rejection. J Heart Transplant 6:281–285
16. Stevenson LW, Donohue BC, Tillisch JH, Schulman B, Dracup KA, Laks H (1987) Urgent priority transplantation: when should it be done? J Heart Transplant 6:267–272
17. Weber KT, Janicki JS, Jain MC (1986) Enoximone (MDL 17043), a phosphodiesterase inhibitor in the treatment of advanced, unstable chronic heart failure. J Heart Transplant 5:105–112
18. McAleer MJ, Copeland J, Fuller J, Copeland JG (1985) Psychological aspects of heart transplantation. J Heart Transplant 4:232–233
19. Herrick CM, Mealey PC, Tischner LL, Cherilyn S (1987) Combined heart failure transplant program: advantages in assessing medical compliance. J Heart Transplant 6:141–146

29. Blood Pumps as a Bridge to Cardiac Transplantation: Characteristics and Development

R. De Paulis and D. B. Olsen

Introduction

After the first pioneering clinical attempts with blood pumps by Dr. Cooley in 1969 and 1981 [1, 2], continued research with animal implantations has led to improvement in the design, techniques of fabrication, choice of materials, and reliability of mechanical components of blood pumps, which have reached a level of practicality high enough for limited clinical application.

Temporary mechanical replacement of the natural heart is now a clinical reality. Results of clinical implantation during 1986 demonstrated that total replacement of the heart with artificial ventricles can satisfactorily bridge the patient until cardiac transplantation [3–8]. As of 31 March 1987, 68 total artificial heart (TAH) implantations had been clinically performed in the United States, Austria, Canada, France, Sweden, and West Germany: 5 as permanent devices and 63 as a temporary bridge to cardiac transplantation. The underlying diseases conditions that led to a need for a TAH were: end-stage cardiomyopathy in 70% (idiopathic, ischemic, viral, or postpartum), acute transplant rejection in 14%, and impossibility of weaning from cardiopulmonary bypass (CPB) in 11% (Table 1) [8].

Application of the TAH has demonstrated several advantages over other forms of mechanical circulatory assistance such as a ventricular assist device (VAD) [9]. The VAD is clinically useful in cases where myocardial disease is thought to be potentially reversible. Even though cardiac failure is nonreversible (e.g., patients on a transplant list), the VAD can be used temporarily while a donor is being sought. Advantages of the VAD include the possibility of avoiding CPB, as well as reduced time and simplicity of implantation. Disadvantages include the increased risk of infection with extended implantation time, as well as bleeding from the cannulation site. Furthermore, if a biventricular assist device is needed, either by first choice or because application of a left VAD may unmask right ventricular failure, risks may be doubled. For these reasons, plus the fact that the time of bridging might be prolonged, the TAH is a better choice. Despite a few complications that have occurred (stroke, infection, bleeding), the TAH's reliability and safety have encouraged more precise definitions of its use in patients who need acute mechanical support.

Assisted Circulation 3
F. Unger (Ed.)
© Springer-Verlag Berlin Heidelberg 1989

Table 1. All TAH bridging to transplantation

Diagnosis	No. of patients	Time (days)	Number trans-planted	Deaths on TAH/ after Tx	Alive	Alive after TAH (%)	Alive after trans-plant (%)
Cardiomyopathy	6	12.5	4	2/3	1	17	25
Idiopathic	11	14.0	9	2/1	8	73	89
Ischemic	17	14.1 +	14	2/8	6 (1)	41	50
Viral	8	11	8	0/3	5	63	63
Postpartum	2	3.5	2	0/1	1	50	50
Transplant rejection	9	95 +	4	4/3	1 (1)	22	50
Congenital heart disease	2	9	1	1/0	1	50	100
Unknown	1	7	1	0/1	0	0	0
Nonweanable CPB	7	5	6	1/4	2	29	33
Total	63		49		25[a] (2)	43	55

( ) = on the TAH

[a] TAH was implanted twice in two patients

Design

The characteristics of pneumatically powered blood pumps, like the VAD or TAH, are quite similar since both have blood–material interfaces. The focus of this presentation will be directed mainly to characteristics of TAHs developed at the University of Utah. Several individual factors influence the final characteristics of blood pumps, and each factor will be analyzed. Clearly, their mutual integration is another important variable that needs to be taken into account.

External Features

A wide range of particulars must be considered in designing a blood pump. First, there has to be a good balance between anatomical and functional design in order to facilitate implantation without impingement of the surrounding vascular structures and surrounding organs, while simultaneously providing adequate stroke volume and optimal internal flow patterns.

The ideal positioning inside the chest should utilize only the pericardial cavity after the natural heart has been removed. Thus, in a small recipient or in recipients without a previous cardiomegaly, the pericardial space could prove inadequate. In this situation, the TAH might be positioned to infringe into the left pleural space [10], resulting in compression of the lower lobes of the lung and thus leading to impairment of the respiratory function, particularly in subjects already compromised.

The shape, weight, and size of the TAH are key features involved in proper positioning and fit. Anatomical fit must provide ease of implantation for a wide range of recipients, with proper angulation between inflow and outflow ports of the ventricle, atria, and the great vessels. Compression, distortion, or kinking of the vascular and cardiac remnant structures can be avoided by careful and meticulous surgical techniques after optimum design has been realized. In this laboratory's experience, each time that distortion of the cardiac and vascular struture was present, fibroproliferative tissue (pannus) formation and intimal flaps developed at the level of either the atrial cuffs or the vascular grafts, with consequent impaired filling and/or emptying of the ventricles. This condition was similar to problems with pannus that was consistently found at the inflow port of the ventricle if a sharp-angled connector were used. Modification to a round, smooth angle totally eliminated this problem [11, 12], underlining the importance of avoiding turbulent flow in order to eliminate abnormal deposits and tissue growth, and, as will be addressed later, thrombus formation.

After gaining experience through years of animal experimentation with the Jarvik-5 [13, 14] and Jarvik-7 (Jarvik-7 and Jarvik-5 artificial hearts are registered trademarks of Symbion, Inc.), artificial hearts were designed expressly to fit into the human chest. Presently, the Jarvik-7 artificial heart and its scaled-down version, the Jarvik-7-70 artificial heart, are clinically the most widely used. The Jarvik-7 artificial heart has a stroke volume of 100 ml and a spherical shape, limiting the utilization of the craniocaudal space inside the chest. This space between the vertebral bodies (T10) and the sternum has been identified as the critical dimension in the human chest. The 100-ml stroke volume heart with a spherical shape results in difficulty in fitting the device in patients weighing less than 75 kg or patients with less than 2 m^2 of body surface area [15]. The scaled-down version, the Jarvik-7-70 artificial heart, reduced this problem, but with a detrimental 30% reduction in stroke volume.

These problems stimulated the development of the Utah-100 artificial heart, which allows better fit without compromising the 100-ml stroke volume (Fig. 1). Its original elliptical shape was expressly designed to optimize the craniocaudal space inside the human chest. In effect, this new shape allowed a significant reduc-

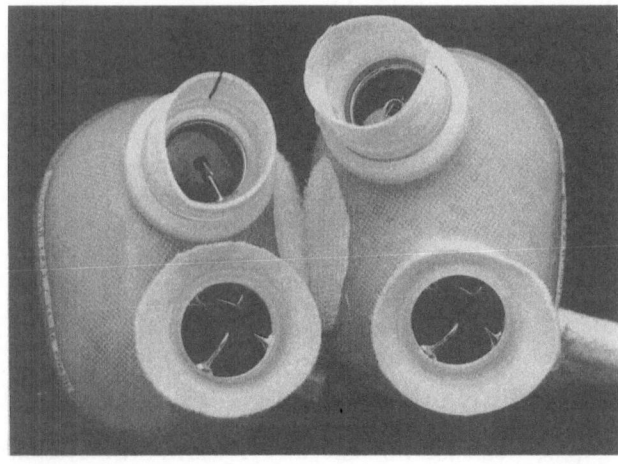

Fig. 1. The cylindrically shaped Utah-100 TAH

tion in the length of the ventricle, permitting implantation into calves weighing less than 50 kg [16]. The actual ventricles consist of a soft, segmented polyurethane (Biomer) housing and a polyurethane (Isoplast) base, bonded together with Biomer.

Another external feature simplifying implantation is the quick connectors that allow simple suturing and inspection of the anastomoses, as well as connecting easily between the TAH and atrial cuff and vascular grafts after they have been sewn to the cardiovascular structures. The quick connectors available on the Jarvik-7 and Jarvik-7-70 artificial hearts are of a snap-on type. They consist of a soft, segmented polyurethane glued to the atrial cuff or to the vascular graft, and stretched over a rigid valve-holding ring incorporated into the housing. The fit must be tight to avoid bleeding or gaps. Maneuvers required to snap them on can result in stretching and torsion to the cardiovascular structures. Furthermore, once the connections have been made, it is impossible to rotate them without disconnection in order to establish optimal orientation and positioning inside the pericardial cavity.

To overcome these problems, a new screw-type connector system has been designed [17] which permits easier and quicker connection, as well as the capability of gently rotating the ventricles once they have been connected, before the screws are tightened.

Internal Features

As previously mentioned, modifications of the external design to obtain a better fit into the pericardial cavity must not compromise an idealized internal design of the ventricle. This means that the flow pattern inside the housing, regardless of the external shape, must be acceptable. The residual volume should be minimal to reduce the time the blood remains within the ventricle. The presence of an excessive residual volume could result in stagnation areas with prolonged blood–material exposure leading to an increased chance of thrombosis.

Threat of thromboembolism is still a primary concern with the artificial heart. Thromboembolism occurs when a thrombus breaks loose from an attached thrombus inside the artificial ventricles or valve-holding system. Even though the chemical, physical, and electrical properties of biomaterials (chemical composition, surface structure, property, etc.) are related to thrombus formation [18], a good design is also important in its prevention. During fabrication, avoidance of impurities and dust, as well as maintenance of the appropriate temperatures and humidity in the prosthetic laboratory (clean room), has eliminated further variables. The hydrodynamic pattern inside the ventricles and connectors remains a most important factor in thrombus formation, regardless of the use of anticoagulation therapy. Contact time of the blood with the biomaterial surfaces leads to activation of the coagulation factors. Longer contact time can be due either to a low flow rate or to the presence of areas of stagnation. Furthermore, vortices and turbulence, plus a higher rate of shear stress, have also been identified as favoring the thrombotic process.

All these considerations underline the importance of the internal features of the artificial ventricles. Any gap between components, any crease in the material,

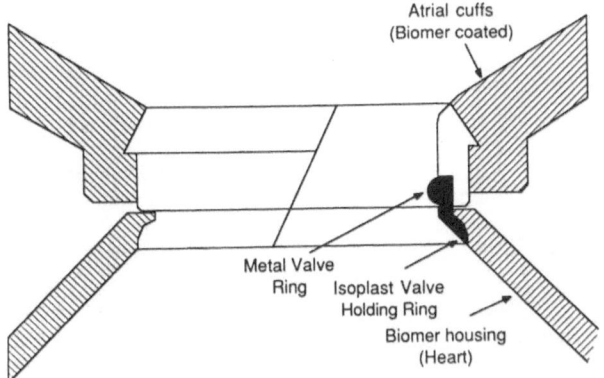

Fig. 2. The snap-on type quick connector

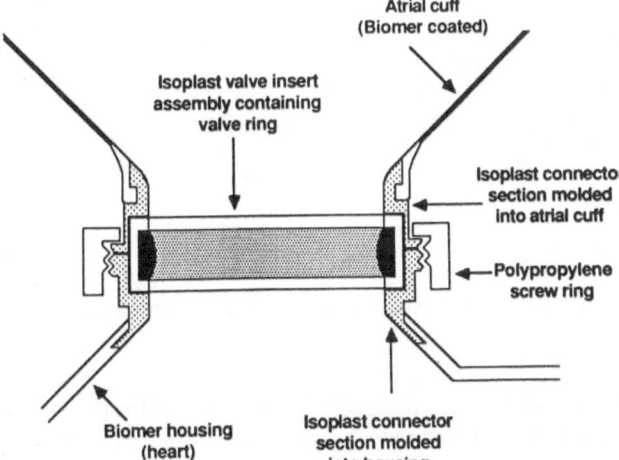

Fig. 3. The new screw-type connector system now in use on the Utah-100 TAH

and any area with a low rate of blood flow should be eliminated. Three critical points have been considered: the quick connector junction, the valve–ring junction, and the high flexing diaphragm–housing (DH) junction. Junctions at the quick connectors are created (a) between the valve and valve-holding ring and (b) between rigid rings of the inflow and outflow ports of the ventricles, and soft rings attached to the atrial cuffs and vascular grafts (Fig. 2). Variations during the fabrication procedure make it difficult to completely avoid gaps between the connectors, leading to potential sites for thrombus formation. The new screw-connector system features a different junction because the two halves of the machine's connector system fit together at the level of the valve ring, and are fastened by means of an external screw ring (Fig. 3). The number of junctions are reduced with this new connector [17].

Thrombus occasionally forms in the highly flexible DH junction area, where the blood is at a lower flow rate when compared to the other areas of the ventricular cavity. Fabrication imperfections, like creases or bubble entrapment in this area, lead to incorporation of plasma protein which subsequently mineralize and

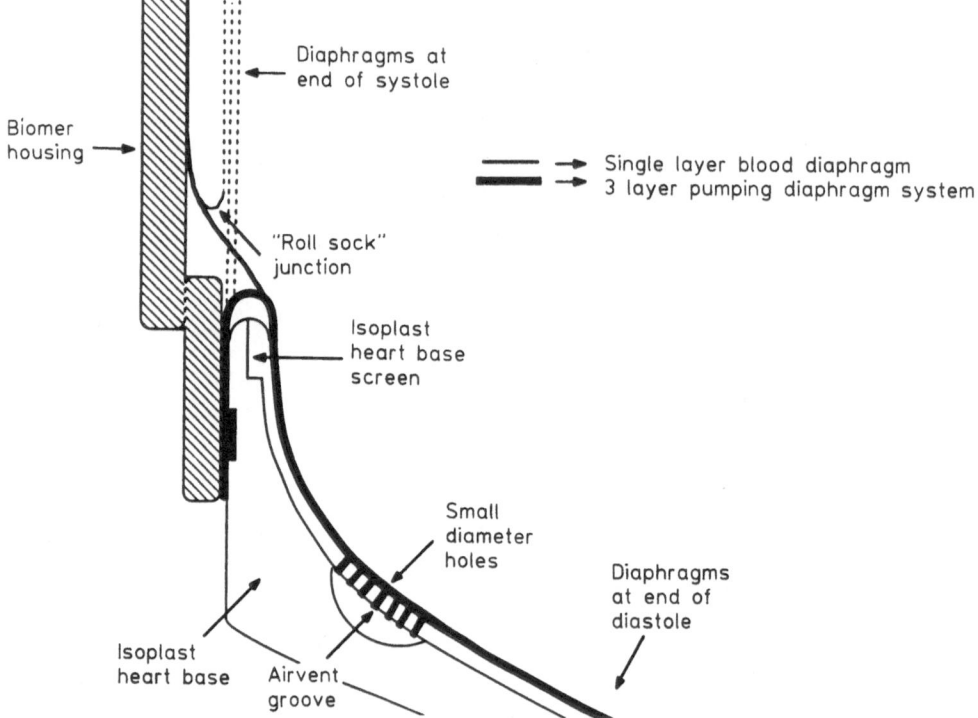

Fig. 4. The newly designed roll-sock junction that assures a better washout and reduced stress on the DH junction

may lead to thrombus buildup. However, microcracks and microfissures that consistently occur when a single thick-layer membrane is used are now avoided in the multiple, thin-layer diaphragms.

The blood diaphragm has a smooth continuity with the polyurethane covering the inner wall of the ventricle. The DH junction area represents the point of maximum stress since it is continuously flexing (46 million heart beats per year) and forms a sharp angle with the rigid housing wall. A new roll-sock junction (Fig. 4) was designed to minimize the stress at this very critical area and maintain improved washout.

It is noteworthy that the quick connectors and the DH junction were identified as predilection sites of thrombus formation in some of the first human recipients [19, 20].

Fabrication

The design of a ventricle must also take into consideration the manufacturing process. Very complex designs make difficult the solution casting of the soft polyurethane over stainless steel molds and hinder subsequent removal from the molds. The Utah-100 heart was designed to be fabricated eventually by injection molding.

Table 2. Utah-100 artificial heart durability test data

Ventricle number	Valves	Durability (years)	Results
U100–L3	BS/BS	0.5	No failure
U100–L2	BS/BS	2.5	Ongoing
U100–R8	D16/D16	0.8	Ongoing
U100–R19	BS/BS	2.1	Ongoing
U100–L22	MH/MH	0.6	Ventricle failed[a]

BS, Björk-Shiley valve; D16, Medtronic-Hall D16 valve; MH, Medtronic-Hall valve
[a] Improper positioning of the base during manufactured

Durability

Limited durability of the flexing diaphragm was overcome by incorporating a thin, four-layer diaphragm system which totally eliminates passage of air into the blood in the event of membrane fracture. The continuous blood-contacting surface of the ventricle and diaphragm was fabricated by pouring polyurethane through the inflow and outflow ports of the ventricles over a concave, stainless steel mold. The blood diaphragm was attached to the housing upon its removal from the mold [21]. The other three diaphragms were fabricated individually, lubricated between layers with graphite, and glued at the base. This diaphragm system acts as an integral layer to pump the blood and combines the qualities of flexibility, strength, and durability (Fig. 4).

An important design consideration is the influence of the shape of the ventricle on the way the membrane will flex. The circularly shaped membrane tends to flex along different lines at every beat (random pattern), while the elliptical or cylindrical shape tends to flex along the same lines. This is true when the ventricle is in a static position, but when the position is changed (with respect to gravity), the flexion pattern changes as well. Once the TAH has been implanted it is subject to continuous position changes. This "pseudorandom" pattern of flexion should achieve a durability similar to the circular shape of ventricle (Table 2).

Physiology of the Blood Pump

Replacement of the function of the natural heart demands that artificial ventricles be capable of pumping all the blood that returns to them from the systemic and pulmonary circulation (preload). Since preload changes continuously with the different metabolic needs, the artificial heart must correspondingly modify its cardiac output. In the pneumatically powered artificial heart, this was achieved either by automatically modifying the heart rate while the artificial ventricles maintained a constant stroke volume (full fill, full eject of each beat) or by having a variable stroke volume with a constant heart rate. Once the proper parameters have been set to obtain complete ejection and partial filling of the ventricle, the

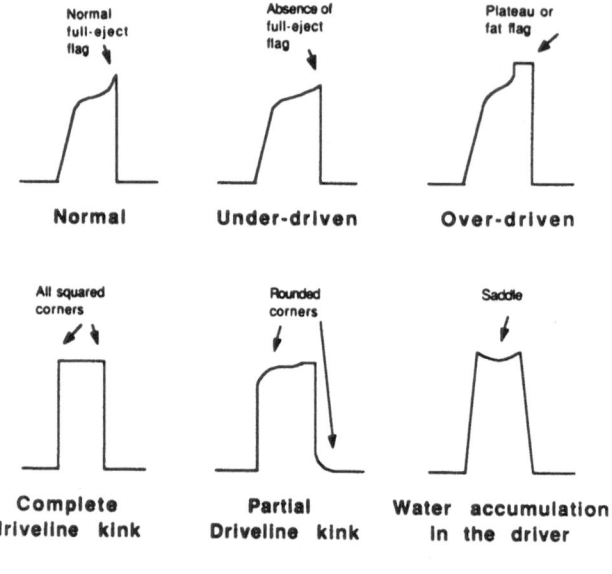

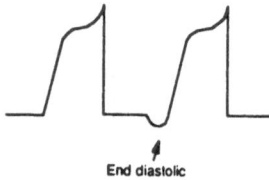

Fig. 5. Drive line pressure waveforms in normal and abnormal conditions

heart can accomodate additional filling in response to increased preload. This capability is known as the Starling law for the artificial heart, and within certain limits the relation between atrial pressure and cardiac output is quite similar to the curve for the natural heart [14].

Complete ejection of the ventricles is achieved by increasing the pneumatic driving pressure to obtain an identifiable spike on the drive line pressure waveform (Fig. 5). This spike indicates that the membrane is completely stretched; therefore, all blood has been ejected. To minimize diaphragm stress, the drive pressure used to pump the blood should be slightly more than is needed to empty the ventricles completely. This slight overdriving of the ventricle accommodates small increases in pulmonary or systemic resistances without compromising the cardiac output, i.e., mild heart failure. Before a more sophisticated monitor and diagnostic device was developed, the pressure waveform was used to evaluate pumping performance of the ventricles.

Figure 5 shows how it is possible to detect some of the problems with the pneumatic TAH or driver. A variable stroke volume with a fixed heart rate is the pumping mode used in all of the University of Utah experiments, and most of the human implantations to date.

Another characteristic of the physiology of the TAH regards the systole–diastole ratio within the cardiac cycle. In the resting natural heart, the systolic time is about one-third the total cycle. In the TAH, systole occupies between 40% and 50% of the total cycle. This prolonged systole permits the use of a lower pressure–time radio (dP/dt), which reduces hemolysis. However, with the shorter diastolic time, it is sometimes necessary to apply a small amount of vacuum during diastole to facilitate ventricular filling. Such a vacuum is rarely needed in animals, but has proven valuable at times in humans to maximize filling at a very low preload [19].

When the ventricle is properly driven, every time the recipient has a higher metabolic requirement, such as during exercise, the cardiac output will automatically increase [22].

Diagnostics

As mentioned previously, the drive line pressure waveforms can be used to monitor the TAH performance. A more sophisticated monitoring system was developed to assess the performance of the blood pump as well as the hemodynamic condition of the recipient: the COMDU^{tm} cardiac monitoring unit (COMDU^{tm} cardiac monitoring unit is a trademark of Symbion, Inc.). This noninvasive, computer-based device measures and graphs the amount of air that leaves the ventricle during diastole. The amount of air is directly proportional to the amount of blood that enters the ventricles [23]. Since the ventricle must always be driven to totally eject the blood during each systole, the filling volume is equal to the stroke volume. Thus, cardiac output can easily be calculated (stroke volume times heart rate). Besides the capability of continuously and noninvasively measuring cardiac output, the COMDU^{tm} cardiac monitor's best feature is diagnostic analysis of the filling waveform. Depending on the shape of this waveform, it is possible to identify and diagnose several mechanical malfunctions (driver failure, stiffening of the membrane, air trapped below the membrane, sticking valve, broken valve) and several hemodynamic conditions (hypovolemia, hypervolemia, pulmonary and systemic hypotension or hypertension, and the presence of atrial contraction), as well as the presence of thrombi (inflow or outflow obstruction inside the housing) and some surgical complications (malpositioning of the ventricles or cardiac tamponade in TAH patients).

In experimental animals, open-port monitoring lines are used to measure the pressures in the atrial and vascular compartments, but the risk of infection is greatly increased. Clinically, it would be helpful to continuously monitor the left atrial pressure to detect and prevent pulmonary stasis. The goal of noninvasively monitoring atrial pressures will soon be realized [24].

The Blood and the Blood Pump

Minimal damage to the blood cellular components is caused by the pneumatic TAH in animals. The hematocrit (Hct), lactic dehydrogenase (LDH), hemoglobin

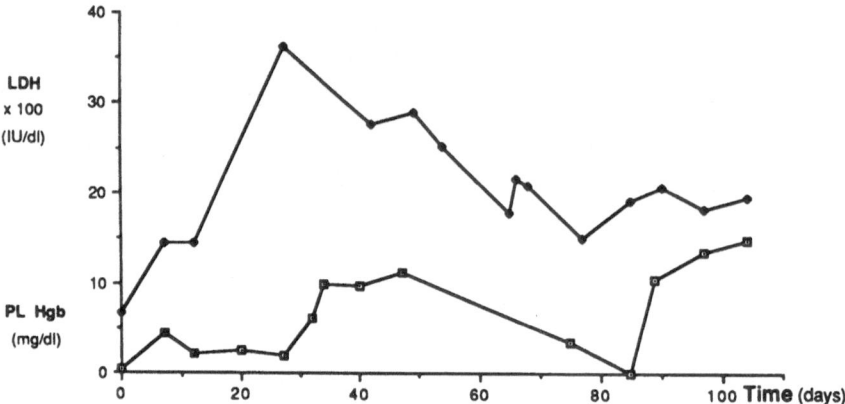

Fig. 6. Hematological data (PHb and LDH) over implantation time in an animal implanted with a Utah-100 TAH

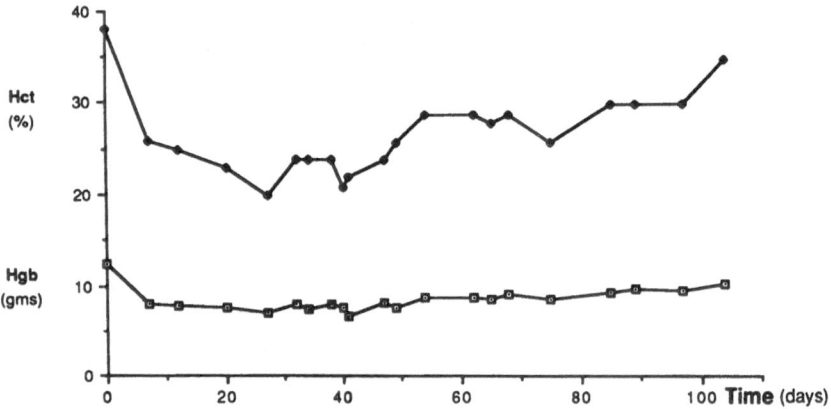

Fig. 7. Hematological data (Hct and Hb) over implantation time in an animal implanted with a Utah-100 TAH

(Hb), and plasma free hemoglobin (PHb) were monitored to evaluate the level of intravascular hemolysis [25]. These parameters remained within the normal range. The Hct decreased after CPB and then reached a plateau that remained constant. The plateau probably represents the younger blood cell, as older cells are more often damaged or destroyed. The PHb and LDH returned to, or were below, preoperative levels, and a low level of hemolysis was easily compensated (Figs. 6, 7). In our experience, blood transfusions are not needed except in cases of obvious postoperative bleeding. Furthermore, the lower Hct level could depend upon CPB and hemodilution effects due to perturbation of atrial natriuretic peptides and alteration of the fluid regulation mechanisms [26]. This aspect is under further study and evaluation. In the human, the degree of hemolysis was clinically significant when the ventricles were powered by pulses of compressed air delivered at a high dP/dT, and has been greatly reduced with the reduction of the dP/dT. The use of hearts with a smaller stroke volume (such as the Jarvik-7-70) did not result in greater hemolysis [27].

Transient impairment of renal and hepatic function immediately after surgery returns to normal until the animal overgrows the artificial heart, with consequent multiorgan failure due to inadequate cardiac output. In clinical experience, renal and hepatic insufficiency has been described as reversed within a few days after the TAH implantation [6].

Areas for further investigation include the activation of some of the blood constituents that are thought to be extremely important in initiating the process of thrombus formation, i.e. platelets, leukocytes, and perhaps complement. Initially, when an artificial material is exposed to flowing blood, a thin layer of protein is deposited. If this is not albumin (fibrinogen or γ-globulin) it may eventually led to platelet adhesion. The consequent release of platelet constituents favors the aggregation of other platelets and forms a white thrombus. In some circumstances, this white thrombus may initiate the formation of a red thrombus. Second, when leukocytes are activated they may play an important role in thrombosis. They have been found on the border of low flow areas (beaching phenomenon) where deposition of fibrin strands attaches [28]. Third, complement is known to be activated by exposure to several biomaterials and to mediate cellular adherence to artificial surfaces [29, 30]. It has been well documented that complement components are involved in several processes like chemotaxis, anaphylotoxin production, immunoadherence, and opsonization – the more generally known inflammatory responses. Still uncertain is the significance of its activation, particularly when it is incomplete or inappropriate.

Conclusion

It is speculative to question whether it will ever be possible to develop a material that will be permanently and completely biocompatible. The experiences over the last few years certainly lead to the affirmation that materials have been greatly improved but that further improvements can be achieved. From this perspective, the temporary use of such blood pumps as a bridge to cardiac transplantation will become more common and widespread. The problem of thromboembolism remains the most serious factor in the use of a mechanical assist or replacement device, other factors being anatomical fit in the chest and the potential for infection. Several modifications in shape and size of the blood pumps have already improved the anatomical fit and will probably make the problem of secondary importance. The surgeons will have several choices on the shelf, depending on patient size and particular chest anatomy.

Once the problem of thrombus formation is overcome, infection will remain the only limitation. Even for temporary support of the circulation while waiting for a suitable heart donor, a totally implantable artificial heart is desirable.

Acknowledgments. This work was performed at the Artificial Heart Research Laboratory, Institute for Biomedical Engineering and Division of Artificial Organs, University of Utah, Dumke Building (535), Salt Lake City, Utah 84112. Reprints may be requested from Don B. Olsen, D.V.M., Director, at this address.

Funding for this work has been supplied in part by grants or contracts from: State of Utah Center of Excellence grant; NIH grant 1RO1 HL32816-02; Symbion, Inc. teaching contract; and the Artificial Heart Laboratory Development fund, University of Utah, to which contributions have been made by many generous donors.

References

1. Cooley DA, Liotta D, Hallman GL et al. (1969) Orthotopic cardiac prosthesis for two-staged cardiac replacement. Am J Cardiol 24:723
2. Cooley DA, Akutsu D, Norman JC et al. (1981) Total artificial heart in two staged cardiac transplantation. Bull Texas Heart Inst 8:305
3. Magovern JA, Pennock JL, Campbell DB et al. (1986) Bridge to heart transplantation: the Penn-State experience. J Heart Transplant 5(3):196
4. Joyce LD, Pritzker MR, Kiser JK et al. (1986) Use of the mini-Jarvik-7 total artificial heart as a bridge to transplantation. J Heart Transplant 5(3):203
5. Griffith BP, Kormos RL, Wei LM et al. (1986) Use of the total artificial heart as an interim device: initial experience in Pittsburgh with four patients. J Heart Transplant 5(3):210
6. Levinson MM, Smith RG, Cork R et al. (1986) Three recent cases of the total artificial heart before transplantation. J Heart Transplant 5(3):215
7. Joyce LD, Johnson KE, Pierce WS et al. (1986) Summary of the world experience with clinical use of a total artificial hearts as support devices. J Heart Transplant 5(3):229
8. Olsen DB, Riebman JR, De Paulis R et al. (1987) Registry and tabulation of orthotopic total artificial heart in man. Trans Am Soc Artif Intern Organs 33(3):182
9. De Paulis R, Riebman JR, Deleuze P et al. (1987) The total artificial heart: indications and preliminary results. J Cardiac Surg 2:2
10. Kolff J, Deeb MG, Riebman JR (1983) Preliminary study of a pneumatic artificial heart. J Heart Transplant 3:60
11. Jarvik RK, Kessler TR, McGill L et al. (1981) Determinants of pannus formation in long-surviving total artificial heart calves and its prevention. Trans Am Soc Artif Intern Organs 27:901
12. Mochizuki T, McRea J, Kim S et al. (1980) Study of the mechanism of pannus heart formation and inhibitors in the total artificial heart. Trans Jpn Soc Artif Intern Organs 9:87
13. Fukumasu H, Iwaya F, Olsen DB et al. (1979) Surgical implantation of the Jarvik-5 total artificial heart. Trans Am Soc Artif Intern Organs 25:232
14. Olsen DB, Fukumasu H, Iwaya F et al. (1978) Living one-half year on artificial hearts. Proc 8th World Congr Cardiol. Excerpta Medica, Amsterdam, pp 1019
15. Jarvik RK, DeVries WC, Semb BKH et al. (1986) Surgical positioning of the Jarvik-7 artificial heart. J Heart Transplant 5(3):184
16. Taenaka Y, Olsen DB, Murray KD et al. (1985) Development of an elliptical total artificial heart for smaller size recipients. Abstr Int Soc Artif Organs
17. Holfert JH, Riebman JB, Dew PA et al. (1987) Early preliminary results of a new total artificial heart connector system. Trans Am Soc Artif Intern Organs 33(3):151
18. Imachi K (1986) Long-term use of artificial heart without anticoagulation. In: Progress in artificial organs. Isao, Cleveland, p 319
19. Levinson MM, Smith RG, Cork RC et al. (1986) Thromboembolic complications of the Jarvik-7 total artificial heart: case report. Artif Organs 10(3):236
20. Griffith BP, Hardesty RL, Kormos RL et al. (1987) Temporary use of the Jarvik-7 total artificial heart before transplantation. N Engl J Med 316(3):130
21. Olsen DB, Kessler TR, Pons AB et al. (1981) Fabrication, implantation, and pathophysiology of the total artificial heart in calves for six months. In: Pierce WS (ed) US-USSR joint symposium on circulatory assistance and the artificial heart. NIH publication no 80-2032, p 3155
22. Chiang BY, Olsen DB, Gaykowski R et al. (1984) Evaluation of treadmill exercise on total artificial heart recipients. Trans Am Soc Artif Intern Organs 30:514

23. Willshaw P, Nielsen SD, Nanas J et al. (1984) A cardiac output monitor and diagnostic unit for pneumatically driven artificial hearts. Artif Organs 8(2):215

24. Blaylock EC, Nielsen SD, Morgan DL, Lioi AP, Morgan JM, Olsen DB (1986) The artificial heart: pursuit of a noninvasive method for determining atrial pressures. Artif Organs 10(6):489

25. Myhre E, Rasmussen K, Anderson A (1970) Serum lactic dehydrogenase activity in patients with prosthetic heart valves: a parameter of intravascular hemolysis. Am Heart J 80(4):463

26. Westenfelder C, Baranowski RL, Kablitz C et al. (1986) Atrial natriuretic peptide release in calves with artificial hearts. Kidney Int 29:389A

27. Levinson MM, Copeland JC, Smith RG et al. (1986) Indices of hemolysis in human recipients of the Jarvik-7 total artificial heart: a cooperative report of fifteen patients. J Heart Transplant 5:236

28. Grevelink JM, Mohammad SF, Cho CS et al. (1985) Pulmonary artery to pulmonary artery (PAPAS). Trans Am Soc Artif Intern Organs 31:377

29. Chenoweth DE (1986) Complement activation produced by biomaterials. Trans Am Soc Artif Intern Organs 32

30. Herzlinger GA, Cumming RD (1980) Role of complement activation in cell adhesion to polymer blood contact surfaces. Trans Am Soc Artif Intern Organs 26:165

Part IV
Total Artificial Heart

30. Toward the Totally Implantable Artificial Heart

F. UNGER

The ultimate goal in designing artificial hearts has been a totally implantable device consisting of ventricles and integrated energy and control systems. In 1982 the first permanent implantation was performed clinically. Since then, six human beings have received a permanent pneumatically driven artificial heart, whereby the driving and monitor system has been extracorporeally located. One patient, Mr. Heydon, lived over 400 days. The most severe limiting factor is thrombus formation within the ventricles at the various sites of transition such as suture lines, valve-supporting rings, and quick connections and caused by the biomaterial itself. Infection along the driving lines also complicates the course, as does inflammation inside the mediastinum due to the constant movement of the heart chambers. These severe complications have put a halt to further implantations.

The artificial heart driven pneumatically exists in two variations of the same basic design. There are five designs currently in use (Jarvik, Ellipsoid heart, Berlin, Pierce, Vasku), with basically **two main differences**: the artificial heart consist of a blood chamber with a moving membrane, a reinforced housing, and the gas chamber with a rigid heart base so that the air can move the membrane; this displaces the blood, resulting in an ejection. The blood chamber has two inlets; the flow is directed by artificial valves. The artificial heart has to fit exactly inside the chest, without kinking the vessels or compromising the surrounding structures, and must allow a cardiac output of up to 10 l/min to maintain adequate perfusion of the body.

The design of the blood chamber is important. Stagnation areas must be avoided. To facilitate easy construction Kwan-Gett presented a very imposing technique for assembling an artificial heart using a separate housing, a moving membrane, and a rigid base. This system has been developed, and the concepts of Jarvik, Vasku, Kolff, Nose, and Shumakov are refinements of it. Despite the developments by Jarvik, the junction between the membrane and the housing remaines (Fig. 1 a), and this junction is the source of constant thrombus formation. W. J. Kolff introduced an improvement in the way of production by vacuum formation of the components. The design and technique are similar to those of Bücherl and Wolner. In their designs, however, the junction remains, and the problem is not solved.

To overcome this problem, i.e., to eliminate the junction, Pierce and Unger designed ventricles with one membrane, with the housing and the heart base attached to it (Fig. 1 b). The production is more difficult, but thrombus formation on the membrane within the ventricles is avoided.

Assisted Circulation 3
F. Unger (Ed.)
© Springer-Verlag Berlin Heidelberg 1989

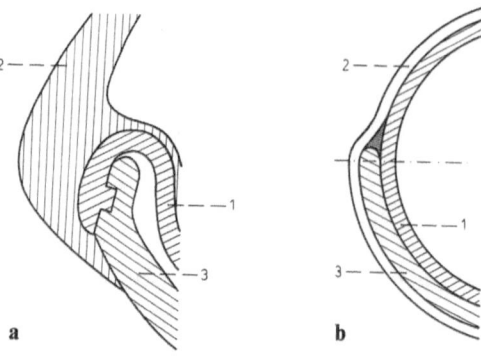

Fig. 1 a, b. Diaphragm housing junctions. **a** Junction of a diaphragm-type membrane in end-diastolic position; **b** junction of a one-piece membrane in end-diastolic position. *1*, Membrane; *2*, housing, *3*, base

The pneumatically driven artificial hearts are feasible only for temporary support and are contraindicated for permanent implantation due to the complications mentioned above. The mechanical blood pumps, driven electrically, are steps toward permanent implantation.

The artificial hearts work physiologically as bridges to transplantation. The long-term results obtained in calves have shown pannus formation and biodegradation of the membrane to be limiting factors.

This chapter presents exciting results from Dr. Semb, of Sweden, who used a Jarvik heart as a permanent implant. His patient died, however, of thromboembolism and pannus formation in the atria. He also performed a successful bridging operation.

Dr. Vasku, from Brno, describes his extensive studies and evaluations of the pathophysiological findings in calves that received TAHs. The artificial heart made of smooth polyurethane is driven pneumatically. The basic design is similar to that of the Jarvik heart. Since Dr. Vasku wrote his paper, three clinical bridging operations have been performed in Czechoslovakia. Dr. Vasku's considerations are important for further experiments in the area of artificial heart research.

Dr. Rosenberg, from the Hershey group led by Dr. Pierce, introduces an implantable mechanical heart. The Hershey pump is driven electrically; the membrane is actuated by moving pusher plates with a roller screw system. The system has been implanted in calves for up to 222 days. The limiting factors are related to the mechanical parts. This mechanical pump is larger than pneumatically driven pumps and can produce a cardiac output of up to 8 l/min. Bench tests have shown reliability of up to 2 years.

Dr. Shumakov, from Moskow, presents the USSR artificial heart, which is based on the Jarvik heart. He describes the design requirements and the experiments done with calves. This design has been used clinically as a bridge.

Dr. Liotta is convinced that the right heart is not a definite necessity, and shows why he thinks it feasible that a univentricular heart can fulfill all the criteria for optimal perfusion. The left heart is filled via the lung, in the manner of a direct shunt between the right atrium and the pulmonary artery. Dr. Liotta presents various physiological responses to support his thesis that an orthotopic univentricular total artificial heart has the same potential for perfusion as two ventricles.

Dr. Fukunaga, from Hiroshima, reports on attempts that have been made to produce a completely implantable artificial heart. The pumps are sacs made of Biomer, and they use a brushless DC motor. Following several bench tests, his group has performed some acute experiments.

The design and extensive testing of artificial hearts for permanent use require dedication and patience on the part of the scientist and a great amount of financial support. The only devices that can be considered are mechanically driven blood pumps. At present, these devices are very bulky and susceptible to failure of their mechanical and electrical components. In addition, biodegeneration of the biomaterial is at present an important problem. But progress has been made in the use of these devices for temporary support; why should the scientist give up now? I personally feel sure that, in small steps, the target of permanent use will be reached, but not today or tomorrow. It depends on the commitment of the universities to basic research, and on public support.

31. The Use of the Total Artificial Heart

B. K. H. Semb

Pumping devices to assist or replace cardiac pumping activity have been in use for more than 20 years. As early as 1963 a left ventricular assist device (LVAD) was implanted in a patient, and after further research left ventricular assistance was performed in a small series of patients in 1966 and 1967 at Baylor University in Texas by Drs. Elliot, DeBakey, and co-workers [1]. Among the numerous LVAD and total artificial heart (TAH) designs, the air-driven pump has to date been the most successful in the clinical total replacement of the failing heart. As early as 1921 Dale and Schuster described a device for the pumping of blood that involved a squeeze mechanism. It consisted of a flexible bladder extending into a rigid blood-filled container [2]. The most common design now is the diaphragm pump with blood on one side of the diaphragm and liquid or gas on the other. The diaphragm concept was further developed by Kolff and his group at the Cleveland Clinic in the mid-1960s. This heart consisted basically of two pumps, one for each side of the heart, where a flexible elastic sac was contained in a rigid outer case. The Kantrowitz auxiliary ventricle had blood passing through a tube which was externally compressed and promoted forward by ligating the aorta between the inlet and outlet of the pump. The traditional membrane pump from Baylor University is quite similar in principle to the presently commercially available Jarvik-7 heart [3].

Much of the more recent research on the pumps focused on the development of unbreakable materials with surface characteristics which avoid clotting and blood destruction. These requirements were partially met by the development of modern polyurethanes. Hence after extensive animal experimentation the first permanent TAH implantation was performed in 1982 [3]. The heart that was used was the Jarvik-7 TAH, which consists of the heart pump itself and a drive system with a cardiac output monitoring and diagnostic unit. The Jarvik-7 heart consists of two halves, each containing a diaphragm pump (Fig. 1). On one side of the diaphragm is blood, on the other side air. During diastole blood flows via the mitral or tricuspid valve into the blood compartment of the pump. This occurs passively by means of the central venous pressure or the left atrial pressure but can also be accelerated by using a vacuum on the air compartment of the pump. When the heart has been filled with blood, air is pumped in under pressure; the membrane then expands, the inlet valve closes, and the outlet valve opens to produce a systolic ejection. To some degree a Starling mechanism is provided by this pump by running it at a level of incomplete filling. Thus when the filling pressure increases, the membrane will collapse further and increase the stroke volume of the pump (Fig. 2). For practical purposes about a 20% increase in cardiac output can

Assisted Circulation 3
F. Unger (Ed.)
© Springer-Verlag Berlin Heidelberg 1989

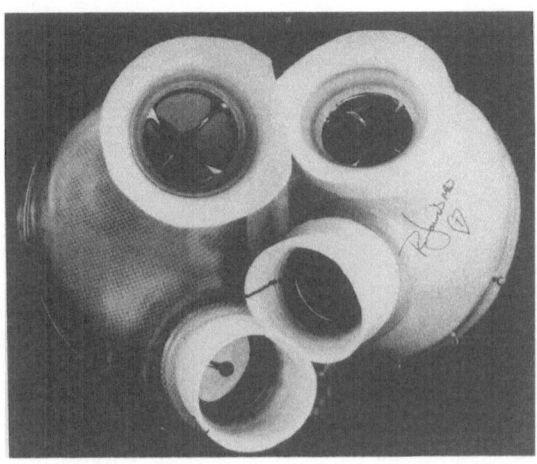

Fig. 1. The two halves of the Jarvik-7 heart with the outlet and the inlet valves and the quick connecting Dacron cuffs

occur via this self-regulatory mechanism (Fig. 3). The drive unit consists of a console containing a back-up system and multiple alarms as well as a computer. The stroke work of the pump is determined by varying the air pressure, the rate, and the duration of the ejection and filling phases.

The principle of pumping is that of complete ejection to empty the blood compartment of the heart and avoid stagnation and clotting. The pressure of the left heart cavity is naturally much higher than that of the right heart cavity, and the balance between right and left pressures is one of the most important aspects following implantation because too high a pressure on the right side will immediately result in pulmonary edema. In order to avoid this, maximum operation of the left heart is employed. The right heart is pumped carefully in order to avoid overflowing of the lungs and then gradually increased until an adequate cardiac output is obtained. A computerized picture of the filling of the heart is valuable in assessing the filling forces. The aim is to have an autoregulatory reserve with incomplete filling of the heart and the potential for increasing cardiac output if necessary. The computer gives a fair assessment of the stroke volume and the cardiac output of the right and left heart. It is possible to follow the cardiac output over a prolonged period, as seen in Fig. 3, which illustrates the increase in cardiac output during exercise.

Apart from the stationary drive unit console, there is a portable compressor. It is battery driven and can be used for several hours before changing the battery. Also this unit contains a back-up system in the form of a second compressor system. It can be programmed for heart rate and stroke volume (Fig. 4).

One of the main problems after implantation of this and other types of artificial heart is the incidence of the thrombosis. In animal experiments the thrombosis has a tendency to localize around the inlet and outlet of the heart valves and on the Dacron cuffs adjacent to the atria and the pulmonary artery and aorta.

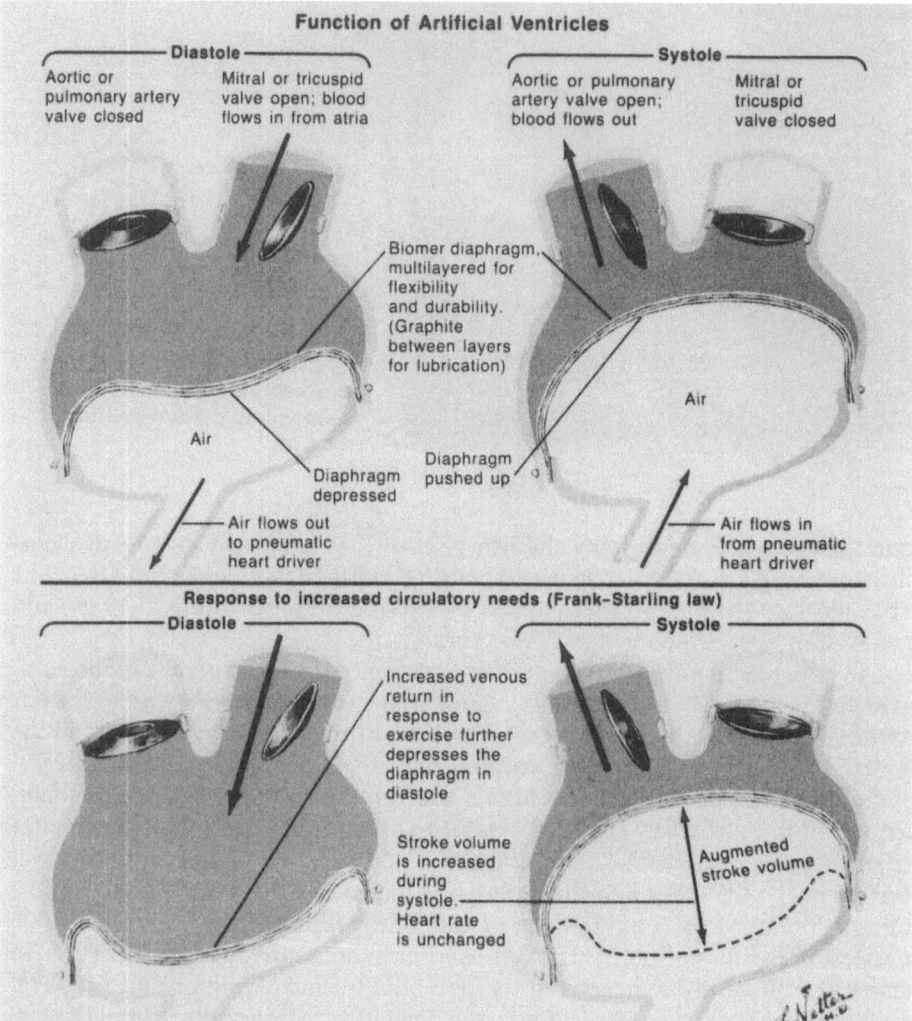

Fig. 2. The principle of pumping is incomplete filling and complete ejection. In the case of increasing venous pressure, a further filling of the heart can occur during diastole and thus increase the cardiac output

The Stockholm Experience

The clinical implantation of the artificial heart essentially follows the principle of cardiac transplantation. However, one is interested in keeping a little more of the atrial structures by excising the heart slightly distal to the atrioventricular groove. This provides solid tissue for anchoring the Dacron cuffs that are necessary to connect the artificial heart. Figures 5 and 6 show Dr. Frank Netter's illustrations of the atrial cuffs as well as the cuffs on the aorta and pulmonary artery sutured

Figs. 2, 5, and 6 are reproduced by courtesy of Ciba-Geigy.

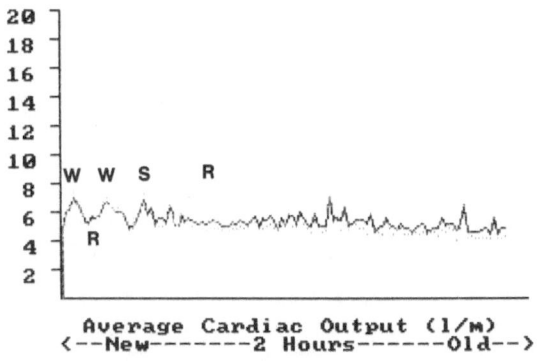

Fig. 3. Average cardiac output during a 2-h period. During rest (R) the cardiac output is around 5.1; when the patient stands upright (S) or walks (W) it increases by about 20%

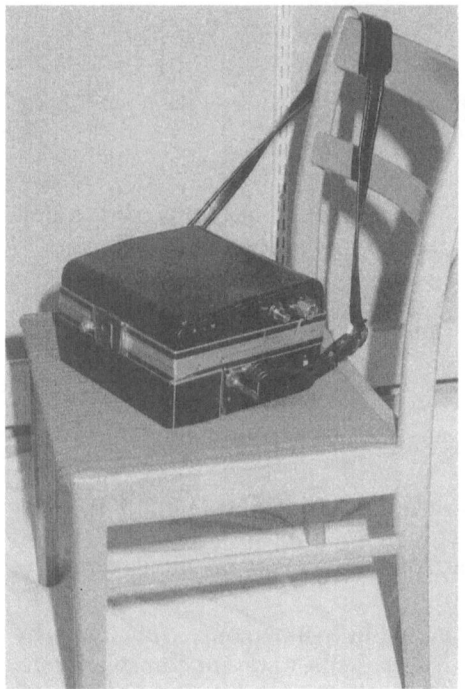

Fig. 4. The portable Heimes compressor

in place. These cuffs consist of a Dacron vascular graft with a quick connect device so that the ventricles of the heart can be snapped on. During the operation one of the main problems is the positioning of the heart. Repositioning is possible by detachment of the heart by means of the quick connects, but the manipulation usually precipitates considerable bleeding which may be difficult to control. In positioning the heart the main problem is to avoid kinking of the left pulmonary veins and the inferior vena cava and distortion of the pulmonary artery. The drive lines for the compressed air have to be taken out on the abdomen, and this presents another serious problem since ascending infection along the drive lines is quite common. A special Teflon button inserted subcutaneously reduces this

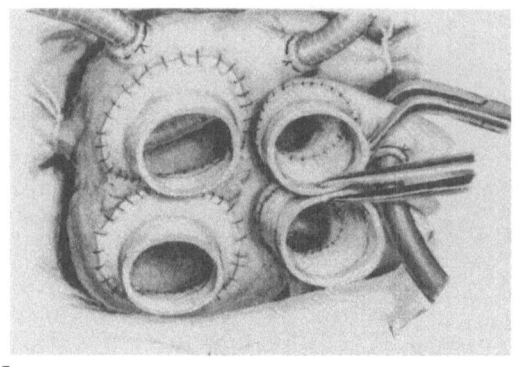

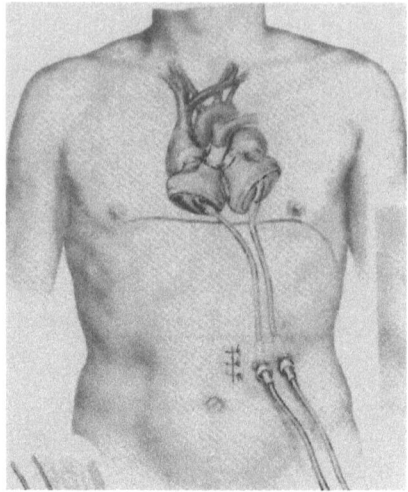

5

Fig. 5. Frank Netters illustration of the atrial
and arterial cuffs   6

Fig. 6. Frank Netter illustrations on the completion of the implantation of the Jarvik-7 heart.
Note the Teflon buttons at the exit of the drive lines on the abdomen

problem. In the postoperative phase continuous attention has to be paid to sterility of the skin exit of the drive lines in order to avoid ascending infection.

Discussion

For the present, there are three main possible indications for use of the TAH:

1. As a permanent substitute for a failing heart where cardiac transplantation is not possible in a dying patient
2. As a temporary substitute in a patient awaiting heart transplantation, when life-threatening deterioration occurs before a donor heart is available
3. Cardiogemic shock or failure to wean from extracorporeal circulation after heart surgery.

Permanent implantation has been attempted in five patients – four times by deVries' group and once by us in 1985. The patients were not transplantable. Usually they developed problems of a thromboembolic nature very soon after artificial heart implantation, leading to massive neurological changes. In our patient we were quite successful in avoiding such complications for a long time, although within the first 3 weeks the patient suffered a minor embolic episode of no clinical consequence. He received massive anticoagulation treatment consisting of both heparin and warfarin, and for a prolonged period even dipyridamole and acetylsalicylic acid. Needless to say, this type of arrangement demands very close supervision in order to balance avoidance of thromboembolism against bleeding. With the combination of warfarin and heparin our impression was that the best parameter to monitor anticoagulation was factor X, since the prothrombin complex also seemed to be somewhat affected by the simultaneous heparin infusion. Heparin was used as a continuous infusion and was monitored most

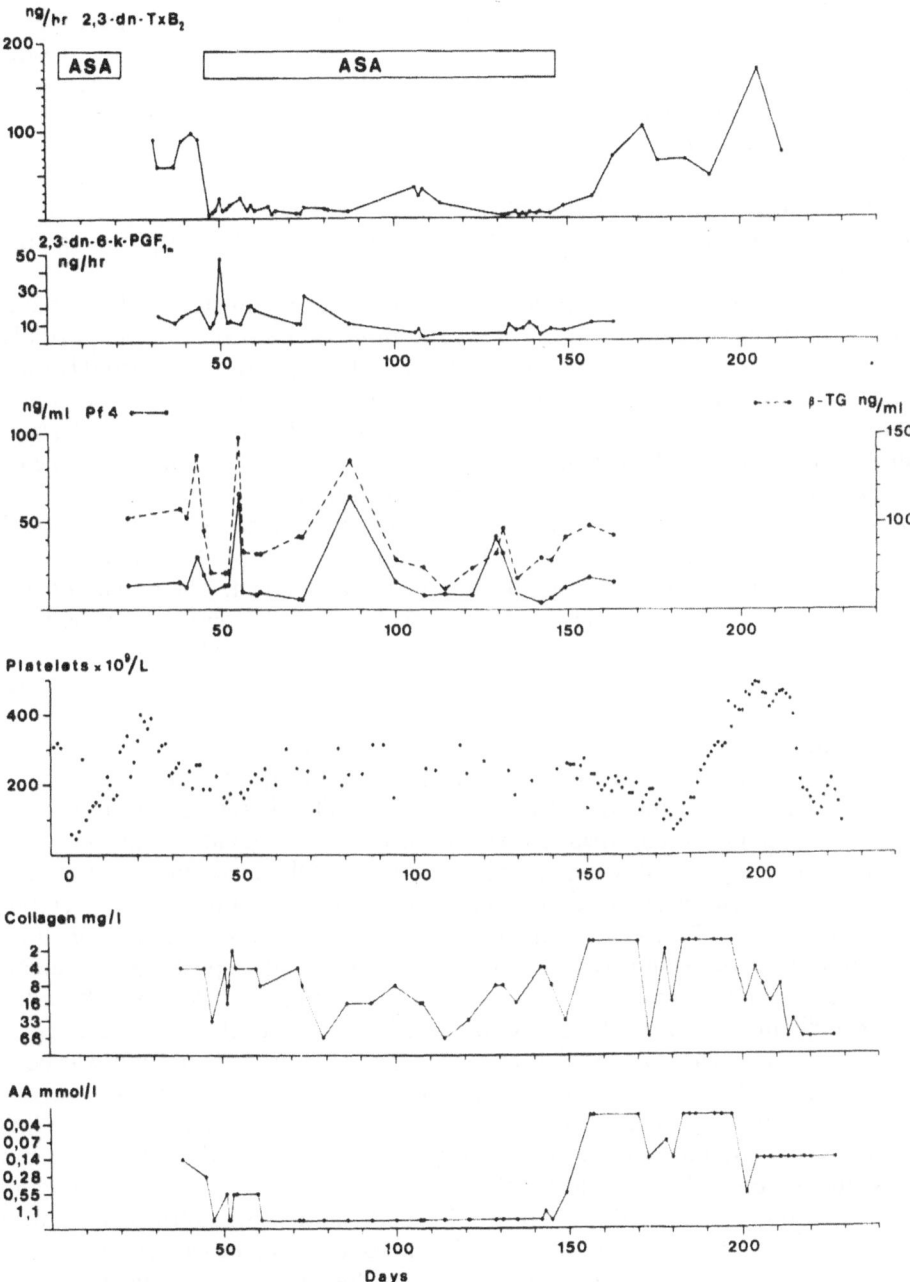

Fig. 7. The *upper part* of the figure depicts the thromboxane B_2 metabolism, which became normal during acetylsalicylic acid medication (*ASA*), indicating that the ongoing platelet activation was suppressed during this period. Both prostacyclin and β-thromboglobulin (*β-TG*) showed atypical changes during the postoperative course. The platelets were generally raised in number, particularly during the period when no acetylsalicylic acid was given. The *lower part* of the figure shows that platelet activation was suppressed by acetylsalicylic acid when arachidonic acid (*AA*) was used as substrate but was not clearly suppressed when collagen was used. *pf 4*, platelet factor IV

safely by means of multiple APTT determinations. Antiplatelet aggregatory drugs were used because continuous platelet stimulation occurred. Acetylsalicyclic acid had a pronounced effect in that it inhibited the platelet stimulation, at least when arachidonic acid was used as substrate. Also interesting was the fact that the thromboxane B_2 metabolism, which was increased after implantation, normalized when acetylsalicylic acid was administered (Fig. 7). Other platelet parameters like β-thromboglobulin, platelet factor IV, and fibrinogen were of no help in assessing the ongoing platelet stimulation after implantation of the artificial heart.

Our first patient with permanent implantation was completely mobilized and became fairly active over a period of several months. By means of the portable drive system he could move around quite freely. Although liver failure and kidney failure (two of the factors contraindicating a transplantation) improved somewhat, he never became a good candidate for transplantation. Eventually he succumbed after an embolic episode with subsequent cerebral hemorrhage. One of the practical problems of his long-term anticoagulation treatment was a very fluctuating tolerance to heparin. During some periods minute doses of heparin would produce complete anticoagulation, whereas during other phases massive doses had to be given over long periods to obtain the same effect. The impact of this massive anticoagulation could not be reversed very easily, and during the final embolic episode several days were needed before a more normal clotting situation could be obtained by means of multiple transfusions and by discontinuing anticoagulants.

At autopsy in patients having had a Jarvik-7 heart for a prolonged period, considerable overgrowth of tissue has been found at the atrial suture line between the atrial Dacron cuff and the natural atrial tissues. This, in retrospect, could have been expected, given that atrial tissue cannot grow into the atrial cuff, which is massive and does not allow any ingrowth of tissue. Obviously this is one of the factors that should be changed in order to avoid this important source of embolism. The interior of the heart pump itself, however, is little affected by even long implantation periods and usually only shows some fibrin deposits on the membranes or the inner lining of the blood compartment of the heart. Another area of thromboembolism is at the inflow and outflow valves of the ventricles.

The idea of using an artificial heart as a bridge to transplantation was conceived shortly after the first human transplantations were performed. As early as 1969 Liotta and Cooley implanted an artificial heart of a similar type to the Jarvik-7 in a patient who was transplanted with a biological heart after 2 days but subsequently died. The next attempt was made in Houston in 1981, and again after a period of 2 days on the artificial heart the patient was transplanted with a fatal outcome. In the meantime several types of artificial heart were developed for use as a bridge to transplantation, e.g., the Phoenix heart, the Pennsylvania State heart, and the Ellipsoid heart developed by Unger in Salzburg and by Bucherl in Berlin, as well as the Jarvik-7 heart. Most experience has been gained with the latter artificial heart, although very encouraging observations were made with the other types also. The first successful bridge to transplantation with a Jarvik-7 heart was performed in the United States in August 1985, when the patient was transplanted after 9 days and subsequently could return home.

In Europe the first bridge to transplantation, was performed by Unger in Austria. The first longtime survivor came from our clinic in a 53 year man in May 1986. This patient went into cardiac failure after his sixth myocardial infarction. After a period of 10 days with an artificial Jarvik-7 heart he was transplanted and eventually was able to return home and later to take up his work. Even after such a short time, at transplantation this patient was found to have developed non-symptomatic thrombosis at the site of the left atrial suture line, which indicates the importance of redesigning the atrial cuffs.

Up to October 1987 a total of 69 patients had been bridged for transplantation with the Jarvik-7 heart. The mean age was 41 years (range: 15–59) and the duration of the bridging period was 17 days. Fourteen of the patients died while on the artificial heart and prior to transplantation. Presently three patients are being supported by the TAH and awaiting transplantation. Hence 52 patients were transplanted, and of these 52, 20 died following transplantation. In total, 32 patients are living and of these, five are still hospitalized while 27 have been discharged from hospital and 12 have returned to work. Altogether about half the patients who have undergone bridge to transplantation with the Jarvik-7 heart and subsequent transplantation have survived this procedure. The mortality is clearly higher than in ordinary heart transplantation, pointing very much to the complexity of the procedure and also probably reflecting a more desperately sick patient population than in ordinary heart transplantation.

Most of the problems of artificial heart implantation have been caused by bleeding problems, which are accentuated by the need for continuous anticoagulation, and by multiple organ failure. After bridging the patient might improve to the extent that it would seem natural to give higher priority for transplantation to other patients without an artificial heart. Nevertheless, the danger of embolism and infections in patients with artificial hearts needs to be taken into account. Also it seems that the regulatory mechanisms of the circulation are somewhat changed in patients on an artificial heart and that the best outcome of the treatment is to be expected in patients in whom the bridging period is no longer than 2–3 weeks. Even with these limitations the TAH as a bridge to transplantation is a valuable adjunct to a heart transplantation program, particularly under circumstances where great fluctuations in the number of donor hearts exist. The use of the TAH as a permanent implant should await the development of better artificial heart systems, as our experience to date shows that the available technology is better suited for short implantation periods.

References

1. DeBakey ME (1971) Left ventricular bypass pump for cardiac assistance. Am J Cardiol 27:3–11
2. Myers GH, Parsonnet V (1969) Engineering in the heart and blood vessels. Wiley-Interscience, New York, pp 137–159
3. Joyce LD, Johnson KE, Pierce WS, DeVries WC, Semb BKH, Copeland JG, Griffith BP, Cooley CA, Frazier OH, Cabrol C, Keon WJ, Unger F, Bucherl ES, Wolner E (1986) Summary of the world experience with clinical use of total artificial hearts as heart support devices. J Heart Transplant 229–235

32. A Contribution to the Assessment of Pathophysiology in Long-Term Total Artificial Heart Recipients

J. Vašků

Introduction

The implantation of total artificial hearts (TAHs) has become an ever more important tool of cardiosurgery in saving the lives of potential recipients of biological transplants when a donor organ is not immediately available. Clinical experience with this bridging procedure is now accelerating. In addition, some clinical experience with permanent TAH implantation has been gathered [1, 2]. This knowledge is advancing methodological procedures concerning the implantation technique, the construction of TAH devices and control and driving units, and the postoperative management of patients. Also, for the first time we can learn of the subjective feelings of TAH recipients. Thus, future clinical development is now a well established branch of TAH research and research into heart transplantation in general. On the other hand, some basic problems concerning permanent TAH implantation in humans have to be solved; these problems derive from the technical equipment and/or from the physiology of the organism with the TAH implanted.

Further technical development will have to involve the construction of reliable portable or totally miniaturized drivers which will allow the patient maximum mobility. This is an inescapable requirement for improving the quality of life of the permanent TAH recipient.

At the same time, we must also pursue ways of adapting living organisms to the implanted device. The implantation of an artificial pump represents extensive intervention in all the basic functions of the organism. Immense experience has been obtained in many centers throughout the world with regard to the general physiology and pathophysiology of TAH recipients. This experience has preponderantly been collected in healthy animals [3–9, 49–52]. These animals eventually became sick in different ways, especially during the later stages of survival. In patients, i.e., in subjects who suffer from different kinds of cardiomyopathy, TAH implantation must, first of all, induce profound relief and restoration of the basic functions of organs (particularly the kidneys, lungs, and liver, or the whole gastrointestinal tract) damaged by the protracted cardiac pathology. Another important task for TAH research workers is to avoid thrombogenesis and thus the possibility of strokes.

If these requirements are fulfilled, then we can expect TAH implantation as a bridging procedure to be beneficial for the patient, especially if enough time is allowed (perhaps 2–4 weeks) for the TAH to improve the patient's general condition and restore the disturbed functions of his organs. However, under the cir-

Assisted Circulation 3
F. Unger (Ed.)
© Springer-Verlag Berlin Heidelberg 1989

cumstances of permanent TAH implantation, some complications must be expected after the initial stabilization. These stem mainly from new functional relations established after several months between the function of the TAH and the TAH recipient. These complications can eventually grow progressively, depending on the prolongation of survival. Of course, sometimes technical problems can also complicate the situation. Therefore, animal experiments with long survival are still an important and necessary tool for deepening our knowledge relevant to the clinical management of long-surviving patients, and for extending our experience and knowledge of the general physiology and pathophysiology of organisms with a TAH. If we could find some suitable form of experimental cardiomyopathy in the calf, and possibly in the goat and sheep, and carry out TAH implantation, our experimental model would be nearly perfect from the point of view of comparison with clinical situations.

In any case, it is possible to say that a new branch of physiology and pathophysiology is already well established. It can be called physiology and pathophysiology of the TAH – a new section of basic medical science.

Some Remarks Concerning the Hardware Used in Our Recent Experiments with the TAH

According to Atsumi and his school [10], we can differentiate two large problem areas in artificial heart research: TAH hardware and TAH software. Whereas the TAH hardware comprises mainly the TAH and the necessary equipment, driving and control units, etc., the software is the complex area of a biological individuum, where neural, humoral, and hormonal regulation is extremely important, including the feedback systems which may participate in proper TAH regulation. In my opinion, we must agree with Atsumi's proposal and take into consideration both these areas of TAH research.

As regards hardware, we started our research with two kinds of blood pump, a Soviet TAH of the "Kedr" type and the US Jarvik 3. Later we constructed our own device, the TNS-BRNO II, which was made of polymethyl methacrylate and produced mechanically. Only the kinetic components of this artificial heart, i.e., the driving diaphragm and valves, were made of polyurethane [4, 5, 11]. The volume of the device was 100 ml, and the motion of the driving diaphragm was concentric. The diaphragm movements were oriented strictly concentrically according to the central line of the blood chamber, where the diaphragm movements were maximal. The mechanical mounting of the TAH housing with the diaphragm could not avoid sharp angles at the diaphragm–housing (DH) junction. This fact, together with the decrease in velocity of blood streaming on the outer circumference of the diaphragm, was the main cause of the frequent occurrence of thrombi in these particular areas of the TAH blood chamber [31]. The two different materials at the sites of valve fixation (i.e., polymethyl methacrylate housing and polyurethane valves), and perhaps the difference in material between the diaphragm and housing at the DH junction, delivered different surface electrical potentials, and thus the most suitable conditions for thrombocytic adhesion and aggregation were present at the sites of contact. Thrombi at these sites were also very common findings in the experiments with the TNS-BRNO II.

Nevertheless, the polymethyl methacrylate housing could be used repeatedly, and only polyurethane diaphragms and valves were exchanged in each experiment. The longest survival obtained with the TNS-BRNO II was 175 days, and the above-mentioned thrombotizing tendency was one of the important factors limiting long survival. Another limiting factor was that on its outer circumference the diaphragm became "broken" and came into full contact with the inflow valve during the pumping cycle. If its surface became covered with thrombi or calcified particles, they could be easily removed by the repeated contact and transported as microemboli to the kidney and also to other vital organs by the bloodstream [5, 12–14]. The most dangerous situation was represented by central nervous microembolization. Two long-surviving calves (calf no. 53, Florian, and calf no. 65, Achmet) died from this complication. In spite of these setbacks related to the TNS-BRNO II design, in many long-term experiments with this TAH we were able to learn a great deal from the surgical procedure and from the postoperative care of the calves. Simultaneously, we could evaluate the excellent durability of our inflow and outflow valves. No experiment was terminated because of valve failure [31].

Our experiences with the TNS-BRNO II, which have been described in detail elsewhere [5, 15, 16], necessitated the construction of a new device without the deficiencies of polymethyl methacrylate versions. After several attempts to construct a TAH totally made of polyurethane, we were generally satisfied with the TNS-BRNO VII model.

Main Features of the TNS-BRNO VII

From the outset the TNS-BRNO VII was constructed in two variations, experimental and clinical, which differ by virtue of the volume of the blood chamber and the localization of drive line connection with the TAH pneumatic chamber.

The main original feature of this pump is the asymmetrical driving diaphragm (Fig. 1) and the axis deviation of the inflow valve [14]. The housing is made of polyurethane, which enables the easy junction with the polyurethane driving diaphragm by sticking. The whole blood chamber is made of one material. Moreover, the sharp angle of the DH junction is eliminated, which contributes to the minimal thrombus formation.

The asymmetrical driving diaphragm removes the setbacks of the driving diaphragms of the previous type. In these previous types, the "breaking" of the outer circumference of the diaphragm during the transition from the systolic to the diastolic position and vice versa was a major disadvantage. Laminar blood streaming was seriously disturbed, further cavitations occurred, and the diaphragm performance was overloaded.

The top of the asymmetrical diaphragm in the TNS-BRNO VII heart is thus transferred away from its center. The site of its primary deformation during the pumping cycle is situated opposite to the mouth of the inflow tract. Thus, the stretching of the diaphragm is markedly decreased in the first stage during tran-

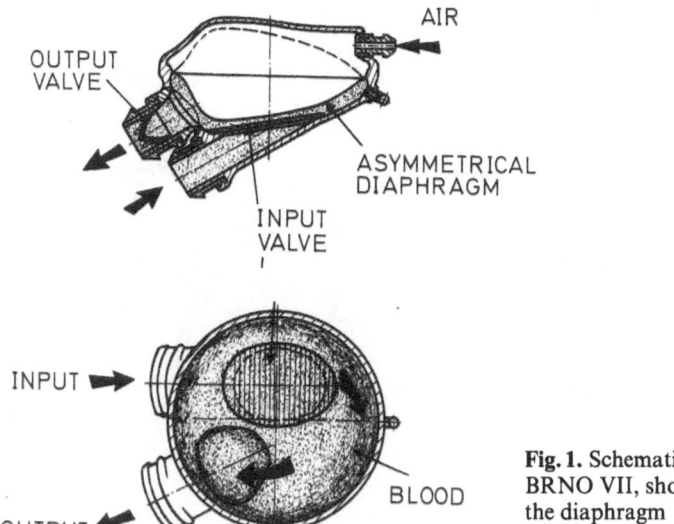

Fig. 1. Schematic drawing of the TNS-BRNO VII, showing the asymmetry of the diaphragm

sition from systole to diastole, and in this way the sensitivity of the whole system to the inflow pressure is increased and the filling of the blood chamber is simultaneously enhanced. The "breakage" of the diaphragm on the outer circumference is removed, which markedly contributes to its long-term durability.

In early diastole, when the change of pressure gradient on the inflow valve occurs, and the valve movement opens the inflow tract, the driving diaphragm moves not to the flap of the inflow valve directly at this site. This minimizes the space between the valve flap and the diaphragm. During the diaphragm movement from diastole to systole, the last point to move is the top of the diaphragm, which stays at this time opposite the inflow tract; the blood movement is accelerated and the diaphragm undulated (Fig. 2). This evacuation regimen markedly

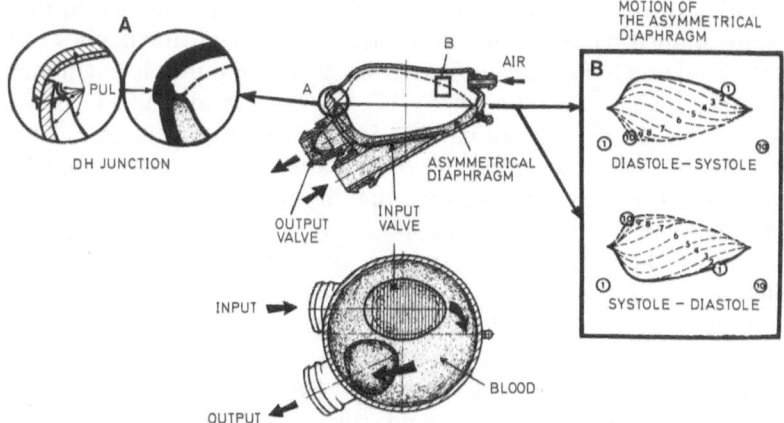

Fig. 2. Schematic drawing of the TNS-BRNO VII, showing a detailed view of the DH junction (*A*) and the mode of diaphragm motion (*B*)

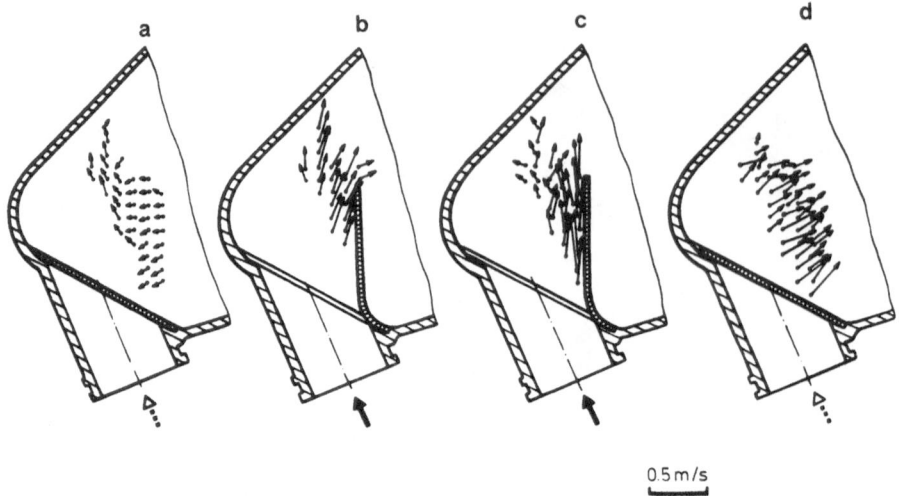

Fig. 3 a–d. An example of the velocity field in the part of a blood chamber in the 120-ml TNS-BRNO VII situated near the inflow valve. Measurements were performed by laser-Doppler ane-mometry. **a** t/T = 0.35 – the inflow valve is still closed; the ejection phase is terminating. **b** t/T = 0.45 – the inflow valve is opened; the filling of the blood chamber starts. **c** t/T = the inflow valve is opened; the filling phase is terminating. **d** 0.15 = the inflow valve is closed; the ejection phase goes on. The measurements were performed in the Institute of Hydrodynamics, Czechoslovak Academy of Sciences, by ing. F. Klimeš and co-workers

enhances the effectivity of pumping and the evacuation of the blood chamber is essentially fast and complete, which is a decisive point in the antithrombogenicity of this type of TAH (Fig. 3). Simultaneously, the contact of the diaphragm surface with the surface of the inflow valve flap during the pumping cycle is reduced as much as possible. The likelihood of removal of calcified particles from the diaphragm surface is also reduced to a minimum, which is very important in the later stages of the experiments.

The above-described functions of the asymmetrical diaphragm and of the inflow valve were studied painstakingly at the Institute of Hydrodynamics of the Czechoslovak Academy of Sciences in Prague by means of pulsatile anemometry and laser-Doppler anemometry (Figs. 4, 5) [17]. These methods make possible simultaneous study of the diaphragm motion and the motion of the inflow valve (Fig. 6). By these methods the superiority of this kind of undulating diaphragm motion over the classical types of concentric diaphragm motion currently used in the majority of artificial hearts was completely confirmed. Its advantages were decisive in prolonging the survival times in our experimental animals and for the complete elimination of thrombus formation in the experiments and also in clinical implantations (Fig. 7). Nevertheless, it is still always essential to prevent infection, because in such a situation the formation of bacteriologically induced thrombi is almost inevitable, and this cannot be avoided even by ideal design of the pumping system and supplementary anticoagulation treatment.

The Chirasist TN-3 stationary system of control and driving units was used and is still used in our experiments without essential changes. Up to now tests

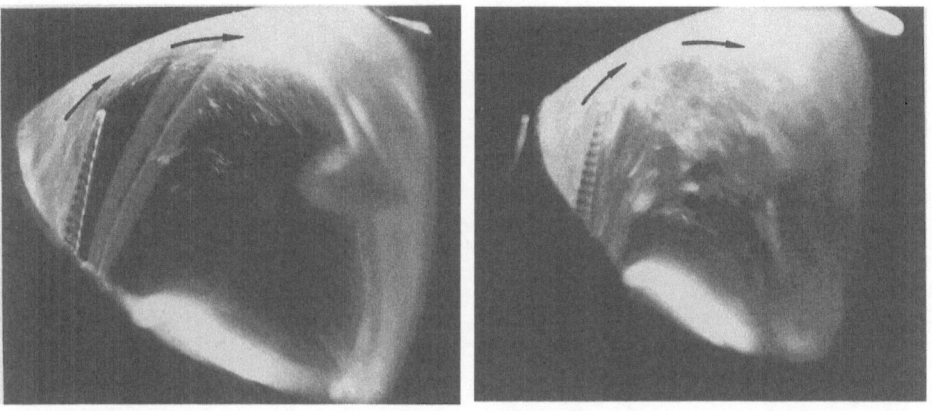

Fig. 4a, b. Visualization of the fluid streaming in the 120-ml TNS-BRNO VII. There is sudden opening of the inflow valve, with fluid ejection into the blood chamber, which begins to fill. Output A = 11 l/min. Laser-Doppler anemometry. Courtesy of F. Klimeš

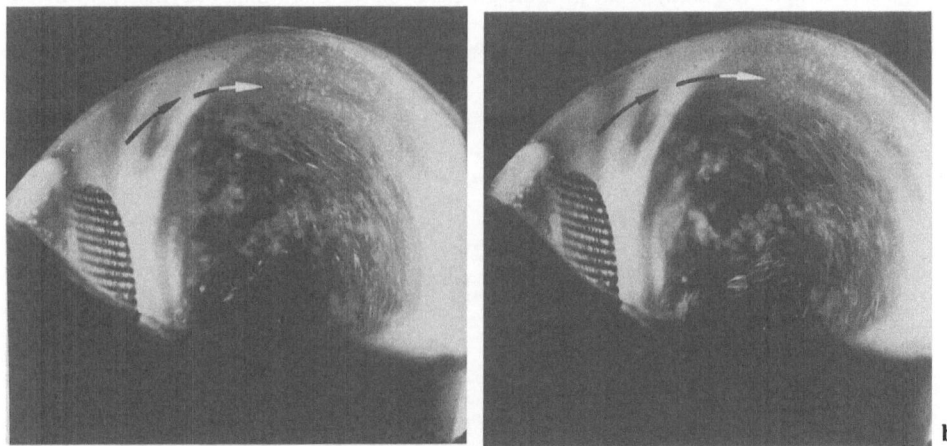

Fig. 5a, b. Visualization of the fluid streaming in the 120-ml TNS-BRNO VII. The inflow valve is opened and the filling phase is proceeding. Output A = 11 l/min. Laser-Doppler anemometry. Courtesy of F. Klimeš

have revealed the quality of these drivers to be excellent. The technical features of this system have been described in more detail elsewhere [18].

Our further research in this area led to the construction of two portable systems (Fig. 8) [19, 20].

A Brief Survey of Experiences with the TNS-BRNO VII TAH in Experiments

To date we have performed 40 long-term experiments with survival periods of 31–226 days (the average being 103.6 days). In these experiments the following TAH

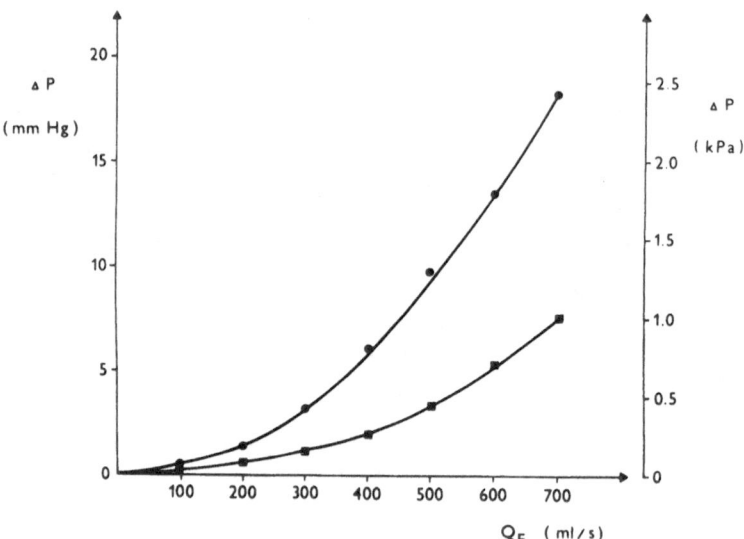

Fig. 6. A comparative study of the pressure gradients on the Björk-Shiley (●) and TNS-BRNO VII (■) inflow valves. Measurements were performed by Dr. Nabel, Division of Artificial Organs, Department of Internal Medicine, Rostock

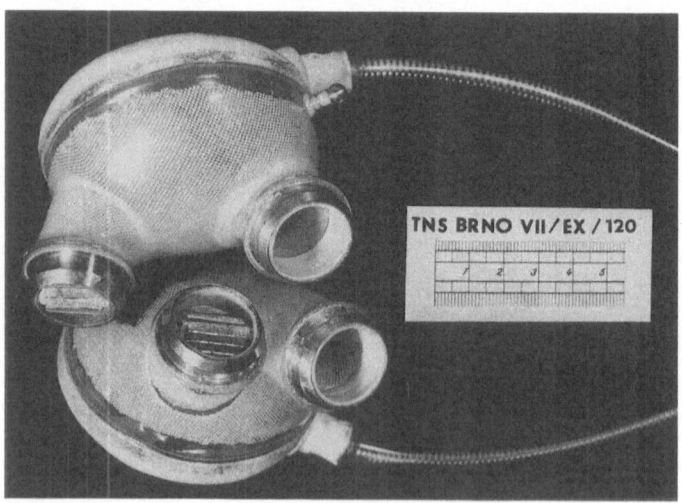

Fig. 7. A general view of the 120-ml TNS-BRNO VII

models were used: the TNS-BRNO II (polymethyl methacrylate, 23 experiments), the TNS-BRNO III (polyurethane, one experiment), the TNS-BRNO VII (13 experiments), and the Rostock artificial heart based on cooperation between Brno and Rostock research centers (three experiments).

The 13 experiments with the TNS-BRNO VII TAH were terminated for the following reasons: infection (three calves), right circulatory insufficiency (three

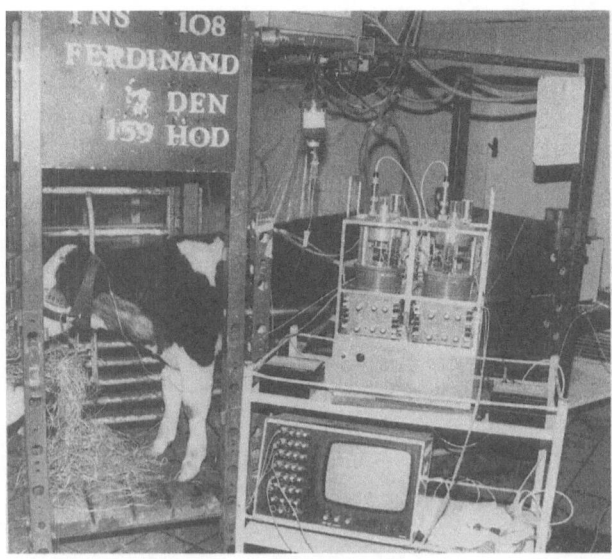

Fig. 8. BRNO portable driver
in the calf experiment

calves), thromboembolization (two calves), diaphragm and air leakage (three calves), and further cerebral hypoperfusion and lung edema of cerebral origin (two calves). Three experiments with the Rostock TAH were terminated because of thromboembolism, infection, and diaphragm leakage. The average survival with TNS-BRNO VII and Rostock hearts, i.e., with polyurethane and Pellethane devices, was 109.4 days.

According to the cadaver studies with the 80-ml version of the TNS-BRNO VII (KL/80), this TAH fits perfectly into the human chest (Fig. 9). This version is aimed at use in human patients as a bridge to transplantation when a donor heart is not immediately available. The experimental results with the TNS-BRNO VII have already been partially described [14]. A more detailed description of the results of these experiments is being prepared in the third monograph devoted to the artificial heart research development in Brno Research Center.

Essentially we can say that the experiments with the TNS-BRNO VII increased the average survival of the calves to 104.1 days (this figure includes one calf that received the TNS-BRNO III) in comparison with 99.2 days in the 23 calves that received the TNS-BRNO II. Also the longest survival was attained using the TNS-BRNO VII, i.e., 218 days in calf no. 110, Haakon (Fig. 10); the longest survival with the TNS-BRNO II was 175 days.

In the group of calves with Rostock artificial hearts, very good results were obtained, the longest survival being 226 days in calf no. 107, Harald (Fig. 11).

Problems Concerning Both the Hardware and Software in the TAH Experiments

These problems concern the close interaction between the device and the organism and relate to the material used and the design.

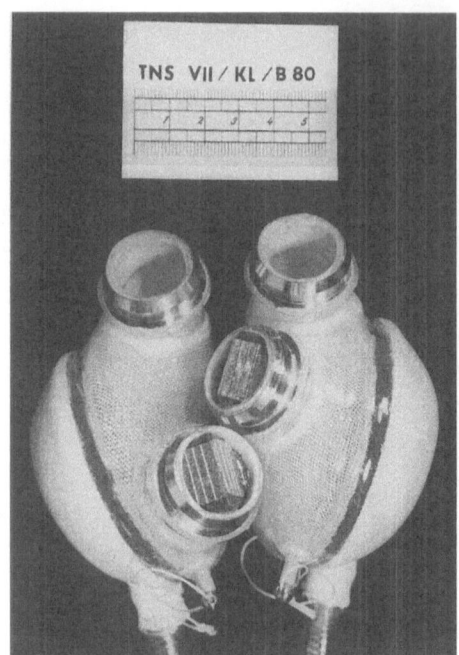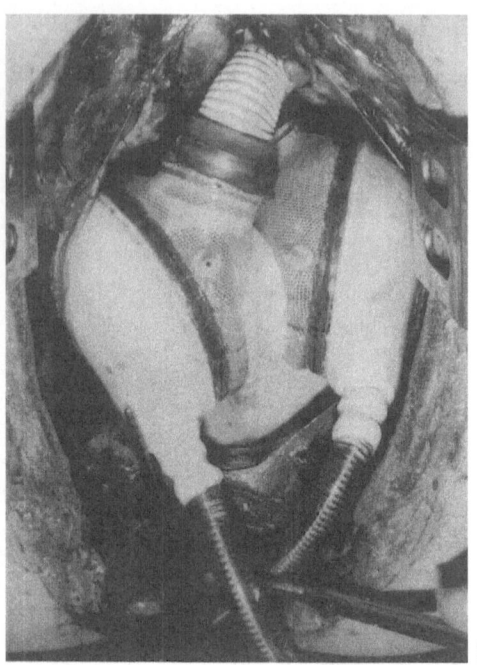

a   b

Fig. 9. a A general view of the 80-ml TNS-BRNO VII designed for human implantation. **b** 80-ml TNS-BRNO VII implanted in the human chest; cadaver study

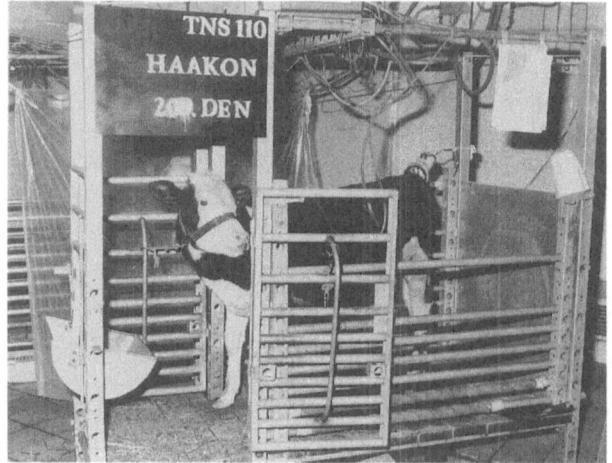

Fig. 10. Calf no. 110, Haakon, which survived for 218 days with the TNS-BRNO VII

Thromboembolism

If we compare our main devices, the TNS-BRNO II and the TNS-BRNO VII, which are made of different materials and constructed differently (as already stated, the former is made of polymethyl methacrylate, has polyurethane diaphragm and valves, and has a symmetrical housing and diaphragm design,

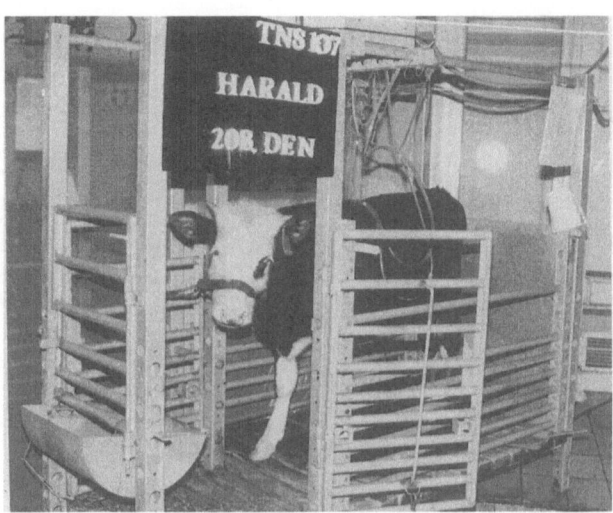

Fig. 11. Calf no. 107, Harald, which survived for 226 days with the Rostock TAH

while the latter is a totally polyurethane device with asymmetrical housing and diaphragm design), the superiority of the TNS-BRNO VII in reducing thromboembolism was evident in the long-term experiments. This superiority was due essentially to the use of one material to construct the whole blood chamber and all its components, and to the undulating diaphragm motion, which eliminates dead corners and secures complete emptying of the blood chamber. The hardware was thus markedly improved. We were now able to omit anticoagulation entirely after 1 month of pumping, and only antiaggregation therapy consisting of acylpyrin and dipyridamole was used.

Another question is the problem of individual species reactivity. Our experiences testify that if the calves were kept without any infection, no thrombi were found in the device. The same was true after 184 days of pumping in the goat, in which the clinical type of TAH was implanted intrathoracically: upon termination of the experiments both blood chambers were without marked thrombotic deposits (Fig. 12) (J. Vašků, 1987, unpublished observations from the experiment in the goat). It is possible to presume that a similar marked benefit would be seen with the clinical application of this type of TAH as a bridge to transplantation.

Mineralization

Another problem, which is very serious, is that of calcification of the driving diaphragms. The occurrence of calcifying deposits can be explained most readily in cases of primary thrombus formation with subsequent calcification of the thrombotic mass, which is a typical example of the dystrophic type of calcification (Fig. 13) [5, 21, 22].

A more intricate entity, from the point of view of pathogenesis, is so-called primary diaphragm calcification, i.e., cases in which there has been no formation of thrombotic deposits, and the nucleating calcification process starts as a pri-

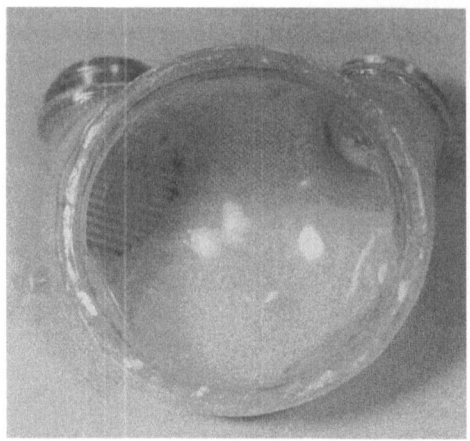
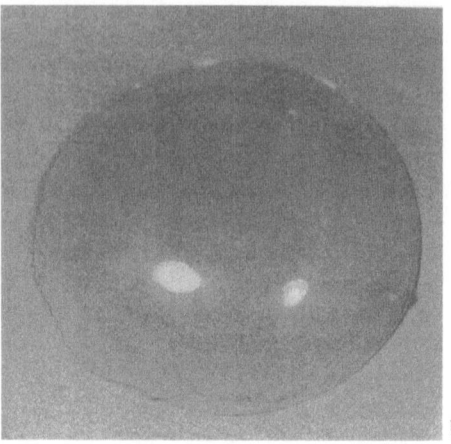

a
b

Fig. 12. a A clinical version of the BRNO TAH, the 80-ml TNS-BRNO VII, implanted intra-thoracically in the male goat no. 113, Hanibal. The right driving diaphragm is in situ, fully transparent, and without marked macroscopic thrombotic and mineralized deposits after 184 days of pumping. **b** The left driving diaphragm from the same experiment, without macroscopic signs of thrombotic or calcifying deposits, after 184 days of pumping

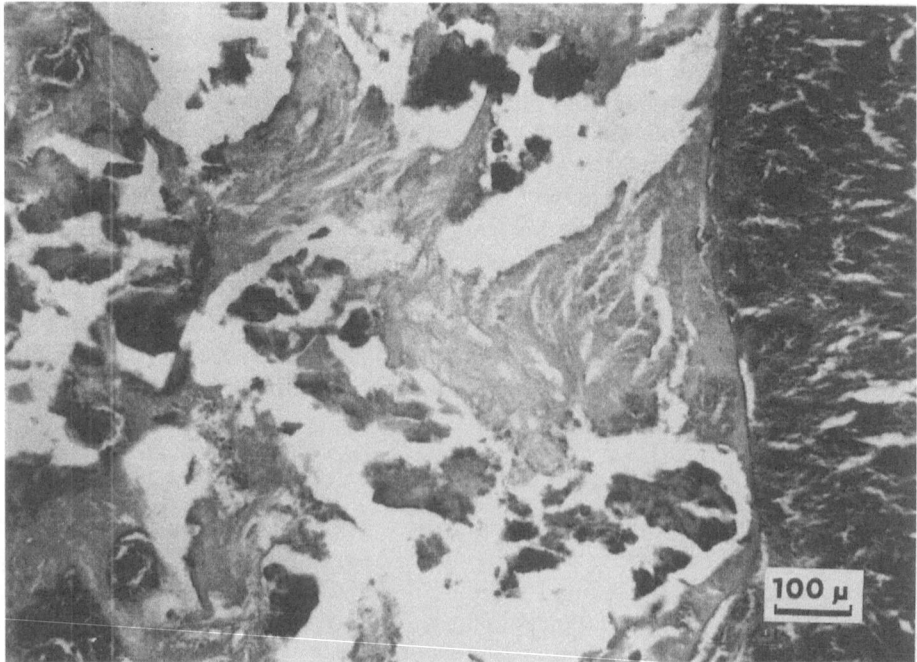

Fig. 13. Mixed calcified and thrombotic deposits on the surface of the driving diaphragm after 155 days of pumping. Calf no. 53, Florian

mary process directly on the diaphragm surface. This form of calcification can be documented by the evidence obtained in our experiments. Once calcificiation nuclei have formed on the diaphragm, its uneven surface can lead to increased thrombocyte aggregation and to what is termed secondary thrombus formation [5, 12, 13].

The structure of calcification plaques, observed in atherosclerotic processes on the vascular wall, resembles the deposits detected in the TAH diaphragms. The chief component seems to be octacalcium phosphate (OCP), in both crystalline and amorphous forms, which, however, dissolves quickly. Tomazic et al. [23] rule out the presence of dicalcium phosphate dihydrate (brushite) or hydroxyapatite. OCP has about five times the amount of water contained in hydroxyapatite. At any rate, amorphous calcium phosphate (ACP) is the first step in the calcification process occurring on the diaphragm. Study of ACP-OCP conversion suggests that it is the surface of amorphous spheroid-like ACP formation where the initial nucleation of OCP takes place. Once the crystals of OCP, i.e., calcification nuclei, have formed, they grow further by the direct addition of Ca^{2+} and PO_4 ions from the liquid phase. OCP nuclei proliferate and make up masses of diminutive, submicron crystals, not big ones. The crystal proliferation thus occurs via the mechanism of an autocatalytic process which, once the crystals have attained a certain size, stimulates the formation of new crystals rather than their further growth. Electron microscopy reveals a mixture of ACP and OCP on the diaphragm, with OCP clearly dominating (Fig. 14) [22].

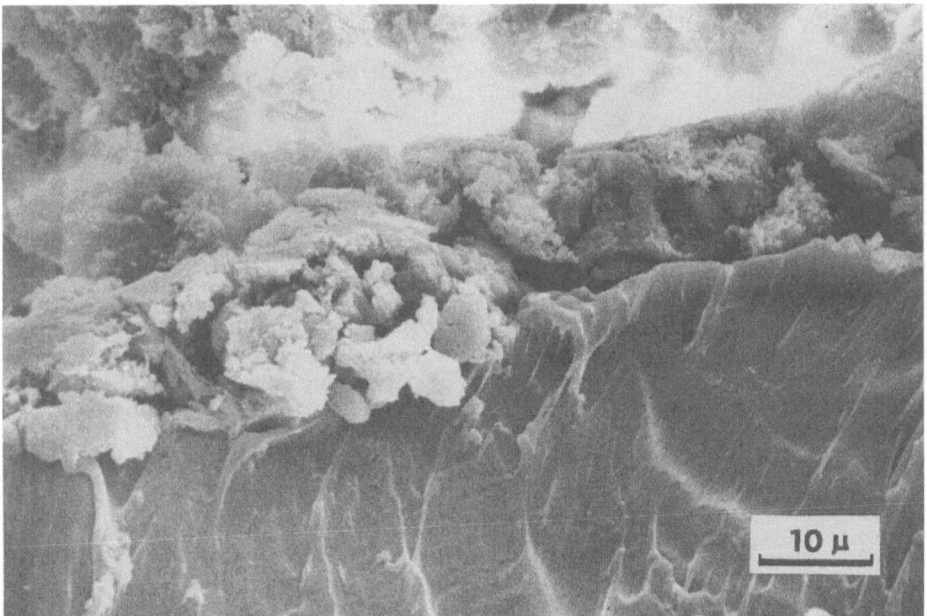

Fig. 14. Scanning electron microscopy of the driving diaphragm from calf no. 93, Hakim, after 147 days of pumping. The cutaway preparation shows the diaphragm surface with mineralized deposits represented by calcium phosphate concretions which markedly deformed the diaphragm surface and invaded the diaphragm

Once calcification has started on the diaphragm, it is crucial to find out whether nucleation can occur immediately on the material, i.e., polyurethane, or whether a phospholipid layer, to which specific protein molecules are fixed, must first form. Three proteins were studied that exhibit considerable affinity to calcium and OCP nucleation. It is quite possible that one of these proteins, osteonectin (osteocalcin), with a molecular weight of 32 000, forms a link between collagen and the mineral phase. Conceivably, this protein may play its role as part of a phospholipid layer arising in polyurethane mineralization [24, 25].

Under a theory holding that calcium and phosphorus ions permeate the diaphragm, with the subsequent occurrence of nucleation, it seemed necessary to cover the diaphragm surface with dense carbohydrate to make the diaphragm completely impermeable. This adjustment was carried out in cooperation with the laboratory of Dr. Stephen Bruck in Bethesda. Surprisingly the result was just the opposite, since the calcification process was accelerated and enhanced. In the calf studied, within 71 days of pumping the diaphragm became markedly mineralized on both sides and by 123 days it was totally mineralized, with the mineralization masses being 5–6 mm thick [14, 22]. It was very interesting to compare the effect on the red blood component of the totally mineralized diaphragms in two differ-

Pathophysiological effects of totally calcified driving diaphragms in two different types of BRNO total artificial heart

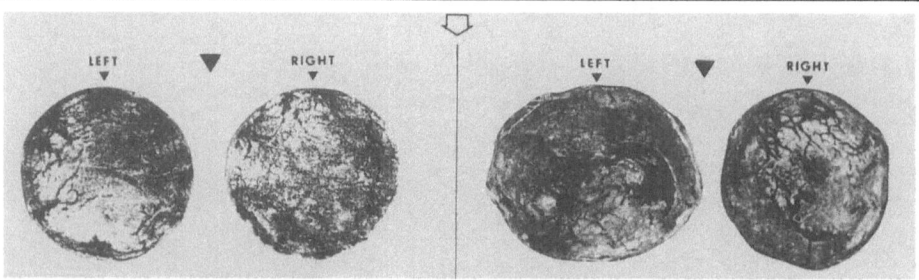

Exp. no. 76 „Kazan"
Left and right driving diaphragms
TAH: TNS-BRNO II (volume 100 ml)
PMM housing, PUL diaphragm + valves ∗
Full contact of the diaphragm with the inflow valve – concentric motion of the symmetrical driving diaphragm ∗
Survival → 123 days

Exp. no. 110 „Haakon"
Left and right driving diaphragms
TAH: TNS-BRNO VII/exp. (volume 120 ml)
PUL housing, PUL diaphragm + valves ∗
Very slight partial contact of the diaphragm with the inflow valve – undulating motion of the asymmetrical driving diaphragm ∗
Survival → 218 days

Values of the red blood elements on the last day of pumping:

Total Hb	Hct	Erythrocyte count	He	Total Hb	Hct	Erythrocyte count	He
19.9 g/l	13%	2.54 mil/mm^3	0.41 g/l	91.8 g/l	28%	4.98 mil/mm^3	0.12 g/l

Fig. 15. A comparative picture from the driving diaphragms of two different types of the BRNO TAH. Under the same conditions of extensive diaphragm calcification on both sides in both types of TAH, a condition far more compatible with longer survival was evident using the TNS-BRNO VII with the asymmetrical diaphragm motion (*right*). *PMM*, polymethyl methacrylate; *PUL*, polyurethane; *He* hemolysis

ent types of TAH, the TNS-BRNO II and the TNS-BRNO VII. In the TNS-BRNO II there is complete contact between the inflow valve and the driving diaphragm, which markedly increases the hemolysis and, moreover, to a great extent removes the calcified deposits from the diaphragm surface, which was also the cause of death in the above-mentioned animal after 123 days of pumping. The same extent of diaphragm calcification in the TNS-BRNO VII caused neither hemolysis nor removal of calcified microemboli, and the calf in question died after 218 days for a technical reason. Thus, our concept of an asymmetrical diaphragm which avoids full contact with the inflow valve and evacuates blood by means of an undulating diaphragm motion seems greatly superior to our older TNS-BRNO II design and secures much longer survival (Fig. 15).

Our experience has shown that while mechanical stress can play a limited role in the development of calcification, by no means can it be considered the factor triggering the mineralization process [22].

We observed great differences in the diaphragm calcification in individual calves. In animals in which the primary organ calcification was extensive, i.e., calcification in the arteries, veins, GI tract, kidneys, and other organs, the extent of the diaphragm calcification was correspondingly marked (Figs. 16, 17). Conversely, where the primary organ calcification was very restricted or almost completely absent, the diaphragm was mostly macroscopically unaffected by the calcifying process (Fig. 18). This correlation has been repeatedly confirmed in many animals [12–14, 22]. We can see that the individual tendency to calcification is so different in various animals that this situation can be assumed to be a certain form of natural calciphylaxis [26, 27].

To explore further this phenomenon, it was necessary to carry out experiments using other animal species. Having conducted preliminary studies, we felt

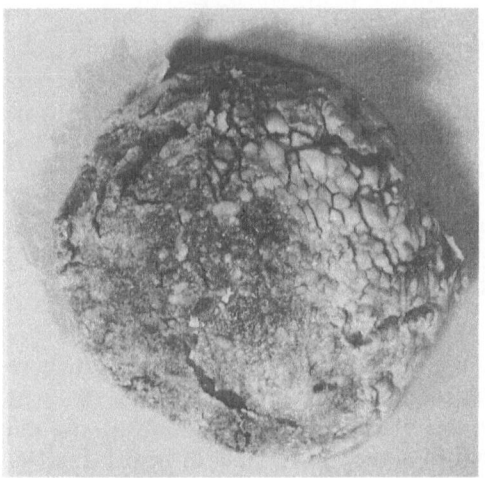 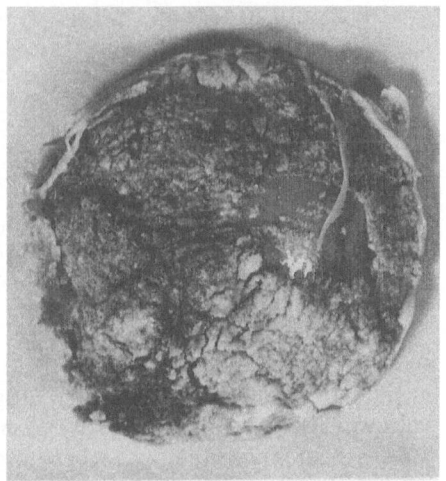

a   b

Fig. 16. a The right driving diaphragm in calf no. 110, Haakon, after 218 days of pumping with the 120-ml TNS-BRNO VII. **b** The left driving diaphragm from the same experiment. In spite of extensive calcification, the transport of calcified microemboli to vital organs did not cause the death of the calf, which expired for a technical reason

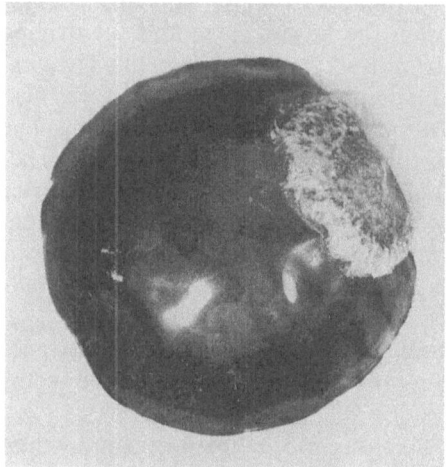
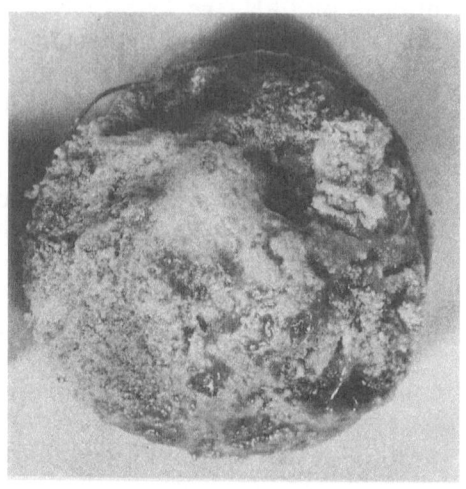

a   b

Fig. 17. a The right driving diaphragm of the Rostock TAH. The Pellethane driving diaphragm is composed of two layers on the right side. The inner layer is massively calcified only in one place, opposite the inflow port. Calf no. 107, Harald, survived for 226 days and the experiment was terminated for a technical reason. **b** The left driving diaphragm from the same experiment is totally calcified after 226 days of pumping

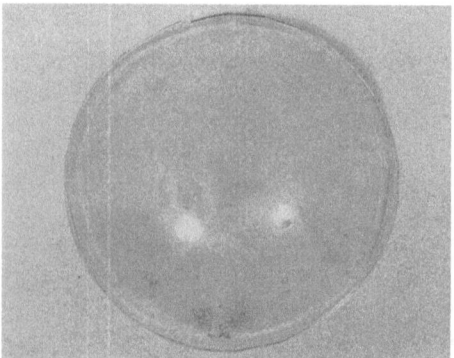
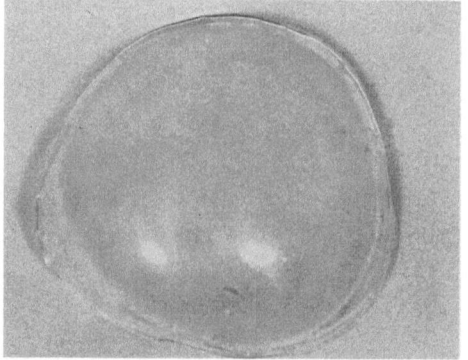

Fig. 18. The right and the left driving diaphragms from the experiment with the 120-ml TNS-BRNO VII in calf no. 100, Armand, after 153 days of pumping. Both diaphragms are absolutely clean, without macroscopic signs of thrombotization or mineralized deposits

ready to implant an artificial heart into a goat. It should be noted that nowhere in the world has the intrathoracic implantation of an artificial heart in the goat yet been successful. As far as we know, our group was the only one among the TAH research workplaces to keep a goat in a very good state of health for 184 days with an intrathoracically implanted TAH – the clinical form of the TNS-BRNO VII (Fig. 19). The experiment was terminated due to severe anemia, acidosis, and signs of hypoperfusion. But both diaphragms were macroscopically free, without marked signs of calcification or thrombotic deposits. This was an

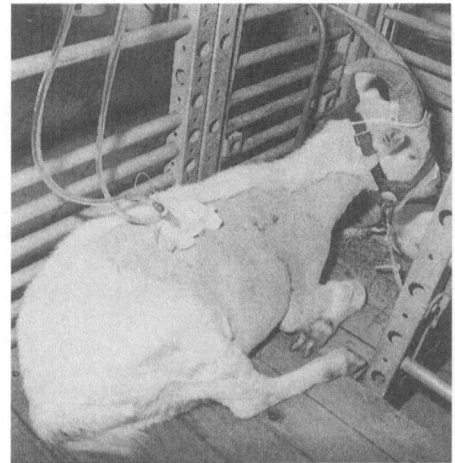

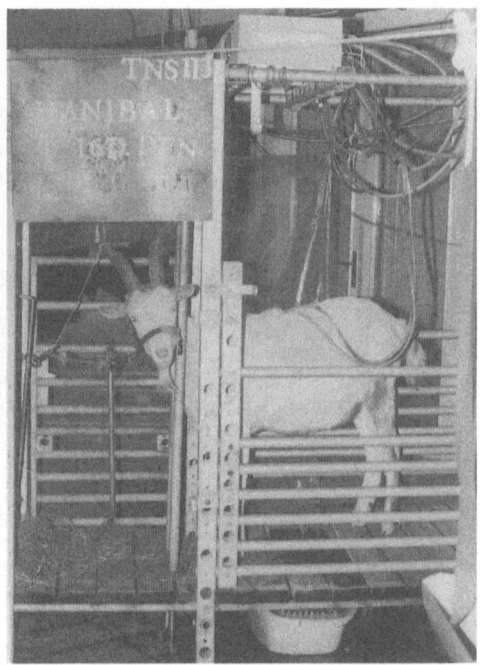

Fig. 19 a, b. The male goat Hanibal, which survived for 184 days of pumping with the intrathoracically implanted clinical version of the TNS-BRNO VII

excellent test for evaluating the clinical form of the TNS-BRNO VII (see Fig. 12) (J. Vašků, 1987, unpublished observations from the experiment in the goat).

Nevertheless, the Japanese group of Atsumi did observe some calcification in extrathoracically implanted blood pumps in goats, and this calcification affected the whole area of the blood chamber [28]. Thus, the results hitherto gained in another animal species, the goat, vary, and more exact comparative study is needed, with the evaluation of a greater number of experimental animals. TAH calcification has also been described in another experimental species, sheep.

Nevertheless, regardless of the individual variations in calcification within one species or between different species, it is reasonable to assume that the surface adjustment will enable us to slow down the mineralization or prevent it altogether. To achieve this it is necessary to employ primarily the well-known inhibitors of calcification and to prevent effectively, by their systemic or local application, the process of biomaterial calcification; of course, this must be done without altering the mechanical properties of the diaphragm, especially its flexibility and compliance while in motion [29] (J Benedict, 1987, personal communication).

The claim by some authors that the application of anticoagulations such as Coumadin can prevent calcification has not been verified in a single one of our experiments [30]. Similarly, we were unable to confirm the hypothesis that vitamin K can stimulate calcification since, even in those cases in which we had to administer extremely high doses of vitamin K to combat massive bleeding, mineralization was not enhanced.

Exploration of this very important field of prevention of calcification is above all necessary for the future permanent clinical implantation of TAHs. As in the

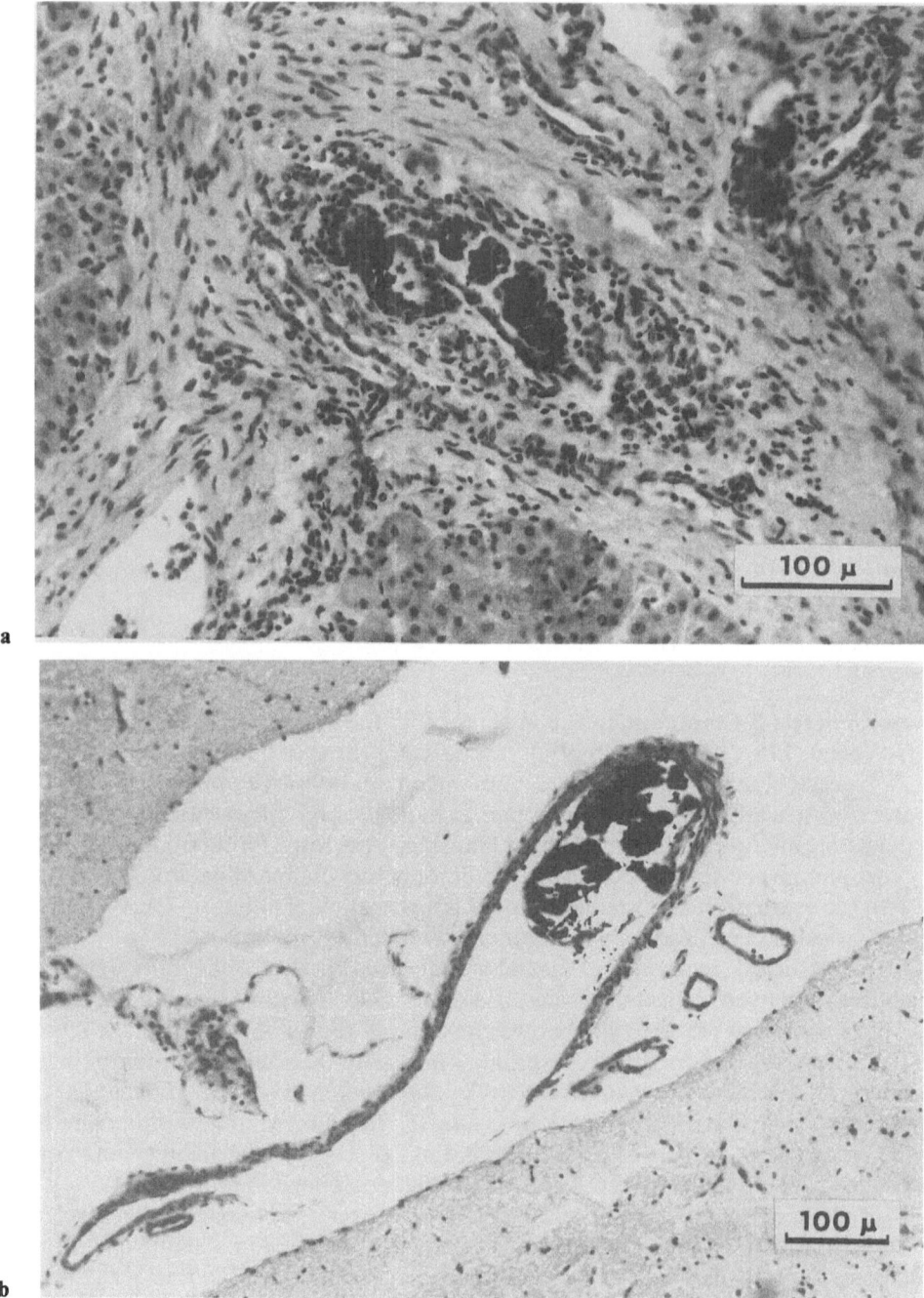

Fig. 20 a, b. Calcified microemboli in the vital organs. **a** Calcified microembolus in the liver in calf
no. 111, Lena, which survived for 137 days with the 120-ml TNS-BRNO VII. von Kossa stain.
b Calcified microembolus in vessel of pia mater. Calf no. 106, Leon, which survived 127 days with
the clinical 80-ml version of the TNS-BRNO VII. von Kossa stain

animals, some individual variations may be presumed, but we must count with this possibility, particularly in elderly patients in whom there are contraindications to a biological transplant. The calcification process poses three main risks for the organism:

1. Mechanical damage of the diaphragm caused by hard concretions of calcium-based compounds resulting in perforation
2. A markedly diminished pumping effect
3. As already mentioned, the detachment of calcified particles from the diaphragm surface and their transport as microemboli to other vital organs (Fig. 20)

Means of totally preventing calcification are currently being studied in our center.

Problems Concerning Predominantly the Software in the TAH Experiments

The resection of biological ventricles removes from the vasomotoric field of the organism the vast area of ventricular mechanoreceptors which participate in the complex cooperation between vasopression and vasodepression shifts during the physiological activity of the organism.

Irrespective of the type of TAH, the vasomotoric dysregulation regularly starts to become evident from about the 50th day of pumping, when the increase in central venous pressure (CVP) begins (Fig. 21) [14, 32–34]. In the cardiac ventricle a receptor area exerts reflex circulatory responses. Primarily they seem to be activated by the distention of the ventricular wall, preponderantly of the left ventricle, resulting from either an increased outflow resistance or an increased diastolic filling [35]. These circulatory responses elicited from the unmyelinated

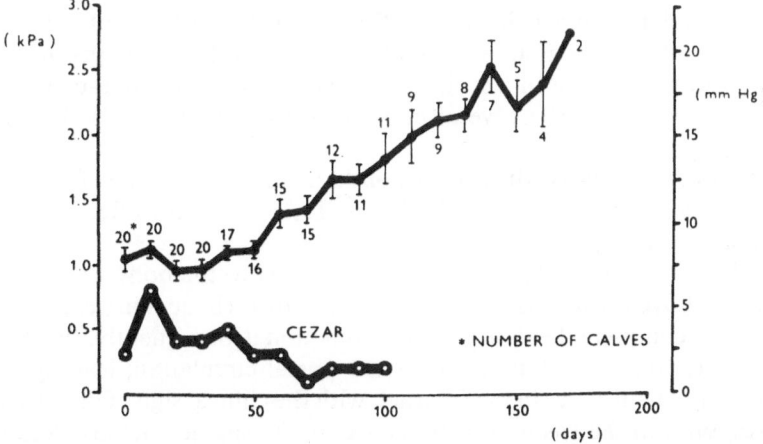

Fig. 21. The increase in CVP in calves with TAHs. Only in one calf was hypotension observed

neural endings are characterized by a marked fall in blood pressure, bradycardia, and generalized vasodilatation involving both resistance and capacitance vessels. These effects are very similar to those induced by the activation of arterial baroreceptors (arcus aortae and sinus caroticus). In both cases, the marked reflex venodilatation occurs with approximately the same order of magnitude as in the resistance vessels.

Experimental knowledge on the influence of the atrial receptors on the veins is less than that on the influence of the ventricular receptors. But these experimental data support a capacitance reflex influence by the stimulation of atrial receptors more in the excitatory venoconstricting direction [35].

Immediately after the ventricular resection the marked venodilatation receptor area is cut off. Due to temporary impairment of the blood supply to the atrial wall, all the neural elements disappear at once after the TAH implantation. Later, with the restitution of the collateral blood supply to the atrial wall, atrial neural regeneration appears and within 50 days the atrial neural endings are completely renewed (Fig. 22).

At first the arterial and venous blood pressure is maintained within the normal values particularly by the arterial depression baroreceptors. The baroreceptors in the sinus caroticus and arcus aortae are sufficient to maintain venodilatation for the normal CVP values, because the vasoconstricting atrial neural elements are absent and cannot interfere. This situation lasts for 50 days of pumping, until the nervous supply in the atrial wall is fully regenerated and starts to elicit its effects in the area of vaso- (veno)constriction (Fig. 23). In response to reflex stimuli, the splanchnic capacitance vessels behave like the resistance vessels of the splanchnic area, muscle, and kidney, constricting and dilating by the same magnitude [36].

The splanchnic organs, especially the liver, are greatly affected by the increased venoconstriction, which maintains the CVP at an elevated level. The marked increase in CVP is transferred to the hepatic microcirculation, where in the terminal hepatic venules the pressure increase slows the regular inflow from the hepatic sinusoids, which in turn receive blood from the terminal portal venules. Thus, the whole very sensitive hepatic microcirculation is affected by venular hypertension, marked slowing or even cessation of the blood-stream in the hepatic microvenular system, a decrease in fluid resorption into the blood bed from Disse's spaces, and finally tissue edema. Degenerative cellular changes, hemorrhage, and a gradual increase in fibrous tissue represent a very characteristic picture of the liver histology after several months of pumping (Fig. 24) [37, 38, 48].

Electron microscopy reveals diffuse mitochondrial damage to the hepatic cells [5]. Hepatomegaly is a regular autopsy finding in TAH recipients after several months of pumping (Fig. 25).

The hepatic index, i.e., the relation of the liver weight to the body weight, is markedly elevated above the normal limit [14]. Serious disturbances in hemocoagulation regularly accompany the damaged liver function. Consequently, the disturbance in the liver microcirculation affects the portal circulation, leading to edema of the mucous membranes in the GI tract, with the clinical sign of diarrhea. An adequate response to the vasomotor influence on the splanchnic area seems to be of utmost importance for cardiovascular stability [39].

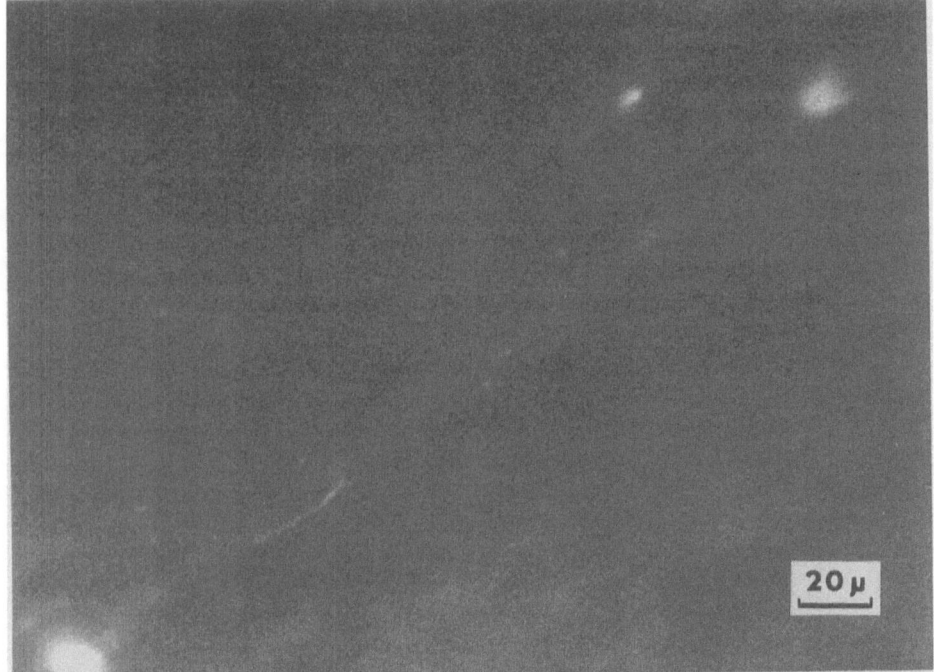

a

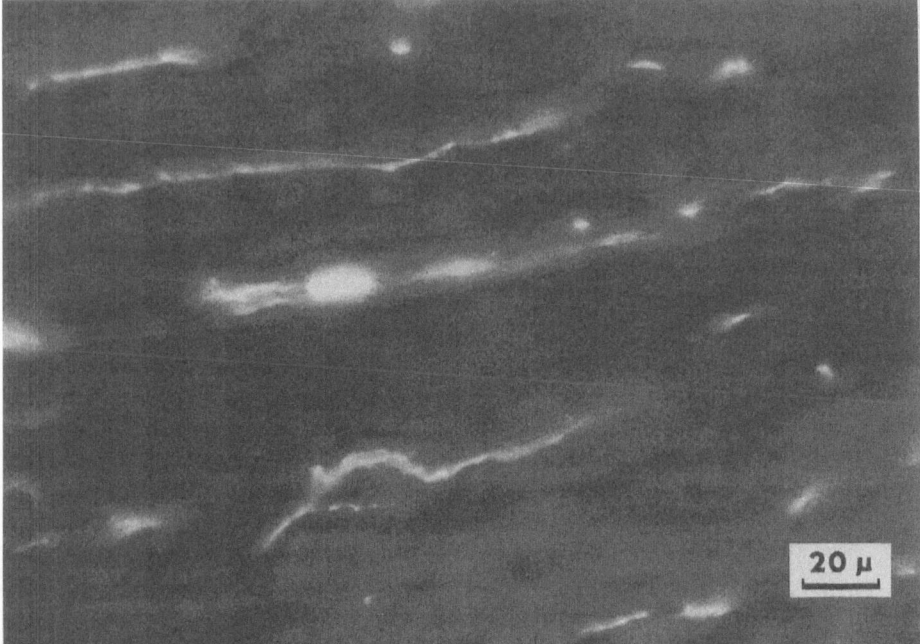

b

Fig. 22 a, b. The histochemistry of the monoamine nerve terminals in the atrial stumps. **a** Disappearance of the fluorescence of the monoaminergic nerve terminals following the resection of biological ventricles 2 days after TAH implantation (the three points with weak fluorescence are mast cells). Calf no. 113, Gunnar. **b** Complete regeneration of the monoaminergic nerve terminals after 137 days of pumping. Calf no. 111, Lena. Formalin-induced fluorescence technique, performed by Dr. S. Doležel

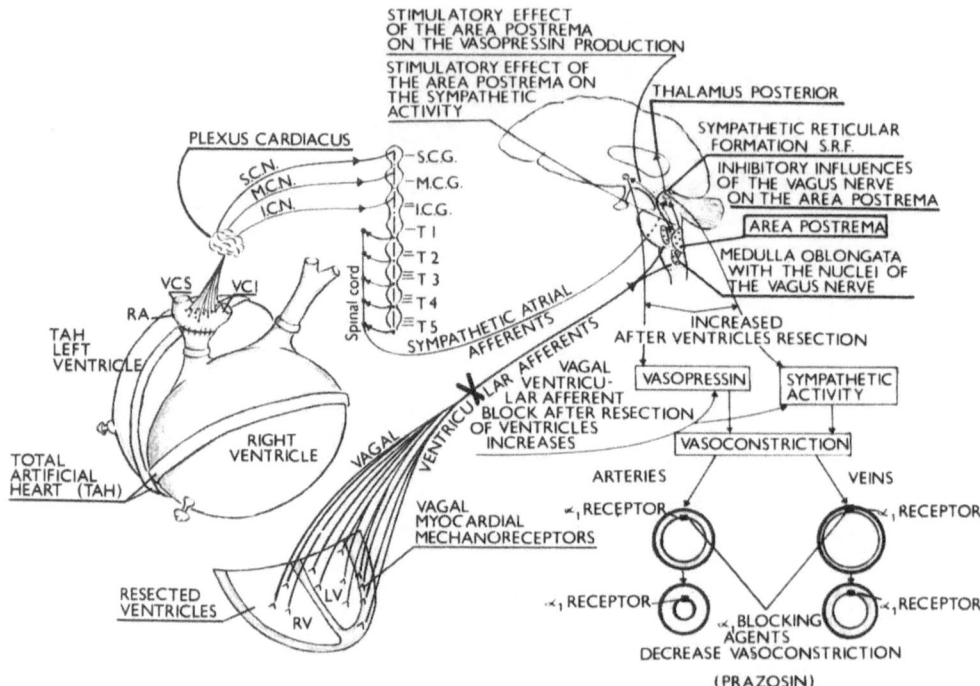

Fig. 23. Schematic drawing of changes in vasomotoric regulation after TAH implantation. After resecting the biological ventricles, vagal ventricular afferents are cut off. The activity of nuclei of the vagus nerve in the medulla oblongata is decreased; thus the inhibiting influence of the vagus nerve on the area postrema is decreased and the latter exerts an increased stimulation on the sympathetic activity, which is markedly strengthened after 50 days of pumping. By this time the sympathetic atrial afferents are fully restored, increasing the vasopression stimulation of the brain stem reticular formation. Simultaneously, the stimulation of vasopressin secretion is enhanced by the stimuli from the area postrema. An overall tendency toward vasoconstriction is then increased markedly. *S.C.N.*, superior cardiac nerve; *M.C.N.*, middle cardiac nerve; *I.C.N.*, inferior cardiac nerve; *S.C.G.*, superior cervical ganglion; *M.C.G.*, middle cervical ganglion; *I.C.G.*, inferior cervical ganglion; *VCS*, vena cava superior; *VCI*, vena cava inferior; *RA*, right atrium; *RV* right ventricle; *LV*, left ventricle

The steady increase in the CVP after ca. 50 days of pumping can be attributed to the steady increase in the constrictive impulses, originating in the atrial receptor field, and the gradual decrease in the vasodilating influence from the arterial baroreceptor fields due to "resetting" of the arterial barodepressive sensors following the loss of the vast ventricular field of the depressoric mechanoreceptors [40].

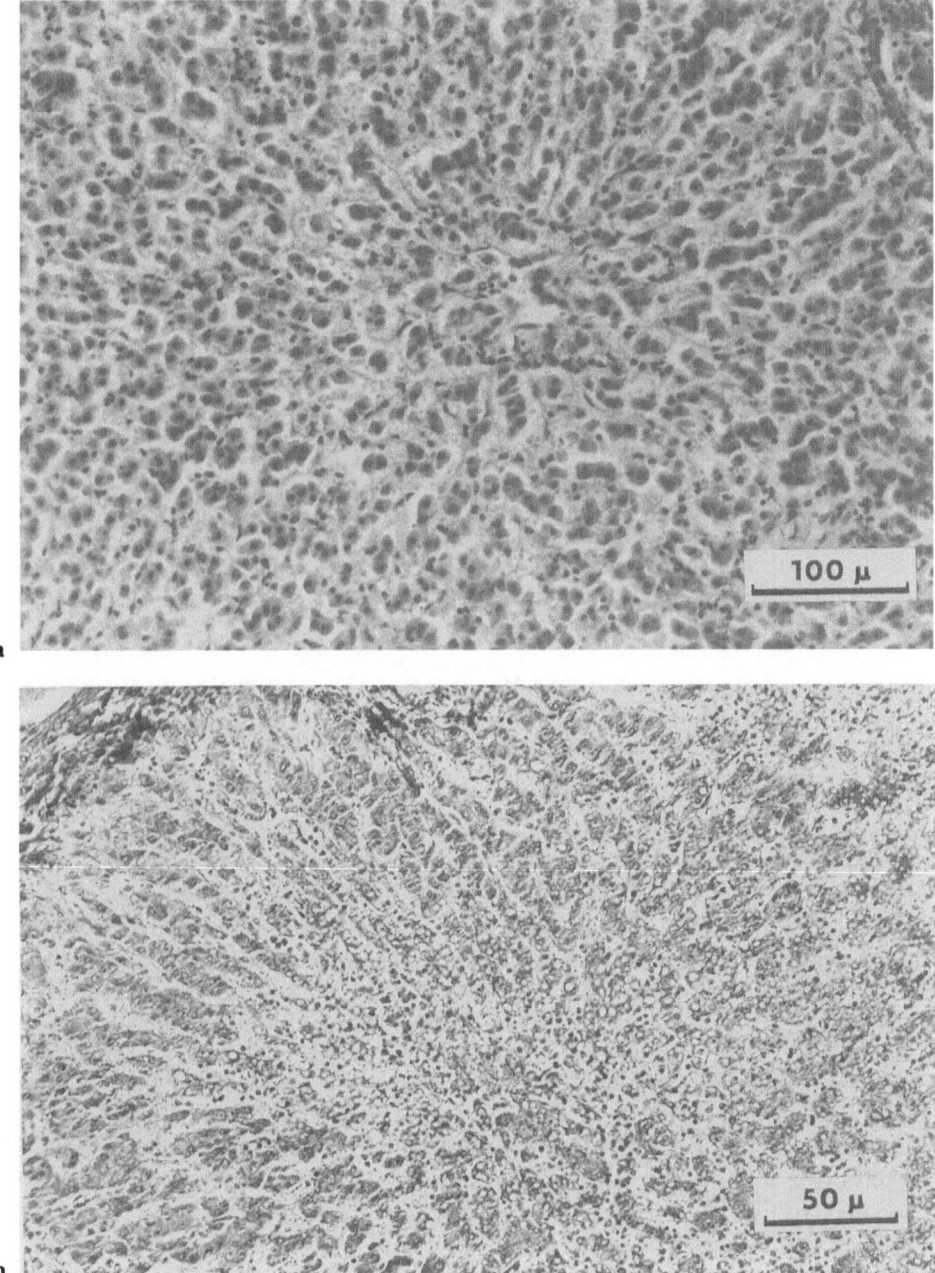

Fig. 24. a Calf no. 102, Pascal, which survived for 78 days with the Rostock TAH. Histology of the liver shows marked dystrophic changes with venostasis in the vicinity of the central vein. HE stain. **b** Calf no. 111, Lena, which survived for 137 days with the 120-ml TNS-BRNO VII. Extensive dystrophic vacuolization of the cells of the liver parenchyma is seen. HE stain

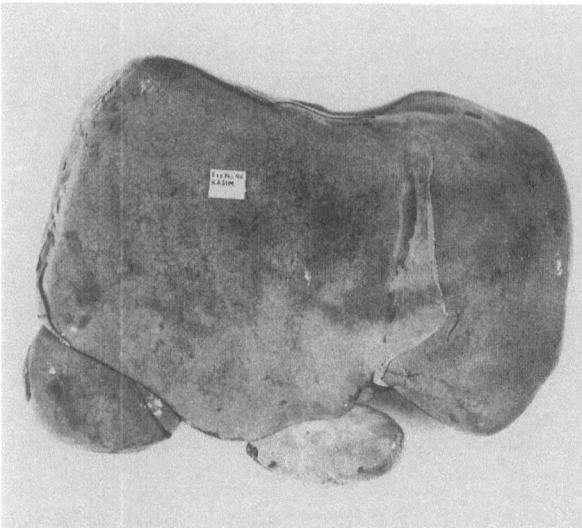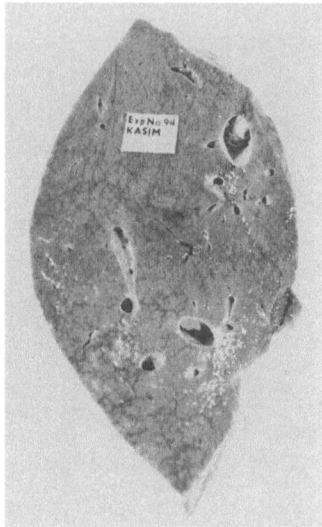

Fig. 25. Marked hepatomegaly after 95 days of pumping in calf no. 94, Kasim, with the 120-ml TNS-BRNO VII. *Left*, general view of the enlarged liver. *Right*, cutaway picture, revealing the typical nutmeg structure of the tissue of the enlarged liver

Experimental Confirmation that Vasomotoric Dysregulation Is Caused by the Cardiac Receptor Imbalance After the Resection of Biological Ventricles

In calf no. 85, Cézar, atrial monoaminergic innervation was markedly decreased or even absent – probably for genetic reasons – and between the 50th and 98th day of pumping the CVP was extremely low, reaching values below 0.5 kPa (3.75 mmHg) and thus representing venous hypotension. Accordingly, all the basic hemodynamic driving parameters were decreased. With the decreased heart rate, underperfusion led to ischemic changes in the central nervous system; these changes were confirmed histologically and were clinically manifested by quadriplegia and ultimately brain edema. At autopsy all the organs were normal, particularly the liver (as already mentioned, in other long-surviving animals hepatomegaly was found regularly, with a simultaneous increase in the hepatic index). Thus, in Cézar we lacked the typical triad observed in all the other calves after 50 days of pumping, i.e., regenerated abundant atrial monoaminergic innervation, marked liver enlargement with an increased hepatic index and extensive histological lesions, and a high increase in CVP [14].

The case of this calf confirmed fully our previous suggestion that the atrial innervation which is mainly represented by the receptor area and which facilitates in the brain stem reticular formation the increased trend toward vasoconstriction, is, after its regeneration, an important pathogenetic factor in the increase in CVP. The most important site of the atrial wall is the entry of the venae cavae into the right atria.

As a result of our experience with calf no. 85, Cézar, we have concluded that there are the following possible ways to interfere with and perhaps prevent the CVP increase with all its pathophysiological sequelae:

1. By means of α_1-blockers or by interfering with the catecholamine metabolism using false catecholamine transmitters
2. Intraoperative chemical and pharmacological treatment of the atrial walls
3. Surgical intervention into the sympathetic cervical ganglia
4. Surgical interventions into the plexus cardiacus

Our first attempt in this direction concentrated on pharmacological treatment [34]. In six calves surviving over 100 days we regularly administered prazosin (an α_1-blocking agent), in some cases together with an angiotensin convertase inhibitor (Capoten) and α-methyldopa (Dopegyt–false transmitter), in order to attain a decrease in the CVP curve and to keep the CVP values within acceptable limits as far as possible (Fig. 26). In these six calves three types of the TAH were used; the TNS-BRNO VII in four calves, the TNS-BRNO II in one calf, and the Rostock TAH in one calf.

The survival times in these animals were as follows:

Calf no. 106, Leon: 127 days (TNS-BRNO VII)
Calf no. 111, Lena: 137 days (TNS-BRNO VII)
Calf no. 112, Olaf: 151 days (TNS-BRNO II)
Calf no. 100, Armand: 153 days (TNS-BRNO VII)
Calf no. 110, Haakon: 218 days (TNS-BRNO VII)
Calf no. 107, Harald: 226 days (Rostock)

In all these calves the CVP started to increase from the 50th day of pumping, undoubtedly based on the above-described functional mechanisms leading to vasomotoric dysregulation. In five calves this functional component was later complicated by mechanical components like dislocation of the TAH, thrombus at the right outflow or right inflow port, and pannus formation in the left inflow port; only in one calf (no. 107, Harald) was the CVP increase purely functional until the last stage of the experiment. In calf no. 100, Armand, the increased CVP could be assumed to be preponderantly functional for the majority of the survival time, but in the final stage the CVP increased primarily because of dislocation of the right ventricle, i.e., for a mechanical reason. The administration of prazosin and α-methyldopa proved absolutely effective in calf no. 107, Harald, which survived for 226 days. The steep slope of the CVP curve was retarded by the drugs named above (Fig. 27). Especially before the termination of the experiment large doses of these drugs markedly decreased the CVP value. The experiment was terminated in Harald after 226 days of pumping because of left diaphragm leakage. There was no liver enlargement, no histological changes typical for other calves with hepatomegaly, and the hepatic index was completely normal (Fig. 28). Thus, we can assume this experiment to be the classic confirmation of our functional theory of CVP pathogenesis being based on vasomotoric dysregulation [34].

Although in the other calves from this treated group the functional pathogenesis factor was complicated by mechanical factors, the pharmacological intervention temporarily lowered the steep slope of the CVP; in addition the hepatic index

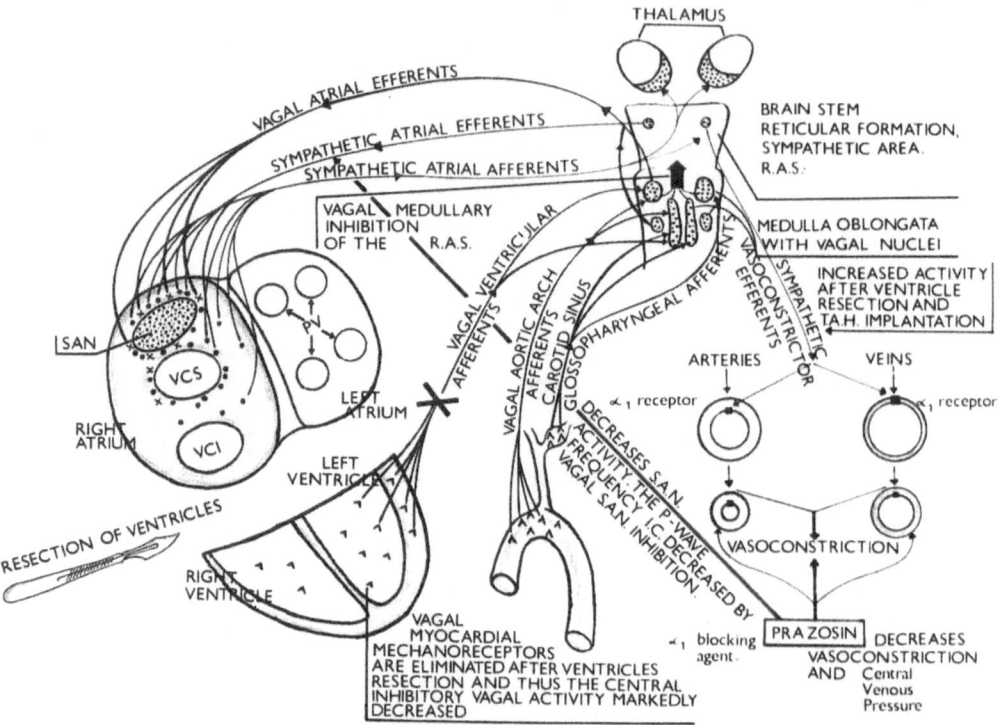

Fig. 26. Schematic drawing of the influence of the α_1-blocking agent, prazosin, on the CVP and P-wave frequency. After the resection of the biological ventricles the vasodepressive activity is maintained by the vagus and glossopharyngeal nerves from the arcus aortae and sinus caroticus. The effectivity of the central vasodepression area is decreased by the elimination of ventricular vagal vasodepressor mechanisms. After the regeneration of the atrial sympathetic vasoconstricting receptor field after 50 days of pumping, sympathetic atrial afferents increase the stimulation of the brain stem reticular formation, ultimately with increased sympathetic and vasoconstricting efferentation to the vessels and to the sinoatrial node. The administration of vasodepressive drugs decreases peripheral vasoconstricting effects in the arteries and veins, and simultaneously decreases the activity of sympathetic atrial efferentation. This mechanism enhances the influence of vagal atrial efferents and thus the decrease in CVP is simultaneously accompanied by a decrease in P-wave frequency. *SAN*, sinuatrial node; *VCS*, vena cava superior; *VCI*, vena cava inferior; *PV*, pulmonary veins

was significantly lower (i.e., nearer the normal values) in the treated calves than in untreated calves (Figs. 29, 30). For example, in calf no. 110, Haakon, in which the initial functional increase in CVP was later complicated by pannus formation (Fig. 31) treatment vasodepressors effectively decrease the CVP for about 50 days before the experiment was terminated due to minute TAH air leakage (Fig. 32).

An interesting correlation has been observed between the magnitude of the CVP increase and the atrial P-wave frequency. The atrial P-wave frequency slightly decreases from the time of implantation. But the administration of α_1-blocking agents regularly induced a more marked decrease in the P-wave frequency with a simultaneous decrease in the CVP value [34, 41–44]. It is very prob-

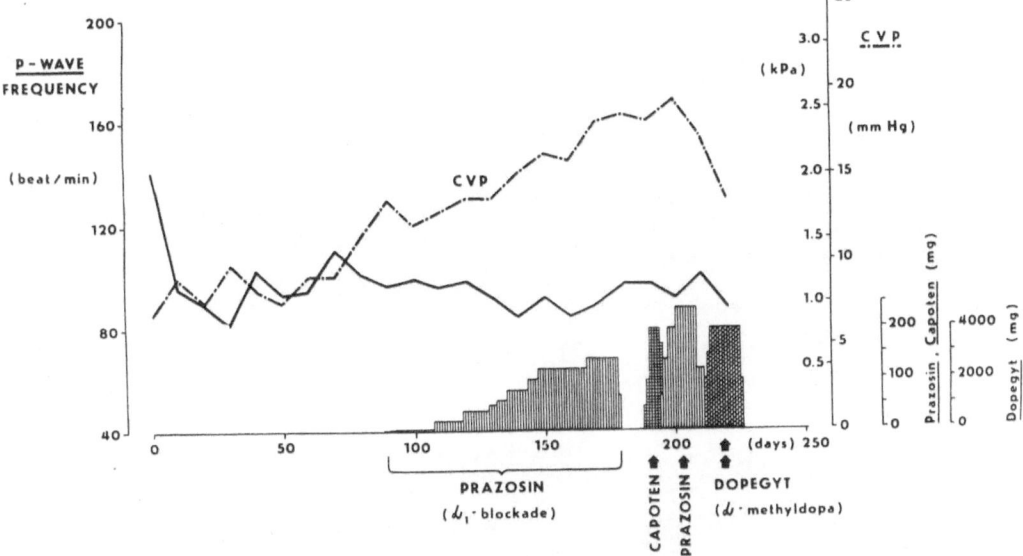

Fig. 27. CVP and P-wave frequency curves in calf no. 107, Harald. The increase in CVP is of functional vasomotoric origin. Large doses of prazosin and Dopegyt after 200 days markedly decreased both CVP and P-wave frequency

able that hormonal factors, aldosterone, vasopressin, and atrial natriuretic factor, also participate in this complex problem of the CVP increase (Fig. 33) [9, 34, 41, 42, 45, 46, 53].

An increase in CVP has been observed by the Japanese authors in the goat as well [47]. Our experience with the goat, with an intrathoracically implanted clinical version of the TAH, was similar, i.e., we could also confirm the CVP increase in this animal species. Shortly after implantation, a sudden, steep increase in CVP occurred, which decreased gradually until the 50th day of pumping. Prazosin was administered only for a short time soon after the implantation. For 120 days the CVP was within normal limits, but from this time it gradually increased until termination of the experiment. It is unclear whether this change was related to the change in the clinical state (i.e., the onset of severe anemia). Prazosin was given again for a short time before the experiment was terminated (Figs. 34, 35).

The experiment with the goat and that with the calf which most probably had an inborn deficiency of atrial monoaminergic nerve terminal regeneration (calf no. 85, Cézar) testify to the lack of any relation between body weight or body growth, and the increase in CVP. Calf no. 85, Cézar, with the marked CVP hypotension, gained weight considerably after TAH implantation whereas the male goat no. 113, Hanibal, was a 3-year-old, fully mature animal with terminated body growth. Nevertheless, the CVP increase occurred in this mature animal too, even if the CVP curve differed in its characteristics from the CVP curve in the calf. A more detailed analysis of the experiments with the six treated calves and of the whole complex problem of vasomotoric dysregulation in TAH recipients leading to CVP increase is provided elsewhere [34].

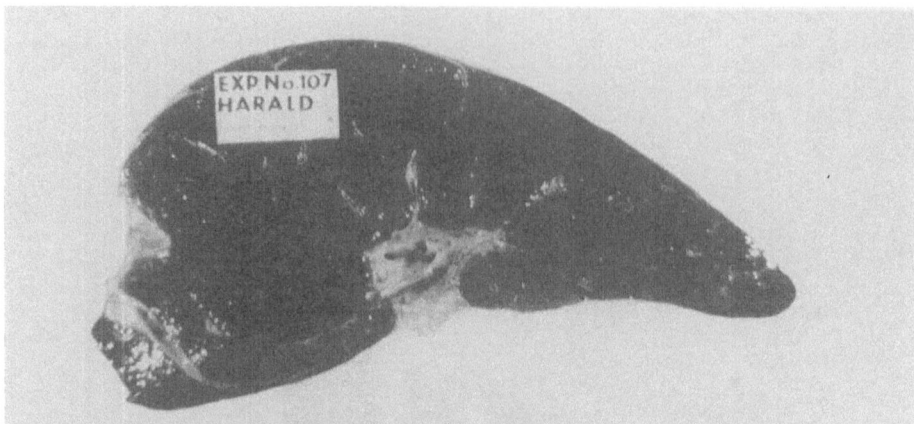

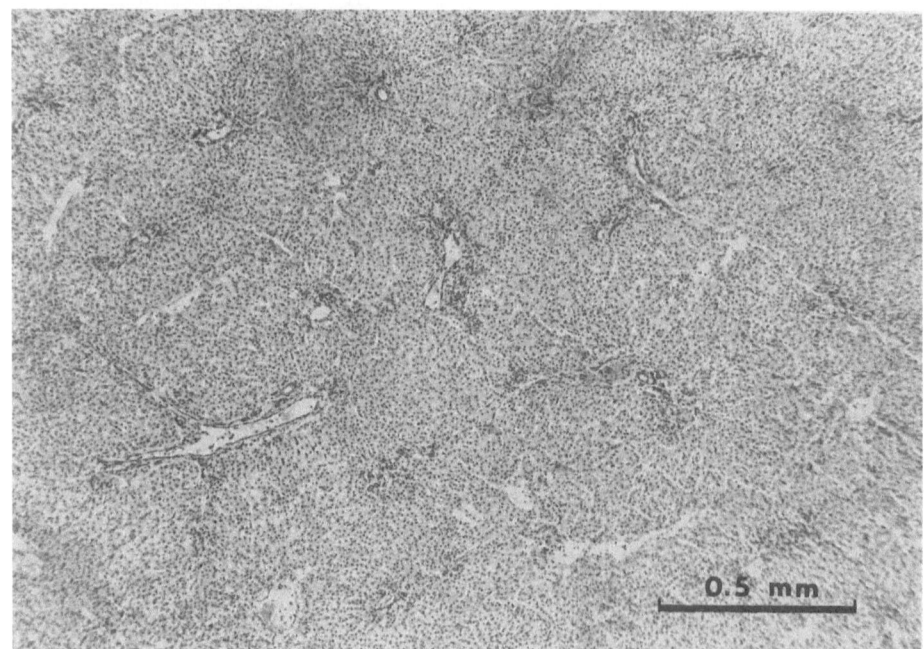

Fig. 28. a Normal appearance of liver tissue after 226 days of pumping with the Rostock TAH in calf no. 107, Harald. **b** Normal histological appearance of the liver tissue in the same calf after 226 days of pumping. HE stain

Two calves alive at the time of writing (June 1987) – calf no. 114, Arvid, which has spent 175 days with the TNS-BRNO VII, and calf no. 116, Alarich, which has spent 95 days with the Rostock heart – were treated from the 50th day by prazosin, which was later replaced by the continuous administration of α-methyldopa (Dopegyt). The CVP of both these animals is within normal limits or perhaps just slightly increased, oscillating between 1.3 and 1.5 kPa (9.75–11.25 mmHg). The clinical state of both the calves is excellent (Figs. 36–38).

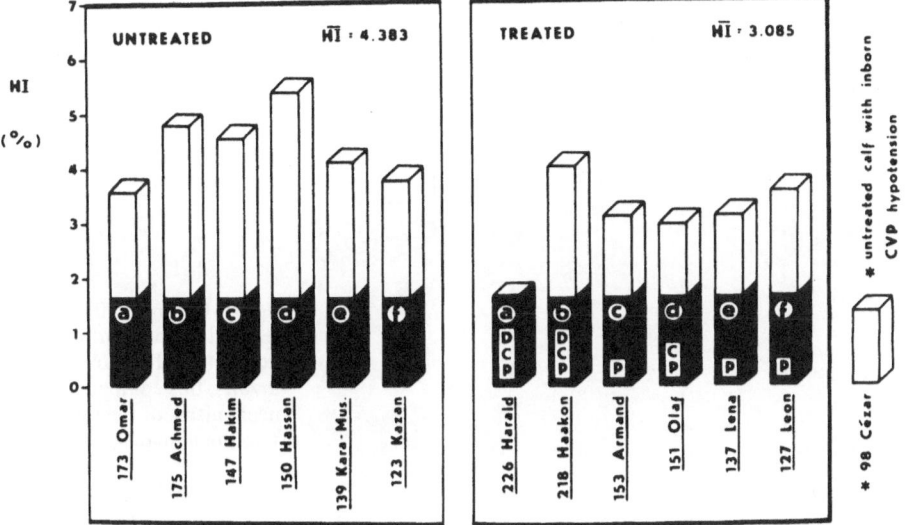

Fig. 29. Values of the hepatic index (*HI*) in six treated (*P*, prazosin; *C*, Capoten; *D*, Dopegyt) calves and six untreated control calves. Where the increase in CVP was only functional, and uncomplicated by different kinds of mechanical obstruction, the vasodepressor treatment kept hepatic index within completely normal limits (Harald). But in all other calves of the treated group, where mechanical obstacles complicated the situation and contributed markedly to the CVP increase, the hepatic index could not be kept within the normal limits. Nevertheless, here too the values of the hepatic index were significantly decreased as compared with the untreated group

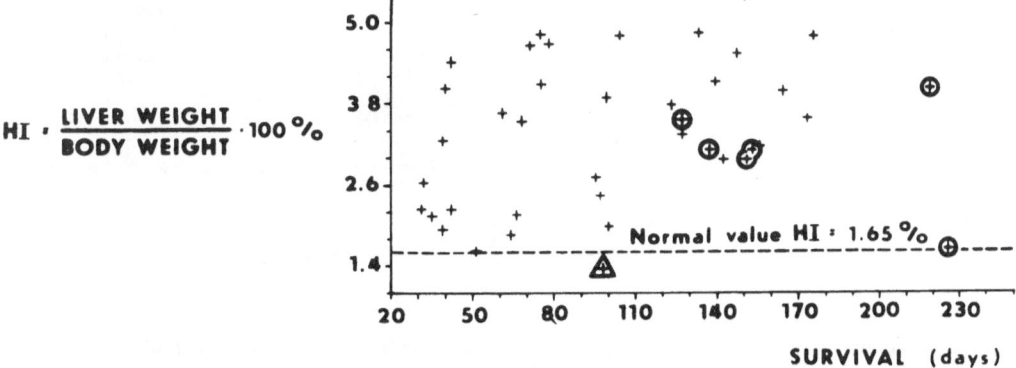

Fig. 30. Values of the hepatic index in 33 untreated calves (+), one calf with inborn CVP hypotension (△), and six calves treated with vasodepressor (○). The calves survived for between 31 and 226 days. After 100 days the hepatic index values in the treated group were significantly within the lower diapazon of the distribution as compared with untreated calves

In closing we can say that all these observations and findings, which mostly concern the software of the TAH, i.e., the regulatory processes of the organism, can serve as a basic data bank which represents an important modelling system for the study of the vascular and metabolic reactions in the organism whose own, biological heart is substituted by an artificial pump. Thus we can observe mech-

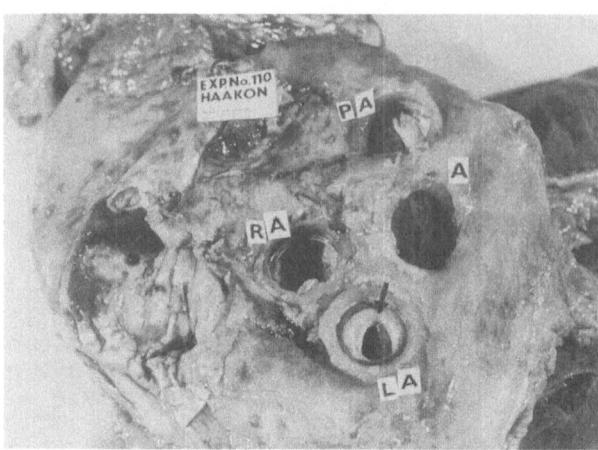

Fig. 31. Calf no. 110, Haakon. Marked pannus formation is seen in the left inflow port (*arrow*); this complicated the mechanisms of the purely functional increase in CVP

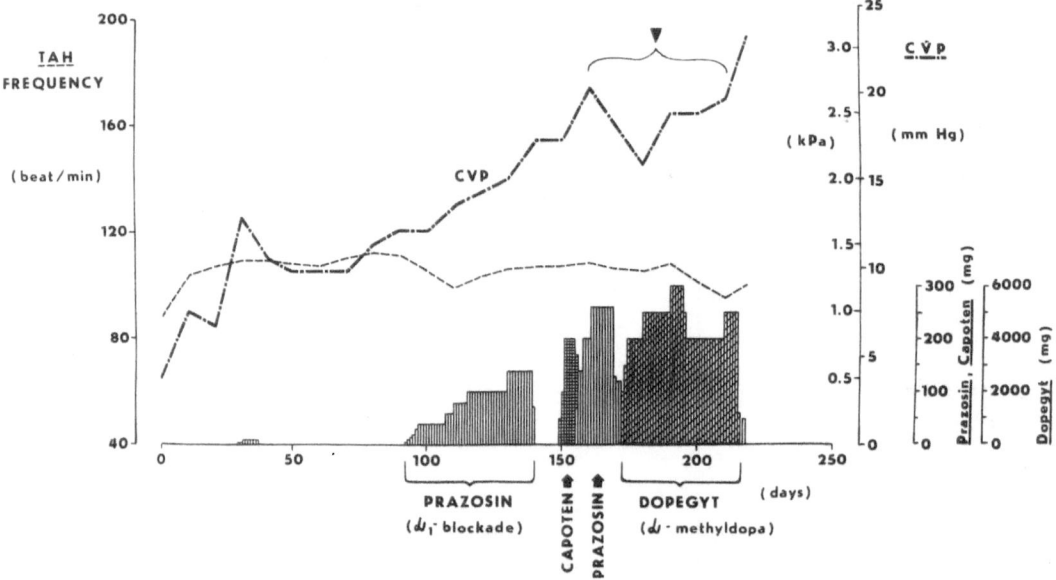

Fig. 32. The course of the CVP curve in calf no. 110, Haakon, with the administration of different vasodepressive agents. In spite of pannus formation (the mechanical factor causing the increase in CVP), the steep slope of the curve around 150 days was decreased for 50 days (arrowhead/brace) by α-methyldopa administration

anisms which are otherwise covered in the intact biological system by the activity of the biological heart. On the one hand, we can enrich our knowledge of new pathophysiological mechanisms, which could prove useful in daily clinical practice, and on the other hand we are continuously building a brand new branch of medical science – the physiology and pathophysiology of the total artificial heart.

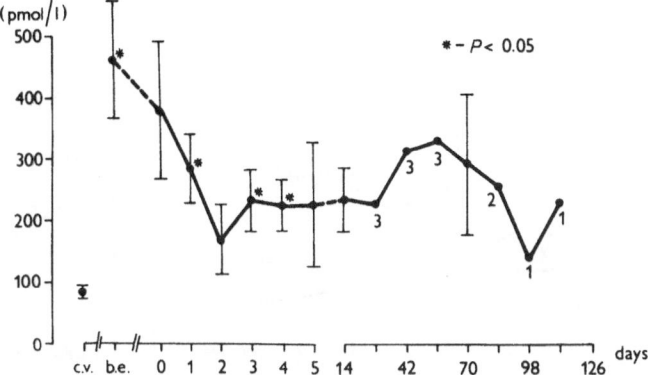

Fig. 33. The serum aldosterone level in the untreated calves with TAHs. At the beginning of the experiment (b.e.) the aldosterone value was several times higher than in normal calves on the farm, which was obviously caused by transport stress. After sudden drop within 2 days after TAH implantation, it increased until 50 days of pumping; then, until 98 days, it decreased markedly. We assume this change to be a compensatory humoral shift accompanied by the increased sodium level in urine. In this way the organism attempts to compensate for the changes in the internal environment caused by the high CVP

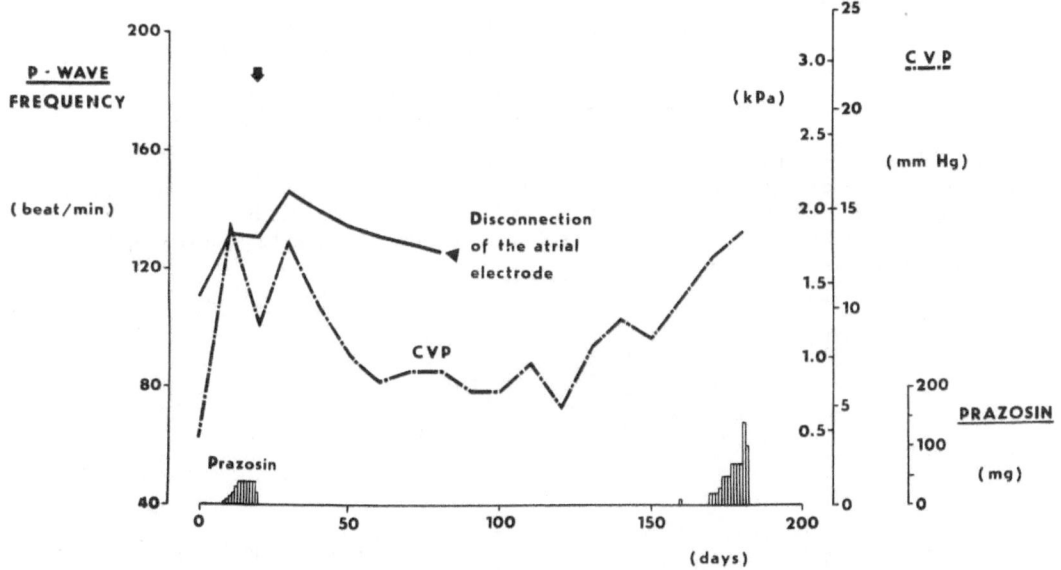

Fig. 34. The curve of the CVP in the goat, Hanibal. The characteristics of the CVP curve in the goat are different from in the calf. The initial increase in CVP was halted by administration of prazosin (*arrow*), but, nevertheless, after 100 days a gradual increase in CVP was observed. The vasodepressor treatment was not intensive enough, because it was more necessary to evaluate the dynamic tendency of the vascular regulation of the gradual increase in CVP

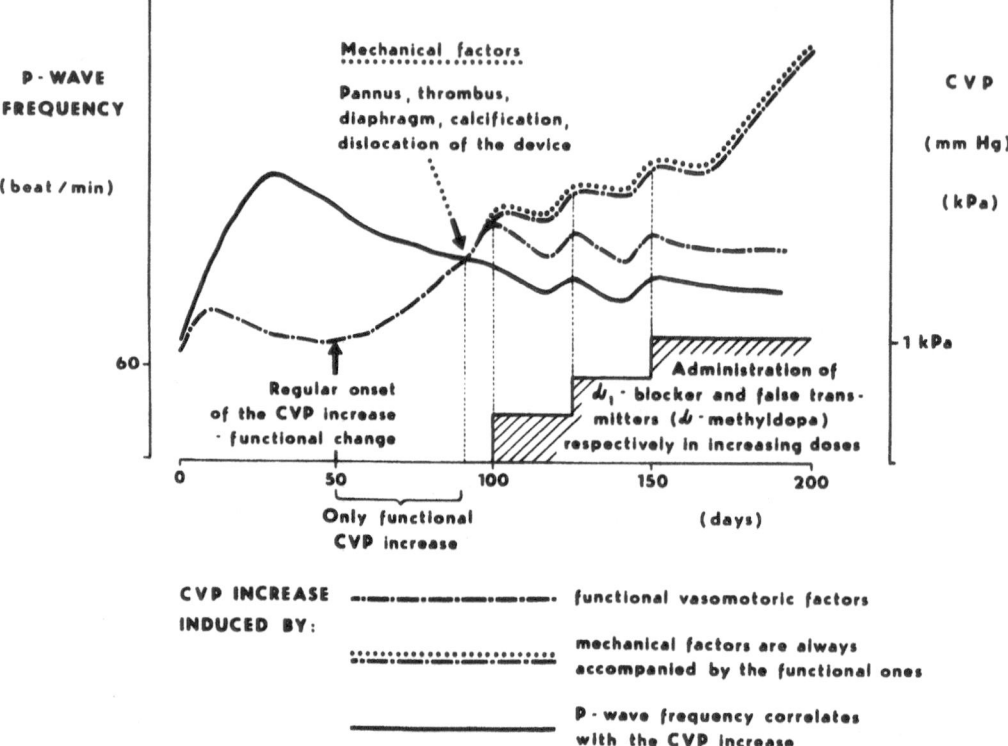

Fig. 35. Schematic drawing showing the possible combination of functional (vasomotoric) and mechanical factors leading to the increase in CVP. The only functional cause of the increase can be totally treated, while the combined functional and mechanical causes can be only partially treated by the administration of vasodepressors. P-wave frequency can also be positively influenced by vasodepressor treatment

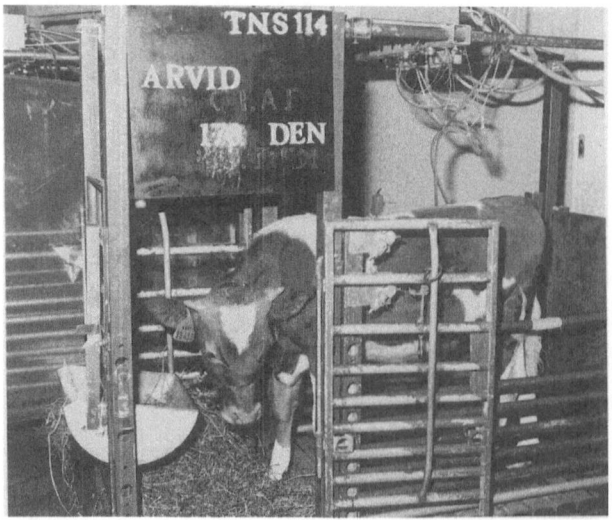

Fig. 36. Calf no. 114, Arvid, treated continuously by vasodepressors from the 50th day of pumping (120-ml TNS-BRNO VII). After more than 170 days of treatment the CVP was essentially very near the normal level. The photograph was taken in June 1987, when survival time was 175 days. Definite survival 190 days

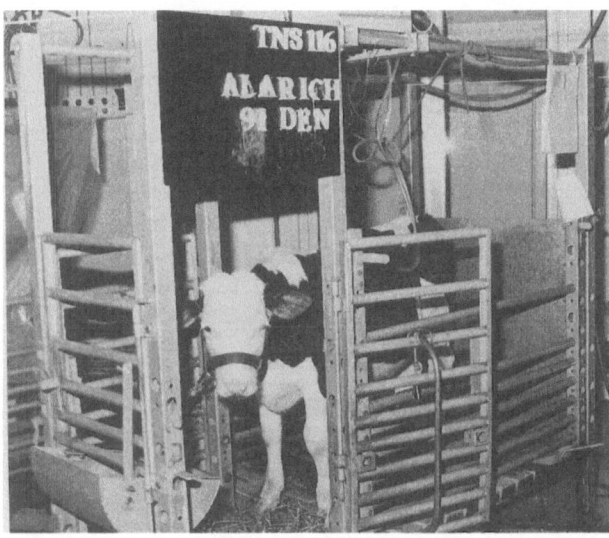

Fig. 37. Calf no. 116, Alarich, also treated from the 50th day of pumping (Rostock TAH) by vasodepressors. After more than 1 month of treatment the CVP was near to normal values. The photograph was taken in June 1987, when survival time was 95 days. Definite survival 104 days

Conclusion

Our increasing knowledge of the relationships between the whole system of the TAH and the organism bearing the TAH suggests that further elaboration of the hardware, i.e., the blood pumps and control and driving units, is required. The development towards miniaturization of the TAH drivers will first involve portable systems based on the principle of pneumatic drive, and most probably subsequent shifts to hydraulic and perhaps electromechanic systems. The development of the blood pumps, in terms of both material used and design, cannot be assumed to be terminated either. From the viewpoint of the relation between the hardware and software, i.e., the functional and regulatory shifts in the organism bearing the TAH, we face two problems: thrombus generation in the TAH and mineralization. Whereas thrombogenesis is a dangerous threat from the day on which the TAH is implanted, mineralization is a problem especially in later stages of TAH pumping. Consequently the elimination of thrombogenesis is a crucial task in short-term TAH implantation, i.e., usually when the TAH is used as a bridge to transplantation. Since no absolutely antithrombogenic material currently exists, it is necessary to devote our attention to adaptation of the surface of the blood chambers and to optimal device design, together with optimal anticoagulation and antiaggregation therapy.

Concerning the problem of mineralization, the local use of inhibitors of calcification is probably of value. The elimination of calcification is very important, especially from the point of view of permanent TAH pumping without a view to later biological transplantation. Our experiences indicate great variability in the intensity and extension of calcifying deposits on driving diaphragms, which is most probably a consequence of different levels of the natural inhibitors of calcification in individual calves.

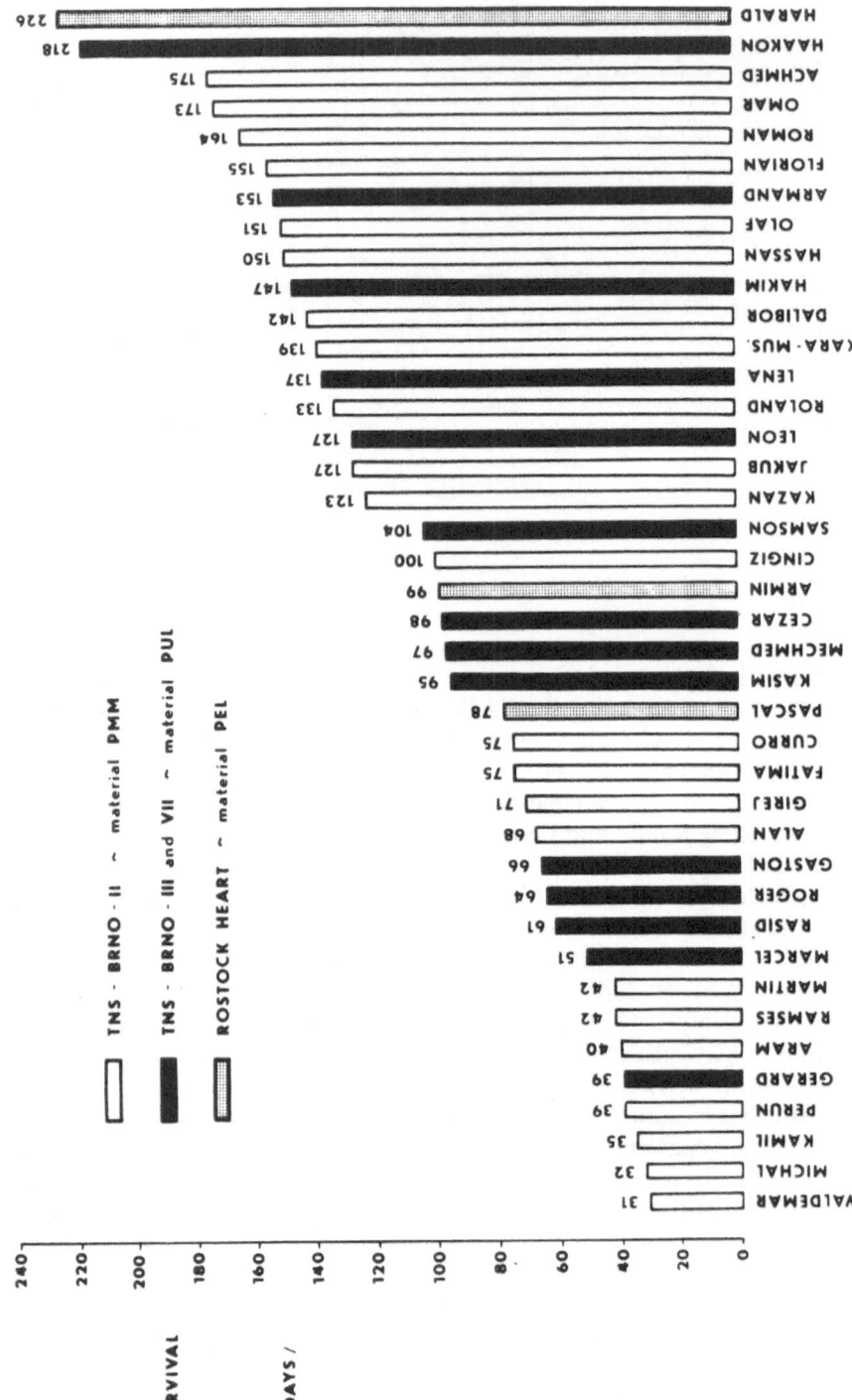

Fig. 38. Survival times in calves in 40 completed experiments with different types of TAH in the BRNO Research Center during 7 years of research. *PMM*, polymethyl methacrylate; *PUL*, polyurethane; *PEL*, Pellethane

The very suitable term coined by Atsumi, i.e., software of the TAH, particularly relates to the processes in the area of neural and neurohumoral regulation of the resistance and capacitance vessels. After resecting the biological atria, a serious imbalance leading to severe regulatory shifts arises, an imbalance based mainly on the lack of vasodepressoric neural impulses. Thus gradually the vasoconstricting situation, with predominant stimulation of α_1-catecholamine receptors, leads to a marked pressure increase in the area of capacitance vessels.

On the basis of important findings in experiments in Brno Research Center, we have elaborated our original hypothesis regarding the pathogenetic mechanism of the increase in CVP. It is very important, because after some time the increase in CVP, leads to functional and morphological destruction of the liver, which markedly influences the life span of TAH recipients.

We have emphasized several possible ways to eliminate the cause of the increased CVP. Pharmacological intervention seemed to be the most feasible approach. Either we blocked α_1-receptors or we decreased the effectivity of catecholamines by intervention in the catecholamine metabolism. In one of six treated calves, we were able to influence the CVP increase markedly, and to keep the hepatic index at a normal value. In the other five animals, in which the initial regulatory imbalance causing the increase in CVP was later complicated by mechanical obstruction on the left or right side, the administration of vasodepressors decreased the values of the hepatic index markedly. Thus we can say that our hypothesis has been confirmed experimentally, and we will extend our studies in this direction.

Last but not least it can be definitely stated that our observations outlined above are of relevance to clinical practice and contribute to the establishment of a new branch of pathophysiology, i.e., pathophysiology of the total artificial heart.

Acknowledgments. The author expresses gratitude to all his co-workers, who contributed more or less directly to the achievement of the results presented and analyzed here. The fast, exact, and effective implantation procedure was the result of cooperation between pathophysiologists and clinical surgeons. The group of clinical surgeons was led by Ass. Prof. Jan Černý, Director of the Department of Cardiac Surgery and Transplantology of the Regional Institute of National Health in Brno.

Very valuable histochemical techniques, developed by Dr. Svatopluk Doležel, made possible the exact evaluation of the degree of neural regeneration processes in the atrial wall.

Electron microscopic preparations were performed in cooperation with the Institute of Histology and Embryology, Faculty of Medicine UJEP in Brno (Director: Prof. Milan Dvořák, Corr. Member of Czechoslovak Academy of Sciences) by Mr. Procházka.

The author is indebted to František Klimeš, Institute of Hydrodynamics, Czechoslovak Academy of Sciences, for exact analysis of flow parameters of the TNS-BRNO artificial heart series.

Histological documentation presented in this chapter was prepared using the technical equipment of Leitz Co., Austria.

For technical help with the preparation of the manuscript, the author expresses sincere thanks to Dr. A. Kobylková and Mr. D. Žerníček.

References

1. Olsen Don (1987) ISAO – International registry bridge to transplant experience with the Jar-vik-7 and the Jarvik-7-70 total artificial heart. Artif Organs 11:63–68
2. Symbion (1987) Clinical update – a current report on use of the Jarvik-7 (100 cc) and Jarvik-7 (70 cc) as a bridge to transplant (April 3). Salt Lake City, Utah, USA
3. Magovern JA, Rosenberg G, Pierce WA (1986) Development and current status of a total artificial heart. Artif Organs 10:357–363
4. Vašků J (1982) Artificial heart. Pathophysiology of the total artificial heart and of cardiac assist devices. University J. E. Purkyně Press
5. Vašků J (1984) BRNO experiments in total artificial heart. Brno, University J. E. Purkyně Press
6. Dostál M, Vašků J, Černý J, Šotolová O, Guba P, Vašků J, Urbánek P, Pavlíček V, Vašků A, Nečas J, Sládek T, Trbušek V, Bednařrík B (1986) Hematological and biochemical studies in calves living over 100 days with the polymethylmethacrylate total artificial heart TNS-BRNO II. Int J Artif Organs 9:39–48
7. Weidemann H (1985) Künstlicher Totalherzersatz. Korrelation klinischer, hämodynami-scher und morphologischer Befunde in vier Entwicklungsphasen (1972–1984). Habilitation Thesis, Berlin, FU, p 207
8. Atsumi K (1986) TAH pathophysiology in the goat. In: Bücherl ES (ed) Proceedings second world symposium artificial heart, vol 1. Vieweg, Berlin 1984, pp 378–383
9. Olsen DB, Westenfelder C, Burns GL, Kablitz C, Baranowski R (1986) Neurohormonal re-sponses in total artificial heart recipients. In: Nosé Y, Kjellstrand C, Iwanovich P (eds) Prog-ress in artificial organs 1985. Isao, Cleveland, pp 112–118
10. Atsumi K (1987) Fundamental studies on implantable total artificial heart (TAH) – guest lecture. Internat meeting on heart transplantation, total artificial heart and assist devices. Brussels 23–25 March 1987 (abstr)
11. Vašků J (1984) Total artificial heart research in Czechoslovakia. In: Unger F (ed) Assisted circulation. Springer, Berlin Heidelberg New York Tokyo, pp 254–269
12. Vašků J (1986) Calcification of the TAH driving diaphragms. In: Bücherl ES (ed) Proceeding of the second world symposium artificial heart,vol 1. Vieweg, Berlin 1984, pp 45–58
13. Vašků J, Černý J, Dostál M, Urbánek P, Vašků J, Guba P, Sládek T, Trbušek V, Vašků A, Hartmannová B, Urbánek E, Doležel S, Pavlíček V, Svoboda P (1985) Calcifying lesions of the driving diaphragms, observed in the total artificial hearts (TAH) TNS-BRNO. II. Life support systems. Proceedings XI annual meeting ESAO-Alpbach, vol 2(1). Innsbruck, Sep-tember 1984, pp 242–244
14. Vašků J (1986) Total artificial heart research in Czechoslovakia: pathophysiological evalu-ation of long-term experiments performed from 1979–1985. In: Akutsu T (ed) Artificial heart. 1. Proceedings of the 1st international symposium on current problems for further de-velopment of artificial heart and assist devices, Tokyo, Aug 2–3, 1985. Springer, Berlin Heidelberg New York Tokyo, pp 161–179
15. Vašků J, Černý J, Vašků J, Urbánek E, Dostál M, Urbánek P, Guba P, Pavlíček V, Sládek T, Smutný M, Úlehla T, Hartmannová B, Trbušek V, Janečková H, Šotolová O, Šotáková E, Wendsche P, Doležel S, Filkuka J, Gregor Z, Bednařík B, Svoboda P (1983) A compara-tive study of a group of eight calves surviving longer than 1 month with the total artificial heart. Artif Organs 7:470–478
16. Vašků J, Černý J, Urbánek P, Vašků J, Dostál M, Guba P, Gregor Z, Svoboda P, Trbušek T, Šotolová O, Wendsche P, Filkuka J, Pavlíček V, Smutný M, Bednařík B, Vašků A, Dole-žel S, Sládek T, Hartmannová B, Urbánek E, Fiala V (1984) Long term evaluation of total artificial hearts in calves. Heart Transplant 4:81–88
17. Klimeš F, Kořenář F, Toman J, Pech P, Gardavský J (1987) The study of the oscillating and pulsating velocity connection of the Newton fluid in the nonelastic tube with symmetrical obstacle and in the blood chamber of the total artificial heart and further the study of the Newton fluid in the elastic tube (numeric, visualization and laser-Doppler anemometry method). Research report – Institute of Hydrodynamics, Czechoslovak Academy of Sciences, Prague 1987, p 41 (in Czech)

18. Vašků J, Urbánek P, Vašků J, Černý J, Smutný M, Urbánek E, Suchánek J, Gregor Z, Dostál M, Guba P, Sládek T, Wendsche P, Pavlíček V, Trbušek V, Šotolová O, Úlehla T, Fiala V (1986) Control and driving of pneumatic total artificial heart TNS-BRNO II and III in long term experiments. Artif Organs 10:145–152
19. Vašků J (1986) BRNO portable driving system. In: Bücherl ES (ed) Proceedings second world symposium artificial heart, vol 1. Vieweg, Berlin, pp 145–148
20. Urbánek P, Vašků J, Úlehla T, Vašků J, Dostál M, Guba P (1986) In vivo testing of electropneumatic portable driving system for the total artificial heart. Life support systems, vol 4, suppl 2. XIII Annual meeting Avignon, pp 44–46
21. Harasaki H, McMahon J, Richards JR, Goldcamp J, Király R, Nosé Y (1985) Calcification in cardiovascular implants: degraded cell related phenomena. Trans Am Soc Artif Intern Organs 31:489–494
22. Vašků J Calcification of the driving diaphragm in a total artificial heart. Czech Med (in press)
23. Tomazic BB, Etz ES, Brown WE (1987) Nature and properties of cardiovascular deposits. Scanning Microscopy 1:95–105
24. Boskey AL, Posner AS (1977) The role of synthetic and bone extracted Ca-phospholipid-phosphate complexes in hydroxyapatite formation. Calcif Tissue Res 23:251–258
25. Eanes ED, Termine JD (1983) Calcium in mineralized tissues. In: Spiro TG (ed) Calcium in biology. Wiley Interscience, New York, pp 203–233
26. Selye H (1962) Calciphylaxis. The University of Chicago Press
27. Vašků J (1967) Calciphylaxis, a new biological phenomenon and its importance. Státní zdravotnické nakladatelství (in Czech)
28. Atsumi K, Imachi K (1984) Guest lecture in the research centre for artificial heart. BRNO, July 1984
29. Tomazic B (1986) Mechanisms of the mineralization processes. Guest lecture – research centre for artificial heart. BRNO, August 1986
30. Hughes SD, Coleman OL, Dew PA, Burns GL, Olsen DB, Kolff W (1984) Effects of Coumadin on thrombus and mineralization in total artificial hearts. Trans Am Soc Artif Intern Organs 30:75–79
31. Vašků J, Černý J, Urbánek E, Trbušek V, Vašků J, Urbánek P, Dostál M, Guba P, Smutný M, Úlehla T, Pavlíček V, Suchánek J, Sládek T, Bednařík B, Svoboda P (1984) Evaluation of the changes in kinetic components of a total artificial heart after several months of pumping. Progress in artificial organs (Isao, Kyoto 1983), vol 1. Isao no 204, Cleveland, pp 204–210
32. Vašků J, Černý J, Urbánek P, Dostál M, Doležel S, Guba P, Vašků J, Smutný M, Sládek T, Filkuka J, Pavlíček V, Trbušek V, Bednařík B (1986) In: Nosé Y, Kjellstrand C, Ivanovich P (eds) Central venous pressure in calves surviving several months with a total artificial heart – progress in artificial organs – 1985. Isao, Cleveland, pp 386–392
33. Vašků J, Vašků J, Černý J, Dostál M, Guba P, Doležel S, Urbánek P, Bednařík B (1986) Changes of vasomotoric regulations in TAH bearers, life support systems, vol 4, suppl 2. Proceedings XIII annual meeting ESAO, Avignon, pp 32–34
34. Vašků J, Černý J, Dostál M, Guba P, Vašků J, Urbánek P, Vašků A, Doležel S (1987) Neurohumoral aspects of total artificial heart. Internat meeting on heart transplant. Total artificial heart and the assist devices, Brussels, 23–25 March 1987, p 43 (abstr)
35. Öberg B (1978) Aspects of reflex control of the capacitance vessels. In: Chermukh AM, Tkachenko BI, Kovach AGB, Biró S (eds) Regulation of the capacitance vessels. Akadémiai Kiadó, Budapest, pp 197–224
36. Shepherd JT (1978) Reflex control of the capacitance vessels. In: Chernukh AM, Tkachenko BI, Kovach AGB, Biró S (eds) Regulation of the capacitance vessels. Akadémiai Kiadó, Budapest, pp 145–196
37. Vašků J (1985) Pathophysiological aspects of the total artificial heart research – new trends in pathological physiology, opuscula pathophysiologica. Acta Fac Med Univ Brun 92:65–74
38. Vašků J, Černý J, Dostál M, Guba P, Vašků J, Urbánek P, Urbánek E, Pavlíček V, Gregor Z, Wendsche P, Sládek T (1985) Total artificial heart (TAH), pathophysiological aspects based on our own observations. Ergeb Exp Med 46:522–532

39. Arndt JO (1986) The low pressure system: the integrated function of veins. Eur J Anaesthesiol 3:343–370
40. Vašků J, Štengold EŠ, Kolmanovskij VB, Naumov VE, Drozdov AD (in press) Patofiziologičeskije mechanizmy venoznoj giperten zii u teljat s iskustvennym serdcom. Doklady Akademii Nauk SSSR (in russian)
41. Vašků J, Vašků J, Dostál M, Černý J, Guba P, Doležel S, Vašků A, Pavlíček V, Urbánek P (1987) Total artificial heart (TAH) – a modelling system for the study of pathophysiology of vascular regulations. 4th IMEKO conference "Advances in biomedical measurement," Bratislava, May 17–20, 1987 (abstr K-6)
42. Vašků J (1987) Recent actual problems on the total artificial heart research in Czechoslovakia, 6th world ISAO and 14th ESAO congress, Munich, September 1987 (abstr)
43. Vašků J, Vašků J, Dostál M, Černý J, Guba P, Doležel S, Vašků A, Mašek J, Urbánek P, Krejčí V (1987) Electric activity of biological atria in total artificial heart (TAH). 4th IMEKO conference "Advances in biological measurement", Bratislava, May 17–20, 1987 (abstr K-11)
44. Vašků J, Vašků J, Dostál M, Urbánek P, Guba P (1987) The relation of atrial P-wave frequency to the central venous pressure (CVP) increase and the administration of alpha-1-blocking agents and alpha-methyldopa in the total artificial heart (TAH) animals. 6th world ISAO and 14th ESAO congress, Munich, September 1987 (abstr)
45. Dostál M, Vašků J, Bílková B, Vašků J, Černý J, Guba P, Doležel S, Vašků A, Nečas J (1987) Changes of hormonal feedback mechanism of calves with the total artificial hearts – 4th IMEKO conferences "Advances in biological measurement," Bratislava, May 17–20, 1987 (abstr K-10)
46. Dostál M, Vašků J, Bílková B, Vašků J, Černý J, Guba P, Doležel S, Vašků A, Nečas J (1987) Study of serum hormone levels (aldosterone, TSH, T_3, T_4) of calves with TAH – 6th world ISAO and 14th ESAO congress, Munich, September 1987 (abstr)
47. Fujimasa J, Imachi K, Nakajima M, Nabuchi K, Tsukagoshi S, Kouno A, Ono T, Takido N, Motomura K, Chinzai T, Abe Y, Atsumi K (1986) Pathophysiological study of a total artificial heart in a goat that survived 344 days. Progress in artificial organs – 1985. Isao, Cleveland, pp 345–353
48. Vašků J (1986) Central venous pressure in the TAH animals. In: Bücherl ES (ed) Proceedings second world symposium artificial heart, vol 1. Vieweg, Berlin, pp 383–394
49. Vašků J (1986) Physiology of metabolism and organ pathology in the calves with total artificial heart. In: Bücherl ES (ed) Proceedings second world symposium artificial heart, vol 1. Vieweg, Berlin, pp 425–435
50. Rosenberg G, Pierce WS, Landis DL, Snyder AJ, Richenbacher WE, Weiss W, Felder G (1985) Progress in the development of the Pennsylvania State University motor driven artificial heart. In: Unger F (ed) Assisted circulation 2. Springer, Berlin Heidelberg New York Tokyo, pp 270–285
51. Imachi K, Fujimasa M, Nakajima K, Nabuchi K, Tsukagoshi S, Motomura K, Miyamoto A, Takido N, Inou N, Kouno A, Ono T, Atsumi K (1984) Overall analysis of the cause of pathophysiological problems in total artificial heart animals by cardiac receptor hypothesis. Trans Am Soc Artif Intern Organs 30:591–593
52. Akutsu T (1984) Current pathophysiological problems with the total artificial heart. Progress in artificial organs (Isao, Kyoto 1983), vol 1. Isao no 204, Cleveland, pp 162–164
53. Herbst WM, Lang RE (1986) Das Herz als endokrines Organ. Ber Pathol 103:571–581

33. Use of an Elliptical Artificial Heart

V. I. Shumakov and N. K. Zimin

Many centers in various countries already have a great deal of experience in developing an artificial heart. Different groups of animals with implanted artificial hearts have survived for several months. The main factors limiting the survival of calves in these experiments are thromboembolism, infection, calcification of the prosthesis, and insufficient output of the artificial heart in relation to the growth of the animals. This last factor has forced researchers to use prostheses that have a large stroke volume (up to 165 ml) but which create significant difficulties in placing the device in the chest cavity.

During the first stage of development in 1968, Akutsu [1] suggested that an oval artificial heart be constructed for intrapericardial placement; this heart, however, did not find wide use in experimental practice. Most authors at that time preferred a round prosthesis [2–4].

Since 1974, experiments at our institute have been conducted on a model of an elliptical artificial heart, the "Poisk," that was developed at the institute [5, 6]. In recent years we have used a modified model of the diaphragm type made from polyurethane (Fig. 1). The mean survival of calves with this implanted heart is 55 days (maximum survival of more than 3 months).

Because of the easy implanting of the elliptical artificial heart, it can be used in calves weighing as little as 60 kg, although it is customary to use animals weigh-

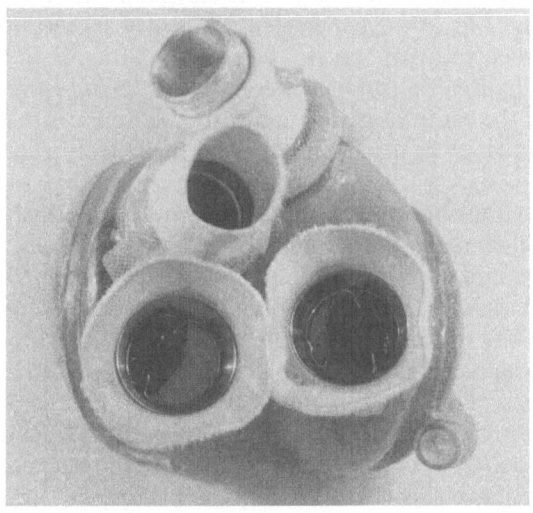

Fig. 1. The Poisk-10M artificial heart

Assisted Circulation 3
F. Unger (Ed.)
© Springer-Verlag Berlin Heidelberg 1989

ing between 85 and 95 kg. The stroke volume of the Poisk model is 90–100 ml, enabling it to reach a productivity of 12–13 l/min. Although the round type of artificial heart is believed by some researchers to create better hydrodynamic conditions, our experience with the Poisk elliptical model having a semirigid case demonstrates a lack of thrombogenesis within the blood chamber (with the exception of the inlet valves) when adequate anticoagulation therapy is maintained. With the Poisk model a low level (not exceeding 6 mg%) of plasma hemolysis is observed in the postoperative period, which we associated with an adequate design and the semirigid case.

In our last five experiments with implantation, we used a noninvasive method to measure stroke volume and left and right atrial pressure. The stroke volume of the artificial ventricle was determined by assessing the curve of air output in the pneumatic line of the left ventricle during diastole. Atrial pressure was based on the diastolic pressure in the pneumatic chambers of the artificial ventricles. Direct measurement of atrial pressure showed a good correlation between these values. An analog computer was used to collect and analyze the data, together with an alarm system to warn of technical breakdowns (e.g., a drop in electrical voltage or changes in pneumatic pressure). This system exhibited high reliability in operation.

Using the current methods for monitoring central hemodynamic parameters, we studied the changes in these parameters at rest and during physical exertion on a treadmill using postural tests (orthostatic, antiorthostatic) (Figs. 2–4).

By unloading the right artificial ventricles at −15 to +10 torr, we were able to construct curves of venous return that characterized the integral value of inflow resistance. By cutting out the right artificial ventricle for several cycles, we were able to measure the level of mean pressure. This method, based on measuring the level of pressure in the pneumatic chamber of the right ventricle, enabled us to substantiate a diagnosis of an impairment in filling. Thus, in one experiment, we observed an increase in inflow resistance of the right ventricle and an increase in mean pressure 2 weeks before the end of the experiment. Autopsy showed a diaphragmatic thrombus on the inlet valve of the right ventricle; 80% of the lumen of the valve was obstructed by this thrombus. In contrast to the invasive method, noninvasive monitoring of the central hemodynamic indices reduces the risk of infection, which is very important in using the artificial heart in clinical practice.

Clinical use of the artificial heart has become a reality in recent years. Such use demands more stringent requirements for the artificial heart as regards reliability as well as ease of implantation and comfort, both of which are determined to a significant degree by the weight and size of the prosthesis. These factors were considered in the clinical variant of the Poisk artificial heart.

The Poisk prosthesis (two artificial ventricles with valves) weighs 210–220 g, and the height of the ventricles (the ventrodorsal dimension) is 70–80 mm. Implantation of this prosthesis in the pericardial cavity of the chest in human cadavers of different physical types, sex, and weight (from 67 to 88 kg) presented no difficulties (Fig. 5). Some authors have reported difficulties in placing the Jarvik-7 artificial heart in the chest cavity of female patients and, for this reason, male patients are preferred. However, even in the operation on Mr. Barney Clark

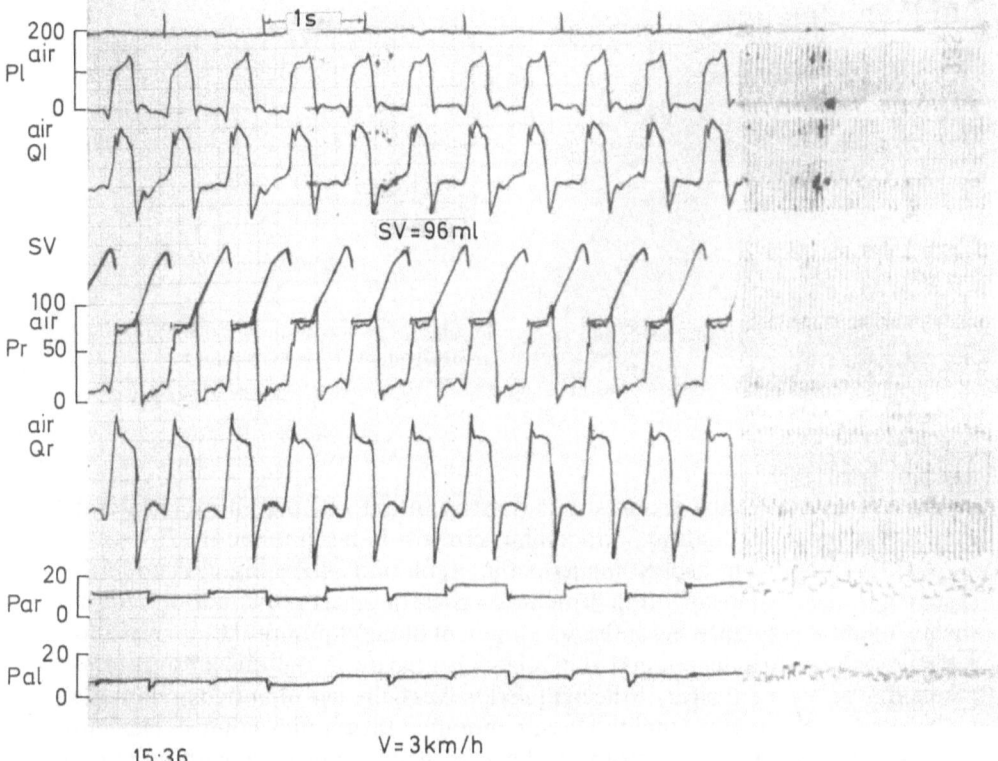

Fig. 2. Pneumatic curve recording during physical load in a calf with an artificial heart. Pl^{air}, pneumodrive air pressure in the left ventricle; Ql^{air}, pneumodrive air outflow in the left ventricle; SV, stroke volume; Pr^{air}, pneumodrive air pressure in the right ventricle; Qr^{air}, pneumodrive air outflow in the right ventricle; Par, right atrial pressure; Pal, left atrial pressure

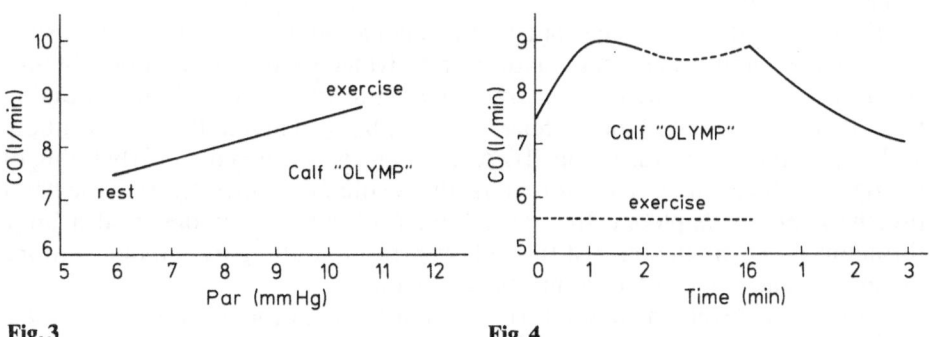

Fig. 3   **Fig. 4**

Fig. 3. Dependence of cardiac output (CO) on right atrial pressure (Par) under physical load

Fig. 4. Dynamics of cardiac output (CO) during physical load

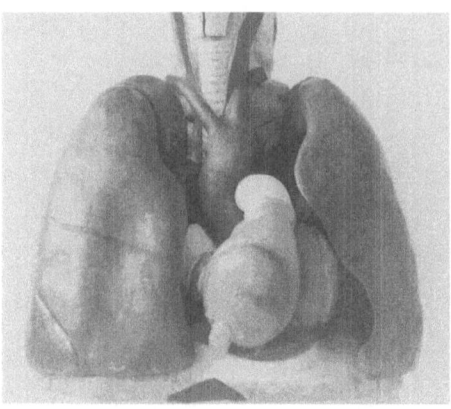

Fig. 5. Placement of the Poisk-10M artificial heart in a cast of a human chest cavity

in the United States, the artificial left ventricle had to be placed more laterally than usual, thus potentiating periodic impairments in heart function [7].

Another important aspect concerns the regulation of the blood coagulating system and the diagnosis of impairment. At present, heart implantation requires the use of anticoagulants. With the development of heart pumps that do not allow a dead zone or turbulence (and this relates primarily to the quick connect elements, the attachment sites of the artificial valves), the use of anticoagulants can be reduced or eliminated totally. Having modified these quick connect elements, American researchers [8], for example, have been able to proceed without anticoagulants after implantation. We are also addressing this question seriously.

"Free" attachment of the inlet and outlet valves is used in the Poisk-10M models, making possible the adjustment of blood flow during the first hours of operation. We also used anticoagulant and disaggregation therapy in our experiments, following the usual scheme of Coumadin, aspirin, and dipyridamole administration. Our methods enable us to diagnose any impairment in the blood coagulation system.

Figures 6 and 7 shows the changes in coagulation indices in the calf Ruslan. These figures show a significant increase in activated partial thromboplastin time (APTT) on day 37, as well as a sharp increase infibrinogen and in prothrombin time (PT), a sharp rise in the numbers of thrombocytes and in their aggregation, and a reduction in antithrombin III. At this time we observed an early filling of the right ventricle and a reduction in its filling volume. In investigating the heart prosthesis after completing the experiment (on day 53), we observed a large thrombus in the air chamber of the right ventricle, resulting from damage to the diaphragm and entry of blood into the air chamber.

At present, developmental efforts are continuing at the institute on a model of the elliptical heart which can be placed intrapericardially (Fig. 8). In patients with different physical types (asthenics, hyperasthenics, etc.), the position of the heart axis differs substantially, and we take this into consideration when constructing the atrial cuffs; these have a conical form that can be modeled in relation to the heart structures (Fig. 9).

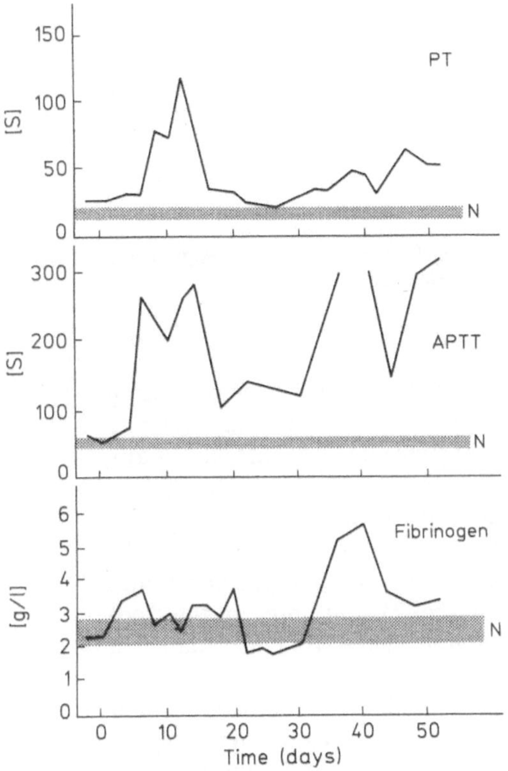

Fig. 6

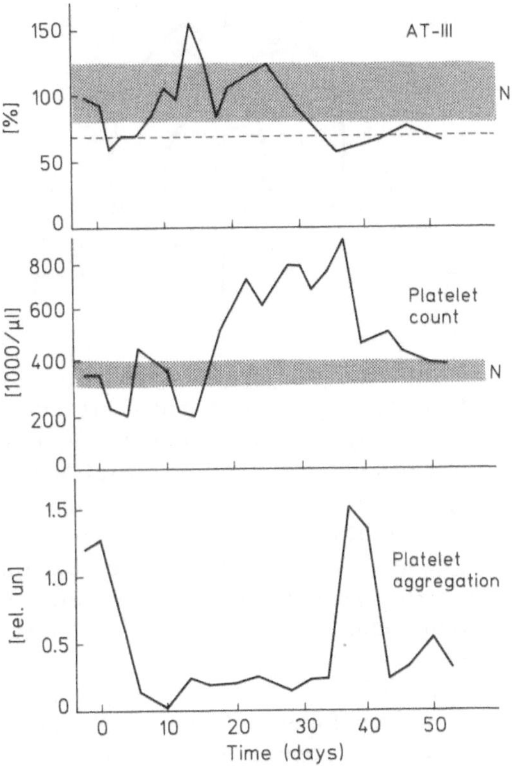

Fig. 7

Fig. 6. Changes in prothrombin time (*PT*), activated partial thromboplastin time (*APTT*), and fibrinogen after implantation of an artificial heart in a calf

Fig. 7. Changes in antithrombin III (*ATIII*), platelet count, and platelet aggregation after implantation of an artificial heart in a calf

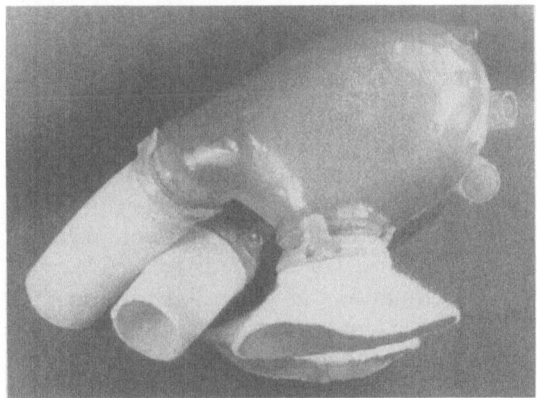

Fig. 8. Variant of the clinical model of the artificial heart

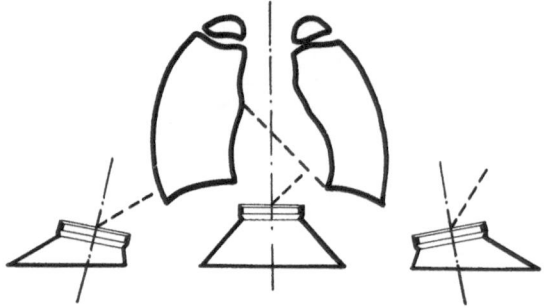

Fig. 9. Variations in the design of the atrial cuff

In planning for clinical application of the artificial heart, we anticipate using a two-stage replacement. The heart pump is implanted in the first stage (lasting up to 30 days). It is important during this stage to prevent the occurrence of any adhesions in the area of the operation so that a second, repeat operation is not jeopardized. Experience has shown that the greatest difficulties arise with anastomoses to the aorta, the pulmonary artery, and the quick connect elements of the atria, which are literally immured by adhesions of the pericardium and lungs. Polyurethane linings to cover these areas for 2–4 weeks help to prevent these adhesions and, thus, significantly facilitate and promote successful performance of the second operation.

A brief description of a clinical case of total artificial heart implantation at our institute follows. Patient K, 55 years old, was delivered to the institute at 6 p.m. on 25 November 1987 with a diagnoses of acute transmural myocardial infarction with an interventricular septum fracture, progressing heart insufficiency, and cardiogenic shock of grade II–III. The patient had two heart arrests. Because of the ineffectiveness of the other methods of treatment we decided to implant the Poisk-10M. The implantation involved severe technical difficulties due to the extraordinarily poor condition of the atrial myocardium. Enormous efforts were required to obtain hemostasis. Because the pericardial cavity was small, the artificial left ventricle was placed in the left pleural cavity (Fig. 10). During the first 24 h postoperatively and under stable hemodynamic conditions (cardiac output: 5.5–6.0 l/min; arterial pressure: 140–120/70–60 mmHg), we noted the development of encephalopathy, oliguria, and, then, anuria. Hence for the treatment we used hemodialysis, hemosorbtion, and after that, semicontinuous hemofiltration. In addition we administered antithrombotic treatment (heparin 30 000–50 000 units/24 h, plus dipyridamole). Up to the end of the seventh 24 h we noted a clear improvement in the clinical condition of the patient. However, during the eighth 24 h the patient's condition suddenly deteriorated rapidly owing to the development of right pneumothorax a rupture of a emphysematic (bulla) provoking extreme hemodynamic deterioration. Despite the elimination of this complication (which took about 20 min), the patient's condition worsened; further active treatment was ineffective and the artificial heart function was stopped. Examining the blood chambers of the prosthesis, we observed small ring-shaped thrombus formations located only in the attachment points of the artificial heart valves.

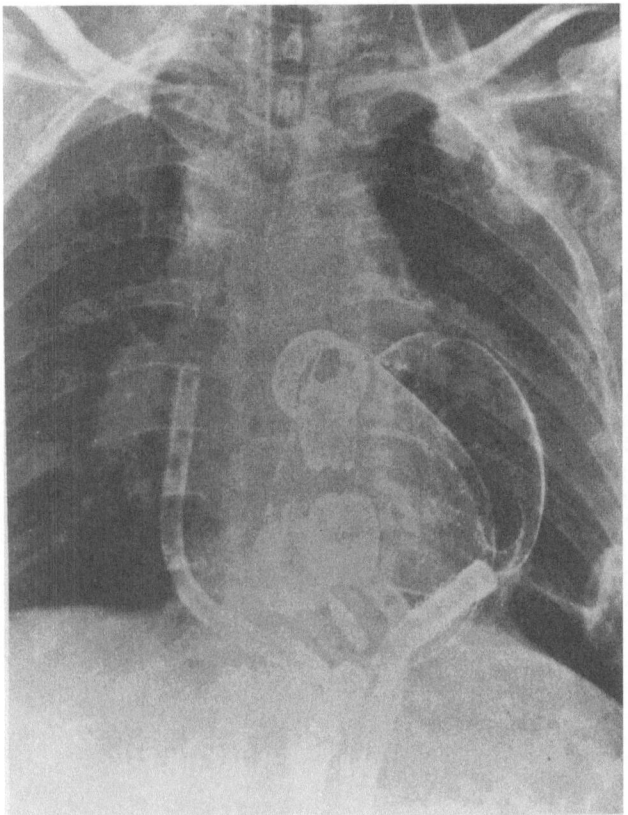

Fig. 10. X-ray film of patient K after the implantation of the Poisk-10M artificial heart

Further improvements to the heart prostheses themselves and to the surgical methods used will enable us in the future to adopt artificial heart implantation as the operation of choice in clinical practice.

Summary

Experiments with the Poisk model of an elliptical artificial heart are reported. Using a modified model of the diaphragm type made from polyurethane, calves survived for a mean time of 55 days, with a maximum survival of 3 months. With adequate anticoagulation therapy, no thrombogenesis was observed in the blood chamber (except for the inlet valves); a low level of plasma hemolysis was observed postoperatively. A good correlation was demonstrated between the stroke volume and left and right atrial pressures. Changes in the blood coagulation indices are reported. Implantation of a clinical variant of this prosthesis into human cadavers demonstrated no difficulties in placing the heart in the pericardial cavity. Developmental efforts are continuing.

References

1. Akutsu T (1975) Artificial heart. Total replacement and partial support. Excerpta Medica, Amsterdam
2. Fukumasu H, Iwaya F, Olsen DB, Lawson J, Kolff WJ (1979) Surgical implantation of the Jarvik-5 total artificial heart. Trans Am Soc Artif Intern Organs 25:232–237
3. Rosenberg G, Phillips WM, Landis DL, Pierce WS (1981) Design and evaluation of the Pennsylvania State University mock circulatory system. Am Soc Artif Intern Organs J 4(2):41–49
4. Vasku J, Cerny J, Hanzelka P, Vasku J, Urbanek E et al. (1981) 150-day survival of a calf with a polymethylmethacrylate total artificial heart: TNS-BRNO-II. Artif Organs 5(4):388–401
5. Shumakov VI, Egorov TL, Itkin GP, Drobyshev VA, Drobyshev AA (1976) A new model of orthotopic prosthesis made of fluorosiloxane gum (in Russian). Med Tekh (4):30–31
6. Shumakov VI, Egorov TL, Drobyshev VA, Drobyshev AA (1978) Problems in constructing the heart prosthesis (in Russian). Proceedings of the international symposium on devices for replacement of the heart and kidneys, Brno
7. Joyce LD, De Vries WC, Hastings WC, Olsen DB, Jarvik RK, Kolff W (1983) Response of the body to the first permanent implantation of the Jarvik-7 total artificial heart. Trans Am Soc Artif Intern Organs 29:81–87
8. Jarvik RK, Kessler TR, Mcgill LD, Olsen DB, DeVries WC, Deneris J, Blaylock JT, Kolff WJ (1981) Determinants of pannus formation in long-surviving artificial heart calves, and its prevention. Trans Am Soc Artif Intern Organs 27:90–96

34. In Vivo Testing of a Roller-Screw Type Electric Total Artificial Heart

G. Rosenberg, W. S. Pierce, A. J. Snyder, W. Weiss, D. L. Landis, W. E. Pae Jr., and J. A. Magovern

Introduction

Work was begun on the development of an electric motor drive total artificial heart at the Pennsylvania State University in 1978. The first systems developed utilized a low-speed high-torque brushless DC motor rotating a triple-track cam mechanism. This mechanism translated a rotary force into a rectilinear motion to actuate alternately the sac type blood pumps located on either end of the motor drive mechanism. The prototype of this system weighed slightly over 1 kg. Implantation of the cam type electric motor driven artificial heart began in 1983 and 222-day calf survival was obtained late in that year [1]. In 1984, work was begun on a roller-screw type electric motor driven artificial heart. The roller-screw device had the advantages of being smaller, lighter, and less expensive to produce. Extensive in vitro testing of the roller-screw device was performed from 1984 through 1986. In mid-1986 implantation of the roller-screw device was begun in calves. Over the next year the device was implanted in six animals with a maximum survival time of greater than 85 days.

The roller-screw device has previously been described [2–7]. The design improvements and results of in vivo testing of the device are presented in the forthcoming sections.

Description of the Roller-Screw System

Figure 1 shows the current roller-screw electric motor driven total artificial heart. Depicted in the photograph are the left and right blood pumps with the associated quick connects for the atria and great vessels. Also shown in the photograph is a 150-cc compliance chamber, and the infusion port which is used for adjusting gas volume within the system [8–11].

Prosthetic Ventricles

Figure 1 shows the roller-screw total artificial heart with the two prosthetic ventricles removed. The left blood pump is shown in the foreground and right blood pump in the background. The prosthetic ventricles are constructed of extremely smooth seam-free segmented polyurethane sacs that are contained within the rigid outer polysulfone or polycarbonate housings. These blood pumps utilize size

Assisted Circulation 3
F. Unger (Ed.)
© Springer-Verlag Berlin Heidelberg 1989

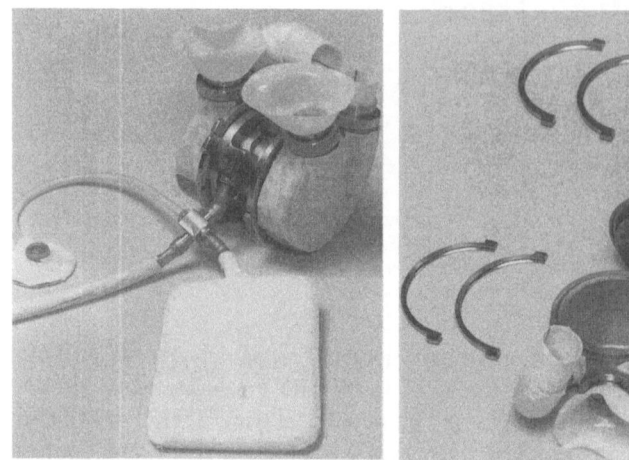
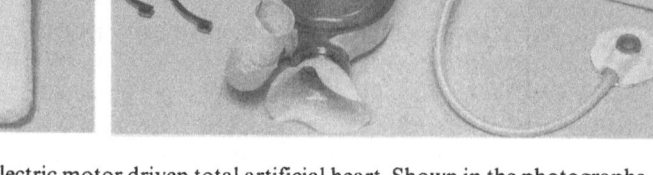

Fig. 1. The roller-screw type electric motor driven total artificial heart. Shown in the photographs are the pumps, motor and linkage, compliance sac, percutaneous lead, and infusion port

29 inlet and size 25 outlet convexo-concave Björk-Shiley Delrin disk valves. Quick connects are provided for both atria and the great vessels. The great vessel connectors are constructed of Dacron graft overcoated with segmented polyurethane. The atrial connectors are constructed of woven segmented polyurethane and polyester cloth. This cloth is also overcoated with a thin layer of segmented polyurethane to impart an extremely smooth blood contacting surface. A more detailed description of the blood pump fabrication may be found in reference [12].

Motor and Mechanical Linkage

Figure 2 is a schematic representation of the brushless DC motor and linkage mechanism employed in the roller-screw total artificial heart. The central component of the system, the roller-screw, consists of a threaded screw shaft, an internally threaded nut, and a number of threaded planetary rollers. The rollers are positioned in the space between the screw shaft and the nut, and mesh with both. When the screw shaft or nut rotates in relation to the other element, the rollers follow a planetary path around the screw shaft. The ends of the rollers are toothed and terminate in cylindrical shaft that seats in guide rings at either end. The roller teeth mesh with a toothed ring located in the nut by pins. Thus the rollers are not subject to sliding during acceleration or rotation. The entire roller-screw system is hardened to minimize wear. The roller-screw has a great number of contact points among which the load is shared, thus providing an extremely reliable system. Efficiency of the roller-screw can be as high as 90%.

Pusher plates are attached to either end of the screw portion of the roller-screw and alternately push on the blood sacs. Two bearings support the roller-screw nut and the attached motor rotor. A guide shaft is attached between the two pusher plates and constrains the pusher plates from rotating.

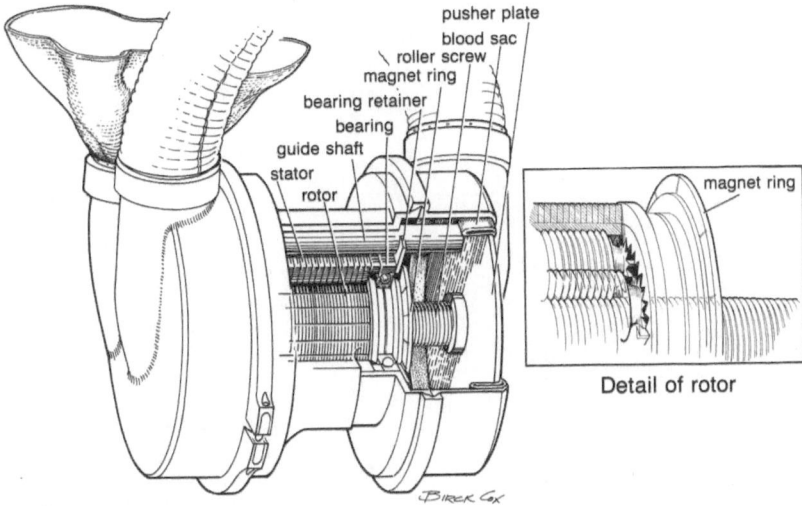

Fig. 2. Cross-sectional view of the roller-screw total artificial heart

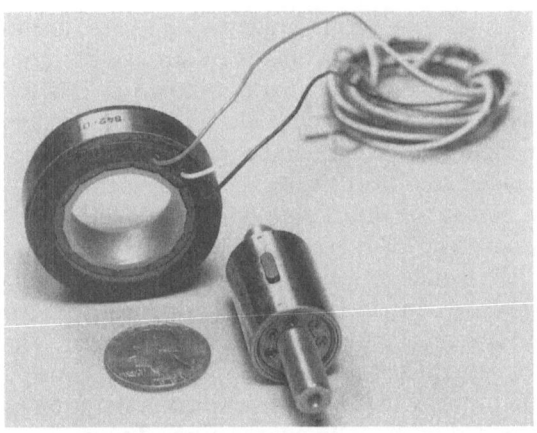

Fig. 3. The current roller-screw and brushless DC motor. The motor is a 14-pole three-phase delta wound motor. The screw is 8 mm in diameter, with a 4-mm lead

Figure 3 shows the current roller-screw motor and roller-screw mechanism. The roller-screw is an 8-mm diameter screw with a 4-mm lead. This screw is constructed of stainless steel. The electric motor shown is a 14-pole fractional slot wound motor that utilizes rare earth cobalt magnets and a vanadium permendur stack. Future motors will utilize neodymium iron magnets. This motor is an electronically commutated three-phase delta wound system.

Electronic Systems

A schematic representation of the roller-screw TAH system as it will be implanted within the human is presented in Fig. 4. The complete electronics system consists

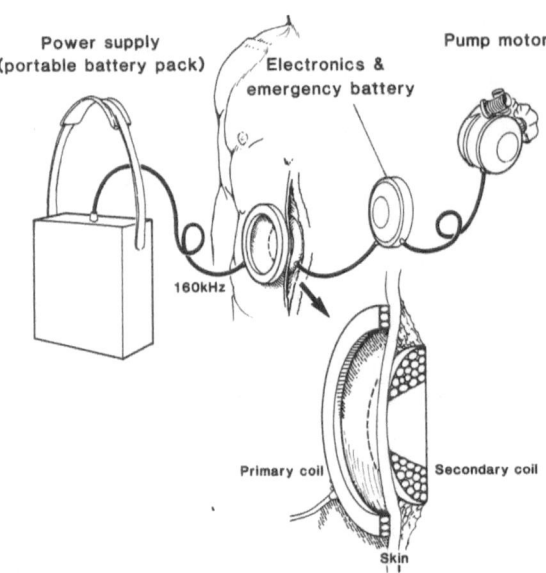

Power supply
(portable battery pack)

Electronics &
emergency battery

Pump motor

160kHz

Primary coil

Secondary coil

Skin

Fig. 4. The transcutaneous energy transmission system as it will be implanted in the human. The portable battery pack will weigh approximately 5 kg and supply energy in excess of 10 h

of a portable external power supply and monitoring system along with an implantable electronics package. The external supply consists of storage batteries and an oscillator that converts the DC energy from the batteries to a 160-kHz RF power signal that is used to drive an external primary coil. The monitoring system keeps watch over the entire system, including the implanted components, to provide diagnostic and emergency management information.

Electrical energy is transmitted across the intact skin from the external primary coil to the internal secondary coil. The 160-kHz electrical energy goes from the secondary coil to the implanted electronics and emergency battery. The internal electronics and emergency battery are contained within a hermetically sealed titanium housing. The 160-kHz signal is then converted back to DC power. The electronic commutation and control system that is contained within the housing automatically controls the operation of the TAH. A more detailed description of each of these subsystems will be provided in the following sections. Figure 5 is a block diagram of the roller-screw electronics system. It shows the architectures of both the external and the internal electronics packages.

Electronic Commutation and Control

The electronic commutation and control system is designed to (a) commutate the brushless motor, (b) track the motor position and cause a reversal at precisely specified and points, (c) control the motion of the motor during each stroke of the pump to limit inertial forces to a satisfactory level, (d) maintain an exact balance between the left and right blood pumps, and (e) vary the cardiac output according to a measure of physiological demand. The controller is located in the internal electronics package, as shown in Figs. 4 and 5. This controller is capable

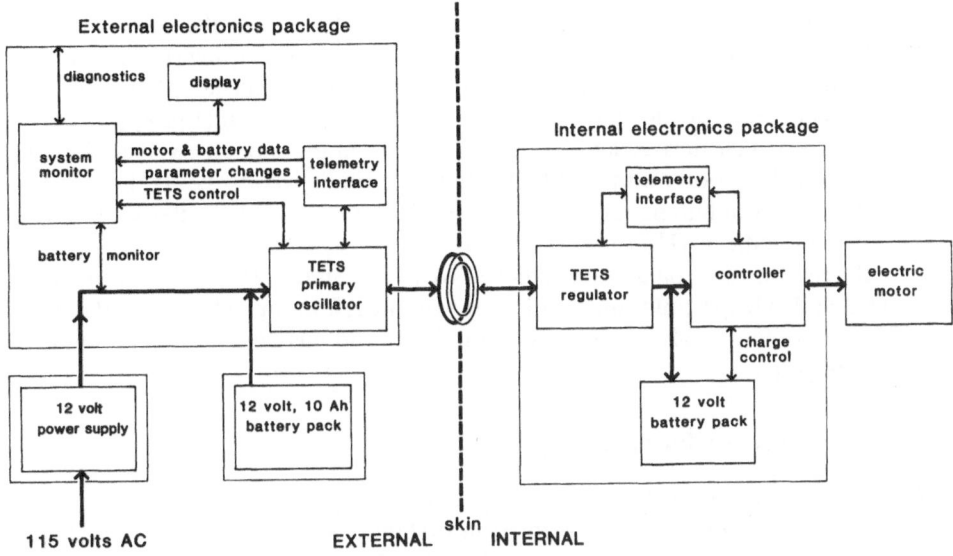

Fig. 5. Block diagram of the roller-screw electronics system

of operating the device given only a source of electrical power, either transmitted across the skin or from the emergency internal battery located within the internal electronics package.

The current controller uses a conventional multichip microprocessor system based upon the GTE65SCOO family. A hardware commutator and pulse width modulator are used. These circuits combine signals from three Hall-effect sensors placed within the motor with pulse width, direction, and dynamic brake signals from the microprocessor system into a commutation code. The commutation code in turn directs the application of the supply voltage by the power switch circuit to the motor windings. The motor commutation sequence is repeated 44 times each half stroke. Upon initial start-up or at any time when the controller senses an illegal sequence, the motor moves with constant voltage excitation towards the left pump end-diastolic position until a signal is obtained from a fourth, end point, Hall-effect sensor, thus providing a reference position. The controller is currently being miniaturized, using a more highly integrated microcomputer and large-scale programmable logic.

For a given stroke speed the controller calculates a desired velocity for each segment of the motor motion. The resultant desired velocity profile corresponds to that which minimizes the peak acceleration of the motor. The controller utilizes a novel motion control method which has been referred to as "adaptive feedforward" control. As motor motion proceeds, the controller provides the motor with a preprogrammed (feedforward) motor voltage for each segment of motion. The controller measures the time required for transition through each segment and records the corresponding motor velocity. Based upon any difference between the desired and actual velocities, the feedforward motor voltage to be used on the next cycle of the pump is revised. This technique allows precise control over stroke and points and tight tracking of the desired velocity.

No implanted pressure transducers are required to control the artificial heart. Based upon a model of the motor and motion translator characteristics, the controller calculates an estimate of the pressure applied to the pusher plate as a function of its position for each left systolic stroke [13]. By analyzing this applied pressure, the controller derives an estimate of the blood pressure, as well as the time required for the blood pump to fill. These two estimates allow control of cardiac output and output balance according to a control philosophy similar to that used for our pneumatic TAH.

Left–right output balance is achieved by manipulating the right pump stroke volume while always pumping a full stroke on the left pump. This method of control has worked reliably in all our calf implants and has been described in detail elsewhere [14].

External Electronics Package

Transcutaneous Energy Transmission System

The transcutaneous energy transmission system that was developed by Thermedics, Incorporated has been adapted by The Pennsylvania State University for use with the roller-screw motor. This adaptation included redesign of the system electronics to allow higher instantaneous peak power than that for which the system was initially designed. The electrical energy is transmitted by a transcutaneous transformer consisting of a pair of loosely coupled coils. The external primary coil has an average diameter of 10 cm and contains three turns of Litz wire. The implanted secondary coil consists of 16 turns of Litz wire in the shape of a truncated cone 7.1 cm in diameter. Each coil is part of a 160-kHz series tuned circuit Although the mean power requirements of the roller-screw artificial heart are typical 10–15 W, the transcutaneous energy transmission system is capable of providing short duration peak power requirement as high as 50 W. Maximum efficiency of the system has measured as high as 75%. The transcutaneous energy transmission system has been fabricated and tested with several roller-screw type electric motor driven ventricular assist devices. The system has functioned satisfactorily in these experiments and when implanted electronics become available the transcutaneous energy system will be utilized with the roller-screw total artificial heart.

Battery Systems

For portable operation the artificial heart will require an external battery supply. At present we are evaluating nickel–cadmium and lead acid batteries for the external supply. Currently silver–zinc batteries have a limited cycle life and are quite expensive. No secondary lithium cells with the require capacity amp hours are available. Our preliminary design system uses a 12 V, 10 A hour rechargeable external battery. This external battery can provide energy to the system until the primary and secondary coils are decoupled. In the event that the coils are decoupled the implanted 450 mA hour battery system contained within the implanted electronics package will supply the necessary energy to run the system in excess of 30 min. We are currently examining nickel–cadmium as well as lithium batteries for the implanted battery systems.

In order to evaluate the various systems for the external and internal batteries, our group has developed an automated battery test unit. This system is a computer-controlled testing device designed to perform various charging and discharging protocols on up to five secondary battery packs. This automated battery test unit is capable of examining various types of battery. The system is based on a Rockwell Aim 65 microcomputer. It can charge and discharge batteries in any preprogrammed manner.

Telemetry System

To have an effective device, a telemetry system is required for bidirectional communication between the implanted and nonimplanted system components. This telemetry system is most critical during the initial start-up phase of the artificial heart. A number of methods have been investigated for such telemetry systems, including the use of infrared light, ultrasound tissue conduction, and separate high frequency inductively coupled coils. The most advantageous method, however, appears to be the utilization of transcutaneous energy transmission coils and circuitry to do the information transfer. This eliminates the need for separate coils or transducers. To transmit information from the external system to the implant, the power oscillator frequency can be shifted without sacrificing transmission efficiency. The normal on-off cycling of the TETS system then serves as a synchronizing signal for each bit change. On the secondary side of this system the demodulated signal is input to a synchronous transmitter receiver which interfaces with the control microprocessor. To transmit information from the implanted secondary coil to the primary coil we modulate the impedance of the internal transcutaneous energy transmission system during the off state. This causes a phase shift of the current in the primary loop, thus yielding phase shift keyed data transmissions. This system of data transmission is just undergoing in vitro testing.

System Monitor

As previously mentioned, the external electronics package will include a system monitor that will continuously monitor the performance of the implanted components, the energy transmission system, and the external battery. The monitor will continually check motor performance and transcutaneous energy transmission system efficiency by determining energy requirements on both sides of the internal–external link. Diagnostic procedures will be established to detect any incipient failure. A liquid crystal display and audible signal will be used to indicate the functional condition of the system. This will include information such as time remaining on a battery pack. The monitor will also provide a link to a more extensive physician's office diagnostics device.

Implantation Techniques

The roller-screw type electric motor driven artificial heart has been implanted in six animals. Figure 6 depicts the roller-screw system as implanted in the calf. The

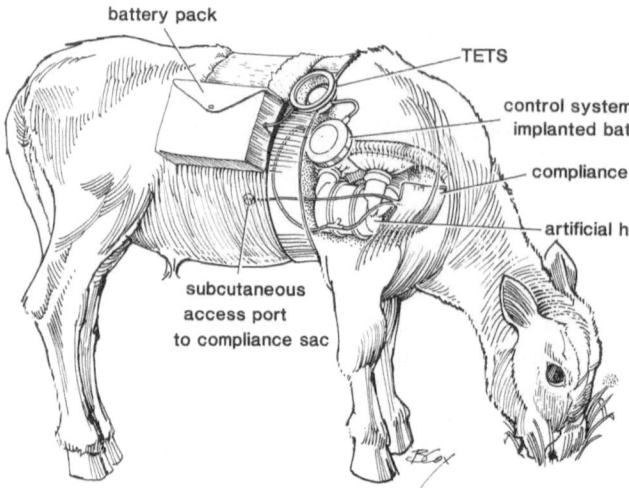

battery pack

TETS

control system and
implanted battery

compliance sac

artificial heart

subcutaneous
access port
to compliance sac

Fig. 6. The roller-screw heart
and electronics as they will be
implanted in the calf. This system, without the implanted
electronics, has been tested in
six calves

systems implanted thus far were all sealed, and utilized the subcutaneous access
port, but a percutaneous lead replaced the transcutaneous energy transmission
system.

The heart is implanted through a fifth interspace thoracotomy. Heparin is administered and an arterial cannula is inserted in the right carotid artery. Superior
and inferior caval cannulas are inserted through the right atrium. Cardiopulmonary bypass is performed using a membrane oxygenator and mild hypothermia.
The heart is excised at the atrioventricular groove and at the level of the aortic
and pulmonary valves. The left atrial connector is sutured into place using a continuous 4-0 polypropylene suture. The pulmonary artery connector is then sutured into place. The aortic connector is positioned in the field, trimmed to length,
and sutured using a continuous 4-0 polypropylene suture. The right atrium is
properly trimmed, and the right atrial connector is again attached with a continuous suture of 4-0 polypropylene. The motor is then positioned within the field
and the connection to the motor ports is accomplished. The system is de-aired
with a modified Swan-Ganz catheter, and pumping is initiated slowly as cardiopulmonary bypass is discontinued.

The postoperative care of the animals with implanted electrically driven hearts
is similar to that which has been employed over the past decade in our pneumatic
artificial heart animals [15]. The animals are maintained on warfarin sodium (prothrombin time between 20 and 25 s), dipyridamole (100 mg every 6 h), and eti-
dronate disodium (20 mg every 6 h).

Results

The roller-screw electric motor total artificial heart has been implanted in six
calves over the past year, beginning in April of 1986. Table 1 lists the results of
these implantations.

Table 1. Implantation of roller-screw electric motor driven total artificial heart

Calf number	Date of operation	Survival time	Cause of death
227 – Jeremy	27 May 86	3 days	Stroke
272 – Milton	8 June 86	8 days	Motor winding failure
354 – Fridge	23 Sept. 86	13 days	Necrotic bowel secondary to long intraoperative hypotension
204 – Alpha	17 April 86	23 days	Pneumonia and poor oxygenation
319 – Casey	4 Nov. 86	52 days	Constriction of inferior vena cava, and tapeworm
415 – Kelly	10 March 87	90 days and ongoing	–

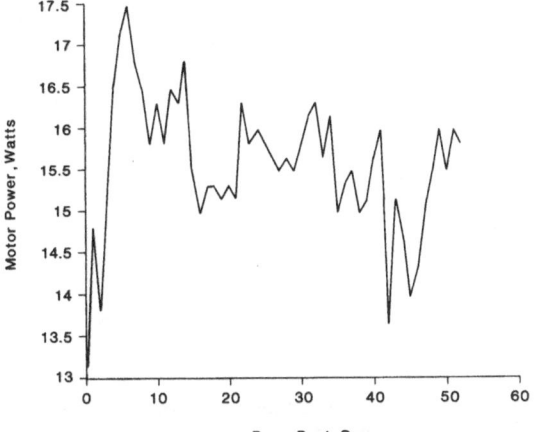

Fig. 7. Mean motor power vs time for calf 319

There was only one system failure, and that was due to a motor winding becoming partially open circuited. This is a very rare failure for electric motors and there was no apparent reason.

All of these animals have had similar hemodynamic performance. Figures 7–10 depict the motor power, the motor beat rate, the cardiac output, and the estimated mean aortic pressure for calf number 319 for the duration of his survival. These curves are typical of the other calves. It should be noted that with the motor power levels depicted in Fig. 9, tissue temperatures at the surface of the implant did not exceed 2 °C above the animal's rectal temperature.

Postmortem examination of calves number 354, 319, and 204 in each case showed encapsulation of the total artificial heart and compliance chamber. There was no apparent tissue damage due to heat rejection from the implanted device.

Average plasma hemoglobin levels for the animals were 8.9 ± 7.8 (mean $\pm$ SD) mg%. The animal's hematocrits averaged $27.8 \pm 7.0\%$.

The postoperative periods of the animals surviving for more than 1 week was quite similar to those of the pneumatic artificial heart animals. The animals were

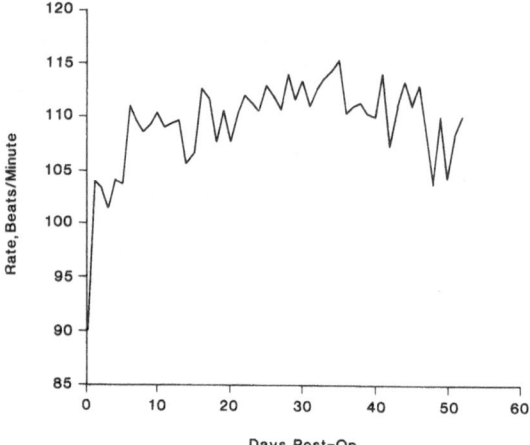

Fig. 8. Artificial heart beat rate for calf 319

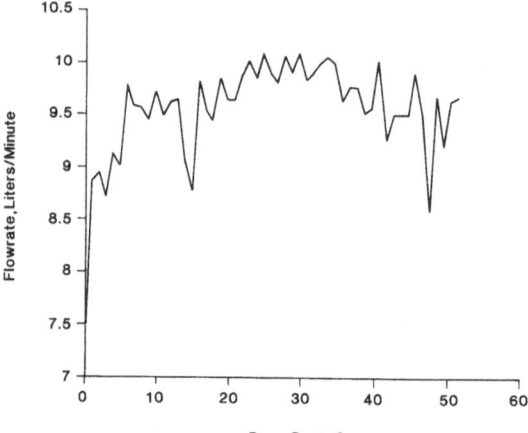

Fig. 9. Estimated blood flow rate for calf 319

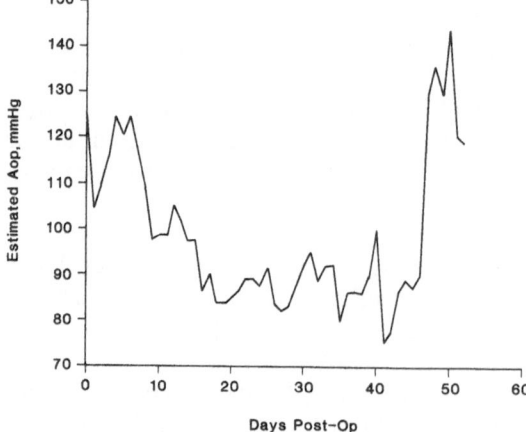

Fig. 10. Estimated mean aortic pressure (*Aop*) for calf 319

able to stand unaided immediately postoperatively and were able to eat and drink at will.

Summary

An electric motor driven roller-screw total artificial heart has been developed at the Pennsylvania State University and implanted successfully in six calves. The longest surviving calf is doing well more than 90 days after implantation. Of the other five calves, one died at 8 days of an electric motor winding failure; the other four animals died of complications following device implantation. One calf suffered a stroke, another calf had a necrotic bowel secondary to long intraoperative hypotension. A third animal died of poor oxygenation secondary to pneumonia, and the final animal died from constriction of the inferior vena cava and the complications of a tapeworm infestation. The calves were able to eat, drink, and tolerate moderate exercise. Further implantations, in the calf, of the roller-screw total artificial heart are planned for the immediate future.

In anticipation of clinical application of the roller-screw device, a smaller, 70-cc stroke volume, pump is under development. This system will be implanted in sheep in a manner similar to the implantation technique that has been employed in the calf. The maximum cardiac output of this device will be 8 l/min, and the overall size and weight of the system will be substantially reduced. It is presently anticipated that implantation of the entire system for clinical application will be as depicted in Fig. 11. Our initial studies in the calf all indicate that the implanted

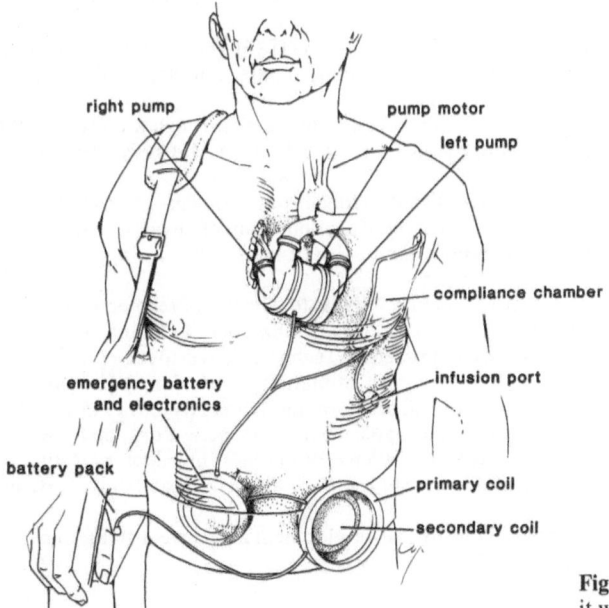

right pump

pump motor

left pump

compliance chamber

emergency battery and electronics

infusion port

battery pack

primary coil

secondary coil

Fig. 11. The roller-screw system as it will be implanted in the human

compliance chamber, infusion port, and transcutaneous energy transmission system have the potential to function satisfactorily for periods in excess of 2 years. Testing of an implanted battery and electronic system is anticipated in the near future. As we establish satisfactory reliability of these components, they will be incorporated into the system to be utilized in the calf. After satisfactory evaluation in vitro and in animals has been accomplished, the device will be ready for clinical application.

References

1. Rosenberg G, Snyder A, Landis DL, Geselowitz D, Donachy JH, Pierce WS (1984) An electric motor-driven total artificial heart: seven months survival in the calf. Trans Am Soc Artif Intern Organs 30:69–74
2. Rosenberg G, Snyder A, Weiss W, Landis D, Geselowitz D, Pierce W (1982) A roller screw drive for implantable blood pumps. Trans Am Soc Artif Intern Organs 28:123
3. Rosenberg G, Donachy JH, Geselowitz D, Snyder A, Landis DL, Pierce WS (1982) Recent progress of the artificial heart. Eur Rev Biomed Technol 4:283–284
4. Richenbacher WE, Rosenberg G, Landis DL, Weiss WJ, Donachy JH, Pierce WS (1983) Development of an implantable electric motor artificial heart. Surg Forum 34:250–253
5. Rosenberg G, Cleary TJ, Snyder AJ, Landis DL, Gaselowitz DB, Pierce WS (1985) A totally implantable artificial heart design. Transactions of the American society of mechanical engineers, 85-WA/DE-11
6. Rosenberg G, Snyder A, Pierce WS, Geselowitz D (1982) Engineering development of the mechanical heart. In: McNeil BJ, Cravalho EG (eds) Critical issues in medical technology. Cravalho. Auburn House, Boston, pp 381–397
7. Gaines WE, Donachy JH, Rosenberg G, Landis DL, Pierce WS (1984) Studies leading to an artificial heart for clinical application. Contemp Surg 24:41–48
8. Jorge E, Snyder AJ, Rosenberg G, Fehr D, Geselowitz DB, Pierce WS (1986) Subcutaneous access port for the compliance chamber of the electric ventricular assist device and total artificial heart. In: Nose Y, Kjellstrand C, Ivanovich P (eds) Progress in artificial organ. Isao, Anaheim, pp 537–540
9. Lee S, Rosenberg G, Donachy JH, Wisman CB, Pierce WS (1984) The compliance problem: a major obstacle in the development of implantable blood pumps. Am Soc Artif Intern Organs 8(1):82–90
10. Reid JS, Rosenberg G, Pierce WS (1985) Transmission of water through a biocompatible polyurethane – application to circulatory assist devices. J Biomed Mater Res 19(9):1181–1202
11. Wisman CB, Rosenberg G, Weiss WJ, Landis DL, Donachy JH, Snyder AJ, Richenbacher WE, Pierce WS (1983) The development and successful application of an intrathoracic compliance chamber for the implantable electric motor-driven ventricular assist pump. Surg Forum 34:253–256
12. Phillips WM, Donachy JH, Rosenberg G, Pierce WS (1980) The use of segmented polyurethanes in ventricular assist devices and artificial hearts. In: Szycher M, Robinson W (eds) Synthetic biomedical polymers; concepts and practice. Technomic, Westport, pp 39–57
13. Snyder A, Rosenberg G, Landis D (1985) Indirect estimation of circulatory pressures for control of an electric motor-driven total artificial heart. In: Langrana NA (ed) 1985 advances in bioengineering. The American society of mechanical engineers, New York, pp 87–88
14. Snyder AJ, Rosenberg G, Landis DL, Weiss W, Pierce WS (1984) Introductory lecture on control. Presented at the second world symposium on the artificial heart, July 3, Berlin, pp 167–190
15. Magovern JA, Rosenberg G, Pierce WS (1986) The development and current status of a total artificial heart. Artif Organs 10(5):357–363

35. Implantable Artificial Hearts *

S. Fukunaga, Y. Hamanaka, H. Ishihara, T. Sueda, and Y. Matsuura

Introduction

While recent progress in heart transplantation has been remarkable, the shortage of donor hearts has become a serious problem in many countries. One solution to this problem is the totally implantable artificial cardiac prosthesis. For such a prosthesis various kinds of implantable artificial hearts have been proposed [1–3]. One of these uses a modified Stirling cycle machine as an actuator [4] and another an electrohydraulic energy converter [5]. Most studies of prostheses, however, treat a variety of artificial hearts utilizing small electric motors.

Artificial hearts with high-speed electric motors and ball screws [6–8] require no reduction gears, but the motors must be able to rotate forward and backward alternately, according to the systolic and diastolic period of the artificial hearts. This results in energy loss owing to acceleration and retardation of the motors. Torque motors and cylindrical cams are also used in artificial hearts [2, 9–11]. Such a driver needs no reversing of the motor, but these torque motors are of low energy density in general.

Two types of motor-driven artificial hearts are being studied at Pennsylvania State University, the drum cam system and the roller-screw system. A survival time of 7 months was reported in the calf with the drum cam driven artificial heart [12, 13].

Yamada et al. reported that linear motors are promising candidates for artificial heart actuators [14], but further improvements are needed to increase thrust force for their totally implantable use.

The present authors developed a new motor-driven artificial heart composed of a flat-type brushless DC motor, Harmonic Drive as a reduction gear, a specially designed cylindrical cam, and polyurethane sacs as blood chambers. The purpose of this paper is to present this new motor-driven artificial heart.

Brushless DC Motor Actuator

The structure of the motor-driven artificial heart is shown in Fig. 1. The high-speed, low-torque rotation of the motor is converted to high-torque, low-speed

---

* With support of a grant-in-aid for scientific research from the Ministry of Education, Science and Culture of Japan.

Assisted Circulation 3
F. Unger (Ed.)
© Springer-Verlag Berlin Heidelberg 1989

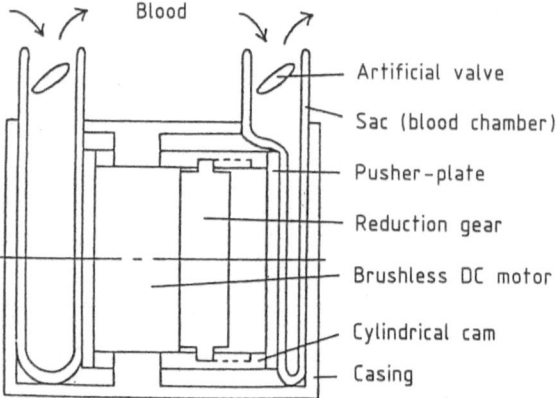

Blood

Artificial valve

Sac (blood chamber)

Pusher-plate

Reduction gear

Brushless DC motor

Cylindrical cam

Casing

Fig. 1. Structure of motor-driven artificial heart

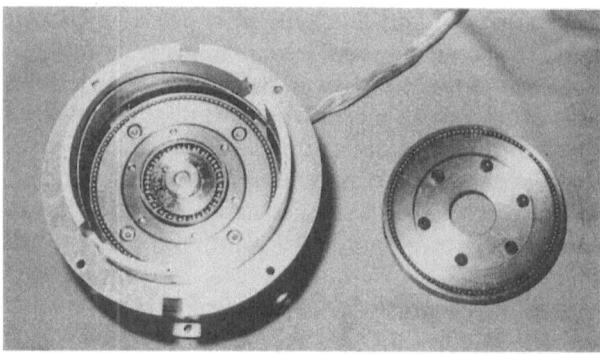

Fig. 2. Harmonic Drive and cylindrical cam

motion by the reduction gear. The cylindrical cam converts this one-way slow revolution into the reciprocation to push the two sacs inside the driver alternately by the pusher plates located at either end of the cam.

A flat-type brushless DC motor is used as an actuator, 69 mm in diameter and 38 mm in length. The speed, torque, and output power of this motor are 5500 rpm, 480 g cm, and 27 W, respectively. The flat-type Harmonic Drive component, 50 mm in diameter and 15 mm in length, is used as a reduction gear. This provides high-gear ratio of 88, with output torque of 0.8 kg m through coaxial input and output shafts.

A specially designed cylindrical cam has an endless groove for cam followers; this convert the one-way rotation into reciprocation without reversing the rotation of the motor. A part of the groove of the cylindrical cam and Harmonic Drive are shown in Fig. 2. As the cam moves from side to side, two sacs inside the artificial heart are pushed alternately by the pusher plates located at either end of the cam. Therefore, the phase of the two sacs, one for the left ventricle, the other the right, is inverted. The percent systole of this driver is fixed at 50% owing to the mechanism.

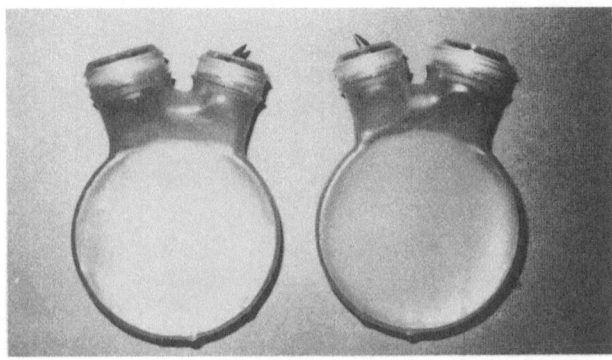

Fig. 3. Biomer sacs with valves

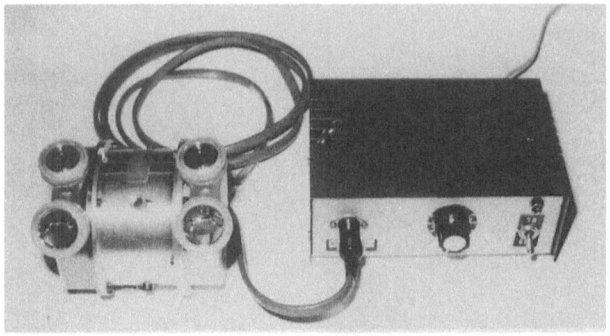

Fig. 4. Artificial heart with controller

Blood Pump

Two sacs are made of Biomer, with design stroke volume of 87 ml (left) and 81 ml (right), as shown in Fig. 3. Björk-Shiley monostrut valves of 29 mm and 25 mm are placed at inflow and outflow of the sacs. An external view of the artificial heart and its controller are shown in Fig. 4. The main body of the driver is made of aluminium alloy and carbon steel. Its maximum diameter, length, and weight are 110 mm, 108 mm, and about 2 kg, respectively.

Measurement

In Vitro Study. A test of the total artificial heart was performed in vitro using a Donovan-type mock circulatory system. A schematic diagram of the mock test is illustrated in Fig. 5. Aortic pressure (AoP), pulmonary arterial pressure (PAP), central venous pressure (CVP), left atrial pressure (LAP), and cardiac output (CO) at aorta were recorded. Electric power consumed by the motor was measured, as was the temperature of the saline water inside the mock circulatory system and that of the surface of the driver. The artificial heart with its controller,

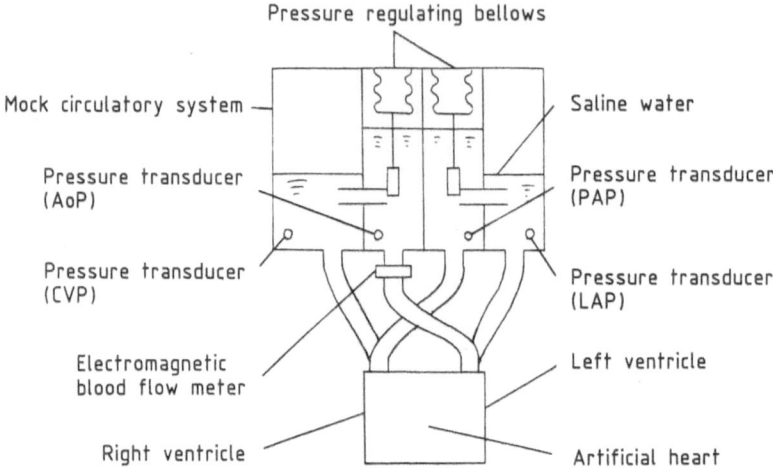

Fig. 5. Schematic diagram of mock test

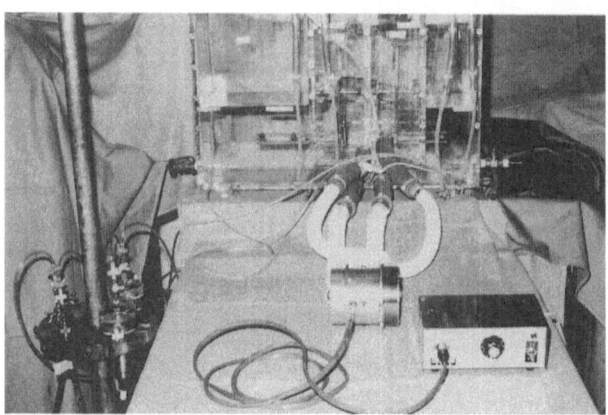

Fig. 6. Photograph of artificial heart on mock circulation

mock circulatory system, pressure transducers, and an electromagnetic blood flow meter are shown in Fig. 6.

The oscillograms of AoP, PAP, CVP, LAP, and CO from the mock test are shown in Fig. 7. Results of the mock test are also summarized in Table 1. The energy obtained by the saline water in the mock circulatory system was calculated, and system efficiency was evaluated, as shown in this table. The artificial heart worked at the driving rate of 39–125 bpm, with CO in the range of 2.9–7.3 l/min. The phase of AoP to PAP is inverted because of the mechanism of this artificial heart. Power consumed by the motor ranged from 15 to 43 W, according to the driving rate, and system efficiency was in the range of 5.3%–7.2%. Temperature increase at the surface of the driver was 3.9 °C, while that of the saline water, about 12 l in the mock circulatory system, was 0.4 °C after about 2 h driving in the ambient temperature of 25 °C.

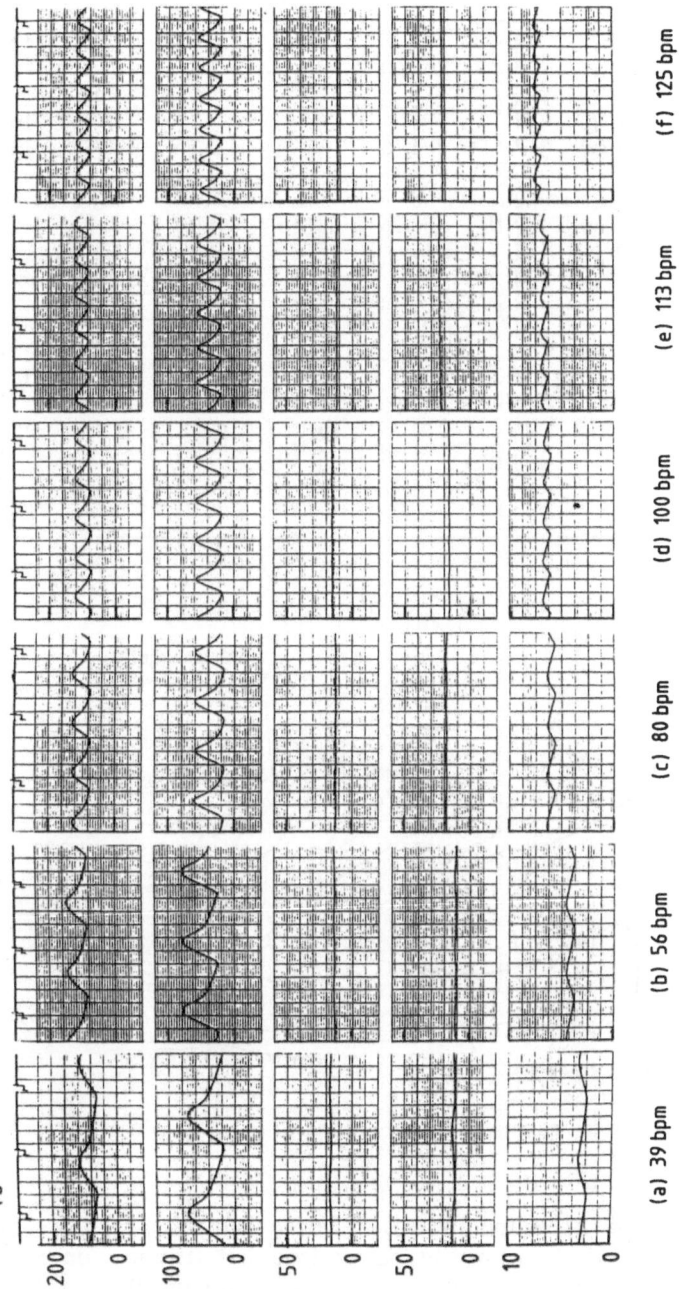

Fig. 7. Data from mock test

Table 1. Results of mock test of artificial heart made of brushless DC motor

Driving rate	(bpm)	39	56	80	100	113	125
AoP							
mean	(mmHg)	84	98	98	96	98	104
max/min	(mmHg)	112/64	144/88	128/90	120/74	120/80	120/84
PAP							
mean	(mmHg)	40	48	34	34	36	36
max/min	(mmHg)	72/18	80/26	60/16	56/18	56/21	54/22
CVP, mean	(cm H_2O)	17	16	13	15	12	12
LAP, mean	(cm H_2O)	12	11	18	16	24	22
Cardiac output	(l/min)	2.9	4.3	6.1	6.5	6.8	7.3
Stroke volume	(ml)	74	77	76	65	60	58
Power consumption	(W)	15	20	25	30	35	43
AoP + PAP, mean	(mmHg)	124	146	132	130	134	140
AoP + PAP, mean	(kPa)	16.5	19.5	17.6	17.3	17.9	18.7
Total flow rate	(ml/s)	48	72	102	108	113	122
Energy obtained by circulating fluid	(W)	0.79	1.40	1.80	1.87	2.02	2.28
System efficiency	(%)	5.3	7.0	7.2	6.2	5.8	5.3

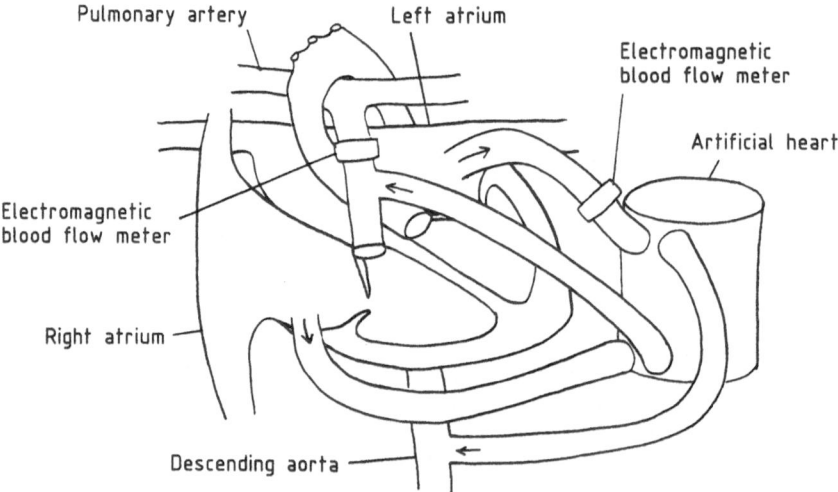

Fig. 8. Biventricular bypass using motor-driven artificial heart

In Vivo Study. An animal experiment was then carried out using a calf weighing 120 kg, as shown in Fig. 8. Blood was by-passed from left atrium to descending aorta and from right atrium to pulmonary artery by the artificial heart. Impraflex grafts of 30 mm were used as withdrawal cannulae and those of 25 mm as return cannulae. Blood flow rate was measured at the pulmonary artery (COPA) and at the withdrawal cannula of the left sac of the artificial heart (COAH). Also recorded were electrocardiogram (ECG), AoP, and CVP simultaneously. A photograph of the animal experiment is shown in Fig. 9.

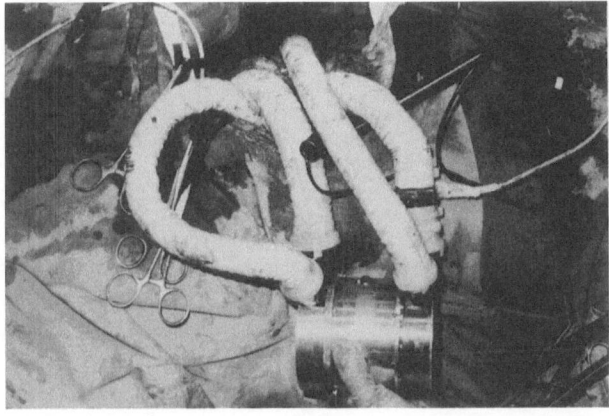

Fig. 9. Photograph of animal experiment

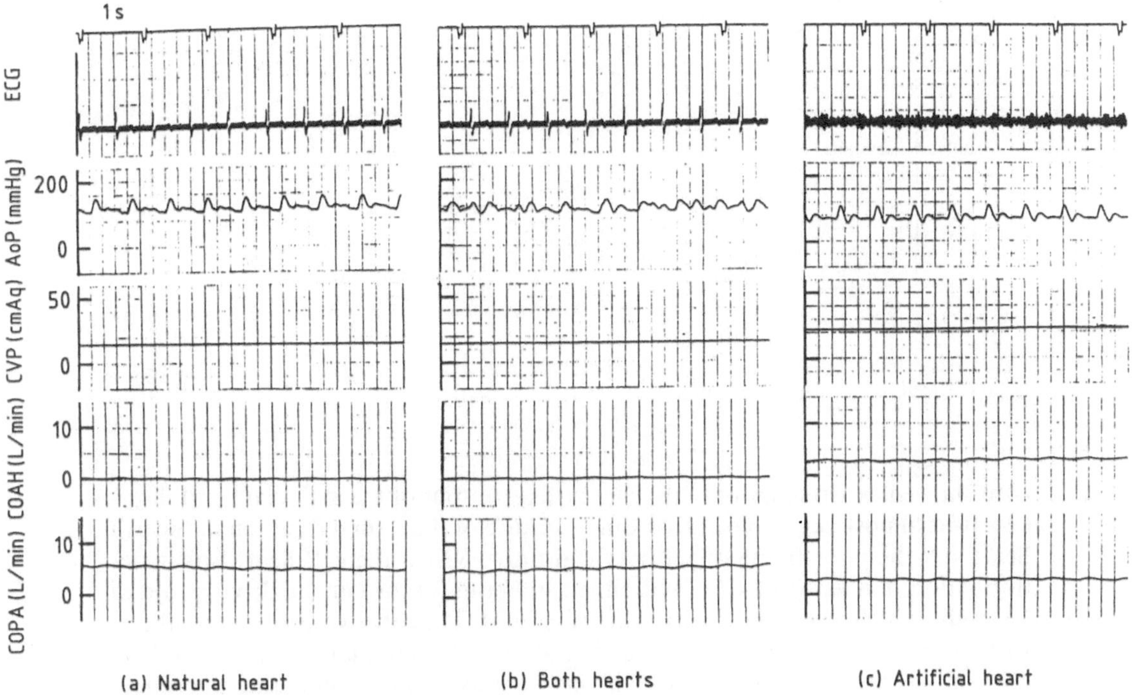

Fig. 10. Hemodynamic oscillogram of animal experiment

(a) Natural heart   (b) Both hearts   (c) Artificial heart

Hemodynamic oscillograms of the animal experiment under anesthesia are shown in Figs. 10 and 11. When the artificial heart was not in operation, the ECG shows that the calf's own heart beat at the rate of about 100 bpm. The value of COPA shows that cardiac output of the calf's own heart was about 6 l/min, while the value of COAH indicates that there was no blood flow in the artificial heart. When the calf heart and the artificial heart worked simultaneously, the AoP re-

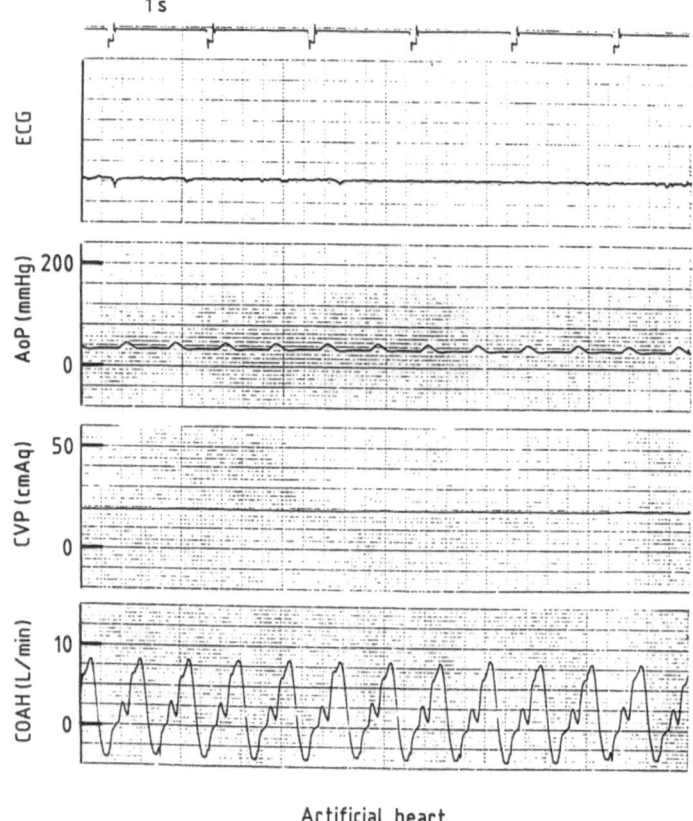

Fig. 11. Result of second experiment

cord showed an irregular pattern. The cardiac output of the artificial heart, however, was almost negligible at that time, because of the strong function of the calf heart and the poor filling of the artificial heart. When the calf heart was under fibrillation, the value of COPA declined to about 3 l/min at the driving rate of 103 bpm, which was equal to the value of COAH. The calf awoke from anesthesia with no indication of brain damage after about 0.5 h circulation by the artificial heart alone, but at this point the calf was sacrificed to terminate the experiment because of the poor chances of long-term survival. In Fig. 11 are shown the ECG, AoP, CVP, and COAH records of another experiment. Insufficient cardiac output resulted here in low AoP and high CVP.

Future Problems

The artificial heart was able to adjust its driving rate in the range of 39–125 bpm on mock test. Cardiac output from the artificial heart varied from 2.9 to 7.3 l/min according to its driving rate. The stroke volume of 58–77 ml was observed at mock test; the efficiency of the left sac was 67%–89% for design stroke volume of 87 ml and that of the right sac was 72%–95% for design value of 81 ml. The flow rate from the left sac was the same as that from the right sac in spite of the different design stroke volume for left and right sacs. The filling of this artificial heart is completely dependent on the left and right atrial pressures, and this device has no active filling aparatus, thus the flow rate between left and right sacs is automatically balanced. As is seen in Fig. 7, percent systole of the artificial heart is fixed at 50%, and the phase of AoP to PAP is inverted. Cardiac output and the waveform of blood pressure, however, seemed to be satisfactory in the mock test. System efficiency of 5.3%–7.2% was evaluated at that time.

Cardiac output of the artificial heart in the animal experiment using a 120-kg calf on an operating table was rather less than expected. The main reasons for this were considered to be severe bending and stricture occurring at the withdrawal cannulae, lack of an active filling apparatus in this artificial heart, and a relatively short diastolic period due to fixed percent systole of 50%.

The major remaining problems in this system consist of improving the artificial heart by equipping it with an active filling apparatus without imbalancing cardiac output between left and right ventricles and increasing system efficiency.

References

1. Pierce WS (1983) Portable artificial heart systems. Trans Am Soc Artif Intern Organs 29:754–759
2. Takatani S (1986) Toward a completely implantable total artificial heart system. In: Akutsu T (ed) Artificial heart 1. Springer, Tokyo Berlin Heidelberg New York, pp 51–57
3. Harasaki H, Sugita Y, Fujimoto L, Sato N, Smith W, Navarro R, Kiraly R, Miose J, White M, Nose Y (1987) Implantable left ventricular assist system. Jpn J Artif Organs 16:183–189
4. White MA (1986) Implantable energy source for artificial hearts. In: Akutsu T (ed) Artificial heart 1. Springer, Tokyo Berlin Heidelberg New York, pp 33–48
5. Moise J, Butler K, Payne J, Wampler R, Smith W, Fujimoto L, Golding L, Kiraly R, Harasaki H, Nose Y (1985) Experimental evaluation of complete electrically powered ventricular assist system. Trans Am Soc Artif Intern Organs 31:202–205
6. Hayashi K, Seki J, Nakamura T, Fukumasu H (1986) Portable drive unit for artificial heart: toward a totally implantable system. In: Akutsu T (ed) Artificial heart 1. Springer, Tokyo Berlin Heidelberg New York, pp 97–102
7. Jufer M (1986) Brushless DC motor for an electrical artificial heart. Proceedings of the international conference on electrical machines, 8–10 Sept., Munich, part 3, pp 1172–1174
8. Steiner HL, Hanitsch R (1986) Electromechanic driving unit for an artificial heart. Proceedings of the international conference on electrical machines, 8–10 Sept., Munich, part 3, pp 1179–1182
9. Takatani S, Takano H, Nakatani T, Kinoshita M, Noda H, Fukuda S, Tsuchimoto K, Akutsu T, Konishi T, Koshiji K, Utsunomiya T (1987) Development of a permanent use motor driven total artificial heart system. Jpn J Artif Organs 16:179–182
10. Gernes DB, Bernhard WF, Clay WC, Sherman CW, Burke D (1983) Development of an implantable, integrated, electrically powered ventricular assist system. Trans Am Soc Intern Artif Organs 29:546–550
11. Takatani S, Tanaka T, Nakatani T, Noda H, Fukuda S, Adachi S, Takano H, Akutsu T (1985) Simultaneously ejecting left-or-right triggered total artificial heart actuated by a single electromechanical system. Trans Am Soc Artif Intern Organs 31:367–371

12. Rosenberg G, Pierce WS, Landis DL, Snyder AJ, Richenbacher WE, Weiss W, Felder G
    (1984) Progress in the development of the Pennsylvania State University motor-driven ar-
    tificial heart. In: Unger F (ed) Assisted circulation 2. Springer, Berlin Heidelberg New York
    Tokyo, pp 270–285
13. Rosenberg G, Snyder AJ, Landis DL, Geselowitz DB, Donachy JH, Pierce WS (1984) An
    electric motor-driven total artificial heart: seven months survival in the calf. Trans Am Soc
    Artif Intern Organs 30:69–74
14. Yamada H, Fukunaga S (1986) Artificial heart actuator using linear pulse motor. In: Akutsu
    T (ed) Artificial heart 1. Springer, Tokyo Berlin Heidelberg New York, pp 77–80

36. The Orthotopic Univentricular Artificial Heart

D. Liotta, J. A. Navia, P. del Río, J. B. Riebman, O. H. Frazier,
O. Lima Quintana, C. Cabrol, I. Gandjbakhch, and D. A. Cooley

Introduction

Biventricular cardiac replacement with a total artificial heart (TAH) has now
moved from the research laboratory into the clinical arena. Years of effort from
several experimental centers have provided the foundation for the development
of clinically applicable TAH systems. Experience with animal TAH implantation
as well as the more recent human implant experience has delineated some problems and limitations of current devices for mechanical biventricular replacement
[1–4]. Patients with small intrathoracic and intrapericardial volumes may demonstrate a poor fit of the TAH, with impingement on surrounding structures or inability to close the chest postoperatively. The problem of maintaining left and
right ventricular balance plagues the TAHs designed with coupled ventricular
pumping mechanisms. The level of energy consumption for a biventricular TAH
also imposes some limitations on the design of a totally implantable TAH system.

Circulatory support with a single ventricle in dogs was reported in 1965 by
Pierce and co-workers, who replaced the heart with a single, internal, left ventricular pump [5]. Successful maintenance of systemic circulation with a single mechanical ventricle finds its origins in the development of the Fontan-Kreutzer
procedure (and its subsequent modifications) for surgically treating tricuspid
atresia in children [6–8].

The Fontan-Kreutzer operation for this and other complex congenital heart
defects is based on the creation of a direct right atrial to pulmonary artery (RA-
PA) shunt by anastomosing the pulmonary artery directly to the right atrium,
completely bypassing the right ventricle. The procedure has proved clinically
since 1971 that life is possible without the right ventricle. Recent reports of the
late clinical results of patients who have successfully undergone this and similar
modified procedures indicate persistence of abnormal hemodynamics at rest and
with exercise, but with the majority of patients having a normal or near-normal
overall functional classification [9, 10]. All patients with right atrial pressure below 14 mmHg postoperatively are excellent. No severe sequelae after surgery
were observed when the preoperative criteria for patient selection were met, when
sinus rhythm was present, and when atriopulmonary anastomosis was perfect,
that is, larger that the normal size of the main pulmonary artery [11]. These clinical data are encouraging and provide a rationale for exploring cardiac replacement incorporating a single mechanical ventricle with a Fontan-Kreutzer type
procedure.

Assisted Circulation 3
F. Unger (Ed.)
© Springer-Verlag Berlin Heidelberg 1989

Circulatory support with a single ventricle has been investigated in goats by Takano et al. [12]. The results of their studies focused on the important role of pulmonary vascular resistance and maintenance of right and left atrial pressures after RA-PA shunt. Experimental evidence indicates that adequate systemic circulation can be achieved with a mechanical left ventricle if the pulmonary resistance is normal and a sufficient right-to-left atrial pressure gradient is present. Maintenance of the left atrial pressure at a positive level prevents collapse of the pulmonary veins with subsequent elevation of pulmonary vascular resistance.

Systemic venous hypertension occurs after the Fontan-Kreutzer procedure in humans as well as in the single ventricle implants described above. If acutely elevated right atrial pressures become prolonged in the postoperative course, the result will be ascites, pleural effusions, edema, and hepatomegaly with hepatic dysfunction. Because of high venous vascular compliance, the abdomen becomes an enlarged venous reservoir. The use of phasic lower body or abdominal compression in the immediate postoperative period in human patients undergoing the Fontan-Kreutzer procedure has been demonstrated to reduce fluid requirements during this period while increasing left atrial pressure and cardiac output [9, 13].

The use of a single ventricle in the orthotopic, univentricular artificial heart (OUAH) procedure presents a number of advantages over mechanical biventricular replacement: reduced required intrathoracic volume for the blood pump, reduced risk of anatomical distortion or compression of adjacent, intrathoracic soft tissue structures, one-half of the number of prosthetic valves and prosthetic surface area exposed to blood, reduced hematological insult, lower power requirements, elimination of right–left pump imbalance, and simpler control and monitoring.

The purpose of this study was to explore the development of the bovine animal model for single ventricle cardiac replacement. Several variations in surgical technique were explored, including the creation of an interatrial shunt. The effect of abdominal compression on postoperative hemodynamics and the clinical course was evaluated.

Materials and Methods

The OUAH was evaluated in 13 short-term (less than 73 h) in vivo studies in calves. The first seven implants of this study were conducted at the Texas Heart Institute, Houston, Texas, utilizing a pneumatically actuated, single-chamber polyurethane (Avcothane) blood pump manufactured by Bioimplant Canada, Inc. and fitted with either St. Jude or Medtronic-Hall valves. This device displaces a volume of 210 cc, weighs 110 g, and provides a stroke volume of 90 cc. The remaining studies took place at the Institute for Biomedical Engineering, University of Utah, Salt Lake City, Utah. The UVAD-85 heart, a vacuum-formed, pneumatic, polyurethane (Pellethane) blood pump constructed at the University of Utah's Artificial Heart Research Laboratory, was used for these studies. This pump is equipped with Medtronic-Hall valves, weighs 85 g, displaces 210 cc, and has an effective stroke volume of 85 cc.

Healthy male Holstein calves weighing 65–90 kg were used for this study. For surgery, the calves were anesthetized, intubated, and prepared for a right lateral thoracotomy. At this time an inflatable, rubber, sack-type abdominal compression girdle (75 cm × 55 cm × 1 cm) was placed around the calves' abdomen and secured in place.

Several variations of the surgical procedure were employed in the studies performed. In each experiment, the blood pump was orthotopically positioned between the left atrium and the aorta, and the right ventricle was eliminated by creating a direct RA-PA shunt. One of three surgical techniques (A, B, or C) was used in each OUAH implant.

A. The natural heart was excised using the current technique for cardiac transplantation [14]. The main trunk and the right branch of the pulmonary artery were opened longitudinally, and a direct RA-PA anastomosis was performed to provide the widest possible shunt area [8]. A 26-mm Dacron, low porosity graft from the left ventricular pump to the aorta was positioned anterior to the RA-PA shunt.

B. This technique differed from the above procedure by preserving the natural orientation between the pulmonary artery and aorta. Only the main trunk of the pulmonary artery was opened, and the RA-PA shunt was created anterior to the aorta using a Dacron or pericardial patch to enlarge the anastomotic area. This technique may prevent compression of the shunt where passing under the aorta in procedure A.

C. The third technique was similar to procedure A, except that the natural heart was removed using the technique for implantation of TAH [15], excising the ventricles from the atrium at the atrioventricular groove and leaving the mitral and tricuspid valve annuli intact for reinforcement at the suture lines. A widely patient, direct RA-PA anastomosis was created without a patch [8], and the aorta was brought anterior to the shunt and connected to the pump by a 30-mm Dacron, low porosity graft. This technique maximized the size of the atrial remnants, allowing for creation of a larger RA-PA shunt and decreasing the risk of shunt compression by the anterior aorta (Fig. 1). This is the elective technique. The posterior approach to place the aortic pulmonary shunt in relation to the ascending aorta offers better immediate and long-term results in the Fontan-Kreutzer operation [11].

The effect of an interatrial shunt was evaluated in two animals by creation of an atrial septal defect (ASD) through the fossa ovalis. One ASD was created with a scalpel cut (4 mm curved incision) and the other with a circular punch (8 mm in diameter). The remainder of the cardiac reconstruction in these animals was as described above in technique C.

After completion of the surgical reconstruction of the heart and insertion of the mechanical ventricle, the animals were slowly weaned off cardiopulmonary bypass. Cyclic abdominal compression was initiated at this time, and an intravenous infusion of isoproterenol was used to maintain pulmonary vascular resistance within normal limits. Crystalloid fluids and blood were infused to maintain right atrial pressure between 12 and 20 mmHg and cardiac output between 3 and 5 l/min. Monitoring lines were placed for continuous recording of aortic and atrial pressures.

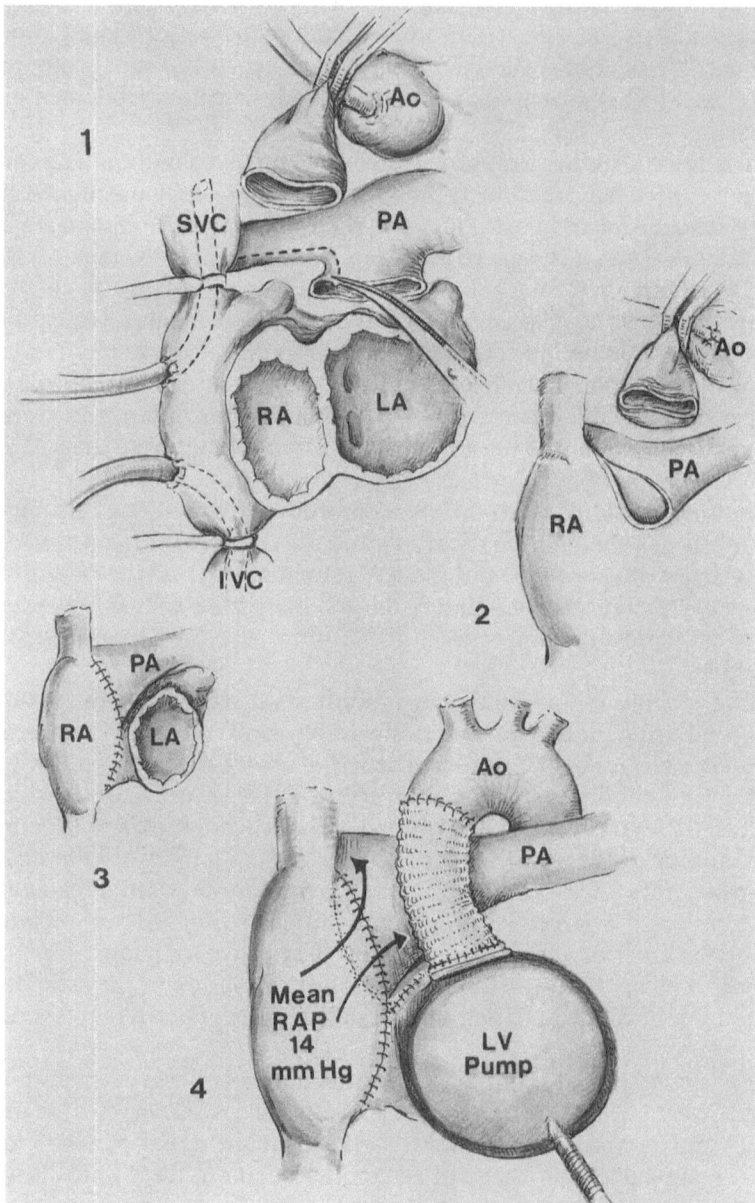

Fig. 1. Surgical technique for implantation of the OUAH. The longitudinal opening of both the main and the right branch of the PA to perform a wide RA-PA anastomosis is illustrated. The anterior position of the aorta, regarding the RA-PA shunt, is emphasized. *Ao*, aorta; *IVC*, inferior vena cava; *LA*, left atrium; *LV*, left ventricular; *PA*, pulmonary artery; *RA*, right atrium; *RAP*, right atrial pressure; *SVC*, superior vena cava

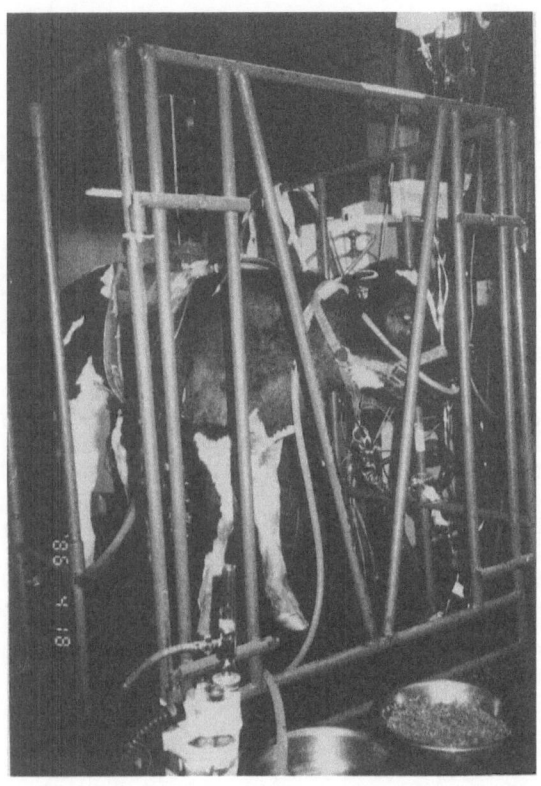

Fig. 2. "Ruggerito," a 74-kg calf, 48 h after OUAH implantation

Postoperatively, the calves were placed in their cages in sternal recumbency, and routine postoperative procedures were followed. Some of the animals were extubated between 1.25 and 8 h after surgery and supplemental oxygen was administered, as needed, by nasal cannula. Transfusions with whole blood and packed cells were given to keep the hematocrit at approximately 30%. Isoproterenol and nitroprusside infusions were used as needed to maintain systemic and pulmonary vascular resistances within normal ranges. Ventricular pump output and air-pressure waveforms from the ventricular driver were intermittently monitored. When possible, the animals were assisted in standing in their cages and were fed hay and water ad libitum. Cyclic abdominal compression was continued through the postoperative period for most animals.

Routine postoperative hematological analysis included the following: pCO_2, pO_2, pH, PVO_2, hematocrit, activated clotting time, complete blood count, and whole-blood and plasma-free hemoglobin. Serum chemistry analysis consisted of electrolytes: Na^+, K^+, Ca^{2+}, and Cl^-.

The duration of each study ranged from several hours to 3 days (Figs. 2–4). Experiments were terminated when the animals expired or were determined to have irreversible hemodynamic abnormalities. Postmortem analysis included careful examination of the reconstructed heart and mechanical blood pump. The

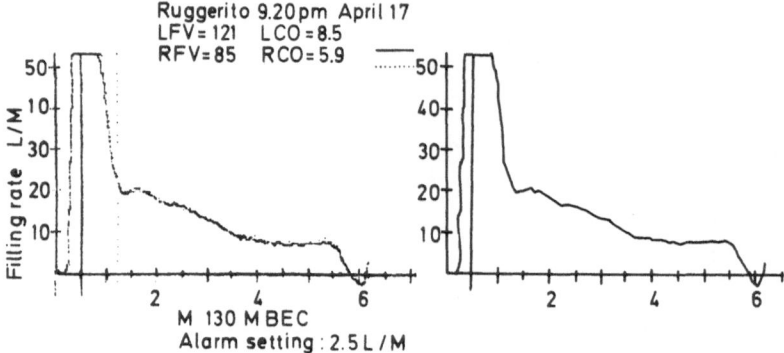

Fig. 3. The cardiac output monitor and diagnostic unit (ComDu) is connected to the exhaust port of the heart driver. A Fleish pneumotachograph is connected in line and its output is a diffepressure transducer. The output of the transducer is sampled and digitized using an A/D interface under the control of a microcomputer and specially designed software. All the data are displayed by the computer on the monitor

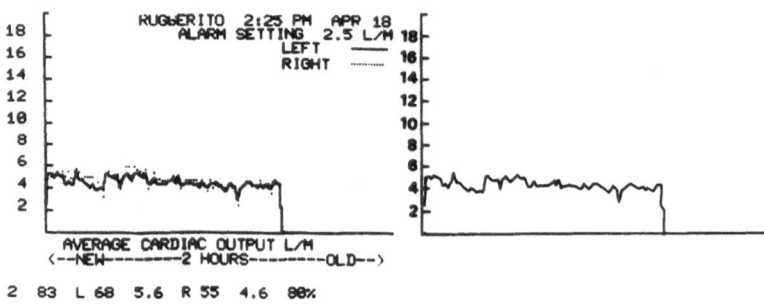

Fig. 4

position of the pump within the chest was analyzed and the RA-PA shunt was examined for signs of distortion or compression. Internal organs were evaluated for congestion, weighed, and sectioned.

Results and Discussion

These studies are by nature very complex experiments, generating data covering many topics. The results presented here for discussion will focus on several specific areas. The relative merits of the various surgical techniques will be discussed, as well as the effect of the ASD. The contribution of phasic abdominal compression to circulatory support will also be reviewed.

In the 13 experimental trials, the results of the three surgical reconstruction techniques were evaluated. Creation of the RA-PA shunt was the most critical step, the outcome of this being dependent on the technique used. The surgical technique C gave the best overall results. By leaving larger atrial remnants and creating a wide RA-PA anastomosis beginning on the superior vena cava just above the right atrium [8], the pulmonary artery could remain in its natural position, and the need for a patch was eliminated. The angulation between the inflow and outflow ports of the mechanical left ventricle was sufficient to prevent compression of the pulmonary artery by the anteriorly placed aorta.

The creation of an ASD allowed direct right-to-left atrial shunting, maintaining a gradient of about 10 mmHg between the atria when the right atrial pressure was above 12-13 mmHg. This permitted the support of left atrial pressure at the level needed to provide adequate cardiac output while decreasing the required mean right atrial pressure and the concomitant venous hypertension. Although a certain degree of arterial desaturation results from this shunting, the impact of inadequate cardiac output (poor organ perfusion, fluid retention, metabolic acidosis, and increased pulmonary vascular resistance) is far more detrimental than a modest reduction in arterial oxygen saturation. The size of the ASD must be carefully controlled to regulate the amount of the shunt flow.

The effect of phasic abdominal compression on central hemodynamics was evaluated at several points in the postoperative course. The hemodynamic benefit from abdominal compression appears to diminish during the first day after surgery. Similar hemodynamic enhancement was seen in most of the experimental trials.

Physiological Basis
of the Orthotopic Univentricular Artificial Heart

The anatomy and physiology indicate that the right ventricle is a volume pump rather than a pressure pump. At rest and during exercise the right ventricle develops volumes per minute similar to those of the left ventricle, although with lower pressure. Mean pulmonary artery pressure increases approximately 1-3 mmHg for each liter per minute increase in flow. Peak systolic pressure during exercise does not exceed 30-40 mmHg.

The right ventricular pump regulates cardiac output equating venous return. In steady-state conditions, venous return and cardiac output must be equal. Intrinsic properties (contractility) and extrinsic factors (heart rate, preload, afterload) regulate venous return and cardiac output [16].

In normal pulmonary circulation both the increase in cardiac output and the increase in pulmonary artery pressure diminish the vascular resistance. Pulmonary resistance falls either by opening of segments of the pulmonary microcirculation (recruitment) or by distention of minute vessels that are already open. The process of recruitment and derecruitment may be either a function of changes in the geometry of the complex microcirculatory network of the lung or the result of the critical opening and closing pressure [17]. The pulsatile character of pulmonary flow also contributes to increase pulmonary circulation.

Another fundamental aspect of right ventricular function concerns the regulation of venous return [16]. The principal element which contributes to venous return is the pressure gradient between the mean circulatory filling pressure (Pms) and the mean right atrial pressure ($\bar{R}\bar{A}^\pi$). The natural resistance of the venous ductal system and gravitational forces oppose venous return (R). The venous return flow ($\dot{Q}$) can be calculated as follows:

$$\dot{Q} = \text{Pms} - \bar{R}\bar{A}\bar{P}/R. \tag{1}$$

The Pms, which was originally reported by Guyton [18], is the mean pressure of the cardiovascular system when the circulation is arrested, i.e., a condition of nonflow. The factors determining Pms are intravascular volume, capacity of the system (heart chambers, arterial and venous beds), and system compliance.

$$\text{Pms} = V - Vo/C. \tag{2}$$

Vo is the volume necessary to fill the system without generating pressure (system capacity), V is the total intravascular volume (Vo + added volume), and C is the system compliance (V/P). The role of the entire venous bed, especially the splanchnic bed, is essential in the Pms, because its compliance is 20–40 times greater than the arterial compliance.

On the other hand, the right ventricle, as a suction pump [19], maintains a low pressure in the right atrium. Mean right atrial pressure is 5 mmHg or less at rest and does not exceed 10 mmHg during exercise. Consequently, the driving pressure of venous return (Pms-$\bar{R}\bar{A}\bar{P}$) depends on both Pms and right ventricular function.

In spite of the aforementioned data, clinical and experimental evidence demonstrates that the right ventricle is dispensable, i.e., the left ventricle alone is capable of maintaining pulmonary and systemic flow. The Fontan-Kreutzer procedure for tricuspid atresia has proven to be an adequate clinical model to study the physiological consequences of acute and chronic exclusion of the right ventricle. Hemodynamic studies during late follow-up show that cardiac output is lower than that of a normal population, both at rest and during exercise. However, cardiac frequency, pulmonary resistance, and LVEDP are normal. High central venous pressure is stable, 15 ± 4 mmHg at rest and 25 ± 3.6 mmHg during exercise. Arterial oxygen saturation is normal and most patients are in NYHA class I functional capacity [9–20].

In summary, after an RA-PA shunt, RA pressure is capable of maintaining adequate forward pulmonary flow. Indirect clinical evidence indicates that forward flow is enhanced by atrial systole [20]. Studies by the Doppler technique demonstrate that flow is biphasic and antegrade even during left ventricular systole. Peak flow is to be expected during diastole, because it is the moment of higher gradient between the right and left atrium.

High central venous pressure in the Fontan-Kreutzer procedure contributes to preload the left ventricle. However, it may limit venous return. In spite of this apparent hemodynamic limitation, a good functional capacity may be reached.

To study right ventricular exclusion, another clinical model is acute right ventricular infarction. Acute right ventricular dysfunction has two effects: low cardiac output and high central venous pressure. The right atrium and right ventricle become a single functional cavity. The diastolic and mean pressures tend to equalize in the right atrium, right ventricle, and pulmonary artery. Loss of right ventricular pump function is evidenced by the fact that increasing diastolic volume is not followed by an increase in the systolic work index. Aditional right ventricular failure rapidly affects left ventricular indirectly demonstrates this phenomenon.

According to Eq. (2), Pms may be increased by a reduction in system capacity (Vo), an increase in total intravascular volume (V), or a reduction in the system compliance (C).

Expansion of intravascular volume in clinical situations such as right ventricular infarction precisely seeks to increase venous return and thereby increases left ventricular preload. This approach is useful but its effect may be transitory. The high Pms is transmitted backwards, 60%–70%, to the splanchnic microvascular bed because arteriolar sphincters regulate hydrostatic pressure more than do the venous sphincters in the splanchnic microvascular bed. The increase in hydrostatic pressure favors edema formation in the small bowel, liver, and pancreas, with resulting ascites. The buildup of a large third space requires further expansion of the intravascular volume with only transitory hemodynamic improvements.

Another way of increasing Pms, when the intravascular volume is kept constant, is by reducing system capacity or system compliance. Hecks and Doty [13] used external phasic compression of the splanchnic circuit and lower limbs with pneumatic antishock trousers for circulatory assistance after the Fontan-Kreutzer procedure. The immediate response was increasing right and left atrial pressures and cardiac output. Hemodynamic stability with less intravascular expansion was the consequence.

We used phasic abdominal compression in 13 calves that underwent OUAH implantation. Pms increased by 70%, from 15 mmHg without abdominal compression to 25 mmHg during phasic compression (during this measurement the blood pump was arrested). The flow increased from 3.95 l/min to 7.05 l/min [21]. Lloyd [22] has shown that when right atrial pressure is high, flow in the inferior vena cava increases with higher abdominal pressure.

After OUAH implantation, Pms and consequently venous return are the most important determinants of forward flow. In the acute postoperative period, massive blood transfusion is detrimental. It is well recognized that a 50% increase in blood volume causes an increase in Pms from 7 to 20 mmHg. After 2 h, however, the blood volume is still 35% above normal, whereas Pms has returned to normal. This phenomenon of vascular stress relaxation is due to an increase in vascular compliance. Assistance of the splanchnic venous circulation with an abdominal compressor (already proposed by Guyton et al. in 1952) [23] decreases the compliance of the vascular system. The hemodynamic benefit from abdominal compression seems to diminish after the first postoperative day.

Pulmonary Circulation After Implantation of the Orthotopic Univentricular Artificial Heart

Immediate after OUAH implantation, pulmonary circulation hemodynamic behavior may be characterized by: (a) a driving pressure across the vascular bed, (b) a pressure-flow relationship, and (c) pulmonary vascular resistance. In 13 short-term (less than 73 h) in vivo studies in calves with OUAH and phasic abdominal compression, the mean right atrial pressure was 18 ± 3 mmHg (SD) while the mean left atrial pressure was 5 ± 2 mmHg (SD). The gradient between RA and LA pressure was then 13 ± 4 mmHg and, at times, as high as 20 mmHg.

Poiseuille's equation relates pressure (P), flow ($\dot{Q}$), longitudinal distance (l), radius of cross-sectional area (r), and viscosity of the liquid (n), assuming a laminar flow, a rigid system of tubes, and homogeneous perfusate. That is, the driving pressure is proportional to flow and inversely proportional to the 4th power of the radius. The latter bears a disproportionately strong influence on pressure. Morphometric analysis shows that the major site of pulmonary vascular resistance is in the small muscular arteries and arterioles.

Another approach to pulmonary vascular behavior after OUAH is to analyze the pressure-flow curve. This relationship shows how a passive change in pulmonary pressure is evoked by the increase in pulmonary blood flow per se (it is assumed that no change whatsoever occurs in vasomotor activity).

Figure 5 illustrates the mean pulmonary vascular pressure ($\overline{PAP}$) as a function of pump output ($\dot{Q}$). Extrapolated to zero flow, this curve theoretically determines the critical closing pressure (CCP) as defined by Burton [24]. In 13 calves after OUAH implantation the pressure-flow slope was 0.10–0.20 mmHg/l/min and the CCP 18 ± 2 mmHg (SD). In several animals such as dogs and pigs and in experiences or isolated lung as well, the pressure-flow relationship appears linear with normal or high blood flows [25, 26]. In man, the pressure-flow slope is

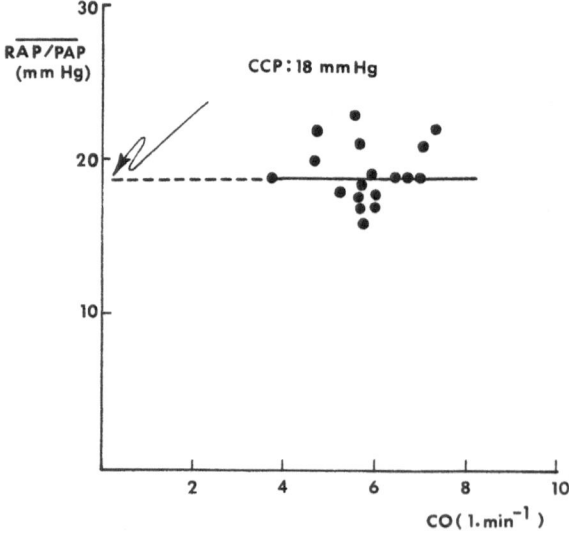

Fig. 5. Pressure-flow relationship after OUAH. *CCP*, critical closing pressure

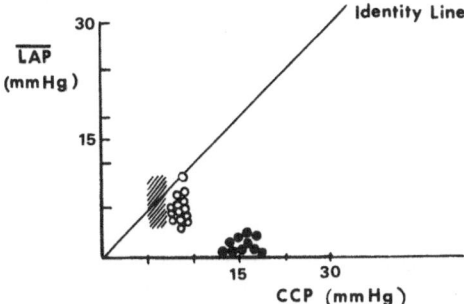

Fig. 6. Relationship between $\overline{\text{LAP}}$ and CCP after OUAH. *Empty circles*, normal CO; *solid circles*, low CO; *shaded area*, CCP corrected

about 1.6 mmHg/l/min/m^2. Physiologically, this incremental resistance means recruitment and distention of pulmonary vessels when facing changes in flow.

IN man, the CCP has been reported to be between 7 and 10 mmHg [27]. Values similar to those appearing in our series have been described in patients with mitral stenosis [27]. *In summary, after OUAH implantation in calves, the pressure-flow curve is characterized by a normal slope and a high CCP.*

It was reported that the pressures responsible for the intrapulmonary distribution of normal pulmonary circulation are $\overline{\text{PAP}}$, alveolar pressure, and pressure in pulmonary veins. In West's lung III zone the driving pressure is set between $\overline{\text{PAP}}$ and vein pressure. According to Starling's model we have been investigating the role of CCP in situations of both normal or high flows and low flow. In both situations CCP is plotted against left atrial pressure ($\overline{\text{LAP}}$) (see Fig. 6). It may be observed that both CCP and $\overline{\text{LAP}}$ look almost superimposed on the identity line. If it is taken into account that CCP is overemphasized [26], it is possible to conclude that, in cases of normal or high flows, the driving pressure is $\overline{\text{PAP}}$-$\overline{\text{LAP}}$. Thus, pulmonary vascular resistance is:

$$R = \overline{\text{RAP}} - \overline{\text{LAP}}/CO.$$

By contrast, in the experiments in which low pulmonary flow was observed, CCP was significantly superior to $\overline{\text{LAP}}$ (18 mmHg vs 3 mmHg), the reason being that the driving pressure was set between $\overline{\text{PAP}}$ and CCP. Thus, pulmonary resistance should be calculated as follows:

$$R = \overline{\text{RAP}} - CCP/CO.$$

Figure 7 shows how isopleth for several CCPs (5, 10, 20, and 30) were calculated as a function of flow. As regards high flows, pulmonary resistance was calculated in the classical form. When cardiac output was either normal or high, pulmonary resistance of 1–2 Wood units shifted along the 10 mmHg CCP isopleth (PAP > Pv > CCP). When the pulmonary flow dropped, resistance increased and shifted along the 20 mmHg isopleth (PAP > CCP > Pv). Our hypothesis suggests that CCP helps to determine the driving pressure through the pulmonary vascular bed as well as the increase in pulmonary resistance with low cardiac output. *A morphological basis for such behavior could be hypertrophy of arteriolar muscle layer.* Without taking into account the hyperreactivity of pulmonary vessels that

D. Liotta et al.

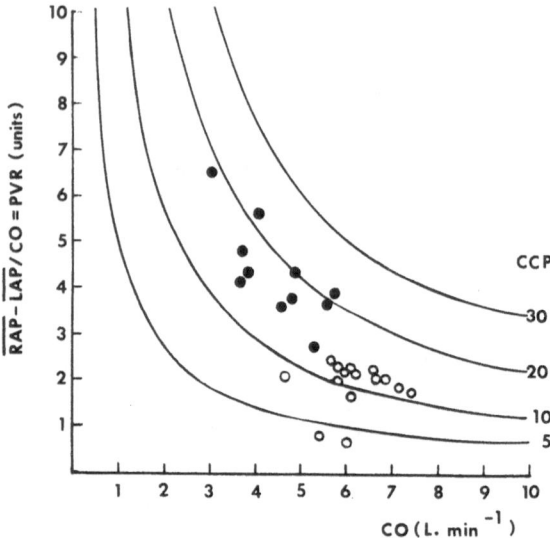

Fig. 7. Pulmonary vascular resistance (*PVR*) as a function of cardiac output (*CO*). *Empty circles*, normal CO; *solid circles*, low CO

calves commonly exhibit in hypoxicemia (i.e., in the case of brisket disease), in this series of animals hemoglobin arterial saturation never dropped below 90%.

During the phasic abdominal compression after OUAH implantation, pulmonary flow was pulse rhythmical. Pulse pressure was lower than preoperative values from 7 to 17 mmHg. Probably, in this situation the predominant mechanism of pulmonary flow increase is pulmonary vessel distention in lieu of recruitment. At the same time, pathological anatomy findings showed basal vascular congestion and interstitial edema (G Burns 1986, unpublished observations).

In summary, increases in CCP elevate pulmonary resistance and diminish the filling of the univentricular prosthesis. In order to maintain normal function of the OUAH, normal pulmonary resistance is essential.

Further experiments in animals other than calves, with less pulmonary vascular reactivity and a lesser splanchnic microvascular bed, are necessary to study the hemodynamics of chronic OUAH implantation.

Acknowledgment. This work was supported by an Alberto Juan Lacroze Grant from the Alfredo Fortabat and Amalia Lacroze de Fortabat Foundation, Buenos Aires, Argentina.

References

1. Olsen DB, Murray KD (1984) In: Unger F (ed) Assisted circulation 2. Springer, Berlin Heidelberg New York Tokyo
2. Kolff J, Deeb GM, Riebman J (1983) Heart Transplantation 3:60–64
3. Joyce LD, DeVries WC, Hastings WL, Olsen DB, Jarvik RK, Kolff W (1983) J Trans Am Soc Artif Intern Organs 29:81
4. Olsen DB, Taenaka Y (1986) In: Bregman D (ed) Critical care clinics: new techniques in mechanical cardiac support, vol 2, no 2. Saunders, Philadelphia, pp 195–207
5. Pierce WS, Morris L, Gardiner BN, Burney RB, Leppik I, Malmud L, Danielson GK (1965) Trans Am Soc Artif Intern Organs 11:271–276

6. Fontan F, Baudet E (1971) Thorax 26:240
7. Kreutzer G, Galindez E, Bono H, de Palma C, Laura JP (1971) Fifth scientific meeting of the Argentinian society of cardiology, August
8. Kreutzer G, Galindez E, Bono H, de Palma C, Laura JP (1973) J Thorac Cardiovasc Surg 66:613–621
9. Laks H, Milliken JC, Perloff JK, Hellenbrand WE, George BL, Chin A, Di Sessa TG, Williams RG (1984) J Thorac Cardiovasc Surg 88:939–951
10. Sanders SP, Wright GB, Keane JF, Norwood WJ, Castaneda AR (1982) Am J Cardiol 49:1733
11. Kreutzer G, Schlichter A, Michelli D, Allaria A, Suarez JC, Román M, Granja M, Rodríguez Coronel A, Berri G, Kreutzer E (1986) Latina Card Inf 2:17, 36
12. Takano H, Taenaka Y, Nakatani T, Umezu M, Matsuda T, Iwata H, Tanaka T, Noda H, Hayashi K, Takatani S, Nakamura T, Seki J, Akutsu T, Manabe H (1984) Trans Am Soc Artif Intern Organs 30:550–554
13. Hecks HA, Doty DB (1981) Circulation 64 [Suppl 2]:118–122
14. Baumgartner WA, Reitz BA, Oyer PE, Stinson EB, Shumway NE (1979) Curr Probl Surg 16:1
15. Olsen DB, Fukumasu H, Kolff J, Nakagaki M, Finch LR, Kolff WJ (1977) Artif Organs 1(2):92
16. Guyton AC (1983) Circulatory physiology: cardiac output and its regulation. Saunders, Philadelphia
17. Fishman AP (1985) Pulmonary circulation. In: Fishman AP, Fisher AB (eds) American Physiological Society, Bethesda, sect 3, vol I, pp 93–165
18. Guyton AC, Polizo D, Armstrong GG (1954) Mean circulatory filling pressure measured immediately after cessation of heart pumping. Am J Physiol 179:261–267
19. Furey SA III, Zieske HA, Levy MN (1984) The essential function of the right ventricle. Am Heart J 107:404–410
20. Shachar GB, Fuhrman BP, Wang Y, Lucas RV, Lock JE (1982) Rest and exercise hemodynamics after the Fontan procedure. Circulation 65:1043–1048
21. Liotta DS, Cooley DA, Navia JA, Frazier OH, Jordana J, del Río PO, Lima Quintana O (1985) Orthotopic univentricular artificial heart. (abstr) Presented ESAO, September
22. Lloyd TC (1983) Effect of inspiration on inferior vena cava blood flow in dogs. J Appl Physiol 55(6):1701–1708
23. Guyton AC, Satterfield JH, Harris JW (1952) Dynamics of central venous resistance with observations on static blood pressure. Am J Physiol 169:691–699
24. Burton AC (1951) On the physical equilibrium of small blood vessels. Am J Physiol 164:319–329
25. Mitzner W, Sylvester JT (1981) Hypoxic vasoconstriction and fluid filtration in pig lungs. J Appl Physiol 51:1065–1071
26. Graham R, Skoog C, Oppenheimer L, Rabson J, Goldberg HS (1982) Critical closure in the canine pulmonary vasculature. Circ Res 50:566–572
27. Mc Gregor M, Sniderman A (1985) On pulmonary vascular resistance: the need for more precise definition. Am J Cardiol 55:217–221

Part V
Heart Transplantation

37. The Artificial Heart as a Complement to Transplantation?

F. UNGER

It is now 20 years ago that Christiaan Barnard performed the first human heart transplantation in South Africa. Following this event, roughly 18 centers performed 180 heart transplants, with disastrous results. Thereafter, only a few centers continued to perform about 50 transplants a year. The introduction of cyclosporin in 1981 made transplantation clinically feasible, and approximately 2000 transplantations were performed worldwide within the past year. The survival rates have improved, thanks to a decreased rate of infection; this is due to triple- and quadruple-drug therapy, whereby cyclosporin and prednisone are reduced in dosage.

To date, over 6800 human beings have received a heart transplant. In 1987, 2200 transplants were performed at 188 centers. The average age of the patients is 42 years (in the heart-lung group the mean age is 32 years); 83% are male. With cyclosporin 85% are alive after 5 years; the actuarial survival curve flattens. For heart-lung recipients the survival is 50% after 1 year and 44% after 2 years.

The etiology of cardiac diseases leading to orthotopic transplantation in the donor-recipient patient cohort is:

- Cardiomyopathy, 55%
- Ischemic heart disease, 40%
- Congenital heart disease, 48%
- Graft rejection, 1%

The 1-year mortality after transplantation is around 27% among patients with congenital heart diseases and graft rejection, 18% in valvular cases, and 10%–12% for patients with cardiomyopathy and ischemic heart disease.

A transplantation is to be considered only when medical therapy does not improve the patient's function class and his or her survival for the next year is estimated at 10%–20%. In cases of acute decompensation the indication can be extended to patients with class-III or -IV disease. Contraindications to transplantation are:

- Age over 60
- Pulmonary vascular resistance of 6–8 WU
- Renal insufficiency
- Shock
- Pulmonary infarction
- Infection
- Severe vascular disease
- Hypertension (diastolic pressure – 105 mmHg)

Assisted Circulation 3
F. Unger (Ed.)
© Springer-Verlag Berlin Heidelberg 1989

- Incapacity to comply with medical therapy
- Diabetes
- Gastric and/or duodenal ulcer
- Malignancy

The main problem is to harvest enough donor hearts, and the waiting lists are growing. As donor availability remains a major problem, older donors are now being accepted. The mean donor age is 25 years (0–53 years). Bridging with an artificial heart reduces the waiting lists temporarily. The need for an alternative, such as an artificial heart for permanent use or a xenograft, is a grave clinical reality. In cases of acute rejection the artificial heart is complementary to a transplantation program.

In this chapter, Dr. Reichenspurner, from Cape Town, reviews the experience of his clinic, which is now headed by Dr. Reichart. In the past 20 years, 112 heart and 14 heart-lung transplantations have been performed. In the former group 51 patients received an orthotopic transplant and 61 a heterotopic transplant. The conclusion reached at the Cape Town clinic is that orthotopic transplantation is the preferable procedure, with a longer survival.

Dr. Tuna, from the Minnesota Heart and Lung Institute headed by Dr. Jamieson, reports their experience with 35 patients who have undergone heart-lung transplantation over the past 6 years. The survival is 70% after 1 year, 58% after 3 years, and 45% after 4 years. The author discusses the indications for and the techniques involved in heart-lung transplantation very extensively and tries to identify predictors of a poor outcome.

Dr. Banner, from the Harefield Hospital headed by Dr. Yacoub, reports on the expanding role of cardiac transplantation. At his institution 488 transplants have been performed, 460 in adults and 28 in children. The techniques are discussed in detail, as is the behavior of the graft. In addition to the surgical techniques for orthotopic transplantation, the roles of heterotopic transplantation, bilateral lung transplantation, domino transplantation, and heart-lung transplantation are discussed relative to the survival rates, which depend in part on the immunosuppressive regimen followed.

Dr. Cabrol, who heads the Department of Cardiovascular Surgery at La Pitie in Paris, relates his experience with regard to the patient- and donor-selection program. At La Pitie over 100 cases a year are treated. Besides the transplant program, Dr. Cabrol has used an artificial heart for bridging in 21 patients.

Dr. Cooper, who was previously in Cape Town and is now in Oklahoma City, discusses the feasibility of a xenograft for transplantation in the sense of an auxiliary heart. He comments on five clinical cases in which he used baboon hearts, based on his experiments. He thinks that a baboon heart might be used as an auxiliary heart to overcome a critical period in cardiac failure.

38. Heart Transplantation in Cape Town – A Review of Twenty Years' Experience

H. Reichenspurner, D. K. C. Cooper, J. A. Odell, D. Novitzky,
P. A. Human, U. von Oppell, E. Becerra, D. H. Boehm, A. Rose,
and B. Reichart

Introduction

Twenty years ago, on 2 December 1967, the first human allogeneic heart transplantation was performed at Groote Schuur Hospital, Cape Town [1]. This operation was based on experimental work by Lower, Stofer, and Shumway [2]. During these 20 years, several notable advances have taken place in this field at Groote Schuur Hospital and elsewhere. The technique of endomyocardial biopsy allowed a precise diagnosis of whether or not acute rejection was present [3]. In 1973, heterotopic heart transplantation was initiated by Barnard and Losman [4]. Since the early 1980s, results of cardiac transplantations have dramatically improved, mainly as a result of the introduction of cyclosporin A and more precise donor and recipient selection [5]. Hormonal therapy for organ donors was introduced in 1983 [6]. In addition, more sophisticated noninvasive monitoring of acute rejection is being undertaken – cytoimmunological monitoring of the peripheral blood and radionuclide scanning of the transplanted heart [7, 8].

In the present study all the mentioned advances are reflected. For the review of the results, our patients were retrospectively analyzed and divided according to the three major immunosuppressive regimens. The respective survival rates and incidence of major complications are compared.

Patients and Methods

Between December 1967 and September 1987, 112 heart and 14 heart-lung transplantations were performed at Groote Schuur Hospital (92% were male and 8% female; the age ranged between 14 and 60 years, with a mean of 40). Sixty-one of the heart transplants were heterotopic and 51 orthotopic.

In 1977, two patients received heterotopic xenografts, one from a baboon and one from a chimpanzee, as emergency procedures, when human donors were not available [9].

In the majority of instances heart recipients had either a dilated cardiomyopathy (48%) or end-stage ischemic heart disease (46%). In others, rheumatic heart disease, endocardial fibrosis, or congenital malformations were a rare indication (6%).

Since 1984, 13 patients have received transplants of the heart and both lungs; two have subsequently undergone retransplantation. The indication for this op-

Assisted Circulation 3
F. Unger (Ed.)
© Springer-Verlag Berlin Heidelberg 1989

Table 1. Indications and outcome in patients after heart and lung transplantation at Groote Schuur Hospital

No.	Pa-tient	Age	Sex	Diagnosis	Date of operation	Results
1	K. St.	27	M	PPH	Feb. 1983	Died 11th p.o. day, acute yellow liver dystrophy
2	A. L.	21	M	PPH	May 1984	Living
3	V. G.	29	F	PPH	May 1985	Reoperation due to chronic obliterative bronchiolitis (May 1986); living
4	L. G.	27	F	Fibrosing alveolitis	June 1985	Died 2 years p.o. from aspergillus septicemia
5	M. F.	19	M	PPH	Aug. 1985	Died after 143 days due to bilateral CMV pneumonia (beginning of the infection 35th p.o. day)
6	S. O.	16	F	After correction of truncus arteriosus, type 1, ES	Jan. 1986	Died on 32nd day due to esophageal fistula, renal insufficiency
7	S. B.	15	M	Double inlet ven-tricle; attempt at correction; pul-monary banding; later on deband-ing, ES	Jan. 1986	Died on 197th p.o. day due to tuberculous pneumonia
8	H. V.	43	M	Lung emphysema	Apr. 1986	Died 4 months p.o. from ruptured false aortic aneurysm
9	G. S.	29	F	After VSD closure, ES	July 1986 (× 2)	Retransplantation, lung dys-function, died on 10th p.o. day
10	F. H.	43	M	Lung fibrosis	July 1986	Living
11	B. G.	44	M	VSD, ES	Jan. 1987	Died 5 weeks p.o., multi-organ failure
12	H. E.	49	M	PPH	July 1987	Died 10 days p.o., multi-organ failure
13	R. E.	27	F	Complete AV-canal; ES	Dec. 1987	Living

CMV, cytomegalovirus; ES, Eisenmenger's syndrome; PPH, primary pulmonary hypertension; VSD, ventricular septal defect; AV, atrio-ventricular

eration was primary pulmonary hypertension in five cases, Eisenmenger's syndrome in five, primary pulmonary fibrosis in one, fibrosing alveolitis in one, and chronic emphysema in one (Table 1).

Until 1985, the number of transplants per year did not exceed ten allogeneic procedures. In 1985, the number of transplants rose to more than ten, and in 1986 23 transplants were done (Fig. 1).

During the 20 years, immunosuppressive medication changed three times considerably. In this review, the patients were divided accordingly (Table 2):

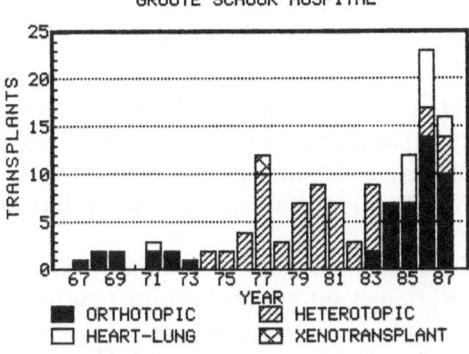

GROOTE SCHUUR HOSPITAL

ORTHOTOPIC   HETEROTOPIC
HEART-LUNG   XENOTRANSPLANT

Fig. 1. Number of heart and heart-lung transplantations per year at Cape Town University

Table 2. Details of the three different patient groups (A, B, and C)

	Group A	Group B	Group C
HTx (*n*)	59	16	37
Pts (*n*)	55	15	32
OHT (*n*)	10	9	32
HHT (*n*)	49	7	5
Immunosuppression	AZA MP ATG	CYA (high dose) MP (high dose)	CYA (low dose) MP (low dose) AZA ATG

ATG, antithymocyte globulin; AZA, azathioprine; CYA, cyclosporin A; HHT, heterotopic transplant; HTx, heart transplantation; MP, methylprednisolone; OHT, arthotopic transplant; Pts, patients

1. *Group A:* "Conventional immunosuppression" (1967–1982): The patients were treated with a combination of azathioprine (2–5 mg/kg/day), methylprednisolone (10 mg/kg/day tapered down to 1 mg/kg/day within 3 months and to 0.5 mg/kg/day within 1 year), and rabbit antithymocyte globulin (RATG, 1–7 mg IgG/kg/day). In this group, 59 transplants were done in 55 patients (10 orthotopic and 49 heterotopic procedures).

2. *Group B:* "High dose cyclosporin A therapy" (1983–1984): This was introduced once cyclosporin A became available. The patients received cyclosporin A in high dosages (18 tapered to 10 mg/kg/day), according to the old Stanford protocol, in combination with methylprednisolone (1.0 mg/kg/day tapered to 0.3 mg/kg/day within 3 months). In this group, 16 heart transplants were done in 15 patients (9 orthotopic, 7 heterotopic transplants).

3. *Group C:* "Quadruple drug therapy" (1984–Sept. 1987): The patients in this group are treated with the following immunosuppressive regimen: cyclosporin A (3–8 mg/kg/day, according to a whole blood trough level of 300–500 ng/ml, radioimmunoassay), in combination with azathioprine (0–2 mg/kg/day) and methylprednisolone (0.3 tapered to 0.1 mg/kg/day) and RATG for the first 4–6 postoperative days (1–4 mg IgG/kg/day, endeavoring to obtain a T-lymphocyte

count of less than 150 cells/mm^3). In addition, RATG is given during severe acute rejections. In this group 37 heart transplants were done in 32 patients (32 orthotopic and 5 heterotopic heart transplants).

Acute rejections were diagnosed by endomyocardial biopsies done when indicated. The results were graded according to a classification by Uys and Rose [10]. Recently, two other noninvasive methods were additionally used: cytoimmunological monitoring of the peripheral blood and radionuclide scanning of the transplanted heart [7, 8].

Chronic rejection as manifested by accelerated coronary artery disease is still a major late postoperative complication. Retransplantation is the only treatment when the cardiac function deteriorates significantly. Repeat procedures were done in ten patients. Three different operative techniques were utilized: Exchange of the organs in heterotopic position was performed in five cases. Replacement of the recipient's heart, leaving the heterotopic graft either in place or removing it, was carried out in three cases. Two third interventions were performed. In these two patients orthotopic transplantation was done by replacing the recipient's own heart and leaving the heterotopic graft in situ. Repeat orthotopic transplants were performed in two patients [11].

Statistical Analysis

In order to compare the outcome and causes of death within the different groups, Fisher's Exact test was used. The survival rates were compared using Log Rank Analysis.

Results

The survival rates of the three patient groups A, B, and C are shown in Fig. 2. For this purpose, the results of orthotopic and heterotopic transplantations were

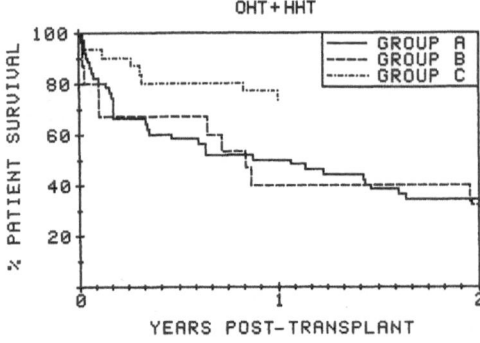

Fig. 2. One- and 2-year survival rates within the different groups A, B, and C. For this calculation, orthotopic (*OHT*) and heterotopic (*HHT*) transplantations were evaluated together. A significant difference in the 1-year survival rate of group C vs groups A and B as evaluated by Log Rank Analysis ($P < 0.05$) is shown

Table 3. Currently used immunosuppressive protocol at Groote Schuur Hospital

Cyclosporin A	3–5 mg/kg/day (whole blood trough level: 300–500 ng/ml)
Azathioprine	0–2 mg/kg/day (WBC > 5000 cells/mm^3)
Prednisolone	0.3–0.15 mg/kg/day
Antithymocyte globulin	2–4 mg IgG/kg/day for 4 days p.o. (T-Ly < 150 cells/mm^3)

combined. The 1- and 2-year survival rates of groups A and B showed no significant difference; at 1 year 48% and 42% of the patients were alive, while after 2 years survival in both groups was 38%. Group C had a significantly better 1-year survival rate than groups A and B (78%, $P < 0.05$). The 2-year survival rate in this group has not been calculated because of small numbers.

In group C, the results within the last 12 months have been analyzed separately. There were 17 orthotopic and 4 heterotopic transplants. Immunosuppressive medication was kept as low as possible (Table 3). One patient died of acute rejection, and a second patient died because of a pulmonary embolus after heterotopic transplantation. Thus, the actuarial survival rate after heart transplantation in the last 12 months (August 1986–September 1987) is 91%.

Orthotopic Transplantations (Fig. 3)

Between 1967 and 1973 and from 1984 until September 1987, 51 orthotopic transplantations were done. Ten transplants were in group A, nine in group B, and 32 in group C. The percentage of patients who are alive and well is significantly higher in group C as compared to groups A and B ($P < 0.05$). One must consider, however, that the follow-up period in groups A and B is much longer than in group C. Groups A and B do not differ significantly with regard to survival. The oldest survivor in group A, 17 years after orthotopic heart transplantation, is presently one of the world's longest living cardiac recipients.

In group A, acute and chronic rejections and infections were the major causes of death (altogether 60%): in group B, unspecific graft failure (10%), infections

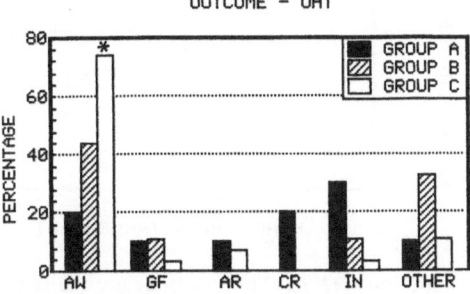

Fig. 3. Results after orthotopic heart transplantation (*OHT*). *AW*, the percentage of patients who are alive and well. The causes of death are as follows: *GF*, graft failure; *AR*, acute rejection; *CR*, chronic rejection; *IN*, infection; *OTHER*, other causes of death, frequently multiorgan failure. *, significant difference from one group to the others as evaluated by Fisher's Exact Test ($P < 0.05$)

(10%), and other complications, particularly multiorgan failure (30%), were the major causes of death. In group C, no prominent cause of death was detected.

Heterotopic Transplantation (Fig. 4)

Sixty-one heterotopic transplantations were done. Forty-nine were in group A. Seven in group B, and five in group C. The percentage of patients in group C who are alive and well is 68% and is therefore significantly higher than in group A or B ($P < 0.05$), although again, groups A, B, and C have different follow-up periods. Within groups A and B, the results do not differ significantly. Acute and chronic rejections and infections were major lethal complications in group A, while complications of multiorgan failure or cerebral emboli were the prominent causes of death in group B. In this respect, group B differs significantly from groups A and C ($P < 0.05$). In group C, no patients have died owing to rejection or infection.

Orthotopic vs Heterotopic Transplantation (Fig. 5)

Orthotopic transplants (groups A, B, and C) are compared with heterotopic procedures (of groups A, B, and C). A similar early 6-month survival rate of 70% was obtained, but in later follow-up the two groups differ significantly: after 2 years 60% of the patients with orthotopic transplantations are alive compared to 42% after heterotopic procedures ($P < 0.05$). Again, one must consider that most heterotopic transplants belong to group A or B.

Acute and Chronic Rejections

Acute and chronic rejection was the major cause of death in group A (30%). The risk has declined to 10% in group B and 6% in group C. Within the last 12

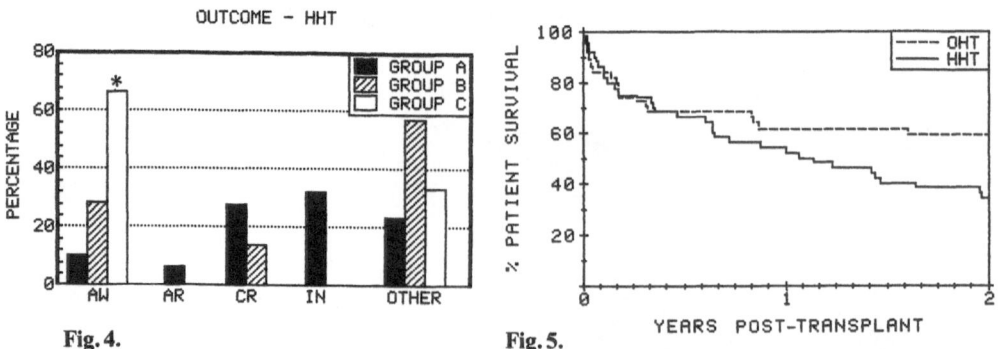

Fig. 4.   **Fig. 5.**

Fig. 4. Results after heterotopic heart transplantation (*HHT*). Abbreviations are the same as those used in Fig. 3. *OTHER*, other causes of death, frequently multiorgan failure and cerebral emboli; * significant difference to other groups ($P < 0.05$)

Fig. 5. Survival rate after heterotopic (*HHT*) and orthotopic (*OHT*) heart transplantation. At 2 years, the two groups differ significantly according to Log Rank Analysis ($P < 0.05$)

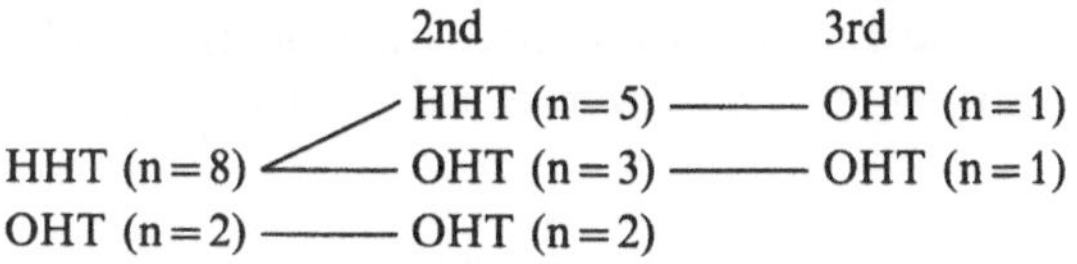

```
          2nd                    3rd
          / HHT (n = 5) ——— OHT (n = 1)
HHT (n = 8) ——— OHT (n = 3) ——— OHT (n = 1)
OHT (n = 2) ——— OHT (n = 2)
```

Fig. 6. Retransplantations at Cape Town University. Operative techniques used in ten patients. *HHT*, heterotopic heart transplantation; *OHT*, orthotopic heart transplantation

months, the rate of acute rejections has dropped to 0.9 per patient per year. When compared to endomyocardial biopsies, radionuclide scanning and cytoimmunological monitoring revealed a sensitivity of 93% and 88% respectively.

Retransplantations (Fig. 6)

Ten heart transplantations were repeated because of severe irreversible chronic rejection. Two interventions were done after orthotopic and eight after initial heterotopic transplantation. Two of these patients had a third intervention. There were no operative deaths. Four survivors are well after the second intervention and one patient after the third [11].

Malignancies

Four patients have developed malignant tumors. Three have died, one from carcinoma of the stomach and two after the diagnosis of Kaposi's sarcoma. One patient with a cerebellar microglioma (after 61 months of immunosuppression) is alive after successful therapy [12].

Complications After Heterotopic Transplantation

Following heterotopic transplantation, thrombus formation within the poorly contracting right or left ventricle of the recipient is not unusual. Therefore anticoagulant therapy is mandatory. Three embolic episodes were fatal. In addition, six nonfatal emboli occurred – three cerebral and three peripheral. However, embolic episodes occurred only in six patients.

Recurrent angina and cardiac arrhythmias in patients with established coronary artery disease of the recipient heart have been very rare following heterotopic transplantation [13].

Heart-Lung Transplantation

Of the 13 patients undergoing transplantation of the heart and both lungs since 1984, eight were weaned from the ventilator and five were discharged from hospital. At present, four patients are alive, 12, 26, and 40 months after transplantation. One of the survivors underwent successful retransplantation after 1 year because of obliterative bronchiolitis in combination with miliary tuberculosis.

The causes of death are listed in Table 1. There were three early deaths resulting from multiorgan failure and six patients died later of infectious complications.

Discussion

The Department of Cardiothoracic Surgery at Groote Schuur Hospital has continued heart and heart-lung transplantation since the first procedure in 1967 done by C. N. Barnard [1]. Disappointing early results were the main reason why most units decided to stop their cardiac transplant program in the late 1960s and early 1970s. However, stimulated by the discovery of cyclosporin A and the improved results with its use, a resurgence of interest in transplantation is occurring [5]. The results have now improved. A 1-year survival rate of nearly 90% is reported from the international registry for heart transplantation [5].

Heart transplantation as a mode of therapy can now be recommended much more liberally than 5 years ago. Basically, the indications for the operation remain much the same as they did in 1967 – namely patients with end-stage heart disease together with a low pulmonary vascular resistance, in whom all forms of medical and conventional surgical therapy have been excluded. In 1987, selection of patients is perhaps less vigorous; e.g., patients in the 6th decade of life may now be considered suitable candidates for the procedure as long as they fulfill the other major requirements for selection, namely in absence of (a) severe irreversible disease of any other major organ, (b) active infection, and (c) severe mental disorders. Insulin-requiring diabetes mellitus is no longer considered an absolute contraindication as patients can be successfully managed without (or with minimal) corticosteroid therapy.

An irreversible pulmonary vascular resistance higher than 5 Wood units is a contraindication for orthotopic heart transplantation, though heterotopic heart transplantation may be performed in the presence of a higher resistance, as long as right ventricular failure has not occurred. In our opinion, heart transplantation is contraindicated if right heart failure is present, because the recipient's heart could not manage with the pulmonary resistance if it exceeds 8 Wood units. In these situations a combined heart and lung transplantation is recommended.

The selection criteria of the donor remain basically unchanged. Male donors over the age of approximately 40 years and female donors over the age of 45 years are excluded unless coronary angiography is normal. No potentially transferable diseases, such as malignancies or infections, should be present. Recently, AIDS is becoming an increasingly important factor in transplantation [14].

Four years ago, hormonal therapy, consisting of triiodothyronine (T_3), cortisol, and insulin, was introduced following extensive experimental work [6]. As a consequence, hemodynamic stability of the donor was nearly always achieved. In some cases, the donor was preserved until the next morning so that the transplantation was then performed as a semielective procedure with the surgical team being rested.

This report analyzes the outcome of three different immunosuppressive regimens. It appeared that cyclosporin A had a major impact only if used in lower dosages. If the results of the "conventional immunosuppression" (group A) were compared with those of high dose cyclosporin A and methylprednisolone (group B), no significant improvement was seen (1-year survival rates of 42% and 48% respectively). Lethal multiorgan failure was more frequent in group B and is probably the result of excessive immunosuppression and cyclosporin A related toxicity. In group C, the dosage of cyclosporin A was therefore drastically reduced by 70% to 3–8 mg/kg/day responding to a whole blood trough level of 300–500 ng/ml. In addition, this drug was combined with azathioprine, low dose methylprednisolone, and an initial course of RATG. As a result, outcome of heterotopic and orthotopic transplantations was significantly improved (1-year survival rate 78%, $P < 0.05$). Within the last 12 months, using a very careful and individualized immunosuppressive protocol (Table 3), the survival rate has been improved to 91%.

Comparing heterotopic and orthotopic transplantation, the latter technique appeared to be the preferable procedure, because the orthotopic technique revealed a significantly better 2-year survival rate. One must consider, however, that most heterotopic transplantations were performed utilizing "conventional immunosuppressive" therapy. In group C (with low dose cyclosporin A), the cumulative 1-year survival rate after heterotopic transplantation has improved to 68%. Presently we would suggest that the following are indications for heterotopic heart transplantation:

1. If only a small donor heart is available for a large recipient who is desperately ill.
2. If irreversible pulmonary vascular resistance of 5–8 Wood units is present (above 8 Wood units, combined heart and lung transplantation is recommended).
3. If acute myocarditis is present. A possibility that the recipient heart might recover then exists; theoretically the donor heart may then be removed because of the risks of immunosuppressive therapy.

Transplantation of the heart and both lungs is restricted to patients with severe pulmonary hypertension, either primary or secondary to congenital malformations (Eisenmenger's syndrome) [15]. In addition, patients with end-stage pulmonary parenchymal diseases and resultant cor pulmonale would also benefit from this procedure. However, the success rate after heart-lung transplantation is still low and in the range of 40%–50% [5, 15, 16].

These initial results of combined heart and lung transplantation show that this procedure has not yet achieved the acceptable results of heart transplantation. An improvement can theoretically be achieved by more careful patient selection, excluding for example, patients with hemodynamically significant tricuspid incompetence resulting in severe, irreversible kidney and liver failure. Pulmonary infections, primarily those caused by *Mycobacterium tuberculosis* and cytomegalovirus (CMV), must be diagnosed early and treated vigorously. CMV infection may be avoided by careful monitoring of donor and recipient antibody status preoperatively. CMV-negative recipients should theoretically not receive organs from a seropositive donor; however, if the recipient is desperately ill, organs can be transplanted if CMV hyperimmunoglobulin is given immediately after transplantation. In order to prevent tuberculosis, which is common in South Africa, isoniazid is given prophylactically to all our patients.

After heart and heart-lung transplantations, acute rejection as a major cause of death is less frequent. This is the result of improved immunosuppression and more sophisticated monitoring, using noninvasive parameters such as cytoimmunological monitoring of the peripheral blood and radionuclide scanning [7, 8]. These techniques allow more accurate timing of endomyocardial biopsies and therefore reduce the number of biopsies necessary to diagnose rejection. In group C, only 0.9 acute rejections per patient occurred.

Diagnosis of rejection after heart-lung transplantation has proved difficult because rejection of either organ may not be synchronous [15, 16]. If present, it is usually encountered early, from the fifth postoperative day onwards. The diagnosis may be suspected clinically by chest radiographs and cytoimmunological monitoring of the peripheral blood. In doubtful cases, endobronchial or, if necessary, open lung biopsies are done.

Chronic rejection remains a major unsolved problem following heart and heart-lung transplantation. Chronic rejection of the heart may manifest as accelerated coronary atherosclerosis and following heart-lung transplantation as obliterative bronchiolitis. This problem is illustrated by two case reports: Patient G.C. had a heterotopic heart transplantation for cardiomyopathy in 1981. In 1983, a retransplantation of the heterotopic heart was done because of chronic rejection. In 1986, again because of accelerated graft atherosclerosis in the second heterotopic heart transplant, the patient was retransplanted by exchanging the recipient's own heart and leaving the heterotopic graft in situ. However, the patient died 6 months later due to a rapid chronic graft rejection in the latest transplanted heart. Another patient, V.G., was retransplanted 1 year after heart and lung transplantation because of chronic rejection, manifested by obliterative bronchiolitis in combination with miliary tuberculosis. At postoperative examination of the heart, high-grade stenotic lesions in the main coronary arteries were additionally found (Fig. 7). One and a half years after the successful retransplantation, this patient again has obliterative bronchiolitis (Fig. 8) and is presently awaiting a third heart and lung transplantation.

The incidence of the development of certain malignant tumors is higher in immunosuppressed patients than in the normal population [17]. In our series, four patients have developed malignant tumors; two patients died of these malignancies. Kaposi's sarcoma led to the death of one patient, in a second patient with this disease, clinical improvement resulted from a reduction of immunosuppression therapy [12]. The patient survived for 3 years but died recently from chronic rejection.

Conclusion

After 20 years, heart transplantation is now an accepted and recommended treatment for end-stage heart failure. It has passed beyond the experimental stage and must now be regarded as therapeutic. The latest survival rate of 91% is encouraging and compares favorably with survival rates after renal transplantation.

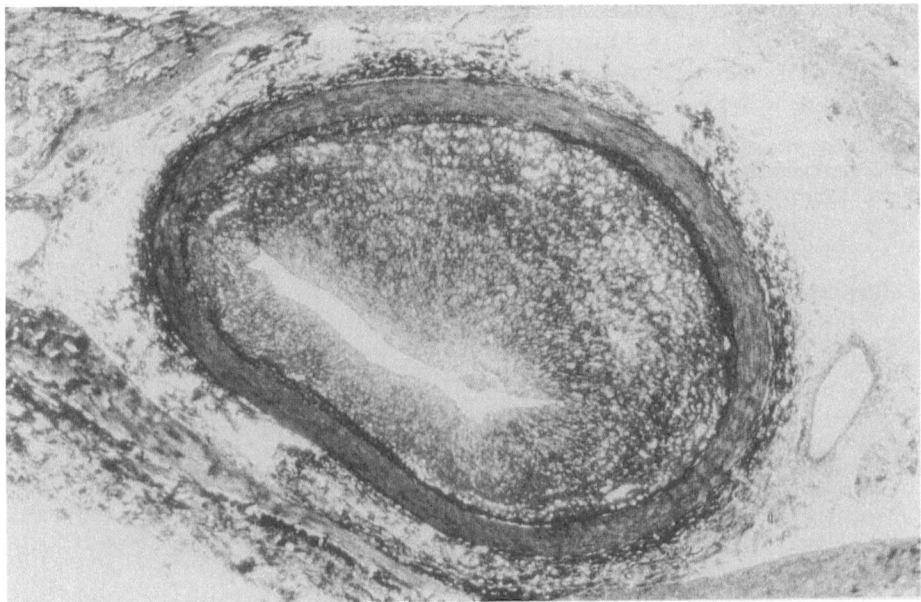

Fig. 7. Chronic rejection of the transplanted heart. Coronary atherosclerosis 1 year after transplantation

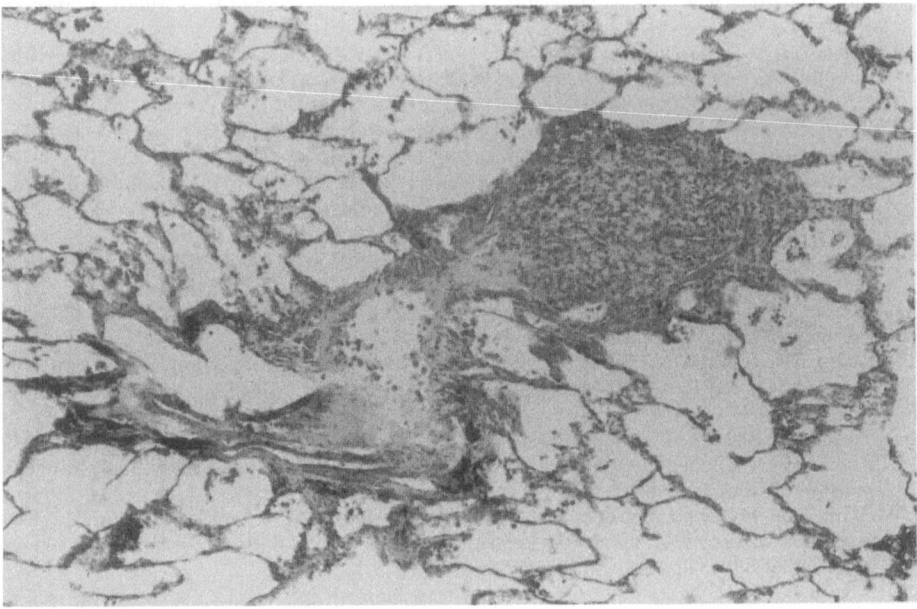

Fig. 8. Another manifestation of chronic rejection is obliterative bronchiolitis in a patient 1 year after heart-lung transplantation

In our opinion, combined heart and lung transplantation is still experimental, but clinically justified in patients who suffer from end-stage pulmonary vascular or pulmonary parenchymal diseases where no other option is presently available.

Acknowledgments. The authors with to express their sincere gratitude to the many members of the medical, nursing, and laboratory staff or Groote Schuur Hospital and the University of Cape Town Medical School who contributed to the care of these patients.

References

1. Barnard CN (1967) The operation, a human cardiac transplant: an interim report of a successful operation at Groote Schuur Hospital, Cape Town. S Afr Med J 41:1271–1274
2. Lower RR, Stofer RC, Shumway NE (1960) Studies on orthotopic heart transplantation of the canine heart. Surg Forum 11:18–21
3. Caves PK, Stinson EB, Graham AF, Billingham ME, Grehl TM, Schumway ND (1973) Percutaneous transvenous endomyocardial biopsy. JAMA 225, 288
4. Barnard CN, Losman JG (1975) Left ventricular bypass. S Afr Med J 49:303
5. Kaye MP (1987) The registry of the international society for heart transplantation: fourth official report – 1987. J Heart Transplant 6:63–67
6. Novitzky D, Wicomb WN, Cooper DKC (1983) Evidence of myocardial and renal functional recovery following hormonal therapy after brain death. Transplant Proc 18:613
7. Reichenspurner H, Kemkes BM, Osterholzer G, Reble B, Reichart B, Hammer C, Steinbeck G, Gokel JM (1986) Particular control of infection and rejection episodes after 4 years cardiac transplantation. Tex Heart Inst J 13:5–12
8. Novitzky D, Cooper DKC, Boniaszczuk J, Isaacs S, Fraser RC, Commerford PJ, Uys CJ, Rose AG, Smith JA, Barnard CN (1985) The significance of the left ventricular volume measurement after heart transplantation using radionuclide technique. J Heart Transplant 4:206–209
9. Barnard CN, Wolpowitz A, Losman JG (1977) Heterotopic cardiac transplantation with a xenograft for assistance of the left heart in cardiogenic shock after cardiopulmonary bypass. S Afr Med J 52:1035
10. Uys CJ, Rose AG (1983) The pathology of cardiac transplantation. In: Silver MD (ed) Cardiovascular pathology. Churchill Livingstone, New York, pp 1329–1352
11. Novitzky D, Cooper DKC, Brink JG, Reichart B (1987) Sequential – second and third – transplants in patients with heterotopic heart allografts. Clin Transplant 1:57–62
12. Bhoopchand A, Cooper DKC, Novitzky D, Rose AG, Reichart B (1986) Regression of Kaposi's sarcoma after reduction of immunosuppressive therapy in a heart transplant patient. J Heart Transplant 5:461–464
13. Cooper DKC (1984) Orthotopic and heterotopic transplantation of the heart: the Cape Town experience. Ann R Coll Surg Engl 66:228–234
14. Rubin RH, Jenkins RL, Shaw BW, Shaffer D, Pearl RH, Erbs S, Monaco AP, Van Thiel DH (1987) The acquired immunodeficiency syndrome and transplantion. Transplantation 44:1–4
15. Reichart B, Blaschke F, Cooper DKC, Novitzky D, Reichenspurner H, Odell JA, Rose AG, Kemkes BM, Klinner W (1987) The transplantation of the heart and both lungs: initial experience of 12 operations in 10 patients. Clin Transplant (in press)
16. Griffith BP, Hardesty RL, Trento A, Paradis J, De Quesnoy RJ, Feen A, Dauber JH, Dummer JS, Thompson ME, Gryfan S, Bahnson HT (1987) Heart-lung transplantation: lessions learned and future hopes. Ann Thorac Surg 43:6–16
17. Penn J (1981) Malignant tumors in organ transplant recipients. Transplant Proc 13:736–738

39. Recent Advances in Combined Heart-Lung Transplantation

I. C. Tuna and S. W. Jamieson

Introduction

Heart-lung transplantation has been successfully applied in the treatment of combined end-stage cardiopulmonary disease for approximately 6 years. Estimates on the number of patients who have undergone heart-lung transplantation during this period range from 100 to 200 persons worldwide, with the most frequent indications for transplantation consisting of primary pulmonary hypertension and end-stage Eisenmenger's complex. The procedure has been successfully performed in both pediatric and adult patients. In the authors' experience, approximately 70% 1-year survival can be expected, with excellent prospects for normal long-term cardiopulmonary function in most patients.

Advances in operative technique and immunosuppressive therapy have resulted in an excellent prospect of immediate benefit from heart-lung transplantation in most patients, but significant long-term morbidity (obstructive airway disease, azotemia, and hypertension) may result in some patients.

Progress towards obviating the undesirable sequelae of heart-lung transplantation, through development of new techniques for the diagnosis of rejection and improved immunosuppressive protocols, as well as recent advances in donor organ procurement, are therefore reviewed below, within the context of clinical heart-lung transplantation as it is currently performed at the Minnesota Heart and Lung Institute of the University of Minnesota.

Historical Background

The evolution of heart-lung transplantation from an investigational endeavor to one of increasing clinical usefulness is summarized in Table 1.

Laboratory investigations begun in the 1950s, and performed in nonprimates, initially suggested that heart-lung transplantation might not prove feasible because of cardiopulmonary denervation and apparent loss of appropriate respiratory drive [1]. Not until 1968, when Cooley performed heart-lung transplantation in a 2-month-old infant (albeit ultimately unsuccessful), was adequate respiratory drive demonstrated in the recipient of a heart-lung transplant [2]. Experience from two additional attempts (unsuccessful) at human heart-lung transplantation by Lillehei and then Barnard, confirmed this observation, and highlighted the inadequacies of available immunosuppressive agents (inhibiting further clinical application of heart-lung transplantations [3, 4].

Assisted Circulation 3
F. Unger (Ed.)
© Springer-Verlag Berlin Heidelberg 1989

Table 1. Historical milestones in heart-lung transplantation

1953–1961	Demikhov, Neptune, Webb, and Lower attempt heart-lung transplantation in laboratory animals (dogs) with limited success
1968	Cooley attempts first human heart-lung transplant
1969	Lillehei performs heart-lung transplantation in man, demonstrates normal, early postoperative pulmonary function
1976	Borel introduces cyclosporin as a potent immunosuppressive agent
1978	First use of cyclosporin in heart transplants in primates
1980	Long-term survival in rhesus and cynomolgus monkeys demonstrated following heart-lung allotransplantation
1981	Long-term success following heart-lung transplantation in man reported

With the introduction of cyclosporin A in 1976, as a potent nonsteroidal immunosuppressive agent, coupled with previous clinical observations, the first successful animal model of heart-lung allotransplantation was developed in primates. Following the demonstration of long-term survival and normal cardiopulmonary function in this model of heart-lung transplantation in 1980, renewed clinical application of heart-lung transplantation was initiated.

After early results in humans with heart-lung transplantation were reported in 1981, subsequent refinements in operative technique (to its present form) and patient selection criteria have optimized clinical results following combined heart-lung transplantation.

Clinical Experience

Current selection criteria, operative technique, and perioperative management of heart-lung transplant recipients at the University of Minnesota Heart and Lung Institute are reviewed.

Donor Selection and Operative Technique

Donor availability has emerged as a major obstacle in the clinical implementation of heart-lung transplantation. The scarcity of adequate donors arises primarily from the dual requirement for both the pulmonary and the cardiac status of potential donors to meet strict criteria for suitability.

Typically, prospective donors have sustained traumatic cerebral injury which in many cases may be accompanied by significant pulmonary injury. Prolonged periods of artificial ventilation also predispose many potential donors to pulmonary infection. Prospective donors therefore undergo screening for significant chest trauma, ideally have undergone artificial ventilation for less than 5 days, and should have no evidence of grossly contaminated pulmonary secretions. Normal chest radiography and arterial blood gases (PO_2 more than 100 mmHg with inspired fraction of O_2 40% or less) are required. On the suitability of a donor

Table 2. Criteria for heart-lung donor selection

Age less than 45 years
No significant chest trauma
Normal chest radiograph
PaO$_2$ greater than 100 mmHg with fraction of inspired O$_2$ less than 40%
Normal peak airway pressures
Normal cardiac status (normal EKG, blood pressure)

has been ascertained, matching with a prospective recipient is performed, based on ABO blood group compatibility and body size. Matching for organ size is most readily achieved by comparison of chest radiographs (taken at comparable magnification), with an ideal match consisting of donor lung fields slightly smaller than those of the recipient. Criteria for heart-lung donor selection are summarized in Table 2.

Donor Organ Harvesting

Donor organs have historically been in an operating room adjacent to that containing the recipient. Long-distance transport is now considered satisfactory for routine use. Final suitability of the donor organs for transplantation (i.e., lack of pulmonary trauma) is ascertained at the time of harvest, by visually examining the heart-lung bloc after exposure through a median sternotomy. Following mobilization of the great vessels, innominate artery, and venae cavae, the trachea is encircled high in the mediastinum (to preserve carinal collateral blood supply), and infusion catheters are placed in the pulmonary artery and ascending aorta. Harvesting of the heart-lung bloc is initiated with division of the inferior vena cava, aortic occlusion, and administration of cardioplegic solution. Simultaneously a modified Collins' solution is infused into the pulmonary artery to aid in pulmonary preservation. With administration of cardioplegic solution (approximately 10 ml/kg) and Collins' solution (60 ml/kg), the aorta and superior vena cava are divided, the trachea clamped high in the mediastinum (with the lungs partially inflated), divided, and the pulmonary ligaments transected. With harvesting completed, the heart-lung bloc is immersed in cold Ringer's solution pending implantation.

Recipient Selection and Operative Technique

Recipients for combined heart-lung transplantation typically possess the general characteristics of cardiac transplant recipients in addition to having terminal pulmonary disease [5, 6]. Ideally suited candidates for transplantation do not have a history of major thoracic or cardiovascular surgery, and are free of ongoing bronchopulmonary sepsis. Selection and exclusion criteria for heart-lung transplant recipients are summarized in Table 3.

Table 3. Criteria for heart-lung recipient selection

Age less than 45 years
End-stage heart-lung disease (New York Heart Association class III or IV)
No evidence of concurrent systemic illness (sepsis, neoplasia, diabetes)
No prior major cardiothoracic surgery
Creatinine clearance > 50 cc/min
Bilirubin < 3.0 g/%

Heart-Lung Transplantation

The technical aspects of the preparation of the recipient for heart-lung transplantation which are critical involve the removal of the native heart and lungs with maintenance of strict hemostasis (recipients typically possess well developed collateral bronchial blood vessels) and preservation of phrenic, vagus, and recurrent laryngeal nerve integrity.

Excision of the native heart and lungs is performed through a median sternotomy, allowing evaluation of both pleural spaces for intrathoracic adhesions. Division of these adhesions prior to the initiation of total cardiopulmonary bypass has proven helpful in the prevention of postoperative hemorrhage. In preparation for transplantation, the native heart is excised as for isolated cardiac transplantation. The left phrenic nerve is preserved on a pericardial pedicle, and the left pulmonary veins mobilized (incorporating the left half of the posterior left atrial wall). The pulmonary ligament is divided, and bronchial collaterals (especially abundant in Eisenmenger's complex) identified and ligated. With division of the left pulmonary artery and main stem bronchus, the native left lung is removed. Resection of the right lung is carried out in a similar manner. Tailoring of the trachea at the level of the carina and excision of pulmonary artery remnants (leaving a small button of tissue in the area of the ligamentum arteriosum to preserve recurrent laryngeal nerve function) complete the preparation of the recipient (Fig. 1).

Implantation of the heart-lung bloc begins with anastomosis of the donor and recipient trachea, at the level of the carina (Fig. 2). Topical cooling is used until donor and recipient atrium and aorta are anastomosed, completing implantation (Figs. 3, 4). Positive pressure ventilation and weaning from cardiopulmonary bypass complete the procedure.

Postoperative Management

Immunosuppressive Therapy
Early postoperative immunosuppressive therapy is aimed at preventing heart and lung rejection while simultaneously promoting healing of the tracheal anastomosis. This can be achieved through the use of high dose cyclosporin A given orally (12–18 mg/kg/day, to achieve serum levels of 200 ng/ml), and azathioprine (1.5 mg/kg/day, adjusted according to white blood cell count). With the exception of parenteral steroids administered on the day of surgery, corticosteroids are

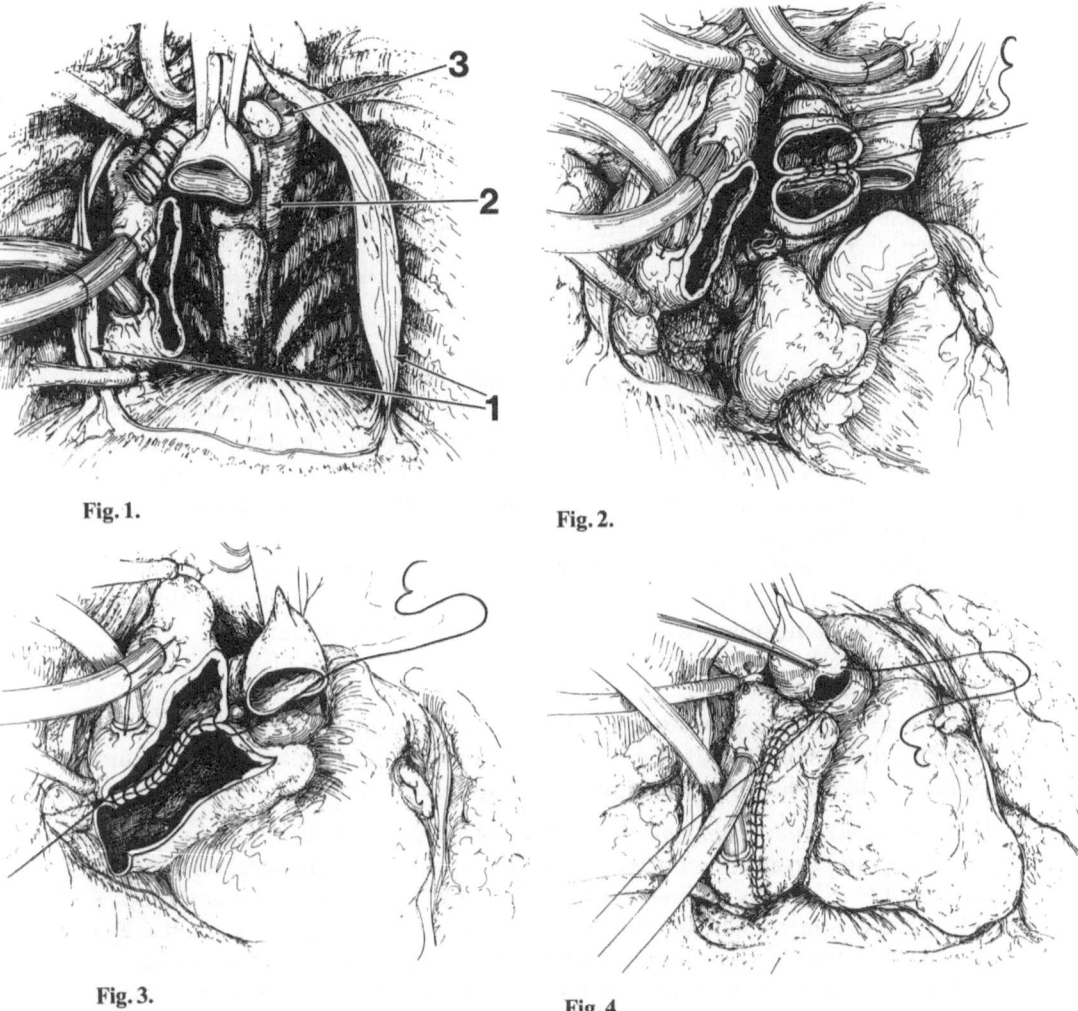

Fig. 1.

Fig. 2.

Fig. 3.

Fig. 4.

Fig. 1. Appearance of the thoracic cavity following preparation of the heart-lung recipient (excision of native lungs and heart), demonstrating (*1*) preservation of the phrenic nerves bilaterally on pericardial pedicles, (*2*) the location of the vagi in the posterior mediastinum, and (*3*) sparing of the recurrent laryngeal nerve by preservation of a small button of pulmonary artery at the level of the ligamentum arteriosum. The aorta, trachea, and right atrium have been tailored for implantation

Fig. 2. Implantation of the heart-lung bloc begins with anastomosis of the trachea, utilizing a single continuous monofilament suture. The donor lungs have been passed beneath the pedicled phrenic nerves into their respective thoracic cavities

Fig. 3. The right atrium is tailored with a curvilinear incision extending from the inferior vena cava towards the right atrial appendage. The donor atrium is then anastomosed to the recipient atrium using a single monofilament suture

Fig. 4. Implantation of the heart-lung bloc is continued with anastomosis of the donor and recipient aorta

Table 4. Immunosuppressive therapy

Early postoperative therapy:
High dose cyclosporin (12–18 mg/kg/day – serum levels 200 ng/ml)
Moderate dose azathioprine (1.5 mg/kg/day)
No corticosteroids

Maintenance therapy
Prednisone therapy added (0.2 mg/kg/day)
Cyclosporin tapered slowly to maintenance levels (trough levels of 150–100 ng/ml)
Continued therapy with azathioprine

---

avoided for approximately 2 weeks following transplantation, in an attempt to promote healing of the tracheal anastomosis. Oral prednisone therapy at 0.2 mg/kg/day is then added to the cyclosporin and azathioprine. The adequacy of immunosuppressive therapy is assessed by daily determination of cyclosporin levels, weekly endomyocardial biopsy, and frequent evaluation of chest radiographs and arterial blood gases.

Evidence of early acute rejection (either heart or lung) is treated with methylprednisone 1 g i.v. daily for 3 days, supplemented by antithymocyte globulin if necessary. Immunosuppresive protocols are summarized in Table 4.

General Medical Care
Abnormalities in early postoperative lung function may represent pulmonary capillary leak, atelectasis, infection, or rejection, with all possibilities requiring evaluation to guide in the selection of appropriate therapy.

Early Postoperative Management. Early postoperative medical care is aimed at preserving and promoting normal lung function. Fluid status is carefully monitored and hydration is minimized since the pulmonary lymphatics have been divided, and the lung tends to retain water. Emphasis is placed on early extubation and the initiation of vigorous chest physiotherapy and breathing exercises.

Close monitoring of renal function is required in the early postoperative period due to a high incidence of postoperative renal failure requiring transient hemodialysis. Renal failure in the early postoperative period may arise as a result of several factors, including the nephrotoxicity of cyclosporin, intentional underhydration in order to decrease lung water, and exacerbation of preexisting renal failure as a result of cardiopulmonary bypass.

Reverse isolation procedures and filtration of room air (to reduce fungal spore and bacterial counts) is also desirable, to minimize the risk of acquired pulmonary infection when high levels of immunosuppressive agents are used in the early postoperative period. Table 5 summarizes the general medical postoperative care of heart-lung transplant recipients.

Late Postoperative Management. The long-term management of heart-lung recipients is directed towards the diagnosis and treatment of acute episodes of heart and lung rejection, and the evaluation of patients for evidence of obliterative bronchiolitis and proliferative coronary vascular disease (probably representing

Table 5. General medical care: early postoperative management

Hydration kept to a minimum
Vigorous chest physiotherapy
Early extubation
Monitoring of renal function (30% incidence of renal failure requiring transient hemodialysis)
Reverse isolation and filtration of room air

chronic lung and heart rejection, respectively). Hypertension or azotemia may also persist late postoperatively, and require additional medical management.

Early clinical monitoring for lung rejection was based on the premise that heart and lung rejection progressed together [8]. Thus results of endomyocardial biopsy were used to evaluate both organs for evidence of rejection. Subsequent clinical and laboratory experience demonstrated that isolated pulmonary rejection could occur in the absence of heart rejection [7]. Therefore, pulmonary rejection must be additionally evaluated through the use of pulmonary function tests, arterial blood gases, and chest radiography. Lung rejection is typically accompanied by a decrease in arterial PO_2. Pulmonary function tests may show an obstructive ventilatory defect superimposed on any preexisting postoperative restrictive changes, with mean expiratory flow (MEF25-75) and PaO_2 appearing to be sensitive indicators of rejection. Forced expiratory volume at 1 s (FEV_1) and the ratio of FEV_1 to forced vital capacity (FVC) also appear decreased with rejection. A 10% change in any of these variables requires further evaluation. Chest radiography, while helpful, appears less sensitive, but may show nodular infiltrates or peribronchial thickening during episodes of pulmonary rejection.

The usefulness of transbronchial biopsy and bronchial lavage for the diagnosis of acute lung rejection remains unclear, and these procedures are not used at our institute.

Late episodes of either heart or lung rejection are treated with high dose oral prednisone therapy, initiated at 100 mg/day. Dosage is gradually tapered to approximately 30 mg/day and maintained there for approximately 1 month.

The late sequelae of heart-lung transplantation may also include airway obstruction secondary to obstructive bronchiolitis, recurrent pulmonary infection, bronchiectasis, and pulmonary fibrosis [9]. Serial evaluation of pulmonary function (as outlined above) is therefore essential. Bronchoscopy with transbronchial or endobronchial biopsy, as well as open lung biopsy, is useful in the diagnosis of obliterative bronchiolitis. With the early detection of deterioration in pulmonary function (when an infectious course has been excluded), high dose corticosteroid therapy should be initiated and may reverse pulmonary abnormalities. With persistence or progression of pulmonary abnormalities following medical management, retransplantation may prove necessary.

Similarly, concentric coronary atherosclerosis may be a late sequela of heart-lung transplantation and can result in fatal myocardial infarction [9, 10]. If significant graft disease is detected by coronary angiography, retransplantation of the heart may be required.

Postoperative hypertension, a well recognized consequence of cyclosporin therapy in heart transplant patients, is common in heart-lung transplant recipients as well, and typically requires treatment with diuretics and vasodilators. Progressive renal dysfunction as a result of cyclosporin is also common and may complicate immunosuppressive management with this agent [11].

Results

The results discussed below are based upon our experience in 35 patients operated on over the past 6 years [12]. Actuarial survival at 1, 3, and 4 years for these patients was 70%, 58%, and 45%, respectively. Factors identified as predictive of poor outcome are discussed.

Perioperative Mortality

Of 36 heart-lung transplants performed (including one retransplantation), eight patients died within 30 days of surgery, representing a mortality of approximately 25%. Four deaths were related to hemorrhage, while two patients died of bronchopneumonia, one of multisystem organ failure, and one of adult respiratory distress syndrome. The four patients with hemorrhage had massive perioperative bleeding from extensive adhesions as a result of prior cardiothoracic surgery. Though this was controlled at the time of operation, the administration of multiple units of blood and blood products resulted in poor pulmonary function, prolonged intubation, sepsis, and death.

Perioperative Morbidity

Early experience with heart-lung transplantation was associated with injury to the recurrent laryngeal nerve or vagus nerve in two of the first three recipients. The operative technique was subsequently modified, with removal of the heart and lungs individually rather than en bloc [6], and no further nerve injuries have been evident.

Long-Term Results

Of 28 survivors of combined heart-lung transplantation (a single patient retransplanted 35 months after initial operation is counted twice), all had normal cardiopulmonary function on discharge from hospital. Subsequently, ten patients developed evidence of airway obstruction and hypoxemia, with a mean time to onset of 11.2 months postoperatively (range 2–35 months). Evidence of obliterative bronchiolitis was found at autopsy or open lung biopsy in seven of these patients. The remaining three demonstrated bronchitis and bronchiolitis on transbronchial biopsy. Obstructive bronchiolitis proved to be progressive in eight of ten patients, of whom four died. One patient was successfully retransplanted. In two patients who developed airway obstruction and hypoxemia, high dose corticosteroid therapy was successful in completely reversing symptoms in one, and partially resolving symptoms in the other.

Table 6. Pulmonary function in uncomplicated heart-lung transplant recipients (% predicted, mean ± SD). (Adapted from [12])

	Early	Late
FVC	64 ± 17	66 ± 14
FEV_1	73 ± 18	71 ± 14
FEV_1/FVC	88 ± 8	84 ± 4
FEF25-75	84 ± 43	74 ± 11
DLCO	77 ± 26	102 ± 6
PaO_2 (mmHg)	89 ± 8	88 ± 7

FVC, forced vital capacity; FEV_1, forced expiratory volume at 1 s; FEF25-75, forced expiratory flow from 25% to 75% of FFVC; DLCO, CO diffusion capacity

Table 7. Hemodynamics pre- and postoperatively in heart-lung transplant recipients. (Adapted from [10])

	Preoperative values	Postoperative values
Blood pressure (mmHg)	89 ± 11	118 ± 17*
Cardiac output (l/min)	4 ± 2	6 ± 2*
Cardiac index (l/min/m^2)	3 ± 3	4 ± 1
PAP (mmHg)	75 ± 19	9 ± 3*
PACWP (mmHg)	6 ± 4	3 ± 2
PVR (Wood units)	18 ± 11	1 ± 1*
PaO_2 (mmHg)	52 ± 23	88 ± 7*
$PaCO_2$ (mmHg)	28 ± 4	36 ± 4*

* $P < 0.05$ preoperative vs postoperative
PAP, pulmonary artery pressure (mean); PACWP, pulmonary artery capillary wedge pressure; PVR, pulmonary vascular resistance

In contrast, the remainder of heart-lung transplant recipient survivors have near normal pulmonary function at a mean of 22.6 months following transplantation (range 4–42 months). A minor restrictive ventilatory defect was seen in all patients, with the remainder of pulmonary mechanics essentially normal (Table 6). In addition, hemodynamic parameters appear normal after transplantation (Table 7).

Discussion

Combined heart-lung transplantation has been demonstrated to be compatible with near normal cardiopulmonary function in man, despite the acute loss of cardiopulmonary innervation, bronchial arterial supply, and pulmonary lymphatic drainage. With careful recipient selection (having identified prior cardiothoracic surgery as a major determinant of postoperative hemorrhage), a significant reduction in operative mortality has been achieved. With improvements in operative mortality, widened applicability of this procedure to other patients with end-stage cardiopulmonary failure should be possible.

While long-term survival and maintenance of normal graft function following heart-lung transplantation is possible, the emergence of postoperative obstructive bronchiolitis as a significant late complication of transplantation requires on-going patient surveillance and therapy, and improvement in techniques for assessing status of lung rejection.

Of seven patients with bronchiolitis who came to necropsy or underwent open lung biopsy, pulmonary arteriolar vessels demonstrated concentric intimal fibrosis (in six) or perivascular lymphocytic cuffing (in three). Additionally, concentric coronary atherosclerosis was seen in five of these patients. Perivascular lymphocytic infiltrates have been associated with pulmonary rejection in animals, while recent work in rats suggests that the early stages of lung rejection may involve infiltration of bronchus-associated lymphoid tissues and pulmonary vessels by host lymphocytes [13]. Thus, obliterative bronchiolitis probably represents the clinical manifestation of chronic low-grade pulmonary rejection, analogous to chronic vascular rejection seen in cardiac transplant recipients.

Consistent with this interpretation is the apparent lack of efficacy in the treatment of bronchiolitis with antibiotics, bronchodilators, or chest physiotherapy. Further, when diagnosed early, corticosteroids appear effective in reversing the otherwise progressive course of this process. Thus, while abnormalities in mucociliary transport, chronic infection, and cyclosporin toxicity have all been implicated in the etiology of obstructive bronchiolitis, chronic rejection would appear to represent the most likely cause. Current immunosuppressive therapy, at least for patients developing this complication, would therefore appear to be inadequate.

Cyclosporin therapy is responsible for significant hypertension and nephrotoxicity following transplantation (with all patients in this series developing some degree of impaired renal function).

The implementation of triple drug immunosuppressive therapy in the long term, consisting of low doses of cyclosporin (to achieve serum trough levels of 50–80 ng/ml), prednisone (0.2 mg/kg/day), and azathioprine (1.5 mg/kg/day) has been demonstrated to ameliorate hypertension and the nephrotoxic effects that accompany conventional immunosuppressive therapy. Improvement in immunosuppressive efficacy is also suspected (reduced incidence of rejection episodes on endomyocardial biopsy among heart transplant recipients), and this may reduce the incidence of obstructive bronchiolitis in heart-lung transplant recipients as well.

Finally, the routine use of improved techniques for distal procurement and prolonged preservation of donor organs is required to expand the availability of suitable donors. Heart-lung perfusion "ex vivo" has been used to prolong donor organ ischemia time for up to 4 h with variable results [14]. Simple techniques such as flushing of the donor organ bloc with cold saline may ultimately prove to extend donor organ protection for up to 6 h following harvest, and are currently being evaluated [15].

In summary, heart-lung transplantation has evolved from a laboratory technique to a clinically applicable procedure for selected patients with end-stage heart-lung failure. While advances in operative technique and immunosuppressive therapy now offer patients an excellent chance for long-term normal cardiopulmonary function, significant morbidity (obstructive bronchiolitis, azotemia, and hypertension) accompanies the procedure for some. Advances in immunosuppressive therapy, techniques for the diagnosis of lung rejection, and improved heart-lung preservation techniques are required before heart-lung transplantation can be considered a routine procedure.

References

1. Haglin J, Telander RL, Muzzaal RE, Kiser JC, Strobel CJ (1963) Comparison of lung autotransplantation in the primate and dog. Surg Forum 14:196
2. Cooley DA, Bordwell RD, Hallman GL (1969) Organ transplantation for advanced cardiopulmonary disease. Ann Thorac Surg 8:30
3. Wildervuur CR, Benfied JR (1970) A review of 23 human lung transplants by 20 surgeons. Ann Thorac Surg 9:489
4. Reitz BA, Burton NA, Jamieson SW, Bieber CP, Pennock JL, Stinson EB, Shumway NE (1980) Heart and lung transplantation: autotransplantation and allotransplantation in primates with extended survival. J Thorac Cardiovasc Surg 80:360
5. Jamieson SW, Stinson EB, Oyer PE, Baldwin JC, Shumway NE (1984) Operative technique for heart-lung transplantation. J Thorac Cardiovasc Surg 87:930
6. Jamieson SW (1986) Heart-lung transplantation. In: Jamieson SW, Shumway NE (eds) Rob and Smith's operative surgery. Mosby, St Louis, pp 594–605
7. McGregor CG, Baldwin JC, Jamieson SW (1985) Isolated pulmonary rejection after combined heart and lung transplantation. Thorac Cardiovasc Surg 90:623
8. Reitz BA, Gaudiani VA, Hunt SA, Wallwork J, Billingham ME, Oyer PE, Baumgartner WA, Jamieson SW, Stinson EB, Shumway NE (1983) Diagnosis and treatment of allograft rejection in heart-lung transplant patients. J Thorac Cardiovasc Surg 85:354
9. Burke CM, Theodore J, Dawkins KD, Yousem SA, Blank N, Billingham ME, VanKessel A, Jamieson SW, Baldwin JC, Oyer PE, Stinson EB, Shumway NE, Robin ED (1984) Posttransplant obliterative bronchiolitis and other late lung sequelae in human heart-lung transplantation. Chest 86:824
10. Dawkins KD, Jamieson SW, Hunt SA, Baldwin JC, Burke CM, Morris A, Billingham ME, Theodore J, Oyer PE, Stinson EB, Shumway NE (1985) Long-term results, hemodynamics, and complications after combined heart-lung transplantation. Circulation 71:919
11. Myers BD, Ross J, Newton L, Leutscher J, Perlroth M (1984) Cyclosporine A associated chronic nephropathy in potentially irreversible renal injury. N Engl J Med 311:699
12. Burke CM, Baldwin JC, Morris AJ, Shumway NE, Theodore J, Tazelaar HD, McGregor C, Robin ED, Jamieson SW (1986) Twenty-eight cases of human heart-lung transplants. Lancet:517
13. Prop J, Wildevuur CR, Nieuwenhuis P (1985) Lung allograft rejection after combined heart and lung transplantation. J Thorac Cardiovasc Surg 90:623
14. Ladowski JS, Kapelanski DD, Teodori MF, Stevenson WC, Hardesty RL, Griffith BP (1985) Experimental use of an autoperfusing heart-lung bloc for organ preservation prior to heart-lung transplantation. Heart Transplant 4(2):128
15. Starkey TD, Sakakibara N, Hagberg RC, Baldwin JC, Jamieson SW (1985) Successful six hour cardiopulmonary preservation with simple hypothermic crystalloid flush. Heart Transplant 4(6):601

40. The Expanding Role of Cardiac Transplantation

N. R. Banner, A. Khaghani, M. Fitzgerald, A. G. Mitchell,
R. Radley-Smith, and M. H. Yacoub

Introduction

Increasing experience in cardiac transplantation has been associated with an improvement in results and a rapid growth in the number of transplants performed for end-stage cardiac failure (Fig. 1). A variety of immunosuppressive regimens based on cyclosporin are now in use. Since September 1982 we have used a regimen of cyclosporin and azathioprine (CYA/AZA) with a policy of minimizing the use of oral steroids and, whenever possible, avoiding their long-term use. The results of this policy have recently been reviewed [1]. It has allowed us to transplant patients in the paediatric and older age-groups and also patients with concomitant diseases which would previously have been considered contraindications to transplantation (such as diabetes or peptic ulceration). The demand for cardiac transplantation continues to exceed the availability of donor organs, and this has led us to explore ways of making optimal use of the donor organ pool by using the hearts from smaller donors for heterotopic transplantation, using bi-

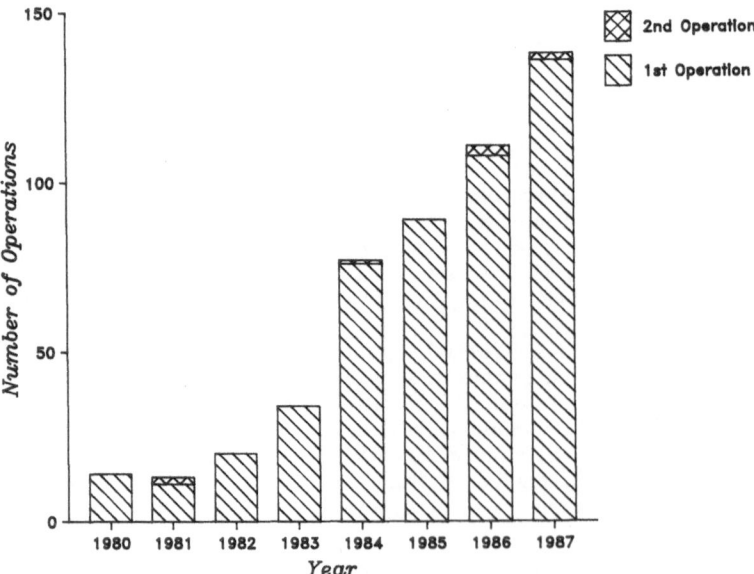

Fig. 1. Number of cardiac transplants per year at Harefield Hospital 1980–1987

Assisted Circulation 3
F. Unger (Ed.)
© Springer-Verlag Berlin Heidelberg 1989

lateral lung transplantation instead of combined heart-lung transplantation for patients with parenchymal lung disease (to allow the use of the donor heart for another recipient) and, more recently, by the "domino" technique of using the heart from a heart-lung transplant recipient for a cardiac transplant candidate.

Indications

The main indication for cardiac transplantation is severe cardiac failure when the patient's quality of life and functional capacity are poor and his life expectancy limited. The common causes for cardiac failure in our transplant recipients are ischaemic heart disease and cardiomyopathy, although a small proportion of patients have undergone transplantation for other indications (Fig. 2). Substantial progress has been made in the drug treatment of advanced cardiac failure [2], and it is important to optimize the transplant candidate's therapy during the assessment and waiting period. The introduction of the CYA/AZA regimen has allowed us to transplant patients over the age of 55 years and to include children in the programme. The first paediatric transplant was performed in August 1984. The age range of patients who have undergone transplantation in our unit is from 9 days to 68 years (Fig. 3).

Patients with medical conditions which were previously considered contraindications have undergone transplantation using the CYA/AZA regimen, including patients with previous peptic ulceration, insulin-dependent diabetes (without nephropathy or retinopathy) and unresolved pulmonary emboli [1, 3]. Patients with a history of systemic hypertension or peripheral vascular disease have been considered operable unless they had evidence of cerebral atherosclerosis. Renal dysfunction secondary to cardiac failure is not a contraindication to transplantation. Patients who have chronic renal failure due to intrinsic renal disease may be considered for combined heart and kidney transplantation. A previous history of alcoholism, depressive illness, ulcerative colitis, autoimmune disease or malig-

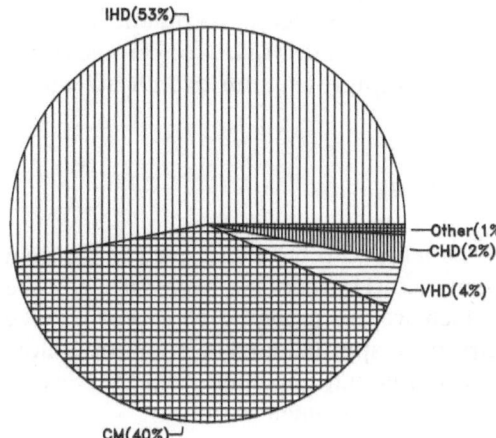

Fig. 2. Indications for cardiac transplantation in 488 recipients. *IHD*, ischaemic heart disease; *CM*, cardiomyopathy; *VHD*, valvular heart disease; *CHD*, congenital heart disease

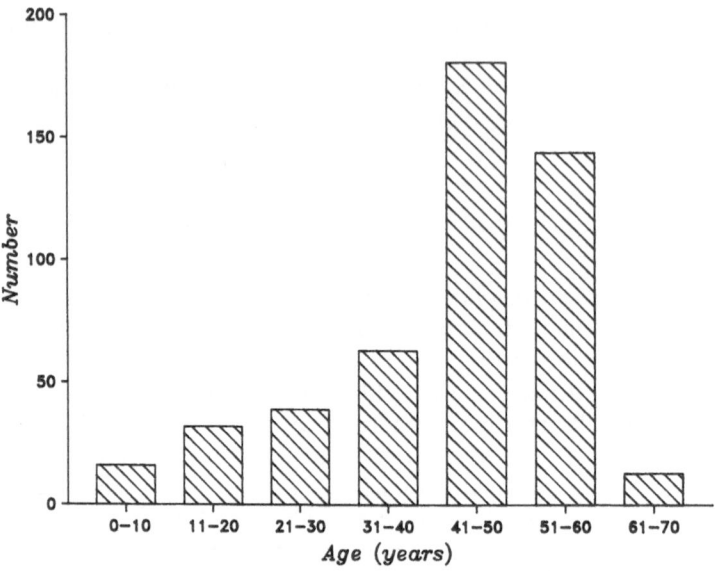

Fig. 3. Age distribution of 488 cardiac transplant recipients

nancy need not be a contraindication to transplantation, providing the condition has been effectively treated. Candidates with chronic liver disease, HBsAg carrier status or anti-HIV antibodies are not considered suitable for transplantation. Candidates must be able to comply with the requirements of drug therapy and monitoring after transplantation.

Donor Selection: Expanding the Donor Pool

The introduction of ventricular assist devices and the total artificial heart as a "bridge" to cardiac transplantation are important advances which may allow the stabilization of transplant candidates whilst a donor heart is being sought. However, until long-term maintenance with these devices becomes a practical proposition, they will not affect the overall shortage of donor organs for cardiac transplantation. This has led us to explore ways of improving our overall utilization of the donor organs available.

Conventional Cardiac Donors: Extended Criteria

The majority of our donors have been patients who have sustained brain-stem death (usually because of trauma or spontaneous intracranial haemorrhage). We have gradually increased the age at which we are prepared to accept cardiac donors for older cardiac transplant recipients – approximately 6% of our donors have been 40 years of age or older [1]. Currently, our upper age limit for conventional donors is 45 years for men and 50 years for women.

The donor's previous medical history is reviewed in as much detail as possible to exclude pre-existing cardiovascular disease and other significant conditions. Long-standing hypertension resulting in left ventricular hypertrophy (based on ECG criteria) is regarded as a contraindication to organ harvesting. Chest trauma, including haemopneumothorax, in the absence of clinical or electrocardiographic signs of myocardial contusion, is not considered a contraindication. Events and procedures during resuscitation of the donor must also be reviewed – short periods of cardiac or respiratory arrest are not, in themselves, considered contraindications, provided there is no evidence of permanent cardiac damage.

A careful examination of the cardiovascular system is required when cardiac output and blood pressure are adequate. Cardiac function is assessed by the adequacy of peripheral and renal perfusion together with the amount of inotropic support required. Infusions of crystalloid and colloid solutions are usually required to expand the circulating volume – a common cause of excessive inotrope requirements is inadequate volume replacement. If very large urine volumes occur as a result of diabetes insipidus following brain death, vasopressin may be used (provided it is acceptable to the renal and liver transplant units involved). The presence of persistent unexplained tachycardia, a third heart sound, and electrocardiographic evidence of myocardial infarction are considered contraindications.

Repolarization changes on the ECG are common after brain death – ST- and T-wave changes alone are not contraindications to organ harvesting. Pathological Q waves and LVH on voltage criteria are not acceptable. Echocardiography, when available at the donor hospital, can help in assessing donor LV function. Preoperative coronary angiography on the donor heart is usually impractical.

Donors are screened for HBsAg and HIV antibodies. We do not use donors from high-risk groups for HIV infection, in order to avoid false-negative antibody results in the "window period" early after infection. Pneumonia and other types of localized bacterial infections are treated with large doses of the appropriate antibiotics. Whenever possible the donor is tested for CMV antibodies – we attempt to use CMV-positive donors only for CMV-positive recipients.

The Potential Role of Bilateral Lung Transplantation

Three patients have undergone bilateral lung transplantation (rather than combined heart-lung transplantation) at our hospital for parenchymal lung disease. This procedure offers the opportunity of using the donor heart for a cardiac transplant candidate. Unfortunately, all three bilateral lung transplant recipients have developed problems with stenosis of the tracheal anastomosis or the major bronchi. Although all three patients are alive, one has required retransplantation (using the combined heart-lung procedure) and a second is awaiting retransplantation. Improvements in the surgical technique for bilateral lung transplantation (perhaps employing the "omental wrap" which has been used for single lung transplantation [4]) will probably allow this procedure to be used more widely in the future and allow donor hearts to be used for cardiac transplant recipients. Single lung transplantation offers the same advantage [4], but it appears that its application will be limited to patients with pulmonary fibrosis.

Living Donors: the "Domino" Transplant

Another approach to the problem is to use the heart from a heart/lung transplant recipient with parenchymal lung disease or pulmonary vascular disease for a cardiac transplant recipient – the "domino" transplant. The heart-lung recipient can undergo detailed cardiac evaluation including coronary angiography (to excluded coronary artery disease) at the time of transplant assessment, and this has allowed us to increase the upper age limit for cardiac donors. The procedure requires a modification of the surgical technique used for heart-lung transplantation (see below). We have used this technique in 25 transplants and the immediate function of the transplanted heart has been excellent in every case. The procedure allows relatively short cold ischaemia times (particularly if both operations are performed in the same hospital), and the donor heart is not exposed to the adverse neural, endocrine and metabolic changes associated with brain death.

Donor-Recipient Matching

The donor and the recipient are matched for ABO blood group and, for orthotopic cardiac transplantation, body size. A direct cross-match between the donor's lymphocytes and the patient's serum is performed whenever possible. A negative cross-match is insisted upon if the patient is known to have cytotoxic antibodies or has undergone previous transplantation. We have retrospectively analysed our data to examine the influence of HLA matching on graft survival in cardiac transplant recipients. It appears that HLA DR (class II) matching is important: the 2-year survival for patients with one DR mismatch was 84%, and for those with two DR mismatches it was 68% [5]. At the present time, prospective HLA matching for cardiac transplantation is usually impractical because of the distance between the donor hospital and our unit and the difficulties associated with performing full tissue typing on peripheral blood samples in the limited time available.

Approach to the Cardiac Transplant Candidate
with an Elevated Pulmonary Vascular Resistance

Increased pulmonary vascular resistance (PVR) is an incremental risk factor for orthotopic cardiac transplantation because of the danger of right ventricular failure in the donor heart. In patients with a high PVR it is essential to exclude irreversible pulmonary vascular disease due to causes such as multiple pulmonary emboli, plexogenic pulmonary arteriopathy (secondary to long-standing left-to-right shunts) or obliterative disease secondary to parenchymal lung disease.

We have used several techniques to cope with a moderately elevated PVR (5–8 Wood units) with no evidence of an irreversible underlying cause. If a donor heart that is larger than that of the recipient becomes available, the donor heart will usually be able to cope with the elevation in PVR. In addition, hearts from donors over the age of 30 years tend to have fairly well developed right ventricles. Heterotopic cardiac transplantation may be used so that the recipient's own right ventricle assists the donor right ventricle in the postoperative period. The recent use of the "domino" transplant technique provides us with a source of donor hearts with secondary right ventricular hypertrophy which appear ideal for this type of transplant recipient.

Patients with irreversible pulmonary vascular disease or severe pulmonary hypertension (PVR > 8 Wood units) require combined heart and lung transplantation.

Heterotopic Cardiac Transplantation

Heterotopic transplantation continues to be of value for a minority of cardiac transplant recipients (approximately 10% of our patients). We have used the procedure when the recipient has been much larger than the available donor, in cases of moderately elevated PVR, and where there seems to be a possibility of a useful recovery in recipient cardiac function. These cases have included patients with a recent onset of congestive cardiomyopathy, those with left ventricular dysfunction following cardiac surgery (which was judged to be at least partly reversible), and patients with ischaemic heart disease who had large myocardial scars or aneurysms, but in whom the remaining myocardium appeared to be capable of providing useful function (in these latter cases, heterotopic transplantation was combined with aneurysmectomy and coronary artery bypass grafting). In addition to the general contraindications to cardiac transplantation, heterotopic transplantation is contraindicated in patients with significant valve disease (which cannot be repaired without the use of prosthetic materials), the presence of a large amount of intracardiac thrombus in the native heart, residual myocardium which cannot be satisfactorily revascularized, or arrhythmias of the native heart which require long-term drug therapy.

Preoperative Care

Patients awaiting cardiac transplantation receive conventional drug therapy for cardiac failure with diuretics and vasodilators [2, 6]. Those who are immobile or who have evidence of intracardiac thrombus on the echocardiogram are at increased risk of pulmonary or systemic embolism and are anticoagulated. Individuals with serious ventricular arrhythmias require appropriate drug therapy and are given priority for early transplantation. Patients who become dependent on intravenous inotropic support are also regarded as priority cases. Central venous catheters are avoided whenever possible because of the potential risk of infection, but they are necessary for administering many vasoactive drugs. Worsening cardiovascular function often reflects deteriorating ventricular function, but remediable factors should be sought (e.g. infection, arrhythmias, pulmonary embolism, adverse response to vasodilators, hypovolaemia due to excessive diuresis). When these measures fail, mechanical circulatory support is required.

Surgical Considerations

Excision of Donor Heart

Organ harvesting is performed at the donor's hospital. Nearly all cardiac donors also provide other transplant organs. This requires co-ordination of the various transplant teams involved both before and during the organ harvesting procedure. Preliminary dissection and preparation for perfusion of the kidneys and liver are normally made before the cardiac procedure begins [7]. Our technique for harvesting the heart differs slightly from that used by most other centres, in that cardioplegia and surface cooling are performed simultaneously after the heart has been excised.

The donor's sternum is split and the pericardium opened. The heart is carefully inspected to confirm that it is suitable for transplantation. At this stage, if heparin has not already been given by the other transplant surgeons, it is administered in a dose of 3 mg/kg. If there is a central venous catheter in situ, either the tip is withdrawn to a point high in the superior vena cava (to lie outside the surgical field) or the catheter is removed completely. The inferior vena cava (IVC) is transected as close as possible to the diaphragm, allowing the heart to empty. Two suckers placed in the pericardium help to keep the surgical field clear during further dissection. The left and right pulmonary veins are then divided as far away from the heart as possible. At this stage the heart is lifted up and the pericardial reflection onto the left atrium is incised to free the heart from the pericardium posteriorly. The aorta is divided near the origin of the brachiocephalic artery and the pulmonary arteries are divided distal to the bifurcation of the pulmonary trunk. Finally, the superior vena cava (SVC) is cut as high up as possible to leave a good length of vein attached to the right atrium (RA).

The excised heart is removed from the operative field and placed in a sterile bowl containing Hartmann's solution at 4 °C. The aorta is then cross-clamped and 1 l of cold crystalloid cardioplegia solution is perfused into the root of the aorta. The advantages of this technique are that it allows simultaneous surface cooling of the heart and perfusion of the coronary arteries and that it removes the cardiac surgeon from the operative field, allowing the other surgeons better access whilst harvesting organs.

When the cooling and perfusion have been completed, the heart, placed in cold Hartmann's solution, is wrapped serially in several sterile polythene bags and packed loosely with crushed ice in an insulated container for transportation.

Orthotopic Transplantation: Conventional Technique

Until recently we have used a technique based on that originally described by Cass and Brock [8] and Lower and Shumway [9], which was subsequently adapted for clinical use [10, 11].

Excision of the Recipient's Heart. The pericardium is opened via a median sternotomy. Cardiopulmonary bypass is established with arterial return to the ascending aorta. The SVC and IVC are cannulated separately via the right atrium, using

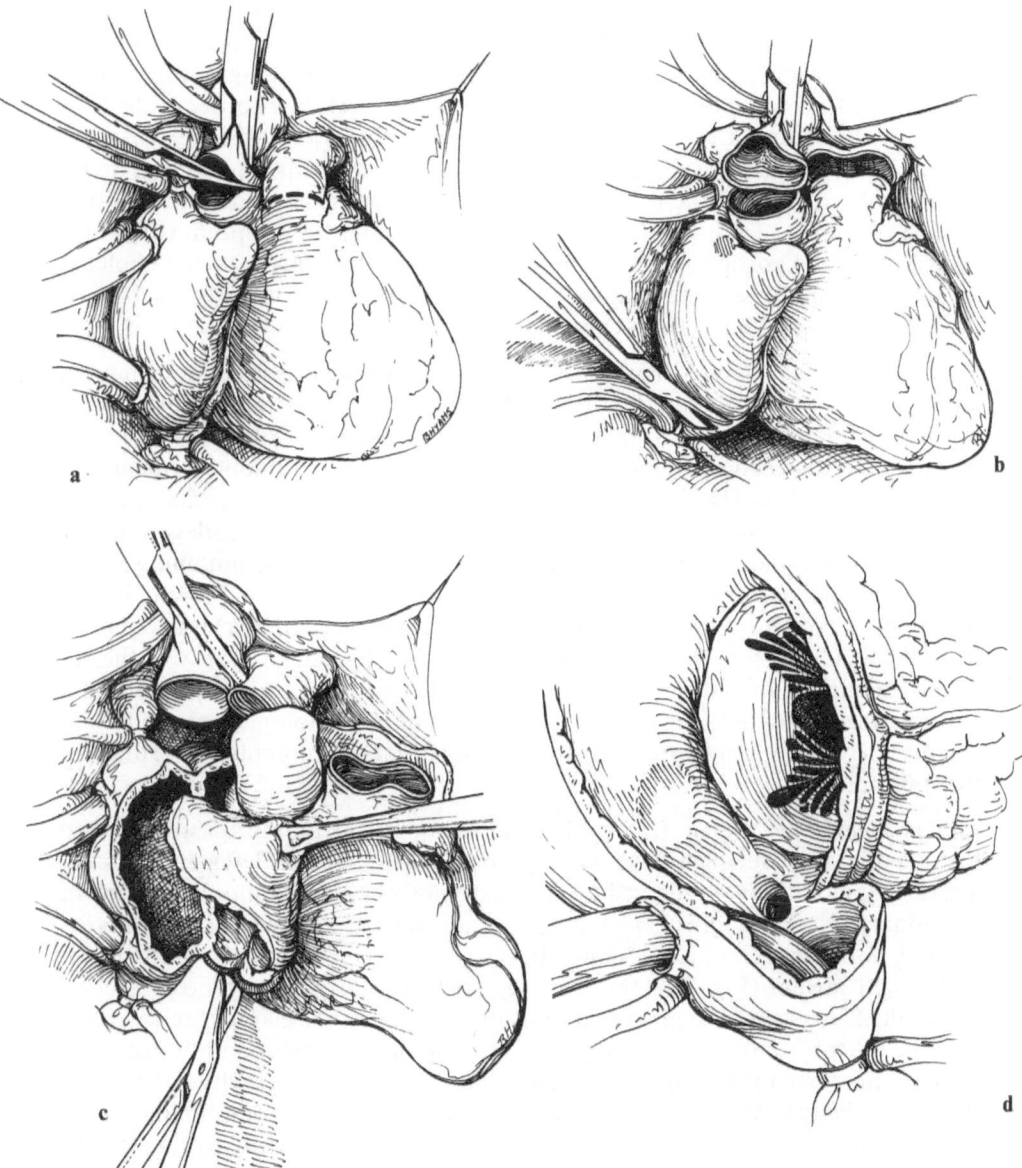

Fig. 4 a–d. Conventional orthotopic transplantation – excision of recipient heart. **a** Division of recipient's aorta; **b** incision in right atrium; **c, d** extension of right atrial incision into coronary sinus

entry points which are located as far posterior as possible near the caval orifices. The heart is fibrillated electrically and the aorta clamped. The diseased heart is then excised, starting by dividing the ascending aorta about 1.5 cm below the aortic clamp (Fig. 4a). The main pulmonary artery (PA) is then transected just above the top of the commissures of the pulmonary valve, avoiding dissection between the aorta and pulmonary artery, as the medial wall of the PA tends to be thin. An incision is then made in the lateral wall of the RA starting at a point between the RA appendage and the SVC cannulation site, extending downwards in front of the IVC cannulation site, to curve around the inferior border of the RA, aiming at the orifice of the coronary sinus (Fig. 4 b). Superiorly, the incision is extended along the medial aspect of the RA appendage towards the junction of the aortic root and roof of the left atrium (LA). The latter is then incised leftwards towards the base of the left atrial appendage. The interatrial septum is then incised as near the aortic root as possible. Excision of the heart is then completed by cutting along the coronary sinus, starting from its orifice, towards the base of the left atrial appendage (Fig. 4 c and d).

Preparation of the Donor Heart. The aorta and pulmonary artery are trimmed, leaving only short segments of aortic and pulmonary arterial wall above the respective semilunar valves for anastomosis. This prevents kinking of the PA and projection of the aortic root into the atria, which could occur if long segments are left behind (particularly if the donor heart is large relative to the recipient). The RA is then incised from the orifice of the IVC towards the RA appendage, curving anteriorly and avoiding the area of the sinoatrial (SA) node and adjoining posterior internodal pathway (Fig. 5 b). The SVC-RA junction is explored. If any thrombus is present (related to a previous central venous catheter) it is removed from the SVC and sent for culture. The SVC is then ligated. A biopsy of the endocardial surface of the right ventricle is then performed through the tricuspid valve and the specimen is sent for histological and immunological examination. Finally, the left atrium is prepared by making an incision joining the orifices of the four pulmonary veins.

Implantation of the Donor Heart. First the donor left atrium is anastomosed to the remnant of the recipient LA, starting from the region of the left atrial appendage (Figs. 5 a, b). This is followed by an anastomosis between donor and recipient pulmonary arteries (Fig. 5 c). The donor aorta is then joined to the recipient's ascending aorta and, finally, the donor RA is sutured to the remnant of the recipient's right atrium (Fig. 5 d). Immediately after the aortic anastomosis is completed the LV is vented to prevent distension, and the aortic clamp is released before the other anastomoses are completed to minimize the period of "warm ischaemia" (time from inserting the the heart into the pericardial cavity to releasing the aortic clamp). After all the anastomoses are complete, cardiopulmonary bypass is continued until cardiac function has recovered sufficiently to support the circulation.

Surgical Considerations in Children. The same surgical technique is employed in children. Slowly absorbable sutures (polydioxanone) are used for all anastomoses to allow for subsequent growth. Careful matching of donor and recipient for size and age is required. Children with even moderately elevated PVR probably require either combined heart-lung transplantation or a "domino" cardiac transplant from a heart-lung recipient with secondary right ventricular hypertrophy (see below).

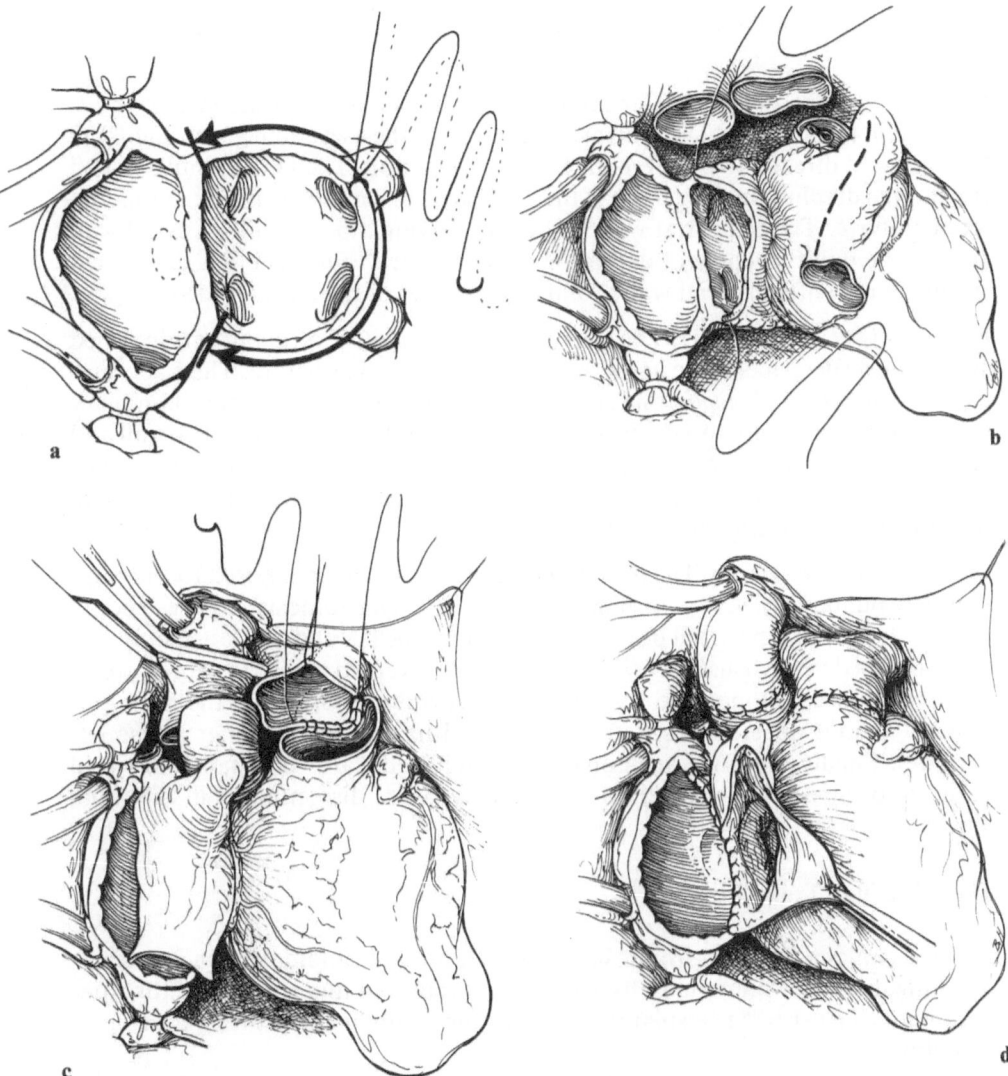

Fig. 5 a–d. Conventional technique – insertion of donor heart. **a** Commencement of left atrial anastomosis; **b** continuation of LA anastomosis onto interatrial septum (*dotted line* marks the incision made in donor RA for the subsequent anastomosis to recipient RA); **c** anastomosis of donor and recipient PA; **d** right atrial anastomosis

An Alternative Technique for Orthotopic Transplantation

We have recently developed and used a technique for orthotopic cardiac transplantation which preserves the atria of the donor heart intact and which may, theoretically, provide better mechanical and electrophysiological atrial function. The separate SVC and IVC anastomoses used in this technique also provide a method for replacing the heart of a heart-lung transplant recipient whose own heart has been removed intact to be used as the donor organ for a cardiac recipient transplant.

Preparation of the Recipient. Cardiopulmonary bypass is established with venous cannulae in the SVC and IVC and arterial return to the ascending aorta. The SVC is cannulated directly to preserve the SVC-RA junction. The IVC cannula is sited close to the diaphragm. The heart is then removed in a manner similar to that described above. The left atrial wall is excised, leaving a 5 mm cuff of atrial wall around the point of entry of each pair of pulmonary veins. The RA is resected leaving 5 mm cuffs of atrial wall around the orifices of the SVC and IVC.

Preparation of Donor Heart. The donor heart is excised, cooled and cardiopleged as previously described. The aorta and PA are prepared as before. The LA is prepared by making an incision on each side joining the upper and lower pulmonary veins to form two common orifices to which the patches of recipient LA wall and attached pulmonary veins will be anastomosed. The openings can, if necessary, be enlarged by making a small incision from the inferior edge of each opening in the direction of the circumflex coronary artery.

Insertion of Donor Heart. The left pulmonary veins are anastomosed to the common left pulmonary venous orifice (Fig. 6 a). This anastomosis requires special care, as its medial aspect will be inaccessible later. The PA and aortic anastomoses are completed in the usual way (Fig. 6 b). The LV is vented before the aortic crossclamp is released. Donor and recipient IVC are anastomosed and the right pulmonary venous anastomosis is then completed in the same manner as the left (Fig. 6 c). Finally, the SVC anastomosis is completed, care being taken to avoid damage to the SA node. Cardiopulmonary bypass is discontinued in the usual way.

The "Domino" Transplant

In this technique the heart from a heart-lung transplant candidate with parenchymal lung disease or pulmonary hypertension is removed intact and used for a patient requiring cardiac transplantation when the combined heart-lung transplant is performed.

Removal of the Heart from a Heart-Lung Transplant Recipient. Cardiopulmonary bypass is established (see "Alternative Technique – Preparation of Recipient" above), the heart fibrillated and the aorta cross-clamped. The IVC is divided as close to the RA as possible, care being taken to leave enough IVC behind for subsequent anastomosis with the the IVC of the heart-lung block. The pulmonary veins are divided well away from the LA (Fig. 7 a). The heart is lifted anteriorly and freed from the posterior pericardium (Fig. 7 b). The right and left pulmonary arteries are divided as far laterally as possible. The aorta is divided just below the cross-clamp, which has been positioned to leave an adequate length of ascending aorta on each side of the division for subsequent anastomosis. The SVC is divided close to the RA, but care must be taken to leave enough SVC attached to the RA to avoid damage to the SA node. The heart is then removed from the pericardial cavity (Fig. 7 c) to be surface cooled and cardiopleged as previously described.

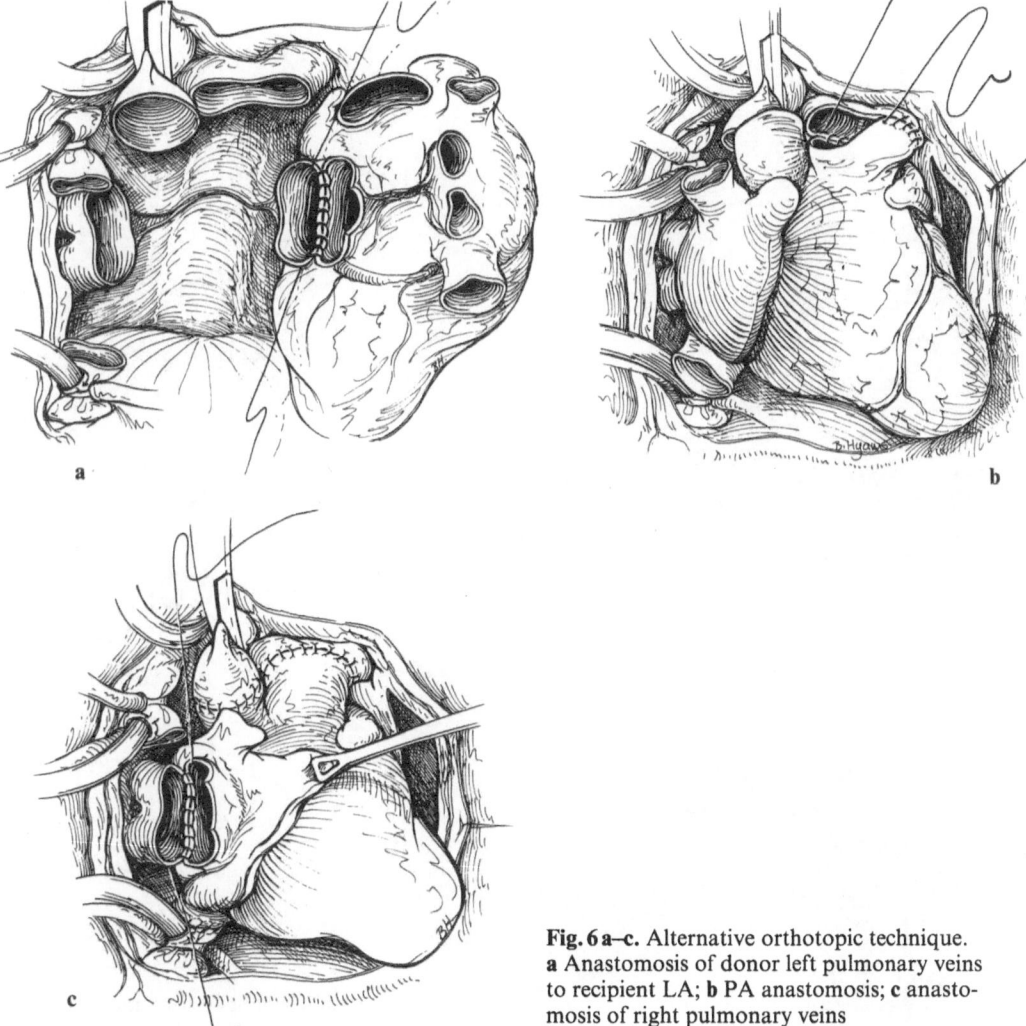

a

b

c

Fig. 6 a–c. Alternative orthotopic technique. **a** Anastomosis of donor left pulmonary veins to recipient LA; **b** PA anastomosis; **c** anastomosis of right pulmonary veins

The lungs are subsequently removed through lateral incisions in the pericardium prior to inserting the heart-lung block.

Implantation of the "Domino" Heart. The heart is prepared by oversewing the orifice of the SVC with a 4/0 polypropylene monofilament suture, taking care to preserve the SA node. Subsequent preparation and insertion are as described in the section "Conventional Technique." If an ASD is present in the donor heart it is repaired before implantation.

Modifications in the Heart-Lung Procedure. Our conventional technique for inserting the combined heart-lung block is based on that developed at Stanford [12].

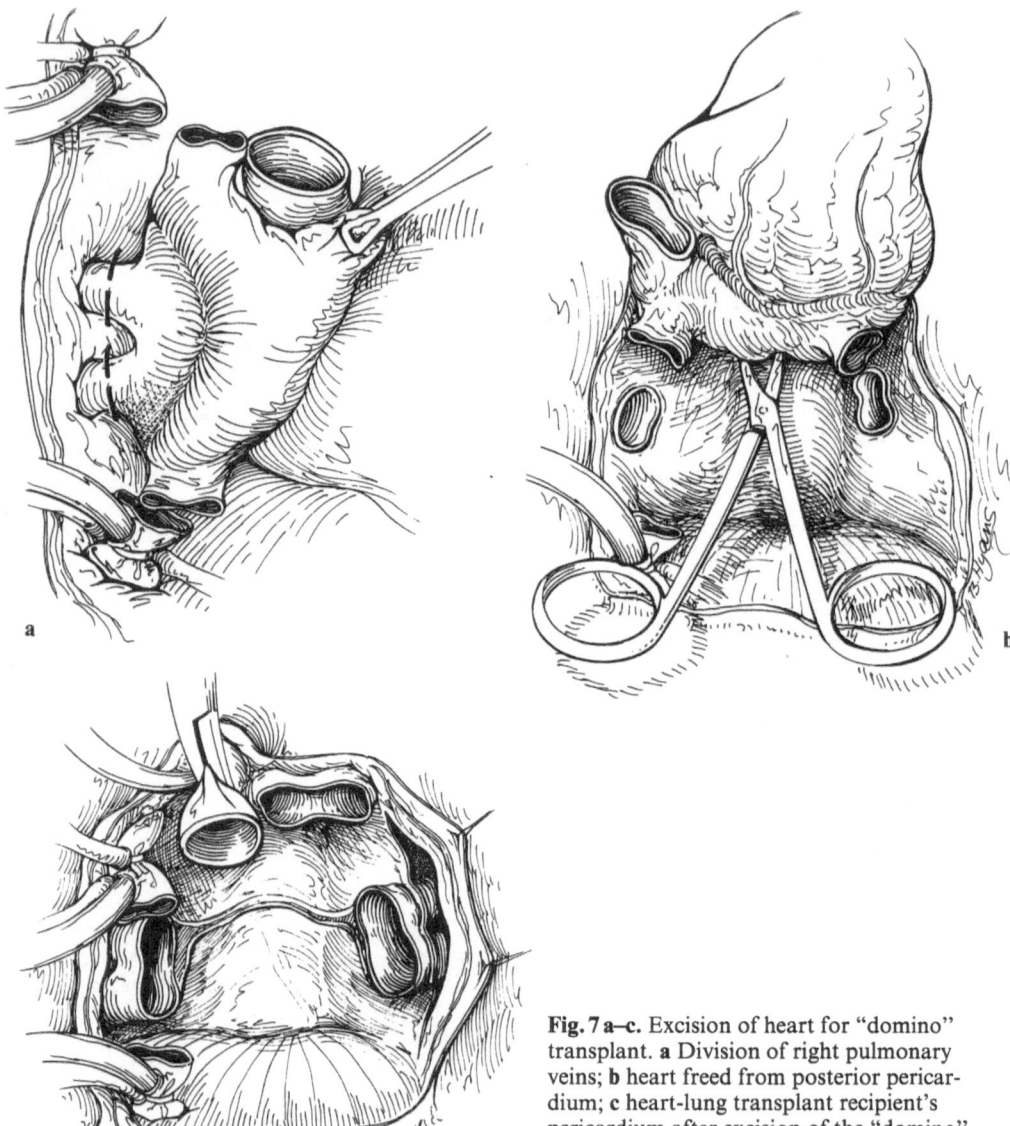

Fig. 7 a–c. Excision of heart for "domino" transplant. **a** Division of right pulmonary veins; **b** heart freed from posterior pericardium; **c** heart-lung transplant recipient's pericardium after excision of the "domino" heart prior to removal of the lungs

The "domino" technique requires separate SVC and IVC anastomoses to be made as described above under "Alternative Technique."

Heterotopic Transplantation

Heterotopic cardiac transplantation was first used clinically in Cape Town in 1974 [13], and variations of the surgical technique were subsequently described [14]. The procedure we use is as follows:

Preparation of the Donor Heart. The orifice of the inferior vena cava is sutured closed. Long segments of aorta, pulmonary artery and superior vena cava are preserved for anastomosis to the recipient. The posterior wall of the left atrium is prepared by joining the orifices of the four pulmonary veins.

Recipient Operation. After establishing cardiopulmonary bypass, with venous cannulae in the SVC and IVC and the arterial cannula in the ascending aorta, the right pleural cavity is opened widely and the pericardium reflected posteriorly to form a pleuro-pericardial flap based on the phrenic nerve, which is carefully preserved. The recipient heart is electrically fibrillated. A vent is inserted in the apex of the recipient's left ventricle (LV). The donor left atrium is anastomosed to a long incision in the recipient's LA which extends from a point posterior to the interatrial groove, just behind the IVC, to the roof of the recipient's LA (Fig. 8 a). The donor superior vena cava is then incised posteriorly and the stoma created is anastomosed to a large T-shaped incision in the recipient's SVC (this connection is important, as it provides access to the donor right ventricle for endomyocardial biopsies (Fig. 8 b); the donor LV is vented at the apex and the donor aorta is then anastomosed to the side of the recipient's ascending aorta using a side-occluding clamp. Finally, the donor PA is anastomosed to the recipient's PA or RA. A PA anastomosis is used when there is poor recipient RV function (Figs. 8 c, d). We prefer not to use prosthetic material to extend the donor PA for anastomosis with the recipient's PA, and occasionally, when extra length has been required, a section of donor aorta has been used for this purpose.

After completion of the transplant procedure the recipient's heart is repaired and revascularized when necessary. After deairing of both hearts through the LV vents cardiopulmonary bypass is discontinued as before.

Early Postoperative Care

Postoperative care of cardiac transplant recipients is similar to that of other cardiac bypass patients with the additional concerns of immunosuppression, rejection, increased risk of infection and renal dysfunction (related to cyclosporin). During the first 24 h patients receive full reverse barrier nursing in isolation rooms with laminar airflow systems. Once ventilation has been discontinued and mediastinal/chest drains have been removed, simple contact precautions are followed. Central venous catheters are removed as soon as possible – prophylactic antibiotics are administered while they are in place (see below).

Bradycardia of the donor heart is not uncommon initially, and an isoprenaline infusion or atrial pacing may be required. Right ventricular (RV) dysfunction secondary to an elevated PVR can often be managed by volume expansion and an epoprostenol (prostacyclin) infusion, together with inotropic support.

Renal perfusion is promoted by a dopamine infusion (2–4 µg/kg/min). Mild renal dysfunction often responds to a reduction in cyclosporin dosage. In more serious cases cyclosporin is temporarily discontinued and oral or intravenous steroids are substituted (see below). If significant metabolic or fluid balance problems arise from renal dysfunction, haemofiltration (combined, if necessary, with dialysis) is used.

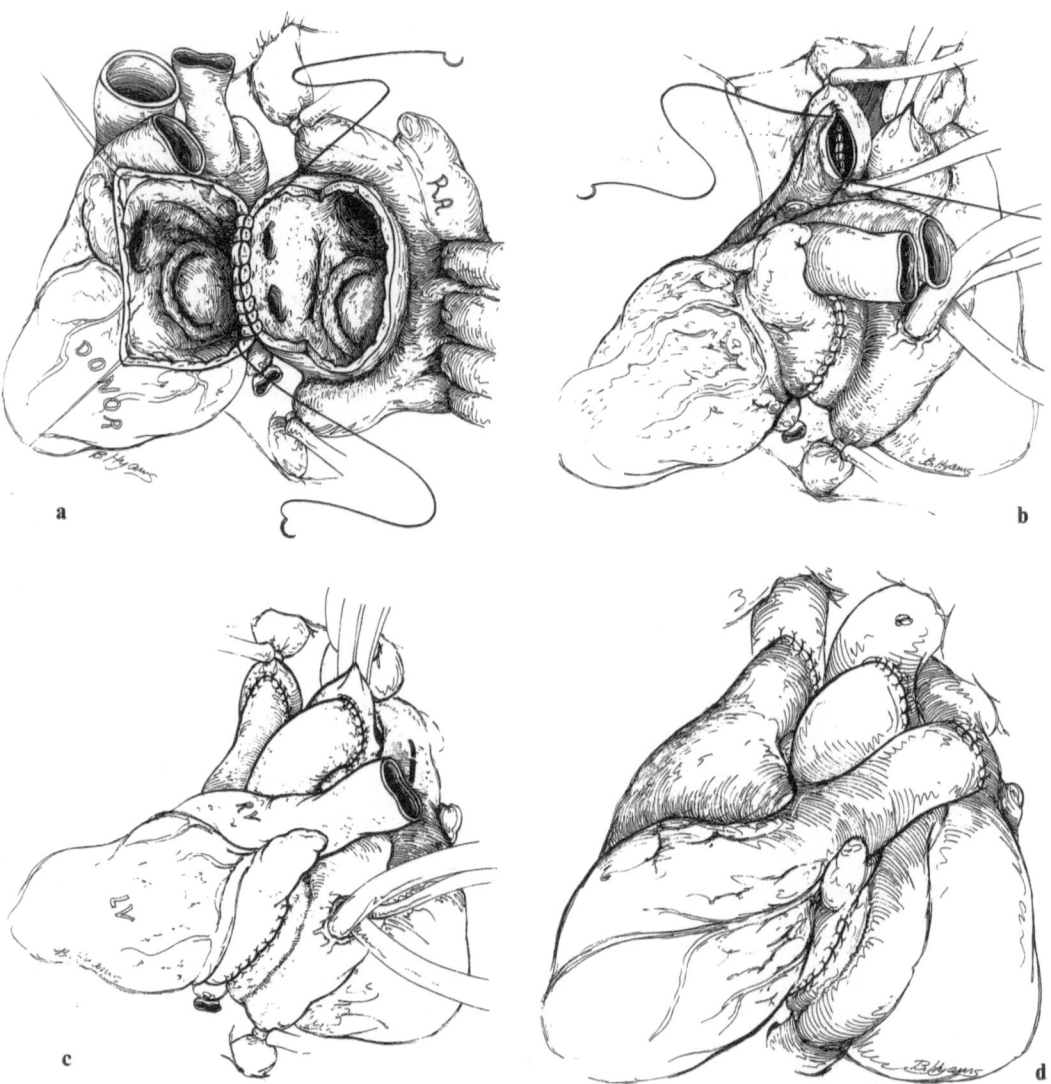

Fig. 8 a–d. Heterotopic heart transplant. **a** Left atrial anastomosis; **b** anastomosis of donor SVC to the side of the recipient SVC; **c** potential location of PA anastomosis (donor PA usually requires extension); **d** completed heterotopic transplant

Immunosuppressive Regimen

Cyclosporin was introduced at our hospital in September 1982. Over the subsequent 5 years there has been a progressive reduction in the doses of cyclosporin used. Our current regimen consists of a preoperative dose of 2–10 mg/kg cyclosporin orally (with a lower dose used when there is renal or hepatic dysfunction) and azathioprine 2 mg/kg orally. Intraoperatively, 1 g of methylprednisolone is given intravenously following the release of the aortic clamp. Postoperatively, cyclosporin is given orally twice daily in a dose of 2–40 mg/kg/day (children require larger doses to achieve the same plasma levels as adults). The dose is adjusted according to the trough plasma level (determined by radioimmunoassay) and the recipient's renal function. We aim to maintain a level of 400–500 ng/ml during the first month and 100–200 ng/ml subsequently. Azathioprine is given in a dose of 2 mg/kg/day (the dose is reduced or omitted if the patient's white cell count falls below 3.5×10^9/l). Oral steroids are not used routinely, but they are used temporarily if the patient has recurrent or persistent rejection or develops postoperative renal dysfunction [1]. Although short courses of steroids are used during the first year, less than 15% of patients are receiving oral steroids 1 year after transplantation [1].

Patients are monitored clinically for signs of rejection (e.g. fluid retention, development of a third heart sound) and noninvasively with serial ECGs (to detect voltage changes and arrhythmias) and echocardiographic determination of indices of left ventricular systolic and diastolic function and wall thickness, together with Doppler assessment of left ventricular diastolic function. We have not been able to substitute noninvasive tests for endomyocardial biopsy in adult transplant recipients. Endomyocardial biopsies are performed routinely on the third and seventh day postoperatively and once a week for the first month, fortnightly up to 3 months and monthly until 6 months after operation. Biopsies are then performed every 2 months up to 1 year and every 6 months thereafter. Additional biopsies are performed when rejection is suspected, either clinically or on the basis of noninvasive tests. Histologically diagnosed rejection is treated with intravenous pulses of methylprednisolone or anti-thymocyte globulin.

Endomyocardial biopsies are not used in children under 5 years of age; rejection is diagnosed clinically and on the basis of ECG and echocardiographic/Doppler criteria. Children between 5 and 12 years of age are now biopsied only when rejection is suspected clinically or on the basis of the noninvasive tests.

Survival

The actuarial survival curves for patients undergoing cardiac transplantation are shown in Fig. 9. The introduction of cyclosporin (1982) was associated with an improvement in survival, and results have continued to improve despite the inclusion of children, patients over the age of 55 years, and those with concomitant medical diseases in the programme. The projected 1-year survival for patients who underwent transplantation in 1987 is 78%.

Complications Associated with Immunosuppression

The problems associated with cyclosporin nephrotoxicity have decreased with the use of lower cyclosporin levels [15]. Hypertension is present in about half the transplant recipients 1 year after operation [1], but it usually responds to treatment with vasodilators (such as nifedipine), sometimes in combination with a

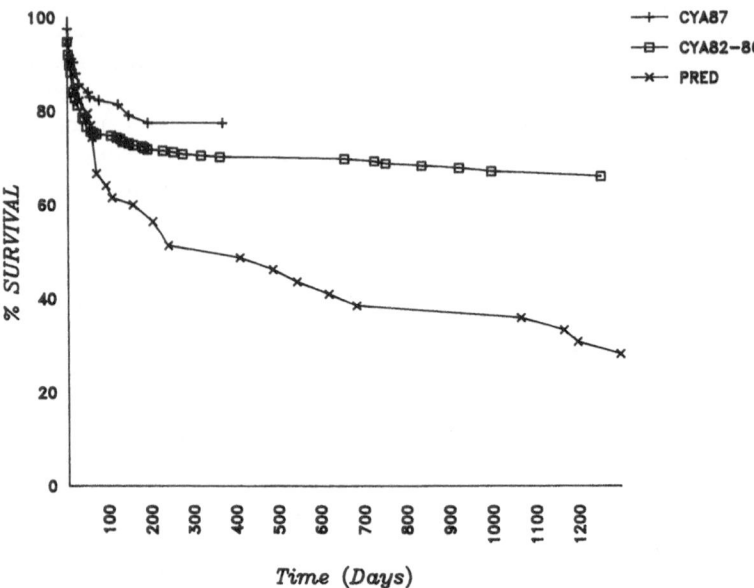

Fig. 9. Actuarial patient survival for cardiac transplant recipients at Harefield Hospital. *PRED*, Patients transplanted between January 1980 and July 1982 using prednisone and azathioprine ($n = 39$); *CYA82-86*, patients transplanted between September 1982 and December 1986 using cyclosporin and azathioprine immunosuppression ($n = 313$); *CYA87*, patients transplanted during 1987 using cyclosporin and azathioprine immunosuppression ($n = 136$)

diuretic. Cardiac transplant recipients are routinely given flucloxacillin and cefotaxime antibiotic prophylaxis during the perioperative period (aminoglycoside antibiotics which can potentiate cyclosporin nephrotoxicity are avoided). Bacterial infection in patients on the CYA/AZA regimen who receive this antibiotic prophylaxis are infrequent and normally respond well to appropriate antibiotic therapy [16].

Acyclovir (200 mg orally four times daily) is given for the first 3 months postoperatively to reduce the incidence of herpetic infections and in an attempt to decrease the risk of the development of Epstein-Barr virus-associated lymphoproliferative disorders. Three cardiac transplant recipients have developed lymphoproliferative disorders (all within 6 months of transplantation). In all three cases the lesions resolved completely following treatment with intravenous acyclovir and a reduction in the level of immunosuppression [1].

Nystatin suspension (100 000 units orally, four times daily) is given for the first month to reduce the incidence of fungal mucosal infections which may predispose to systemic infection.

Coronary Artery Disease in the Transplanted Heart

The development of coronary artery disease in the transplanted heart is a potentially serious late complication after cardiac transplantation. It would

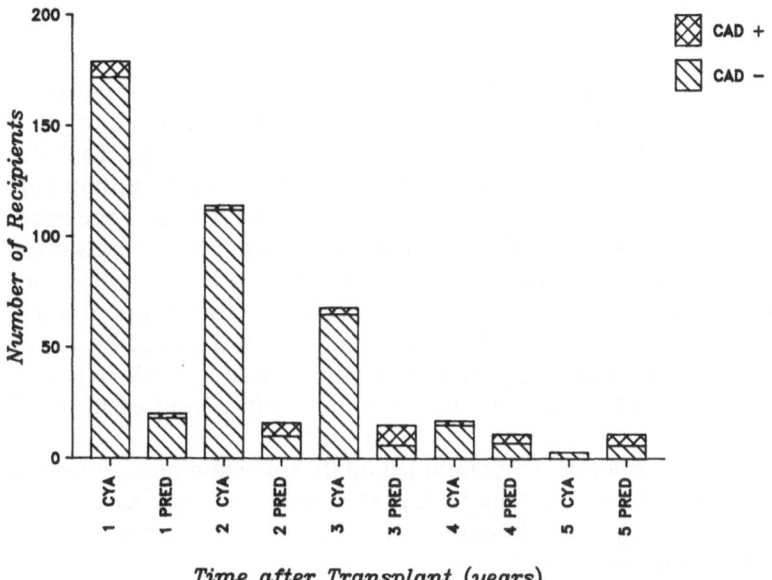

Fig. 10. Number of patients with coronary artery disease [*CAD*+] (narrowing >50% of lumen area) compared with number without coronary disease [*CAD*−] at coronary angiography each year after transplantation. *PRED*, treated with prednisone and azathioprine; *CYA*, treated with cyclosporin and azathioprine

seriously hamper a cardiac transplant programme if a sizeable proportion of recipients required retransplantation because of accelerated coronary artery disease.

Figure 10 shows the incidence of angiographically determined coronary artery disease (>50% reduction in lumen area) in patients who were treated with prednisone and azathioprine compared with that in patients treated with cyclosporin and azathioprine. These figures underestimate the size of the problem because they represent a survivor group, and coronary angiography is known to be less sensitive in detecting coronary artery disease in the transplanted heart than it is in detecting conventional coronary artery disease. However, in addition to the improved survival in the cyclosporin and azathioprine group, the risk of coronary artery disease is less during the first 4 years after transplantation in these patients than in patients who receive prednisone and azathioprine. This is a retrospective analysis of patients treated during two different time periods, with a marked difference in the number at risk in each group, and the results may be affected by many factors; however, the improvement may be due to more effective immunosuppression with cyclosporin, preventing "chronic rejection," or to the adverse metabolic effects of long-term steroid therapy.

In addition to the reduced incidence of coronary artery disease, left ventricular function in the cyclosporin group (as determined by radionuclide ejection fraction) appears to be better than in the prednisone and azathioprine group [17].

Paediatric Cardiac Transplantation

The introduction of the CYA/AZA regimen has enabled 28 children (aged between 9 days and 14 years) to receive transplants without the deleterious effect of steroids on growth. The indications were dilated cardiomyopathy, of various aetiologies, in 18 (the youngest of whom was 10 months), restrictive cardiomyopathy in two and hypertrophic cardiomyopathy in three. Five patients were transplanted for congenital heart disease, including three neonates and infants (aged between 9 days and 4 months) who had hypoplastic left heart syndrome. Acute right heart failure was the cause of three of the six early deaths. It appears that in this age-group a PVR of more than 4–5 Wood units is not tolerated by a heart from a donor without pulmonary hypertension (and consequent RV hypertrophy). There have been no late deaths during a follow-up period of up to 40 months.

Postoperatively, the children are maintained on the same immunosuppressive regimen as the adult patients, and long-term oral steroids have not been used in any patient. The dose of cyclosporin required to achieve the same plasma levels is higher in children than in adults.

Quality of Life and Rehabilitation After Cardiac Transplantation

The transplant recipient is committed to lifelong drug therapy and medical surveillance. The impact of cardiac transplantation on survival and quality of life in patients operated on at Harefield and Papworth hospitals was investigated in a study commissioned by the Department of Health and Social Security of the United Kingdom [18]. The effect of transplantation on the recipient's quality of life was assessed using a questionnaire, the "Nottingham Health Profile," to provide a six-dimensioned measure of subjective health status. The results of the study confirmed our clinical impression, i.e. that the majority of cardiac transplant recipients achieve excellent rehabilitation and a marked improvement of quality of life following transplantation.

The exercise capacity of transplant recipients is generally good, but it is less than that of normal subjects matched for age and sex. A recent collaborative study between our hospital and the Toronto Rehabilitation Centre has shown that exercise capacity and estimated maximum cardiac output of orthotopic cardiac transplant recipients can be enhanced by an endurance training programme [19]. One patient from our hospital has successfully completed the Boston Marathon [20].

Conclusions

Although there are still some problems, the results of cardiac transplantation have continued to improve and it is now a well-established procedure for the management of end-stage cardiac failure. The cyclosporin and azathioprine regimen has allowed us to operate on patients in the paediatric and older age-groups, to reduce the number of contraindications to transplantation and to avoid the complications of long-term steroid therapy. The expanded role of transplantation has exacerbated the problem of limited donor organ supply. The development of new techniques, such as the "domino" transplant and bilateral lung transplantation, together with the continued use of heterotopic cardiac transplantation, allows us to have a flexible approach to cardiac transplantation which increases the use of the available donor organs.

References

1. Banner NR, Fitzgerald M, Khaghani A, Aravot D, Reid C, Mitchell AG, Radley-Smith R, Yacoub MH (1987) Cardiac transplantation at Harefield Hospital. In: Terasaki PI (ed) Clinical transplants 1987. UCLA Tissue Typing Laboratory, Los Angeles, pp 17–26
2. The Consensus Trial Study Group (1987) Effects of enalapril on mortality in severe congestive heart failure. N Engl J Med 316:1429–1435
3. Young JN, Yazebeck J, Esposito G, Mankad P, Townsend E, Yacoub M (1986) The influence of acute preoperative pulmonary infarction on the results of heart transplantation. J Heart Transplant 5:20–22
4. Toronto Lung Transplant Group (1986) Unilateral lung transplantation for pulmonary fibrosis. N Engl J Med 314:1140–1145
5. Yacoub M, Festenstein H, Doyle P, Martin M, McClusky D, Awad J, Gamba A, Khaghani A, Holmes J (1987) The influence of HLA matching in cardiac allograft recipients receiving cyclosporin and azathioprine. Transplant Proc 19:2487–2489
6. Cohn JN, Archibald DG, Ziesche S et al. (1986) Effect of vasodilator therapy on mortality in chronic congestive heart failure: results of a veterans administration cooperative study. N Engl J Med 314:1547–1552
7. Rolles K (1986) Management of the multiple organ donor. Hosp Update 12:633–636
8. Cass MH, Brock R (1959) Heart excision and replacement. Guys Hosp Rep 108:285–290
9. Lower RR, Shumway NE (1960) Studies on orthotopic transplantation of the canine heart. Surg Forum 11:18
10. Barnard CN (1968) What we have learned about heart transplants. J Thorac Cardiovasc Surg 56:457–468
11. Stinson EB, Dong E, Iben AB, Shumway NE (1969) Cardiac transplantation in man. Surgical aspects. Am J Surg 118:182–187
12. Jamieson SW, Stinson EB, Oyer PE, Baldwin JC, Shumway NE (1984) Operative technique for heart-lung transplantation. J Thorac Cardiovasc Surg 87:930–935
13. Barnard CN, Losman JG (1975) Left ventricular bypass. S Afr Med J 49:303–312
14. Novitsky D, Cooper DKC, Barnard CN (1983) The surgical technique of heterotopic heart transplantation. Ann Thorac Surg 36:476–482
15. Martin M, Packman D, Kingswood C et al. (1987) Determinants of cyclosporin nephrotoxicity following cardiac transplantation. Transplant Proc 19:2516–2517
16. Khaghani A, Martin M, Fitzgerald M, Shakel M, Aravot D, Yacoub MH (1988) Cefotaxime and flucloxacillin as antibiotic prophylaxis in cardiac transplantation. Drugs 35 [Suppl 2]:124–126
17. Reid CR, Qureshi S, Yacoub MH (1987) Determinants of left ventricular function 1 year after cardiac transplantation. Br Heart J 57:85
18. Buxton M, Acheson R, Caine N, Gibson S, O'Brien B (1985) Costs and benefits of the heart transplant programmes at Harefield and Papworth Hospitals. HMSO, London
19. Kavanagh T, Yacoub MH, Mertens DJ, Kenndy J, Campbell RB, Sawyer P (1988) Cardiorespiratory responses to exercise training after orthotopic cardiac transplantation. Circulation 77:162–171
20. Kavanagh T, Yacoub M, Mertens D (1986) Exercise rehabilitation after cardiac transplantation. Care Crit Ill 2:96–98

41. Heart Transplantation –
Current Experience at La Pitié Hospital, Paris

C. Cabrol, I. Gandjbakhch, A. Pavie, V. Bors, T. Mestiri, E. Solis,
A. Cabrol, P. Leger, J. P. Levasseur, E. Vaissier, F. Simonneau, J. Szefner,
A. Auriol, and B. Aupetit

Introduction

Heart transplantation has become a therapeutic option for patients with end-stage heart disease. With the advances in the detection of early rejection using transvenous biopsy in 1973 and the introduction of cyclosporin in 1980, the results of cardiac transplantation improved dramatically. The current 1-year survival is 78.9%, 76.6% for 5 years [1].

In our own experience (Fig. 1) and according to several other reports [1–4], although improvement is evident in the long-term survival, an important early mortality of 12%–15% persists, which is in part responsible for the total mortality of the method. We believe this early mortality is due to two main factors: improper recipient selection and wrong choice of the donor.

Improper Recipient Selection

Potential candidates for the procedure are patients with end-stage heart disease and limited life expectancy. Absolute age limits are no longer defined, but in general the range is from 5 to 50 years. Patients above and below this range are considered on an individual basis.

Severe pulmonary hypertension remains a contraindication for heart transplantation. Active systemic infection generally precludes transplantation, as do systemic illnesses (collagen disease, vascular disease, malignancies). In general, a recent pulmonary infarction is a relative contraindication for transplantation.

However, because of an increased confidence based on the good results observed, and sometimes because of the insistence of the referring physician, the family, or the patient himself, some of these contraindications are neglected, such as small infections or gastrointestinal disorders. Three of them are now more often neglected and may be the cause of postoperative failure:

1. Non-insulin-dependant *diabetes patients* are being accepted more and more frequently by some groups.
2. *Patients over 55 years* of age; however, according to some statistics, such as those reported in the International Heart Transplantation Registry [1], survival is surprisingly better for this group than for younger patients.
3. With *borderline pulmonary hypertension* and increased pulmonary vascular resistance, the normal heart (as a donor's heart is supposed to be) is unable to adapt itself rapidly.

Assisted Circulation 3
F. Unger (Ed.)
© Springer-Verlag Berlin Heidelberg 1989

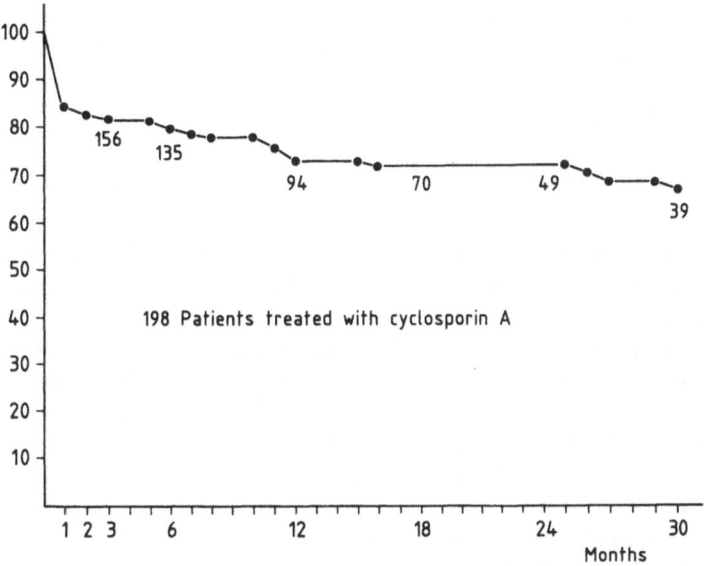

Fig. 1. Actuarial survival curve for heart transplantation at La Pitié Hospital, Paris

In the latter cases, it is not always easy to know if it is reasonable to perform an isolated cardiac transplantation or a heart-lung transplantation. In our experience, when pulmonary artery systolic pressure was higher than 50–70 mmHg, the transpulmonary vascular gradient was greater than 15 mmHg, the pulmonary vascular resistance was higher than 6–8 Wood units, and the pulmonary vascular resistance index more than 6 Wood units, catheterization studies were made with the use of vasodilators: nitroprusside, nitroglycerin, nifedipine, and prostaglandin.

When a 20% diminution of the pulmonary vascular resistance pretest value was observed, a spasm effect was considered predominant and was usually successfully treated and overcome during transplantation. In contrast, when the administration of vasodilators was ineffective and the pulmonary artery vascular resistance remained high, special surgical procedures were discussed.

In cases of pulmonary vascular resistance between 6 and 8 Wood units, orthotopic isolated cardiac transplantation was usually performed without serious problems when a donor heart could be obtained that was oversized in relation to the recipient, that exibited good hemodynamics prior to explantation (with no drugs or with less than 4 g/kg/min dopamine), and with limited ischemic time, as when the donor could be brought into the operating room adjacent to that of the recipient (on-site procurement).

When the fixed pulmonary vascular resistance was more than 8 Wood units, the only possibility besides a heart-lung transplantation, which still has a less favorable early and late prognosis than isolated cardiac transplantation, was to perform (especially in case of ischemic disease) a heterotopic transplantation in which the recipient's right ventricle did most of the work in the early postoperative course. But this method has some drawbacks: a more difficult introduction of the bioptome for endomyocardial biopsy and, as we observed in some cases of native ischemic disease, persistence or reappearance of angina.

Wrong Donor Choice and Management

It has become more and more difficult to obtain a suitable donor due to the increase in the number of transplants performed, as can be seen from the curve of our transplantation activity (Fig. 2).

The shortage is so important that some groups are tempted to neglect some well-defined contraindications. Certain rules for selecting a donor for heart transplantation should be followed. There should be absence of any transmissible disorder or infection, of any possible coronary disease (so the age of the donor must be less than 35 years), and of any other cardiac anomaly, prolonged cardiac arrest, or thoracic trauma. In addition, two compatibilities are needed: an immunologic compatibility in the ABO transfusion groups and the absence of cytotoxic antibodies, (i.e., a negative cross-match between the recipient's serum and a panel of potential donors' lymphocytes, permits distant procurement of a donor heart); a hemodynamic compatibility – i.e., an excellent donor heart – sustaining in the donor a normal blood pressure without, or with a minimal amount of, drugs.

The use of hearts from donors *50 or 55 years old* can be cause of present or secondary severe coronary lesions of the donor heart after transplantation. Another reason for early failure is the choice of a *poorly performing* donor's heart that already requires fairly high inotropic support. Low performance of a donor's heart may be the result of *imperfect preservation* during excision or transportation, in the case – now usual – of distant procurement. Poor performance of the donor heart may also be due, as we mentioned above, to the existence in the recipient of a pulmonary vascular resistance more elevated than expected seen at the last cardiac catheterization of the recipient.

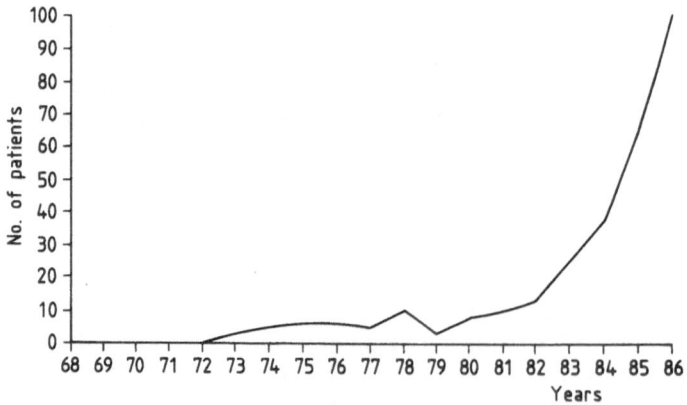

Fig. 2. Number of heart transplantations from 1968 to 1986 at La Pitié Hospital, Paris

So the precise choice of a recipient is very important when a donor is announced, taking into account, not only the immunologic compatibility, but also the hemodynamic compatibility, which depends equally on the condition of the donor and the condition of the recipient.

The shortage of donors should stimulate efforts to improve myocardial preservation for longer than 4 h and thus to ensure the promising future of xenotransplantation.

Early Postoperative Problems

These errors in the selection of recipients and donors explain the important postoperative problems seen after transplantation, such as the early hemodynamic failures observed during the first days or weeks (Fig. 3).

The very poor general condition of long-term bedridden recipients also explains the frequent occurrence during the first month of lethal pulmonary embolism and stress complications (pancreatitis, intestinal necrosis). Early infections seen during this period are the consequence of imperfect preparation of the recipient or of a fever or low-grade infection that was ignored in the donor.

Rejection is a constant threat from the fifth postoperative day to the first year. In our experience, cyclosporin considerably decreased the frequency and the severity of rejection overall. Last year, a new problem appeared in patients treated with cyclosporine: there were acute, severe, and sometimes lethal rejection episodes like those seen with conventional therapy. In spite of a careful inquiry, we were unable to explain this phenomenon, which has also been observed by other groups. In most of the cases cyclosporin suppressed the usual clinical, electrical, and hemodynamic symptoms of rejection. So the early diagnosis of rejection, which is so important to counteract the short- and long-term consequences of such lesions, remains a current problem in cardiac transplantation.

There are three main ways to detect rejection [5–10]:

1. The ideal way: Early recognition of the humoral and cellular changes produced by the rejection episode, by way of so-called immunologic monitoring; this is, in our experience, unreliable.

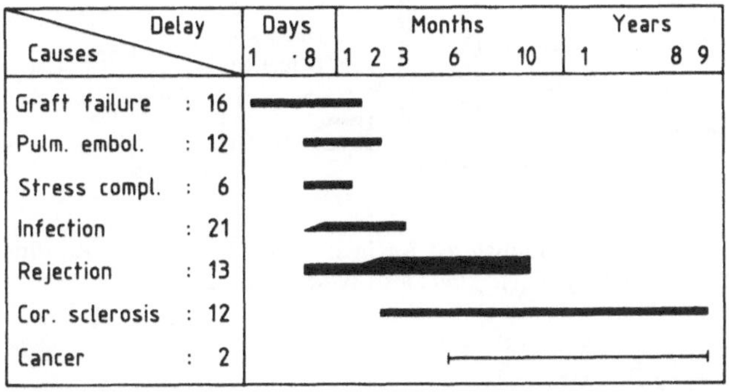

	Delay	Days		Months			Years	
Causes		1 ·8	1 2 3	6	10	1	8 9	
Graft failure	: 16							
Pulm. embol.	: 12							
Stress compl.	: 6							
Infection	: 21							
Rejection	: 13							
Cor. sclerosis	: 12							
Cancer	: 2							

Fig. 3. Causes of death after heart transplant at La Pitié

2. The obvious way: detection of the consequences of rejection on the cardiac function via their clinical, echocardiographic and electrocardiographic symptoms occurs too late.
3. Presently, the only way to be sure of an ongoing rejection is the histologic diagnosis, the golden standard, which, unfortunately, is an invasive method requiring the percutaneous introduction of a cardiac bioptome and the obtaining of a small piece of right ventricular endomyocardium, which shows, under microscopic examination, in case of rejection, important lymphocyte infiltration and myocyte necrosis.

Although they have been lessened by the use of cyclosporin, secondary viral infections remain a problem. A careful screening of the donor is essential in this respect, to avoid the frequent transmission of germs, particularly cytomegalovirus and toxoplasmosis [11].

Another concern with the use of cyclosporin is its nephrotoxicity. This effect can be acute during the first postoperative days. It is more common in patients with functional renal insufficiency due to the long-lasting cardiac failure, who are treated with diuretics. The renal damage develops rapidly, causing oliguria, anuria, and death. This side effect prompted us to follow two principles in immediate immunosuppression therapy: first, delayed use of cyclosporin, which is replaced during the first 2 days by conventional therapy until the renal function and hemodynamic situation of the transplanted patient improve, and second, the use of cyclosporin in low doses (Fig. 4).

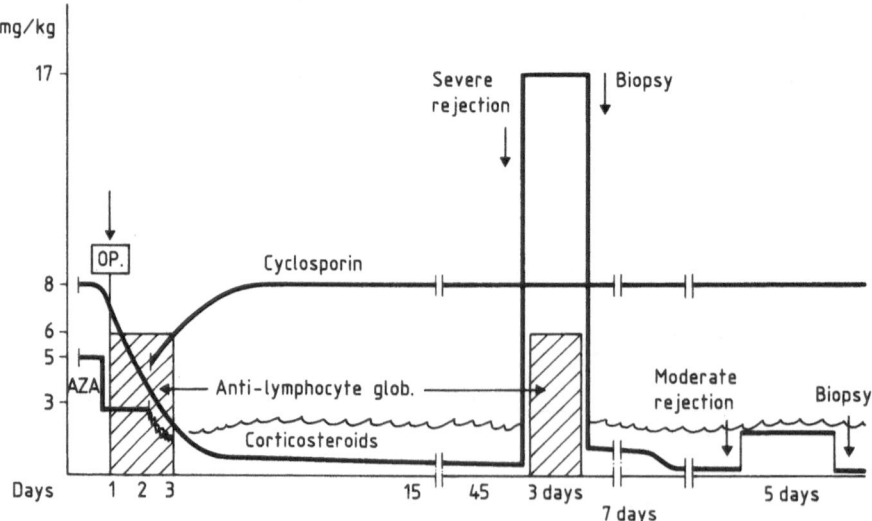

Fig. 4. Present immunosuppressive therapy administered for heart transplantation at La Pitié. *Aza*, Azathioprine; *Op.*, operation; *Anti-lymphocyte glob.*, anti-lymphocyte globulin

Immunosuppressive Therapy

Our present immunosuppressive protocol consists of methylprednisolone (mPred), 8 mg/kg i.v. before and during the operation, azathioprine (Aza) before (5 mg/kg) and after (2 mg/kg) the transplantation, and a 3-day course of rabbit antilymphocyte globulin (ALG) (6 mg/kg/day). When the hemodynamic condition of the patient becomes stable and the hepatic and renal functions are satisfactory. Aza therapy is discontinued and cyclosporin (Cy) therapy is gradually started (3 mg/kg/day–5 mg/kg/day) It is increased progressively to achieve a Cy serum level of 100 ng/ml–150 ng/ml. Corticosteroids are tapered down: 6 mg/kg the first day, 4 mg/kg the second day, 2 mg/kg the third day, 1 mg/kg after the first week.

Two months after the operation, the patients receive a maintenance therapy consisting of Cy and small doses of oral prednisone (Pred, 0.3 mg/kg/day). A third of our patients now also receive small doses of Aza (2.5 mg/kg/day).

In case of rejection, when the episode is severe, corticosteroids are increased (mPred, 17 mg/kg/day) and a 3-day course of ALG is given. Three days later a cardiac biopsy is done, and according to its results, maintenance therapy is resumed or steroids are slowly tapered down to maintenance levels (0.3 mg/kg/day).

In case of a moderate rejection episode, the daily doses of mPred are increased over a 5-day period and a biopsy is performed. Usually, the serum level of Cy is maintained constant.

Lately, new treatments have appeared in immunosuppressive therapy. They use monoclonal antibodies and they increase the doses of Cy in case of rejection; they systematically switch from Cy therapy to conventional therapy after 2 or 3 years to avoid Cy renal toxicity at the time when the risk of rejection becomes lower. So the search for an ideal immunosuppressive is continuing [12].

Late Complications

The precautions taken with the early use of cyclosporin have almost suppressed the early nephrotoxic complications encountered but chronic nephrotoxicity is still observed. This is demonstrated by the elevation of the serum creatinine level, more pronounced in older patients that in younger, and is aggravated by the use of nephrotoxic antibiotics, sometimes needed to treat severe infection. These lesions are characterized histologically by tubular atrophy and interstitial fibrosis without glomerular alteration and can be prevented by using low doses of cyclosporin. If they appear, they are potentially reversible by discontinuation of cyclosporin and a switch to conventional therapy (corticosteroids and azathioprine).

The systemic hypertension observed in almost all patients treated with cyclosporin also remains a threat for the future. In spite of extensive studies made in our group and in others [13], we were unable to find any alteration of the renin angiotensin system or of the aldosterone level, and the only abnormal finding was a constant hypervolemia. This systemic hypertension is best treated by the administration of calcium blockers.

Finally, one of the most intriguing and dangerous problems in cardiac transplantation is the occurrence of occlusive coronary lesions. We must distinguish, in this respect, lesions already present in the donor heart, such as coronary atherosclerosis, or lesions induced during transplantation such as coronary embolism, from three types of coronary artery lesions seen in our series secondary to transplantation. They are early coronary arteritis, late obliterative fibrous arteritis, and late atherosclerosis.

Early coronary arteritis generally occurs between 3 and 18 months after transplantation on small coronary arteries. It is characterized by lymphocyte infiltration, arteritis, and sometimes thrombosis. Its etiology is certainly immunologic and it represents a rejection lesion that is potentially reversible.

Late obliterative fibrous arteritis usually occurs 2 years post-transplantation on large and medium-size vessels. The lesions are essentially fibrosis of the intima, sometimes with disruption of the media, without an important lymphocyte infiltration. It represents possibly the end stage of the previously described lesion, early coronary arteritis, and it is slowly progressive.

Finally, *late atherosclerosis* also appears 2 years post-transplantation on the large coronary arteries. The lesions are essentially fibrotic, with atheromatous deposits similar to the usual coronary atheroma. It represents possibly the same lesions as those previously described (late obliterative fibrous arteritis) in patients with high risk factors for atheroma, now infiltrated these with lipidic plaques. The angiographic aspect is typical, with diffuse multiple distal lesions. These lesions are rapidly progressive. They are silent (without angina) in a denervated heart and detected only by systematic routine coronary angiography. They cannot be treated by coronary artery bypass and require retransplantation. Their frequency and their severity make them a major threat to transplantation and they deserve all the attention of future research.

Treatment of Patients with Acute Irreversible Heart Failure

Treatment of patients with acute irreversible heart failure or those whose condition is suddenly aggravated while they are waiting for transplantation, when a suitable donor heart is not immediately available, is one of the current problems in cardiac transplantation.

At La Pitié Hospital, we decided to use a total artificial heart as a bridge to transplantation in such patients. From April 1986 to May 1987, we implanted a Jarvik 7-type total artificial heart in 21 patients, 18 men and three women. Ages varied from 19 to 56 years. All patients were in terminal congestive cardiac failure, which was secondary to idiopathic cardiomyopathy in seven patients, viral myocarditis in one, postpartum myocarditis in two, valvular disease in one, acute rejection in three, ischemic disease in five, and early failure of the donor heart after transplantation in two. All patients had a life expectancy of a few hours. Hepatic and renal functional insufficiency were present in all cases, subacute pulmonary edema was seen in 16 cases, and a cardiac arrest at the beginning of anesthesia was present in two cases. The cardiac prosthesis used was a Jarvik 7 – 100 cc in nine cases and 70 cc in 12 cases. Mechanical circulatory support lasted from 2 to 32 days. There was no mechanical failure, no hemolysis, and no thromboembolism, and in only two cases was there right ventricular device malposition. Usually, hepatic and renal functions improved in a few days. Left atrial pressure was continuously monitored to avoid pulmonary edema, which disappeared with in a few hours after the implantation. Ten patients died before transplantation, four of infections and six of multiple organ failure. One patient is still on the artificial heart, ten have undergone transplantation. Two patients died after transplantation, one of cerebral lesions and one of fulminant hepatitis. Eight patients remain well and fully rehabilitated. Thus, the total artificial heart is, in our experience, a very safe device; it is easy to run and offers the best treatment for the type of patient who can recover in this way to a stable physiological condition and later successfully undergo transplantation without any emergency.

Mechanical support of the failing heart prior to heart transplantation is a new, developing field. Several questions have been raised regarding its use:

- What patients can benefit from the use of a cardiac-assist device?
- Do these patients take priority for transplantation, condemning the carefully selected candidates to wait in vain for a suitable heart if this practice becomes generalized?
- Do all the patients with an artificial heart need to undergo eventual transplantation, whatever their general condition, if a suitable donor heart is available for them?

In our opinion, the use of an artificial heart or a ventricular-assist device must be reserved for patients with no contraindications for transplantation, in acute (and not chronic) irreversible cardiac failure, and with "reversible" organ dysfunction. Those patients on circulatory support should undergo transplantation only when their condition is satisfactory and stable and without any priority.

Conclusion

After almost 20 years of clinical application, and due to the great progress made during this time by the pioneers of the method, cardiac transplantation is now a safe and reliable treatment for patients in intractable cardiac failure untreatable by other medical or surgical means. Several unresolved problems remain as a challenge for the many active and excellent centers now engaged in this promising field.

References

1. Kaye M (ed) (1986) International society for heart transplantation. Registry 1986. Minneapolis
2. Cabrol C, Gandjbakhch I, Pavie A, Cabrol A, Mattei MF, Leger P (1985) Heart transplantation in Paris, at "La Pitié" Hospital. Heart Transplant 4:476–480

3. McGregor CG, Jamieson SW, Oyer PE et al. (1984) Heart transplantation at Stanford University. J Heart Transplant 4(1):31–32
4. Frazier OH, Cooley DA, Okerebe OUJ, Vanburen CT, Kahan BD (1985) Cardiac transplantation at the Texas Heart Institute: recent experience. Tex Med 81:48–52
5. Carrier M, Perrotta N, Copeland JG, Davis TP, Russell DH, Emery RW (1986) Urinary polyamines are noninvasive markers of heart allograft rejection. J Heart Transplant 5:392
6. Chomette G, Auriol M, Delcourt A, Karkouche B, Cabrol A, Cabrol C (1985) Human cardiac transplants: diagnosis of rejection by endomyocardial biopsy – causes of death (about 30 autopsies). Virchows Arch [A] 407:297–307
7. Billingham ME (1982) Diagnosis of cardiac rejection by endomyocardial biopsy. J Heart Transplant 1:25–30
8. Hammer C, Reichenspurner H, Ertel W et al. (1984) Cytological and immunologic monitoring of cyclosporin-treated human heart recipients. J Heart Transplant 3:228–232
9. Hoshingaga K, Pascor EA, Wood NL, Szentpetery S, Mohanakumar T, Lower RR (1986) Expression of transferrin receptors or lymphocytes and its correlation with rejection in cardiac transplant recipients (abstract). J Heart Transplant 4:589
10. Havel MP, Laczkovics AMD, Preiss PS, Muller MM, Wolner E (1986) Neopterin as a new marker to detect acute rejection after heart transplantation (abstract). J Heart Transplant 4:594
11. Baumgartner WA (1983) Infection in cardiac transplantation. J Heart Transplant 3(1):75–80
12. Oyer PE, Stinson EB, Jamieson SW et al. (1983) Cyclosporin A in cardiac allografting: a preliminary experience. Transplant Proc 15:1257–1262
13. Hunt SA (1983) Complications of heart transplantation. J Heart Transplant 3(1):70–74

42. Clinical Application
of Implanted Natural Auxiliary Hearts

D. K. C. COOPER

Introduction

The implantation of a natural auxiliary heart may be on a permanent basis, or it may be temporary as a means of support while recovery of the patient's own heart is awaited or a more definitive procedure is planned. Considerable clinical experience has now been amassed with auxiliary hearts implanted on a permanent basis [1]; to date, all such hearts have been allografts. Clinical experience of temporary support by an auxiliary heart has been small, and it would seem that it is in this area of transplantation that xenografts may play a future role.

Early experimental work in this area was done mainly by the Russian surgeon, Demikhov [2], but it was not until Barnard and Losman developed their technique of implanting an auxiliary heart in the chest in 1974 [3, 4] that a clinical program was initiated. The technique developed by Barnard and Losman has been clearly described [5]; in brief, it involves anastomoses between recipient and donor right atria, left atria, aortae, and pulmonary arteries (Fig. 1).

Permanent Natural Auxiliary Hearts

Allografts

The introduction of the immunosuppressive agent cyclosporin (CYA), which has significantly reduced the incidence of irreversible acute rejection (leading to permanent loss of donor heart function), has greatly reduced the indications for the implantation of an auxiliary heart – the operation of heterotopic heart transplantation (HHT). In the pre-CYA era, irreversible loss of the heterotopic donor heart did not necessarily lead to death of the patient, as the circulation might be maintained by the recipient native heart until retransplantation could be performed [6–8]. Today, however, irreversible rejection is relatively rare, and so this great advantage of HHT has become less important.

Nevertheless, HHT still has a role in certain specific conditions [1]:

1. Whenever there is any possibility of recovery of the recipient's own myocardium, e.g., in acute myocarditis, then HHT should be preferred.

2. When there is any possibility that initial donor heart function will be less than adequate to maintain the circulation alone. This could be expected most commonly when there is a large discrepancy in body mass between recipient and

Assisted Circulation 3
F. Unger (Ed.)
© Springer-Verlag Berlin Heidelberg 1989

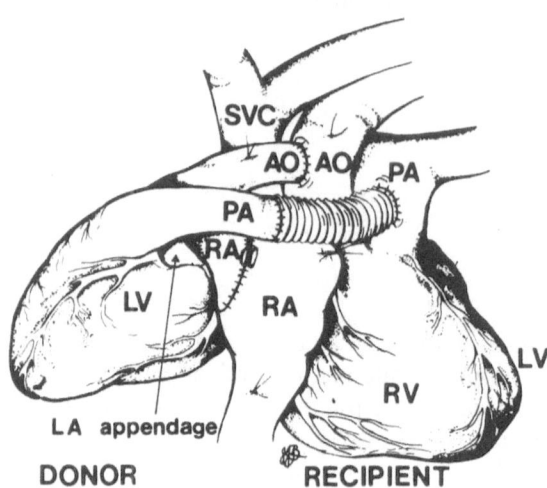

Fig. 1. Heterotopic heart transplantation – the completed operation. *SVC*, superior vena cava; *RA*, right atrium; *RV*, right ventricle; *PA*, pulmonary artery, *LA*, left atrium; *LV*, left ventricle; *AO*, aorta

donor; though a small donor heart will eventually hypertrophy to adapt to the demands made upon it, it might fail in the early post-transplant period unless the recipient heart remained in situ to lend some support. Similarly, when a donor heart has undergone a particularly long ischemic period during transportation and transplantation [9], or for some other reason is deemed less than ideal (and yet the recipient's cardiovascular status is deteriorating so rapidly that survival until the next donor becomes available is not expected), then HHT would again seem to be advisable; the support given by the recipient heart in the early transplant period will allow time for recovery of the donor heart.

3. When the patient is suffering severe anginal attacks unresponsive to full medical therapy and unrelieved (where possible) by myocardial revascularization procedures, yet left ventricular function continues to be good, it seems particularly contraindicated to excise the recipient heart and perform orthotopic transplantation (OHT). Following HHT, a well-functioning transplant would greatly diminish the demands on the ischemic recipient heart, thus reducing the threshold of angina, and yet retain the support given by the recipient left ventricle.

4. A fixed pulmonary vascular resistance (PVR) greater than 6 Wood units (480 dyn/s/cm^{-5}) has longed been considered a contraindication to OHT, as it was anticipated that early failure of the donor right ventricle would occur. When the PVR was fixed greater than 8 Wood Units (640 dyn/s/cm^{-5}) it has generally been assumed that transplantation of the heart and both lungs should be carried out. When the PVR was fixed between 6 and 8 Wood units, and where right ventricular function was not severe, then HHT has been advocated. There have been few cases, however, where this theory has been put into practice and the results clearly documented. Furthermore, the extent of reversibility of the PVR may be difficult to ascertain absolutely before transplantation.

A recent study from New York indicated that, while in some cases elevated PVR correlates with poor outcome form right ventricular failure, high resistance is not an absolute contraindication to OHT [10]. This study demonstrated that there is a very considerable reversible element in PVR (following the infusion of nitroprusside, nitroglycerin, PGE_1, or the administration of 100% oxygen) in the majority of patients awaiting heart transplantation. OHT was successfully performed in such patients even if the PVR remained above 6 Wood units following nitroprusside infusion, though some such patients had transient, but significant, right ventricular failure after surgery. When the PVR had no demonstrable reversible element and remained significantly above 6 Wood units, then HHT could be performed successfully if there was no native right ventricular failure or significant tricuspid regurgitation; one patient underwent successful HHT with a fixed PVR of 15 Wood units.

A second recent study, from Pittsburgh, has suggested that the transpulmonary gradient (TPG) (mean pulmonary artery pressure–pulmonary capillary wedge pressure), and not the calculated PVR, is a more accurate predictor of outcome following OHT [11]. In 187 patients undergoing OHT, neither the PVR (using 6 Wood units as the point of differentiation) nor the peak pulmonary artery systolic pressure (using 50 mmHg as the point of differentiation) significantly influenced early mortality, as judged by 7- and 30-day actuarial survival. The TPG, however, seemed to affect survival in a significant fashion ($P < 0.05$). A TPG of more than 15 mmHg was associated with a higher mortality than was a TPG of between 10 and 15 mmHg; mortality was even lower when the TPG was less than 10 mmHg. This relationship persisted even when patients with known causes of death (infection, hyperacute rejection, technical, bleeding) were excluded from the analysis. There may therefore be a place for HHT in patients in whom the TPG is above 10 mmHg, though the level of TPG above which heart and lung transplantation should be performed remains uncertain.

The indication for HHT in relation to the PVR and/or TPG, therefore, remains controversial, but it would seem that in patients with left ventricular failure from ischemic or cardiomyopathic disease, HHT should be preferred whenever there is serious doubt that the right ventricle of the transplanted heart will be able to support the pulmonary circulation successfully. This would be suggested if the PVR were above 6 Wood units and showed no reversible element whatsoever, or if the TPG remained above 10 mmHg after an attempt had been made to reduce it by infusion of nitroprusside and/or 100% oxygenation of the patient for a period of several minutes. In patients being considered for transplantation for congenital heart disease in whom there is a large left-to-right shunt which has resulted in a high PVR (and, of course, in patients with primary pulmonary hypertension) transplantation of the heart and both lungs will almost certainly be indicated.

Xenografts

Experimental Studies

At the present time, the use of an animal heart as a permanent orthotopic transplant would be a controversial procedure. The experimental evidence is that, with the possible exception of certain nonhuman primate hearts, an animal heart transplanted to man would be subjected to hyperacute (vascular, humoral) rejection with very early graft failure, sometimes within the first 5–10 min following transplantation [12, 13]; primate hearts are likely to be rejected hyperacutely in some instances [14–16] and acutely in others [17, 18]. It is therefore difficult to predict the outcome of a transplant in man using any one primate subgroup as donor.

Cynomolgus monkey hearts inserted heterotopically into baboons are rejected by a cellular (acute) response, which can successfully be overcome by combination immunosuppressive therapy using cyclosporin, azathioprine, corticosteroids, and anti-thymocyte globulin [17, 18]. Hearts from African green (vervet) monkeys, on the other hand, transplanted into baboons, are frequently rejected hyperacutely, and survival is not greatly prolonged by combination immunosuppressive therapy [14–16]; pretransplant total lymphoid irradiation, in combination with pharmacological immunosuppression, does result in longer survival of some hearts but, in this experimental model, has been associated with a very high mortality [16].

Clinical Experience

Evidence from kidney transplants in humans using chimpanzees as donors would suggest that chimpanzee tissue is rejected in a first-set fashion, namely by a cellular response, and that the donor organ may function for several weeks or even months [19]. Baboon kidneys, however, would appear to be subjected to a more vigorous rejection process, with a combination of both acute and hyperacute rejection, resulting in a shorter period of survival [20]. Although these early experiences were made in the pre-CYA days, current opinion is that CYA has little or no effect in preventing or even delaying a hyperacute reaction.

There is no evidence to suggest that hearts (as opposed to kidneys) would be rejected any differently. Clinical experience with cardiac xenografts is limited to only five reported cases [21–24]. Four of these were in the precyclosporin era, and the longest survival was only 4 days, this following the use of a chimpanzee heart as an auxiliary pump [23]. One of the four cases involved the use of a sheep heart, where the likelihood of any useful period of function must have been negligible [22].

The fifth and final case involved the use of a baboon heart in an infant immunosuppressed with a combination of drugs including CYA [24]; survival was 21 days. In this case, it was believed that the lack of a successful outcome was related largely to the choice of a donor baboon that was incompatible with the recipient in regard to ABO blood group; evidence was submitted suggesting that anti-A and anti-B antibodies played a significant part in the development of donor heart rejection.

ABO Compatibility

This conclusion has been supported to some extent by independent experimental work using the vervet monkey as donor and the chacma baboon as recipient [14, 15]. In these studies, early hyperacute rejection (within the first 60 min) was not seen in those cases where ABO compatibility was present between donor and recipient, but it was seen in a significant percentage of cases where incompatibility was present. Mean donor heart survival was also shorter in baboons· receiving ABO-incompatible vervet monkey hearts. These observations were noted in both nonimmunosuppressed recipients and in recipients immunosuppressed with a combination of pharmacological agents.

Comment

Whether pharmacological immunosuppression including CYA will delay or prevent rejection of transplanted primate hearts in man remains uncertain, but it would seem reasonable to expect that chimpanzee hearts will function for at least some weeks or even months under these circumstances. The outlook for baboon hearts would seem less optimistic, though function for 3 weeks has already been shown to be possible in one case [24]. Prolonged function, extending for years, would seem unlikely with either species, as the number and severity of acute rejection episodes and the development of chronic rejection changes (graft arteriosclerosis) will almost certainly be greater following xenotransplantation than after allografting, though again, this point remains unproven. The possibility that graft arteriosclerosis will develop is high, as this is considered to be the result of a low-grade immunological rejection process.

Temporary Natural Auxiliary Hearts

Allografts

The temporary insertion of a human auxiliary heart would seem to have little place in modern cardiac transplantation. It has been clearly demonstrated that temporary support of a failing circulation can be satisfactorily provided by one of the several ventricular-assist devices or artificial hearts which are currently available.

Xenografts

Bridge to Transplantation

The use of an auxiliary (or orthotopic) nonhuman primate heart, however, as a bridge to transplantation would seem feasible for, as discussed above, it seems likely that chimpanzee hearts, in particular, will function satisfactorily for several days and possibly weeks or months. This would allow time for a suitable human heart to be located and inserted (with removal of both the chimpanzee organ and the recipient's native heart, if it is still in situ).

Indeed, this was one possibility in two patients in whom auxiliary cardiac xenografts (one baboon and one chimpanzee) were implanted by Barnard and his colleagues in 1977 [23]. The baboon heart proved of insufficient size to support the circulation, and unfortunately, in this pre-CYA era, the chimpanzee heart was rejected on the fourth postoperative day before a suitable human donor could be found.

Ethical Considerations

Three aspects of this procedure, however, remain for discussion. The first is whether it is ethical to use an animal such as a chimpanzee, which is reputedly in short supply in the world at large, for such a purpose. Almost no one would object to the use of a pig or sheep heart as a temporary natural auxiliary pump, but the chimpanzee, with its close relationship to man, stimulates a far greater emotional response in the public, a significant percentage of whom may object to the use of this animal for this purpose [25, 26].

These objections will probably be particularly vociferous if chimpanzee hearts are used in adults, as adequate mechanical devices for supporting adult patients with failing ventricles are readily available, and, indeed, in many cases insertion has been followed by successful allotransplantation.

Infants and Children

The use of a xenograft as an auxiliary pump as a bridge to transplantation would seem to be indicated particularly in infants and children with complex congenital heart disease, such as hypoplastic left heart syndrome [27], as left ventricular assist devices and artificial hearts have not yet been developed of a size that can be implanted in these small patients. It is probably in this field, therefore, that xenografts will be explored initially. The small volume of the thoracic cavity may prohibit the insertion of an auxiliary (heterotopic) heart, however, and OHT may prove necessary. The complex abnormal anatomy of the recipient's own heart may be another factor making heterotopic transplantation difficult or impossible, again necessitating orthotopic siting of the xenograft. Retransplantation would be performed when a suitable human donor organ became available.

An animal heart inserted heterotopically (or orthotopically) as a bridge to transplantation would have some advantages over a mechanical support device, the most important and obvious being the fact that the animal heart can be totally enclosed within the thoracic cavity, thus reducing the risk of infection. There is, similarly, a reduced possibility of thromboembolism occurring when mechanical parts are not implanted. The complications of anticoagulation will not be avoided totally, however; it would seem wise to anticoagulate patients with auxiliary xenograft hearts (just as it is in patients with auxiliary allografts [8]), as the possibility remains that thrombus formation will occur in the patient's poorly contracting native right or left ventricle, and that embolism to the pulmonary or systemic circulations may take place.

Development of Lymphocytotoxic Antibodies

A second feature of the use of auxiliary xenograft hearts has not yet been fully explored. This relates to whether the recipient will develop lymphocytotoxic antibodies to this heart which will also react with human tissue, thus increasing the difficulty of finding a suitable human heart for subsequent definitive transplantation. This point has not been clarified in the experimental work which has been carried out to date, and it would seem worthy of exploration. If lymphocytotoxic antibodies to chimpanzee cells develop in the recipient, and these also cross-react with human donor cells, then clearly the advantages of the xenograft would be greatly diminished.

Transfer of Pathogenic Agents

The third aspect of the implantation of a natural auxiliary (or orthotopic) primate heart in man (whether temporary or permanent) which requires very careful consideration is the risk of transferring pathogenic agents which may result in serious infection or the development of neoplasia. Primates captured in the wild and, to a lesser extent, colony-bred animals, are known to harbor a host of pathogenic agents [28], of which viruses probably represent the greatest risk to man [29, 30]. This concern regarding the transfer of pathogens is reinforced by the consideration that the transfer of even a naturally mildly pathogenic agent may result in serious disease in an immunosuppressed patient. The simian retroviruses, which include viruses related to the human immunodeficiency virus type-1 that causes AIDS in man, and the herpesviruses must be considered particularly dangerous if transferred to man.

Results of recent studies [30] suggest that primates bred under suitable conditions of management would exhibit a lower tendency toward viral infection. It would appear, therefore, that the use of nonhuman primates as potential organ donors may be possible, provided that these animals are at least free of those infectious agents which are known to pose a serious threat to human health, e.g., *Mycobacterium tuberculosis*, herpesviruses, exogenous retroviruses, and Marburg virus. In this regard, the feasibility of breeding and maintaining specified pathogen-free animals seems worthy of investigation.

New Immunosuppressive Agents
The development of new pharmacological agents such as FK506 (formerly FR900506) [31], particularly when used in low-dose combination with CYA so that the toxic effects of each drug are minimized, may lead to further possibilities in this field, particularly if hyperacute rejection can be successfully prevented.

Comment
We would therefore appear to be at the threshold of an exciting era in cardiac transplantation, where the use of xenografts is explored, initially as bridging devices, particularly in infants and young children. In adults and larger children, it might be wise initially to utilize the heterotopic position for such xenografts if inserted as temporary assist devices. Experience gained in this area may lead to developments which allow xenografts to be used on a more permanent replacement basis.

Acknowledgement. I thank my colleague Dimitri Novitzky for his constructive comments.

References

1. Cooper DKC, Novitzky D, Becerra E, Reichart B (1986) Are there indications for heterotopic heart transplantation in 1986? A 2- to 11-year follow-up of 49 consecutive patients undergoing heterotopic heart transplantation. Thorac Cardiovasc Surg 34:300
2. Demikhov VP (1962) Experimental transplantation of vital organs. Consultants Bureau, New York
3. Barnard CN, Losman JG (1975) Left ventricular bypass. S Afr Med J 49:303
4. Losman JG, Barnard CN (1977) Hemodynamic evaluation of left ventricular bypass with a homologous cardiac graft. J Thorac Cardiovasc Surg 74:695
5. Novitzky D, Cooper DKC, Barnard CN (1983) The surgical technique of heterotopic heart transplantation. Ann Thorac Surg 36:476

6. Novitzky D, Cooper DKC, Rose AG, Barnard CN (1984) The value of recipient heart assistance during severe acute rejection following heterotopic cardiac transplantation. J Cardiovasc Surg 25:287

7. Novitzky D, Cooper DKC, Barnard CN (1984) Reversal of acute rejection by cyclosporin in a heterotopic heart transplant. J Heart Transplant 3:117

8. Cooper DKC (1984) Advantages and disadvantages of heterotopic transplantation. In: Cooper DKC, Lanza RP (eds) Heart transplantation. MTP Press, Lancaster, p 305

9. Wicomb WN, Cooper DKC, Novitzky D, Barnard CN (1984) Cardiac transplantation following storage of the donor heart by a portable hypothermic perfusion system. Ann Thorac Surg 37:243

10. Addonizio LG, Robbins RC, Reison DS, Drusin RE, Smith CR, Reemtsma K, Rose EA (1986) Transplantation in patients with high pulmonary vascular resistance. J Heart Transplant 5:394

11. Kormos RL, Thompson M, Hardesty RL, Griffith BP, Trento A, Uretsky BF, Reddy PS (1986) Utility of preoperative right heart catheterization data as a predictor of survival after heart transplantation. J Heart Transplant 5:391

12. Lexer G, Cooper DKC, Rose AG, Wicomb WN, Rees J, Keraan M, Du Toit E (1986) Hyperacute rejection in a discordant (pig to baboon) cardiac xenograft model. J Heart Transplant 5:411

13. Cooper DKC, Human PA, Lexer G, Rose AG, Rees J, Keraan M, Du Toit E (1988) The effects of cyclosporin and antibody adsorption on pig cardiac xenograft survival in the baboon. J Heart Transplant 7:238

14. Cooper DKC, Human PA, Rose AG (1987) Is ABO compatibility essential in xenografting between closely related species? Transplant Proc 19:4437

15. Cooper DKC, Human PA, Rose AG, Rees J, Keraan M, Reichert B, Du Toit E, Oriol R (1989) The role of ABO blood group compatibility in organ transplantation between closely related animal species J Thorac Cardiovasc Surg (in press)

16. Cooper DKC, Human PA, Reichart B (1987) Prolongation of cardiac xenograft (vervet monkey to baboon) function by a combination of total lymphoid irradiation and immunosuppressive drug therapy. Transplant Proc 19:4441

17. Sadeghi AM, Robbins RC, Smith CR, Kurlansky PA, Michler RE, Reemtsma K, Rose EA (1987) Cardiac xenograft survival in baboons treated with cyclosporin in combination with conventional immunosuppression. Transplant Proc 19:1149

18. Kurlansky PA, Sadeghi AM, Michler RE, Smith CR, Marboe CC, Thomas WA, Coppey L, Rose EA (1987) Comparable survival of intra-species and cross-species primate cardiac transplants. Transplant Proc 19:1067

19. Reemtsma K, McCracken BH, Schlegel IU, Pearl MA, Pearce CW, De Witt CW, Smith PE, Hewitt RC, Flinner RL, Creech O (1964) Renal heterotransplantation in man. Ann Surg 160:384

20. Starzl TE, Marchioro I, Peters GN, Kirkpatrick C, Wilson WEG, Porter KA, Rifkin D, Ogend DA, Hitchcock CR, Waddell WR (1964) Renal heterotransplantation from baboon to man. Experience with six cases. Transplantation 2:752

21. Hardy JD, Chavez CM, Kurrus RE, Neeley WA, Webb WR, Eraslan S, Turner KD, Fabian LW, Labecki JD (1964) Heart transplantation in man: developmental studies and report of a case. JAMA 188:1132

22. Cooley DA, Hallman GL, Bloodwell RD, Nora JJ, Leachman RD (1968) Human heart transplantation. Am J Cardiol 22:804

23. Barnard CN, Wolpowitz A, Losman JG (1977) Heterotopic cardiac transplantation with a xenograft for assistance of the left heart in cardiogenic shock after cardiopulmonary bypass. S Afr Med J 52:1035

24. Bailey LL, Nehlsen-Cannarella SL, Concepcion W, Jolley WB (1985) Baboon-to-human cardiac xenotransplantation in a neonate. JAMA 254:3321

25. Caplan AL (1985) Ethical issues raised by research involving xenografts. JAMA 254:3339

26. Veatch RM (1986) The ethics of xenografts. Transplant Proc 18:93

27. Sade RM, Crawford FA, Fyfe DA (1986) Symposium on hypoplastic left heart syndrome. J Thorac Cardiovasc Surg 91:937

28. Benirschke K (ed) (1986) Primates – the road to self-sustaining populations. Springer, Berlin Heidelberg New York Tokyo
29. Kalter SS (1986) Overview of simian viruses and recognized virus diseases and laboratory support for the diagnosis of viral infections, chapter 46. In: Benirschke K (ed) Primates – the road to self-sustaining populations. Springer, Berlin Heidelberg New York Tokyo, p 681
30. Van der Riet F de StJ, Human PA, Cooper DKC, Reichart B, Fincham JE, Kalter SS, Kanki PJ, Essex M, Madden DL, Lai-Tung MT, Chalton D, Sever JL (1987) Virological implications of the use of primates in xenotransplantation. Tranplant Proc 19:4068
31. Ochiai T, Nakajima K, Nagata M, Suzuki T, Asano T, Uematsu T, Goto T, Hori S, Kenmochi T, Nakagoori T, Isono K (1987) Effect of a new immunosuppressive agent, FK506, on heterotopic cardiac allotransplantation in the rat. Transplant Proc 19:1284

Part VI
Energy Sources

43. New Trends in Energy Sources for Cardiac Assist Devices

F. UNGER

Cardiac assist devices are usually connected to electrical or atomic-energy devices, which are very bulky and require constant monitoring. Atomic energy is sometimes enhanced by heat radiation. From the field of plastic surgery has come the idea of using a muscle as the energy source, mainly the latissimus dorsi. Dr. Andersen, from the Philadelphia group headed by Dr. Stephenson, shows in this chapter that with a stimulated muscle wrapped around a compliance chamber, a device such as an LVAD or a dynamic patch in the aorta can be driven permanently. The problem is muscle fatigue, which can be overcome by a special type of electrical stimulation. The idea originated with Leriche in 1933, who used the pectoral muscle to stimulate a canine heart that had failed due to an infarction. The technique described here is important for the further development of permanent cardiac assist devices. Dr. Khalafalla reports on a similar technique; her system could serve as the energy source for a permanent dynamic aortic patch.

Dr. Chachques, from Dr. Carpentier's group in Paris, reports on cardiomyoplasty. The latissimus dorsi is trained electrophysiologically and then, in a second procedure, wrapped around the heart to assist in the systolic phase. This technique has been applied in seven patients and demonstrates hemodynamic effectiveness. The technique is also being investigated clinically by Dr. Magovern in Pittsburgh.

Dr. Thoma, from Vienna, reports on the problems encountered with driving various cardiac assist devices such as IABP, VAD, and TAH and discusses their safety. He also shows how the TAH can be driven in an automatic mode. The control and drive parameters lead the integrated loops, which are computerized. Special attention is given to the type of patient who is a candidate for such a therapeutic regimen.

Dr. Mitamura, from Sapporo, is engaged in the field of transcutaneous energy transmission. His system consists of a transcutaneous transformer, a power oscillator, an output power conditioning system, rechargeable batteries, and an alarm system. With this system, high amounts of energy can be transmitted through the intact skin to drive an LVAD.

Dr. Fasol, from Vienna, and his colleague Zilla discuss the endothelialization of blood contact surfaces with cultured endothelial cells. This improves survival, and the idea has an impact for other clinical implants in the circulatory system.

Assisted Circulation 3
F. Unger (Ed.)
© Springer-Verlag Berlin Heidelberg 1989

44. Biologic Cardiac Assist: Performance Characteristics [1]

J. S. ANDERSEN, C. R. BRIDGES, W. A. ANDERSON, M. A. ACKER,
R. L. HAMMOND, F. DiMEO, JR., A. CHIN, and L. W. STEPHENSON

Introduction

Currently, the patient with end-stage heart failure has few therapeutic options. These include cardiac transplantation, mechanical assist devices, and medical therapy only. Despite recent advances in all types of treatment, *ideal* therapy for the patient with a failing heart has yet to be offered. Such an option should provide independence from external mechanical attachments, allow for an immunocompetent host, and minimize effects associated with blood-surface interaction. Cardiac assist devices powered by skeletal muscle might meet these requirements.

Skeletal muscle has the capacity to adapt to new patterns of work and become fatigue resistant. These changes occur when skeletal muscle is subjected to low-frequency electrical stimulation for a period of several weeks. We have fashioned pumping chambers from this transformed, or "preconditioned," muscle and demonstrated that the power output generated by these ventricular pumping chambers is sufficient to replace work done by the right ventricle or provide partial replacement or assistance of left ventricular function.

Skeletal muscle-powered cardiac assist devices have been under investigation in several laboratories worldwide. Many different approaches toward harnessing the energy of contracting skeletal muscle have been studied. Our laboratory in Philadelphia has directed efforts toward using skeletal muscle to form pouch-shaped or tube-shaped ventricles which eject blood and function in a manner analogous to that of the native cardiac ventricle [1–7]. We have demonstrated that such ventricles placed in the circulation can pump blood effectively for at least several weeks.

Historical Perspective

In general, there have been two approaches to the utilization of skeletal muscle to augment cardiac function. Skeletal muscle grafts have been applied directly to the beating heart in hopes of improving the collateral blood supply to ischemic myocardium and, in some cases, to directly bolster cardiac contractile function.

[1] Supported by NIH Grant #LB134778, the John Rhea Barton Research Foundation, and the Mary L. Smith Lead Trust.

Assisted Circulation 3
F. Unger (Ed.)
© Springer-Verlag Berlin Heidelberg 1989

The other avenue of investigation has been the formation of skeletal muscle pouches or ventricles that, when stimulated to contract, provide their own pumping function. Most early efforts at exploiting the contractile function of skeletal muscle failed as a result of muscle fatigue.

Muscle Grafts Applied to the Heart

Over 50 years have passed since skeletal muscle was first used in cardiac surgery. In 1933, Leriche and Fontaine applied pectoralis major muscle to the surface of canine infarcted myocardium [8]. Their pioneering work in dogs showed that after 3.5 months, unstimulated pectoralis major muscle grafts appeared viable and well incorporated into surrounding myocardium tissue. During the same period, de Jesus from Puerto Rico reported use of pectoralis muscle to repair a defect resulting from a penetrating cardiac injury in a young man [9].

In 1935, Beck reported that the blood suply to the canine myocardium could be altered by applying pedicled muscle grafts to the epicardium [10]. Following application of these grafts, he gradually occluded both coronary arteries with silver bands. By injecting the extracardiac vascular bed with dye, he was able to demonstrate the development of collateral blood flow from the enveloping graft to the myocardium. He and others subsequently used this technique to treat human patients with symptoms of ischemic heart disease. In his first clinical report, three of four patients who had pectoralis major muscle grafts applied to the heart claimed symptomatic improvement.

In 1961, Petrovsky described the use of nonstimulated pedicled grafts of left hemidiaphragm to treat left ventricular aneurysms in human beings [11]. He sutured these grafts directly to the epicardial surface of the defective left ventricle under enough tension to flatten out and obliterate the aneurysm. His initial results in eight patients were encouraging. A later report in 1966 discussed the results of 100 such procedures [12]. He felt that these grafts were well tolerated, became firmly adherent to the myocardium, reinforced the scarred tissue, and may have improved myocardial blood supply. His operative mortality was 19%, but he reported that 29% of his patients were subsequently freed from chest pain and dyspnea.

Christ and Spira wrapped pedicled latissimus dorsi grafts over partial-thickness defects in the left ventricle. In their studies, the grafts became adherent to the myocardium and neovascularization occurred [13]. Sola et al. placed inlay grafts of skeletal muscle into the wall of the canine left ventricle and found the grafts were well tolerated for many months and aneurysmal dilatation did not occur [14].

Muscle grafts have been used in the treatment of mediastinal infections associated with open sternal defects. As an extension of earlier work by Petrovsky, Shaff et al. described the use of pedicled pectoralis major grafts to treat patients with infected false aneurysms of the left ventricle following repair with Teflon felt [15].

In 1959, Kantrowitz and McKinnon wrapped pedicle grafts of left canine hemidiaphragm around the heart and then stimulated the graft via the phrenic nerve so that the graft would contract in synchrony with cardiac systole [16, 17].

They noted active contraction of the muscle graft but could not demonstrate hemodynamic changes. Later, similar experiments by Kusaba et al. included ligation of the distal left coronary artery to induce heart failure [18]. They noted a 12% increase in left ventricular pressure, a 13% increase in peak femoral artery pressure, and a 4% increase in aortic blood flow. After 15 min of continuous stimulation of the muscle graft, however, these effects were no longer observed as a consequence of muscle fatigue.

In 1974, Spotnitz et al. described an attempt to wrap a rectus muscle cuff around the canine heart [19]. As they stimulated the graft to contract, the animal developed right ventricular distension and ventricular fibrillation and deteriorated rapidly.

Left ventricular inlay grafts of vascularized canine rectus abdominus muscle were constructed in 1980 by Drinkwater and Chiu [20]. While on cardiopulmonary bypass, these grafts were made to contract with an external R-wave synchronous stimulator. This stimulation device provided a train or a rapid succession of stimuli during each contraction instead of a single stimulus. In these acute experiments on cardiopulmonary bypass, the left ventricular pressure increased up to 30 mmHg when the grafts were stimulated.

In 1964, Nakamura and Glenn augmented the right canine atrium with a pedicled graft of right hemidiaphragm [21]. This increased atrial volume to approximately twice normal. The grafts were stimulated acutely via the phrenic nerve and contracted well. At 7 months, the grafts were again stimulated. Rapid rises in right atrial pressure were noted during graft stimulation.

In the same study, Nakamura and Glenn also wrapped both ventricles with pedicled grafts of left canine hemidiaphragm. At 7 months, the grafts were stimulated to contract during cardiac systole at a rate of 160/min. They reported a 20 mmHg (10%) augmentation of systolic aortic blood pressure in one dog. This effect lasted up to 6 min before the muscle succumbed to fatigue. Termet et al. wrapped canine latissimus dorsi muscle around the heart [22]. After 8 months, they stimulated these pedicled grafts via the thoracodorsal motor nerve while fibrillating the heart. They reported that an aortic systolic pressure of 80 mmHg could be generated with each muscle graft contraction during cardiac fibrillation. This effect subsided after 10–15 min as the muscle fatigued.

Following an interest in congenital heart disease, Shephard applied inlay and only grafts of canine diaphragm to the right ventricle [23]. During initial work, she found that denervation atrophy occurred despite an intact blood supply. This was less severe if the nerve supply was preserved and the grafts were electrically stimulated on a long-term basis.

In 1968, Hume wrapped latissimus dorsi muscle around the heart and placed an electrode around the thoracodorsal nerve and connected this to an R-wave synchronous pacemaker [24]. He reported that the skeletal muscle grafts contracted continuously and in synchrony with cardiac systole for up to 2 weeks. However, he did not report on the hemodynamic effects of his work. In 1969, Phillips et al. wrapped canine diaphragm around the heart and preserved the vascular and nerve supply [25]. They described the stimulation of the diaphragm during various induced cardiac arrhythmias. No mention was made of hemodynamic results.

In 1980 Macoviak et al. from our laboratory, reported the use of innervated vascularized pedicled grafts of canine diaphragm to replace full-thickness portions of the right ventricular free wall [26]. These grafts were made to contract by stimulation, directly or through the intact phrenic nerve [26–29]. Echographic study demonstrated graft thickening concurrent with each contraction [27]. When the grafts were stimulated by an implantable R-wave synchronous pacemaker, strain-gauge studies demonstrated active tension development weeks after implantation [29]. Blood flow studies at 1 month demonstrated collateral blood flow between the muscle graft and the adjoining myocardium [28].

The surgical teams of Carpentier in Paris [30] and Magovern in Pittsburgh [31] have recently applied pedicled grafts of latissimus dorsi to the hearts of human beings suffering from various cardiac maladies. These grafts were stimulated by an implantable R-wave synchronous pulse generator. Both groups report improvement in cardiac performance during muscle-graft stimulation.

Most recently, Anderson and co-workers from our laboratory have wrapped latissimus dorsi muscle around the canine heart and stimulated the muscle graft chronically with a totally implantable burst stimulator [32]. At 4 months, the grafts were actively contracting and echographically deforming the left ventricular free wall. The hemodynamic results were variable, however. In one dog, the aortic pulse pressure increased by 40 mmHg while the graft was contracting in synchrony with cardiac systole. In another animal, the systolic pressure dropped significantly during graft stimulation, probably as a result of a tethering effect on the heart. Three of the animals were placed on cardiopulmonary bypass and the hearts were fibrillated. During ventricular fibrillation on bypass, average left ventricular pressure increased by 15 mmHg during each muscle graft contraction.

Skeletal Muscle Pumping Chambers

Pumping chambers or "ventricles" constructed from skeletal muscle have been the other, and perhaps potentially more important, type of biologic cardiac assistance. These muscle pumps have been built from a variety of different skeletal muscles. The latissimus dorsi muscle has been popular owing to its single main blood supply, its single motor nerve, its ease of harvesting, and its minimal donor disability. The latissimus dorsi is large and flat; it is easy to mobilize into the thoracic cavity and can be molded into various shapes. Other muscles used have included the rectus abdominus, quadriceps femoris, pectoralis major, gluteus maximus, psoas, and diaphragm. Working on the concept if diastolic counterpulsation, Kantrowitz wrapped left canine hemidiaphragm around the descending aorta in 1959 [16, 17]. The muscle graft was stimulated through the intact phrenic nerve by an external stimulator to contract during cardiac diastole. He reported a 26.5% increase in diastolic aortic pressure until the muscle fatigued several seconds later.

Kusserow and Clapp adapted quadriceps femoris muscle to power a bellows-type blood pump [33]. The pump functioned effectively for several hours.

In 1974, Spotnitz et al. constructed skeletal muscle pouches from canine rectus muscle [19]. They found their geometry and physical characteristics to be similar to those of the heart, as described by Frank and Starling. They noted that the transmural pressure, developed during active tension, increased as the resting wall tension (preload) was increased. The rectus muscle appeared to be less compliant than cardiac muscle. However, in his experiments with filling pressures of 50–150 mmHg, systolic pressures of greater than 500 mmHg could be obtained.

In 1975, Vachon et al. wrapped denervated pedicled grafts of diaphragm around a fluid-filled balloon pressure transducer and evaluated pressure, flow, and power output as a function of filling pressures and stimulation parameters [34]. The muscle pouches were stimulated directly. With stimulation of 30 V, the muscle pouch generated up to 176 mmHg pressure. Their pouches also produced increased stroke work with increased filling pressures. In addition, during these acute experiments the pouches were able to generate a power output of 50 mW. They reported a calculated power output of the left ventricle of 335 mW and 33.5 mW for the right ventricle. Unfortunately, these muscle pouches fatigued after several minutes. Von Recum et al. also constructed skeletal muscle pouches from diaphragm and stimulated them directly. Those pouches too failed after several hours as a result of muscle fatigue [35].

Juffe et al. constructed pouch-like skeletal-muscle pumping chambers from gluteus maximus muscle dissected free from its insertions [36]. A balloon transducer was introduced into the pouch and the muscle was stimulated via the gluteal nerve by a pacemaker. Pressures as high as 170 mmHg were recorded initially. One animal was followed with this device implanted in the abdomen for 26 days. That muscle pump eventually failed, probably as a result of nerve damage.

A Comparison of Skeletal Muscle with Cardiac Muscle

Skeletal muscle and cardiac muscle share many similarities, but they differ in several important physiologic and histologic properties. Both muscle types are able to convert stored chemical energy to mechanical contractile force. Both exhibit similar behavior in response to stretch and force-velocity generation. In skeletal muscle, active tensions of 1–5 kg/cm^2 cross-sectional area can be obtained. This contrasts with the cardiac papillary muscle, which generates active tension of about 500 g/cm^2 cross-sectional area [37].

Cardiac muscle and skeletal muscle have the same basic ultrastructure. The myofibrils are oriented longitudinally and the sarcomere – the basic contractile unit – is almost identical. Both muscle types have extensive sarcoplasmic reticulum and similar transverse tubular systems [38].

The neuroelectrical pathways of these two muscle types are different, however. Cardiac muscle functions as an electrical syncytium, as electrical impulses travel between cells. Intercalated disks are thought to facilitate the flow of current between cells by functioning as a low-resistance pathway. Cardiac muscle will contract nearly simultaneously as an "all-or-none" unit in response to a solitary electrical stimulus. The strength of contraction is not determined by the electrical impulse, but is more a function of resting tension and other variables. Skeletal muscle fibers are arranged into motor units that contract individually, as each unit contains its own nerve ending. An electrical stimulus applied to a skeletal muscle motor nerve may be sufficient for contraction of some, all, or none of the motor units. In this way, the strength of a contraction is a function of the number of motor units activated as well as of the rate of recruitment.

The process of externally stimulating cardiac muscle and skeletal muscle is different, therefore, owing to the differing intracellular conduction pathways. A single muscle twitch generated by a single electrical stimulus applied through the motor nerve is usually not sufficient to cause skeletal muscle to generate cardiac-type work. This contrasts with the heart, where a single external electrical stimulus precipitates a powerful contraction of the entire myocardium. The work of Chiu, Dewar and associates [39, 40] and our own laboratory [1–4] has shown that burst stimulation of skeletal muscle leads to rapid mechanical summation of motor units and generation of substantial contractile force. The magnitude of the contractile force can be modified by varying the parameters that define burst stimulation. These include burst duration (duty cycle ON), interval between bursts (duty cycle OFF), burst frequency (frequency of impulses during ON cycle), pulse amplitude (impulse voltage), and individual pulse duration. For a given muscle, these parameters govern the force and duration of contraction. Burst frequencies are typically set at 25, 43, or 85 Hz, and increasing burst frequencies correspond with increasing force of contraction. Duty cycles for skeletal muscle ventricles are generally set at 25%–33% ON and 75%–67% OFF. Investigators in our laboratory and others have shown that chronic burst stimulation of skeletal muscle does not generally cause muscle or nerve damage [2, 40–45].

Skeletal muscle and cardiac muscle have differing metabolic demands and consequently differing mechanisms for generating high-energy substrates. The rhythmically contracting heart must function continuously for a lifetime without developing fatigue or pausing for a rest. Skeletal muscle is required to perform mechanical work for relatively brief periods of time with intervening periods of rest. Cardiac muscle has a highly developed mechanism for aerobic metabolism; consequently, the cardiac muscle cell has a large portion of mitochondria – the energy-producing unit of the cell – approximately 30% by volume. These organelles are the primary focus of the process of oxidative phosphorylation. This contrasts with the skeletal muscle cell, which contains from 2% to 5% of mitochondria by volume [38].

Histologically, cardiac muscle cells are relatively uniform while skeletal muscle has differentiated into two basic fiber types. Type-II, or fast-twitch fibers are relatively prone to fatigue and are more plentiful than type-I, or slow twitch fibers. Type-I fibers are relatively fatigue resistant like cardiac muscle fibers. The relative number of each fiber type varies in response to the work with which a particular muscle is required to perform. Muscles which move quickly for brief periods, such as ocular muscles, are composed predominantly of type-II fibers. Postural muscles, such as the soleus, depend on protracted contractile times and are composed of more fatigue-resistant type-I fibers [38]. Type-II fibers generate peak tension more rapidly than the slower type-I fibers. Type-II fibers generate phosphocreatine predominately through anaerobic, glycolytic pathways in contrast to type-I fibers, which depend more on aerobic, oxidative phosphorylation pathways to generate high-energy phosphate bonds. When evaluated histologically, type-II fibers have a large proportion of sarcoplasmic reticulum and a relatively small mitochondrial volume. In contrast, type-I fibers have a smaller amount of sarcoplasmic reticulum and a larger mitochondrial volume.

Histochemical study of skeletal muscle shows specific myosin isotypes correlating with each of the differing fiber types. Type-I fibers have a specific "slow" isoform of myosin, while type-II fibers have an analogous "fast" myosin isoform. Muscles that have been used for cardiac augmentation, including the diaphragm, rectus abdominus, pectoralis major, and latissimus dorsi, are all mixed-fiber-type muscles.

Skeletal Muscles Fatigue and the Process of Electrical Conditioning

Fatigue occurs when the high-energy phosphate reserves of skeletal muscle have been used up and the muscle is no longer able to replenish high-energy phosphates at the rate that they are being utilized. As a result, no matter how many the motor units are recruited, or how rapidly the contractile function diminishes.

In 1960, having noted that motor neurons that innervated fast-twitch muscles exhibited a short after-hyperpolarization and motor neurons which innervated slow-twitch muscles exhibited a longer after-hyperpolarization, Buller et al. sought to determine whether the differentiation of skeletal muscle fiber types was a consequence of the motor neuron influencing muscle or muscle influencing motor neurons [46]. Knowing that all muscles in kittens are slow twitch at birth, their initial cord-isolation studies demonstrated that there was a failure of the normal muscle differentiation process. Later, they conducted a cross-innervation experiment in cats [47]. The motor nerve to the soleus muscle (a predominantly slow-twitch type-I muscle) was switched surgically with the motor nerve to the flexor digitorum longus (a predominantly fast-twitch type-II muscle). After the nerves regenerated, the contraction rate of the soleus reinnervated by the nerve to the flexor digitorum longus was accelerated while the contraction rate of the reinnervated flexor digitorum longus muscles was slowed. This cross-innervation brought about changes in both the contraction time and the relaxation time of the two muscles.

In 1969, Salmons and Vrbova determined that it was actually the pattern of the stimulation through the motor nerve which governed the ultimate differentiation of muscle type [48]. Slow-twitch muscles are subjected to chronic low-frequency stimulation. If fast-twitch skeletal muscle is subjected to chronic low-frequency electrical stimulation, an orderly sequence of changes occurs, which results in the transformation of a fast-twitch muscle into a slow-twitch muscle. This can be demonstrated by histochemical, biochemical, and physiologic criteria. Initially, there is an increase in capillary density during the first week of the new stimulation pattern. By 3 weeks there is a marked change in the sarcoplasmic reticulum. During this initial period, the activity of calcium transport. ATPase, and the rate of calcium uptake are decreased to levels approaching those of slow-twitch type-I fibers. The activities of enzymes involved in anaerobic metabolism, including phosphofructokinase, lactate dehydrogenase, and glycogen synthetase, decrease to levels approaching those of type-I fibers and myocardial fibers [49].

Likewise, there is a dramatic increase in the level of oxidative enzyme activity, including malate dehydrogenase, citrate synthase, and hexokinase. By 6–8 weeks, histochemical myosin ATPase stains show essentially complete conversion of type-II fibers to type-I fibers.

The physiologic properties of the transformed muscle are also altered. The time to peak tension is decreased, as is the relaxation time. There is a decrease in the tetanus-twitch ratio and the rate of tension development. By 8 weeks of electrical stimulation, the maximum velocity of isotonic shortening is significantly reduced.

Work done in our laboratory by Macoviak et al. showed that electrical preconditioning of diaphragm at 10 Hz continuous stimulation frequency (600 impulses per minute) results in 95%–100% conversion of muscle fibers to type-I fatigue-resistant fibers [50]. Perhaps more importantly, we found that preconditioning of the entire hemidiaphragm could be accomplished at a more physiologic stimulation frequency of 2 Hz (120 impulses per minute) [51, 52]. This lower rate is similar to that of the normal canine heart rate. Mannion et al. demonstrated that the latissimus dorsi muscle could be preconditioned at stimulation frequencies of either 2 or 10 Hz [53, 54].

Mannion and co-workers studied canine diaphragm that was stimulated continuously in an indirect manner via the motor nerve, at frequencies of 2 and 4 Hz, for 1 year [55]. At completion of the study, the muscles were contracting vigorously and completely transformed.

Further work by Acker et al. in our laboratory showed that near complete transformation of latissimus dorsi muscle could be accomplished after several weeks of electrical preconditioning using intermittent burst stimulation at a frequency of 25 Hz. The burst was set to last 312 ms and the intervening rest period was set to 812 ms. This yielded a contraction rate of 54/min. In this experiment, the latissimus dorsi was mobilized and formed into a pouch-like skeletal muscle ventricle. The preconditioning process was initially completed by a 6-week period of isometric contractions, followed by a period of contraction against a mock circulation device for measurement of stroke work and power output [1]. A second, similar experiment demonstrated that the preconditioning process could be accomplished while the muscle was performing useful-type work and contracting against the mock circulation device [2].

Clark and co-workers studied the bioenergetics of skeletal muscle using phosphorus-31 nuclear magnetic resonance (P-NMR) [56]. They evaluated the biochemical basis of fatigue resistance during active exercise by comparing electrically preconditioned latissimus dorsi muscle with contralateral unconditioned control muscle. The resting spectra of each muscle were similar, showing ATP and phosphocreatine (PCr) stores, both high energy phosphates, and a pool of inorganic phosphate (Pi). The concentrations of these phosphate moieties were followed during periods of mild, moderate, and intense exercise. The ratio of Pi to PCr (Pi/PCr) was evaluated as an index of energy reserve. An increasing ratio indicated diminishing stores. For control muscles, the tension development reached a plateau while the Pi/PCr ratio continued to increase. In the electrically preconditioned muscle, the increase in Pi/PCr was relatively small. Evaluation of the Tension-Time Index during the same experiment showed that unconditioned control muscle reached a plateau during the most intense exercise period. This study indicated that, in sharp contrast to unconditioned control muscle, the capacity of electrically preconditioned skeletal muscle for oxidative phosphorylation rivaled that of the heart itself.

In a companion study, oxygen consumption and blood flow were measured during a similar exercise cycle [57]. This study showed that preconditioned muscle is also more efficient in its use of oxygen than unconditioned muscle. Preconditioned muscle generates as much as or more isometric work than control muscle while consuming less oxygen per gram of tissue.

Skeletal Muscle Ventricles

Skeletal muscle ventricles (SMVs) can now be constructed and made to pump in vivo either against mock circulation devices or in the circulation for weeks at a time [1–3]. The muscle can be stimulated either directly, by weaving wire electrodes through the muscle body, or indirectly through the thoracodorsal motor nerve. Stimulating the muscle indirectly has many advantages over the direct mode. Nerve stimulation allows complete uniform transformation of the muscle fibers to the fatigue-resistant state by electrical preconditioning, where direct stimulation promotes transformation segmentally in the area of the wire electrode [50]. Studies in our laboratory over a 1-year period of continuous burst stimulation via the thoracodorsal motor nerve have yielded not only 100% latissimus dorsi muscle transformation to type-I fibers, but also normal nerve conduction velocities and normal nerve histology.

Current work with SMVs, which includes construction of SMVs from latissimus dorsi, SMVs in mock circulation, and SMVs in circulation as diastolic counterpulsators, is described in the following sections.

Construction of Skeletal Muscle Ventricles

The surgical technique of constructing a skeletal muscle ventricle is fairly straight-forward [1–7]. The latissimus dorsi is a large, flat muscle overlying the back and flank. Its principal function is adduction of the forelimb. The muscle has attachments to the thoracic spine, the eleventh rib, the platysma, the trapezius, the teres major, the triceps, and the insertion to the humerus. The blood supply comes from the thoracodorsal artery as well as via numerous small arterial branches from the intercostal arteries. The thoracodorsal nerve supplies motor innervation.

The animal is anesthetized and the latissimus dorsi is mobilized through a flank incision extending from the axilla to the tip of the eleventh rib. The lesser blood supply from the overlying skin and the chest wall is divided. The attachments mentioned above are also divided, leaving only the thoracodorsal neurovascular pedicle intact. A specially modified Medtronic pacing lead is placed around the proximal aspect of the thoracodorsal nerve. This lead is connected to a permanent implantable nerve stimulator. The muscle is then wrapped

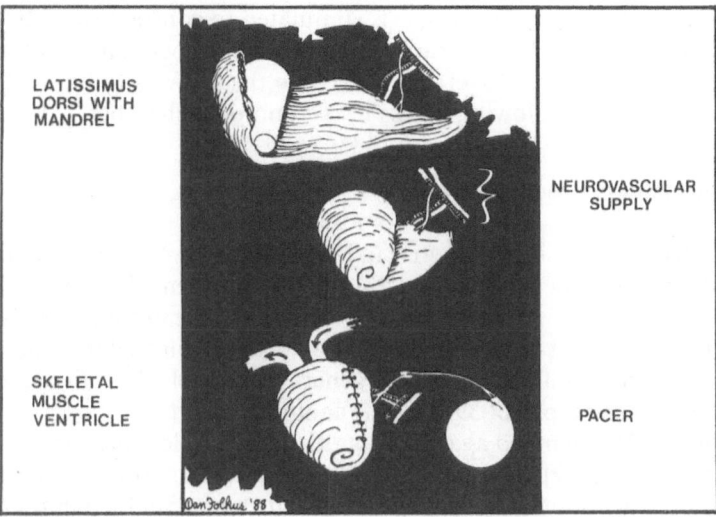

Fig. 1. The latissimus dorsi is a large, flat muscle. The muscle is wrapped around a cone-shaped Teflon mandrel to form a skeletal muscle ventricle. The pacing lead is affixed to the proximal aspect of the thoracodorsal nerve

or rolled around a previously machined Teflon mandrel of a given shape and size (Fig. 1). The mandrel is either conical, when forming pouch-type ventricles, or cylindrical, to produce tube-type or flow-through ventricles. The mandrel also has a Teflon felt collar on one or both ends which ultimately acts as a sewing annulus. The wrapped layers are sutured to each other as well as to the felt collar. The direction of the wrap is always such that the neurovascular pedicle will be on the outside. Generally, 1.5–2.5 muscle wraps are obtained. The SMV can be placed inside the thoracic cavity or left on the chest wall under the skin and subcutaneous tissue. It is sutured to the surrounding tissues to prevent migration or kinking of the pedicle. The subcutaneous tissue and skin are then closed over the SMV.

The SMV is allowed to rest for a 3-week vascular delay period. Although the neurovascular pedicle supplies an adequate blood supply to prevent immediate muscle necrosis at the time of mobilization, division of the small arteriolar blood supply from the intercostal arteries during construction renders the muscle relatively ischemic. Immediately following skeletal muscle ventricular construction, the distal half of the muscle is unable to increase its blood flow in response to the increased demands of exercise. A 3-week vascular delay period, however, allows for recovery of resting and exercise-induced increases in blood flow [4, 42]. The combination of a vascular delay period and electrical preconditioning allows the SMV to be essentially fatigue resistant. Using radiolabeled microspheres, Mannion et al. have demonstrated that all layers of an SMV receive substantial blood flow following the vascular delay period while the ventricles are pumping in the circulation [5].

After completion of the vascular delay process, the SMV can be used immediately or be further electrically preconditioned. The electrical preconditioning process takes approximately 6 weeks. The muscle is stimulated to contract isometrically against the rigid Teflon mandrel at a rate of 54 contractions per min at 25 Hz (duty cycle = 312 ms ON, 812 ms OFF) [1]. At the time the SMV is to be used, the Teflon mandrel is removed, allowing access to the pumping chamber.

Skeletal Muscle Ventricles in Mock Circulation

Skeletal muscle ventricles have been constructed by several investigators, and they have reported encouraging results. Stevens and Brown formed cylindrical pouches from canine rectus abdominus muscle and stimulated the muscle directly [58]. The unconditioned pouches were connected to an external mock circulation device. For several hours the system was able to generate flows of 73% of canine cardiac output and a power output of 39% of the canine left ventricle.

In our laboratory, SMVs pumped against a totally implantable mock circulation device for many weeks [1, 2]. These studies allowed long-term evaluation of the capabilities of SMVs without the potential complexities of actually pumping blood. The SMVs were constructed as described above, using a 17-ml cone-shaped Teflon mandrel. The mock circulation device shown in Fig. 2 consists of two similar polyurethane bladders connected by a rigid conduit. One bladder is placed inside the SMV while the other is contained within a hermetically sealed rigid Plexiglas canister. The pouch and canister bladders and the conduit are filled with saline while the canister is pressurized with air. As the SMV contracts and ejects fluid into the conduit, the ventricular pouch pressure must overcome the

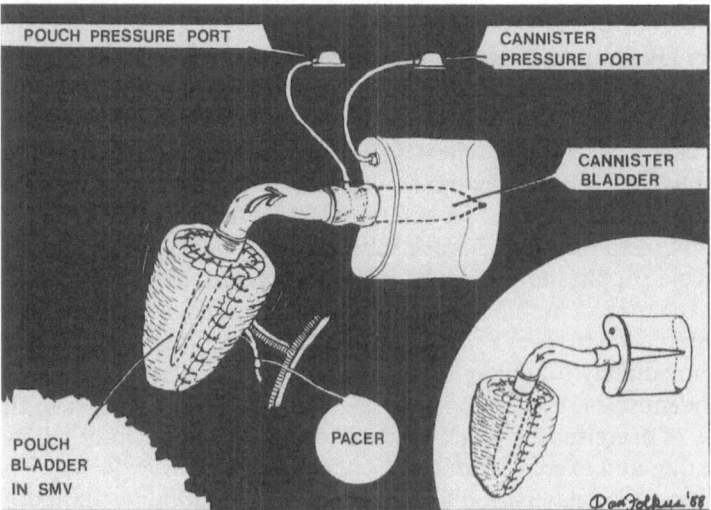

Fig. 2. The mock circulation device allows determination of skeletal muscle ventricular function by varying preload, afterload, and stimulation parameters. The device consists of a pouch bladder and a canister bladder connected by a rigid conduit. The canister bladder is housed within a hermetically sealed canister. The bladders are filled with fluid and the canister is filled with air. Varying the fluid volume controls preload, and changing the canister air pressure controls afterload

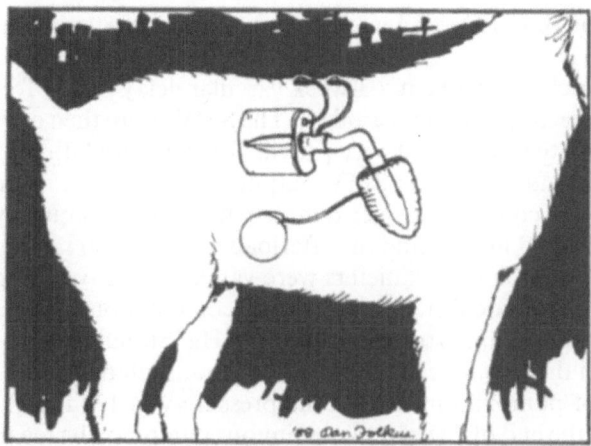

Fig. 3. Totally implantable mock circulation device lies along the lateral chest wall of the animal under the skin and subcutaneous tissue, with no tubes or wires crossing the skin

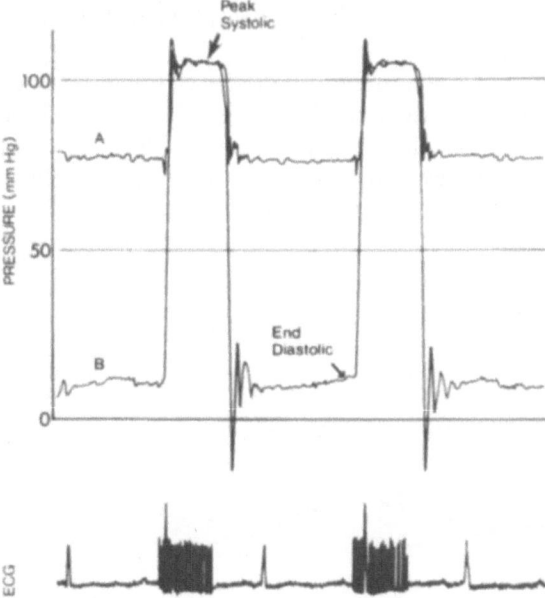

Fig. 4. A typical mock circulation trace obtained at a preload of 10 mmHg and an afterload of 80 mmHg. The burst frequency is 85 Hz. The upper trace (A) represents the pressure within the canister. The lower trace (B) represents the pressure within the skeletal msucle pouch bladder

pressure within the canister before the canister bladder will accept fluid. Thus, the pressure within the resting SMV cavity is the ventricular preload pressure, while the pressure within the canister corresponds to the systemic afterload. Two percutaneous access ports allow for independent manipulation and measurement of the pressures within the bladder conduit and the canister. No tubes or wires crossed the animal's skin during periods of continuous pumping. Animals were able to move about freely and without apparent discomfort or physical disability. Figure 3 demonstrates the device in place.

A typical mock circulation pressure trace obtained after 7 days of continuous pumping is shown in Fig. 4. The SMV in this figure is generating a pressure of

105/10 mmHg at a preload of 10 mmHg and against an afterload of 80 mmHg.
The ventricular output is 190 ml/min.

   In initial studies, the ventricles underwent a 3-week vascular delay period followed by a 6-week electrical preconditioning period [1]. The SMVs were then connected to the mock circulation device. This device provided for manipulation of
both SMV preload and afterload as well as SMV output. The ventricles were
made to contract at a rate of 54 contractions per minute with a burst frequency
of 25 Hz. The preload was set to 40 mmHg and the afterload was set to 80 mmHg
during periods of continuous pumping. Parameters were varied each day during
brief measurement periods to evaluate function at varying combinations of preload from 10 to 60 mmHg and afterload from 60 to 200 mmHg. Stimulation parameters were varied through the implanted stimulator by a transcutaneous pro-
grammer. At the initiation of pumping, mean systolic pressure was 134 mmHg
and flow was 464 ml/min. At the end of 2 weeks of continuous pumping, the mean
peak systolic pressure was 104 mmHg and flow was 206 ml/min. These SMVs
were capable of greater pressures and flows when preload, afterload, and burst
frequency were changed (Figs. 5–7). Skeletal muscle ventricles functioned for up
to 9 weeks.

   A subsequent study was designed to determine functional characteristics of
skeletal muscle ventricles during the electrical conditioning process [2]. These
SMVs were constructed with a 3-week vascular delay period but without a period
of electrical preconditioning. The ventricles were connected to the mock circulation device following the vascular delay period and stimulated to contract im-

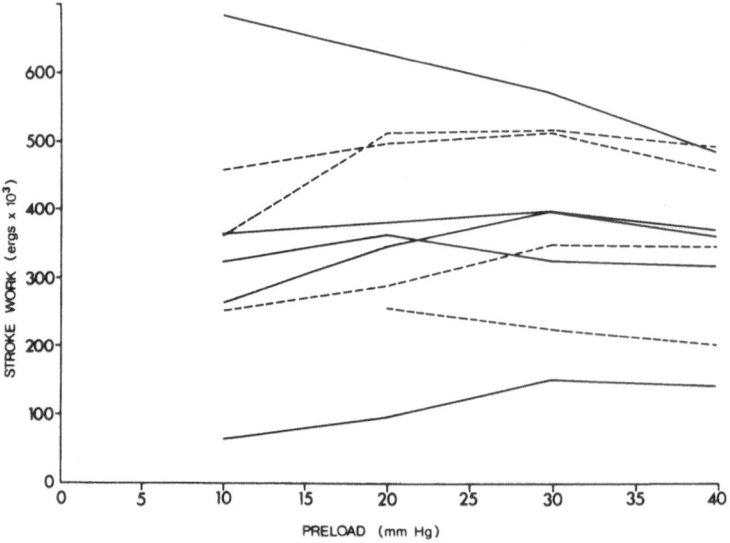

Fig. 5. Stroke work obtained at various filling pressures in SMVs that had been pumping continuously for 48–72 h when these measurements were made. They were stimulated at 85 Hz frequency. *Solid lines* represent electrically preconditioned muscle, *dashed lines* represent SMVs that
were conditioned as they performed work. Average canine right ventricular stroke work is
220×10^3 ergs

mediately. The preload, afterload, and stimulation parameters were similar to those in the initial study. After 2 weeks of continuous pumping these ventricles generated a mean peak systolic pressure of over 100 mmHg and flow over 200 ml/min. In other studies, our laboratory has measured the stroke work of the canine right and left ventricle to be 220×10^3 ergs and 1830×10^3 ergs respectively. After 2 weeks, these SMVs generated mean stroke work of 400×10^3 ergs. This was intermediate between the work of the canine right and left ventricle. Two animals were still generating significant work after 2 months.

Comparing the function of conditioned and electrically preconditioned skeletal muscle ventricles with those being conditioned is of interest. Maximal stroke work performed by SMVs after 48–72 h of continuous pumping against the mock circulation device is shown in Fig. 5. The electrically preconditioned ventricles and those being conditioned functioned at essentially the same capacity. Mean stroke work is greater than that of the native right ventricle (220×10^3 ergs), while optimal stroke work occurs at a preload of 20 and 25 mmHg. This may be indicative of the relatively greater stiffness of SMVs constructed in this present configuration when compared with cardiac ventricles.

During the first week of continuous pumping, performance of electrically preconditioned and conditioned skeletal muscle ventricles is predictable. Since the muscle being conditioned is more susceptible to fatigue than the electrically preconditioned muscle, measurements of continuous function would be expected to show muscle being conditioned performing at a slightly lower level than electrically preconditioned muscle. Examination of systolic pressure and flow during

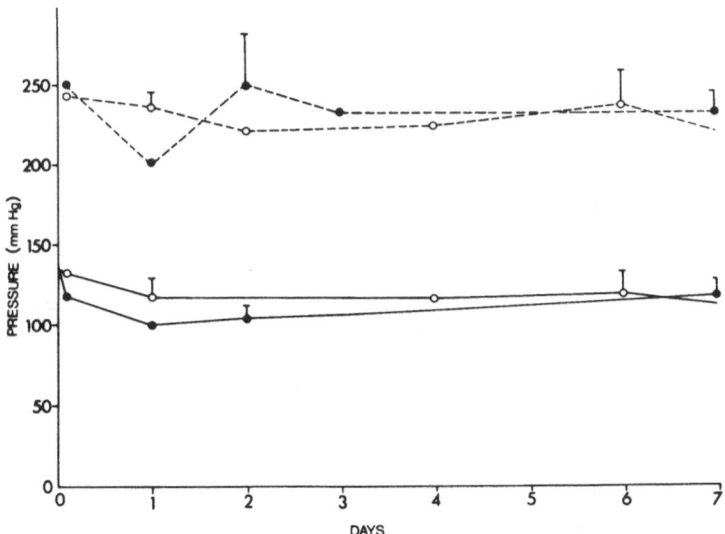

Fig. 6. Continuous pressures were obtained at an afterload of 80 mmHg and preload of 40 mmHg with a burst frequency of 25 Hz. Maximal pressures were obtained at an afterload of 200 mmHg and a preload of 60 mmHg with a burst frequency of 85 Hz. *Open circles* represent electrically preconditioned muscle, *closed circles* represent SMVs in the process of being conditioned. *Dashed lines* represent maximal recordings, *solid lines* represent continuous recordings

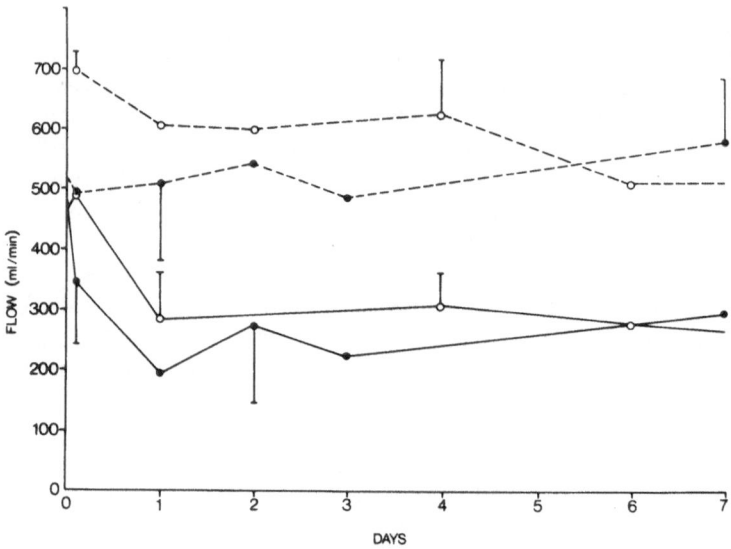

Fig. 7. Continuous flow measurement was obtained at an afterload of 80 mmHg and preload of 40 mmHg with a burst frequency of 25 Hz. Maximal flow was obtained at an afterload of 60 mmHg and a preload of 50 mmHg with a burst frequency of 85 Hz. *Open circles* represent electrically preconditioned muscle, *closed circles* represent SMVs in the process of being conditioned. *Dashed lines* represent maximal recordings, *solid lines* represent continuous recordings

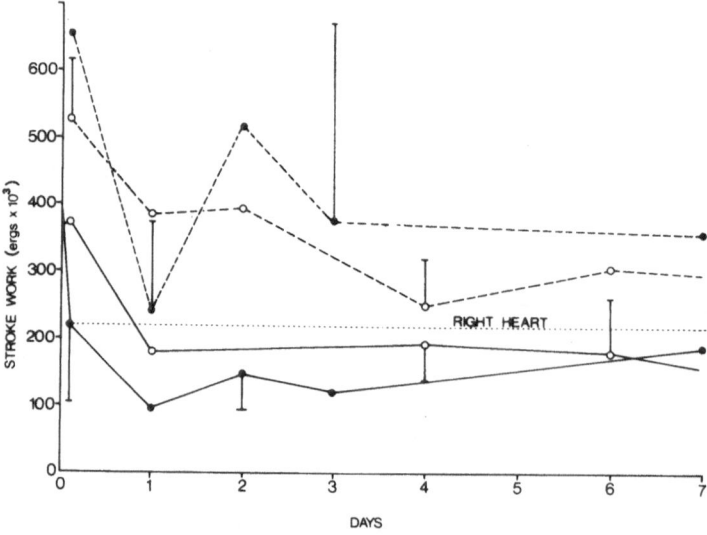

Fig. 8. Continuous work measurement was obtained at an afterload of 80 mmHg and preload of 40 mmHg with a burst frequency of 25 Hz. Maximal work was obtained at an afterload of 60 mmHg and a preload of 50 mmHg with a burst frequency of 85 Hz. *Open circles* represent electrically preconditioned SMVs, *closed circles* represent SMVs being conditioned. *Dashed lines* represent maximal recordings, *solid lines* represent continuous recordings

the first week of continuous pumping shown in Figs. 6 and 7, respectively, reveals the predicted result. It is clear, however, that by the seventh day of continuous pumping, the performance of muscle being conditioned and electrically preconditioned muscle is essentially identical.

Evaluation of stroke work yields similar results, shown in Fig. 8. Of importance is the finding that these ventricles generate stroke work continually at levels comparable to those of the right heart. Maximal stroke work after 7 days of continuous pumping is above that of the native canine right ventricle.

These studies indicate that canine skeletal muscle which has not received prior electrical preconditioning is capable of performing sustained useful work while it is becoming conditioned or transformed. The optimal preload pressures appear to be somewhat higher than normal physiologic levels, but this may be more a factor of SMV design, with respect to wall thickness and chamber size, than an absolute property of skeletal muscle.

Skeletal Muscle Ventricles
as Arterial Diastolic Counterpulsators

Current efforts toward adapting skeletal muscle ventricles as arterial diastolic counterpulsators are not significantly different from the ideas initially developed by Kantrowitz [16, 17]. These SMVs are designed to pump blood, augment aortic diastolic blood pressure, and reduce mean systemic afterload during systole. Presently, the intra-aortic balloon pump (IABP) accomplishes these goals clinically. Although the IABP is effective, its use is limited to acutely ill patients requiring only temporary cardiac assistance. A skeletal-muscle-driven diastolic counterpulsator potentially offers the chronically ill patient a form of cardiac assistance that would be effective on a long-term basis.

Working in our laboratory, Mannion demonstrated that electrically preconditioned skeletal muscle ventricles connected acutely to the descending thoracic aorta as a diastolic counterpulsator were able to function well in the circulation for many hours [4–7]. Stroke work generated by these SMVs was 680×10^3 ergs after 4 h of continuous pumping. This is about three times that of the native canine right ventricle. In other acute studies, Nelson et al. demonstrated improvement in the subendocardial viability ratio when SMVs of their own design were used to power an arterial diastolic counterpulsation device [59].

Acker et al. demonstrated that skeletal muscle ventricles could function chronically as diastolic counterpulsators, pumping blood in the circulation [3]. Latissimus dorsi muscle, tube-shaped SMVs were constructed in dogs. These SMVs were fashioned around a cylindrical Teflon mandrel with a Gortex bladder. This geometry allowed inflow and outflow in a flow-through manner. Following a 3-week vascular delay period, the Teflon mandrel was removed and ringed Gortex conduits were attached to the Gortex-lined bladder (see Fig. 9). With the SMV positioned on the chest wall, the Gortex conduits were brought into the chest via second- and fifth-space thoracotomies. The device was inserted into the circulation by dividing the descending thoracic aorta and re-establishing flow through the Gortex bladder-conduit device. The nerve electrode and an epi-

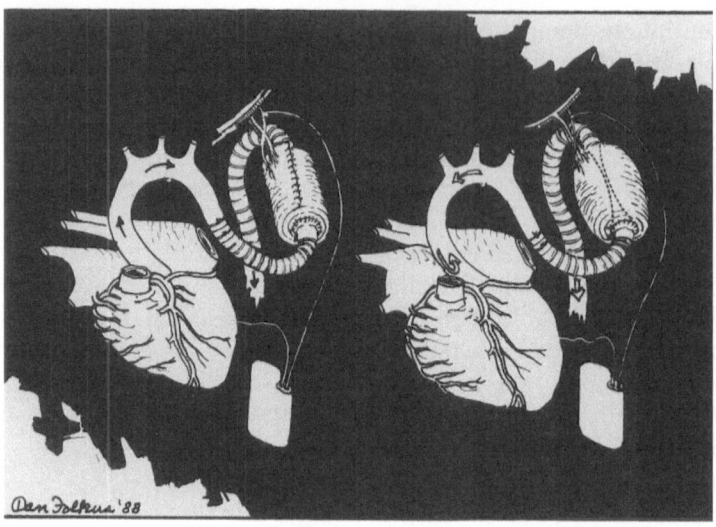

Fig. 9. Skeletal muscle arterial diastolic counterpulsator. The *left* drawing shows the SMV relaxed and the heart ventricles contracting. The *right* drawing shows the cardiac ventricles during diastolic and the SMV contracting. The skeletal muscle ventricle was positioned on the chest wall, with the skin and subcutaneous tissue closed over it

cardial sensing electrode were connected to a totally implantable prototype Medtronic pacemaker. The skin and subcutaneous tissue were closed over the SMV, which was then stimulated to contract during diastole, generally with a synchronization ratio of 1:2–1:3, depending on the native heart rate. The pacemaker delivered burst stimuli of 25–85 Hz with a burst duration of 185–240 ms and a delay of 240 ms from the R-wave. These animals were tether free, in that no tubes or wires crossed the skin barrier. They tolerated the diastolic counterpulsator without apparent discomfort or disability.

Diastolic augmentation is apparent in the arterial pressure trace shown in Fig. 10. This trace was obtained at a burst frequency of 85 Hz on day 12 of continuous pumping. Diastolic augmentation of 50 mmHg was observed on every other beat.

Two-dimensional short-axis echocardiography of the SMV in the same dog after 12 days of continuous pumping is shown in Fig. 11. By altering the burst frequency of stimulation from the chronic setting of 25 Hz to 43 Hz and 85 Hz, the decrease in cross-sectional area at the midpoint of the SMV measured 70%, 90%, and 100% respectively during contraction. Concomitant M-mode echocardiography while the burst frequency was set to 85 Hz is shown in Fig. 12. Thickening of the wall of the SMV is pronounced and the lumen is nearly 100% obliterated.

Pulsed Doppler evaluation of the blood flow through the lumen of the contracting SMV just distal to the outlet end was obtained at burst frequencies of 25, 43, and 85 Hz. Forward (antegrade) blood flow was, respectively, 29%, 40%, and 63% greater during the assisted cardiac cycle than during the unassisted cycle. Evaluation at 85 Hz is shown in Fig. 13.

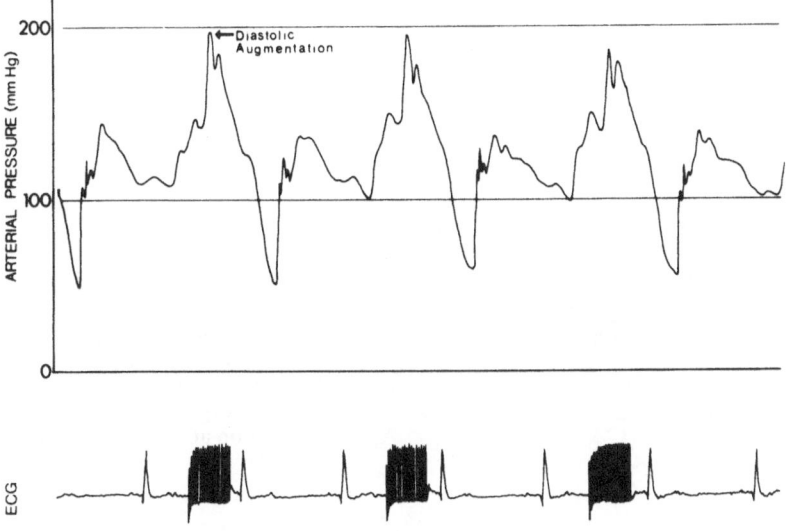

Fig. 10. A femoral aterial trace obtained after the SMV had been continuously pumping for 12 days in the circulation. The device is activated in a 1:2 mode

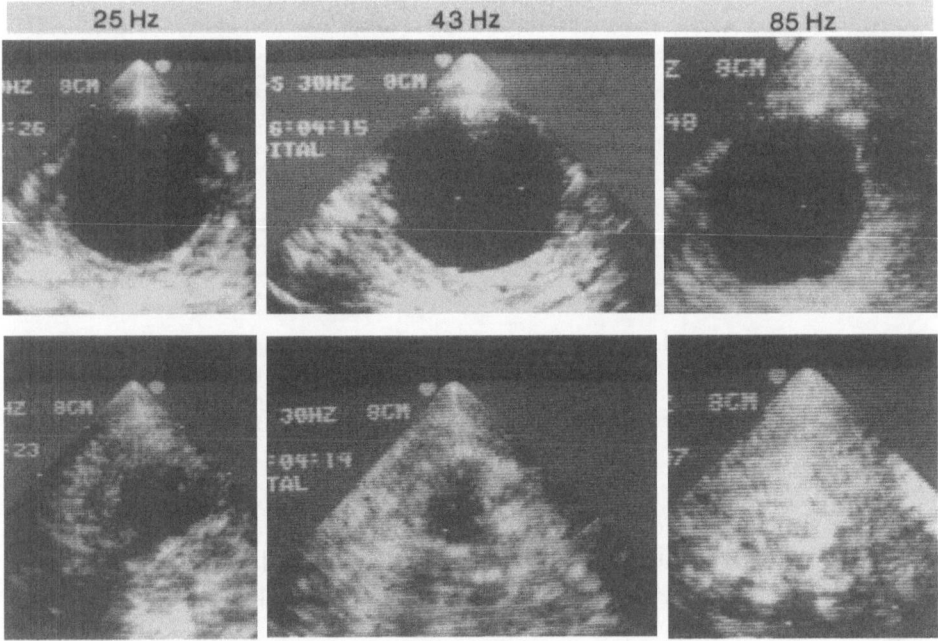

Fig. 11. Two-dimensional echocardiogram, short-axis view, obtained at the midpoint of the skeletal muscle ventricle. This study was obtained with same dog as Fig. 10, after 12 days of continuous pumping as a diastolic counterpulsator. Increasing the burst frequency from 25 Hz to 43 Hz to 85 Hz results in progressively increasing luminal obliteration during contraction. *Upper panels* show the SMV during relaxation, *lower panels* during the corresponding contraction

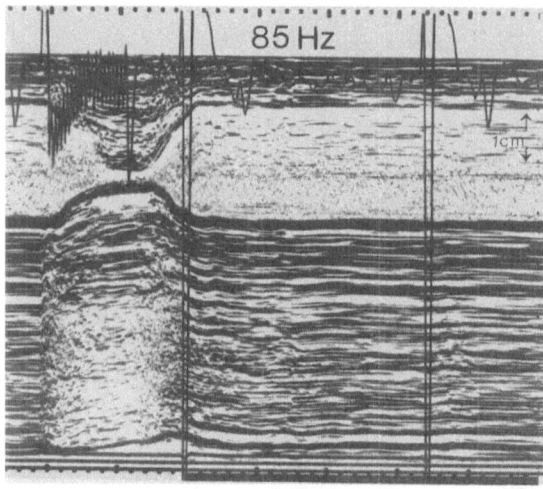

Fig. 12. M-mode echographic examination of the skeletal muscle ventricle in the same dog during contraction demonstrates thickening of the muscle wall as well as nearly complete luminal obliteration at a burst frequency of 85 Hz

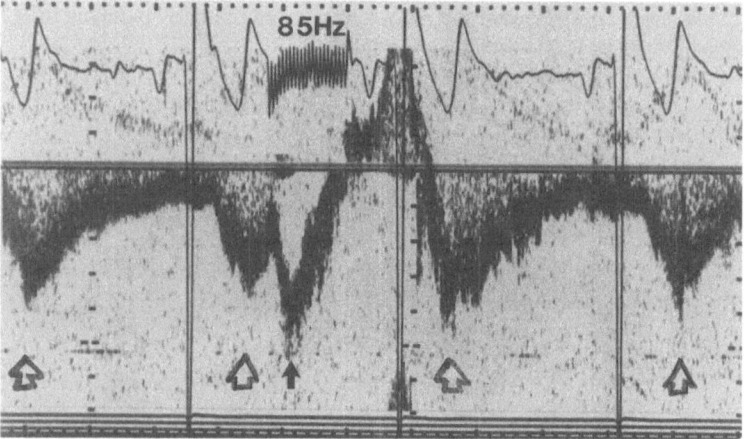

Fig. 13. Pulsed Doppler evaluation of the blood flow through the skeletal muscle ventricle in the same dog on the same day as in Figs. 10–12, near the outlet end after 12 days of continuous pumping. At 85 Hz, forward flow during an assisted cycle, represented by the *closed arrows*, is significantly higher than forward flow generated by the native heart during an unassisted cycle, *open arrows*

These skeletal muscle ventricles functioning as diastolic counterpulsators have generated useful work in circulation for up to 11 weeks [3]. The two longest surviving animals with this device in place both died from complications of renal failure. Autopsy revealed evidence of distal thromboembolism which resulted in multiple renal and splenic infarcts. There was no evidence of proximal embolization in the coronary or cerebral arterial systems. Despite these complications, this study demonstrated the capability of skeletal muscle ventricles to perform significant and useful cardiac-type work in the circulation for an extended period of time.

Summary

Since the first attempts at using skeletal muscle to augment cardiac performance, many obstacles have been overcome. The greatest problem, muscle fatigue, has for the most part been solved by the process of electrical conditioning as well as the practice of allowing for a vascular delay period. Stroke work of ventricles fashioned from skeletal muscle seems to be about equal to or somewhat greater than that of the native right ventricle. Performance of the SMVs can probably be improved by changing design characteristics. In-circulation studies have shown the ability of SMVs not only to pump blood continuously for many weeks, but also to function well at the high preload and afterload conditions of the systemic arterial circulation.

References

1. Acker MA, Hammond RL, Mannion JD, Salmons S, Stephenson LW (1986) An autologous biologic pump motor. J Thorac Cardiovasc Surg 92:733–746
2. Acker MA, Hammond RL, Mannion JD, Salmons S, Stephenson LW (1987) Skeletal muscle as a potential power source for a cardiovascular pump: assessment in vivo. Science 236:324–327
3. Acker MA, Anderson WA, Hammond RL, Chin AJ, Buchanan JW, Morse CC, Kelly AM, Stephenson LW (1987) Skeletal muscle ventricles in circulation: one to eleven weeks' experience. J Thorac Cardiovasc Surg 94:163–174
4. Mannion JD, Hammond RL, Stephenson LW (1986) Canine latissimus dorsi hydraulic pouches. Potential for left ventricular assistance. J Thorac Cardiovasc Surg 91:534–544
5. Mannion JD, Velchik MA, Acker M, Hammond R, Staum M, Alavi A, Duckett S, Stephenson LW (1986) Transmural blood flow of multi-layered latissimus dorsi skeletal muscle ventricles during circulatory assistance. Trans Am Soc Artif Intern Organs 32:454–460
6. Mannion JD, Acker MA, Hammond RL, Stephenson LW (1986) Four-hour circulatory assistance with canine skeletal muscle ventricles. Surg Forum 37:211–213
7. Mannion JD, Acker MA, Hammond RL, Faltemeyer W, Duckett S, Stephenson LW (1987) Power output of skeletal muscle ventricles in circulation: short-term studies. Circulation 76:155–162
8. Leriche F, Fontaine R (1933) Essai experimental de traitement de certains infarctus du myocarde et de l'aneuvrisme du coeur par une greffe de muscle strie. Bull Soc Nat Chir 59:229–232
9. de Jesus FR (1931) Breves consideraciones sobre un case de herida penetrante del corazón. Bol Assoc Med PR 23:380–382
10. Beck CS (1935) A new blood supply to the heart by operation. Surg Gynecol Obstet 1:407–410
11. Petrovsky BV (1961) The use of the diaphragm grafts for plastic operations in thoracic surgery. J Thorac Cardiovasc Surg 41:348–355
12. Petrovsky BV (1966) Surgical treatment of cardiac aneurysms. J Cardiovasc Surg 2:87–91
13. Christ JE, Spira M (1982) Application of latissimus dorsi muscle to the heart. Ann Plast Surg 8(2):118
14. Sola OM, Dillard DH, Ivey TD, Haneda K, Itoh T, Thomas R (1985) Autotransplantation of skeletal muscle into myocardium. Circulation 71:341–348
15. Schaff HV, Arnold PG, Reeder GS (1982) Late mediastinal infection and pseudoaneurysm following left ventricular aneurysmectomy repair utilizing pectoralis major muscle flap. J Thorac Cardiovasc Surg 84:912–916
16. Kantrowitz A, McKinnon W (1959) The experimental use of the diaphragm as an auxiliary myocardium. Surg Forum 9:266–268

17. Kantrowitz A (1960) Functioning autogenous muscle used experimentally as an auxiliary ventricle. Trans Am Soc Artif Intern Organs 6:305–310
18. Kusaba E, Schraut W, Sawatani S, Jaron D, Freed P, Kantrowitz A (1973) A diaphragmatic graft for augmenting left ventricular function: a feasibility study. Trans Am Soc Artif Intern Organs 19:251–257
19. Spotnitz HM, Merker C, Malm JR (1974) Applied physiology of the canine rectus abdominis. Trans Am Soc Artif Intern Organs 20:747–756
20. Drinkwater DC et al. (1980) Cardiac assist and myocardial repair with synchronously stimulated skeletal muscle. Surg Forum 31:271–273
21. Nakamura K, Glenn WWL (1964) Graft of the diaphragm as a functioning substitute for the myocardium. J Surg Res 4:435–439
22. Termet H, Chalencon JL, Estour E, Gaillard P, Favre JP (1966) Transplantation sur le myocarde d'un muscle strie excite par pacemaker. Ann Chir Thor Cardiol 5:260–263
23. Shepherd MP (1969) Diaphragmatic muscle and cardiac surgery. Ann R Coll Surg Engl 45:212–231
24. Hume WI (1968) Construction of a functioning accessory myocardium. Trans Southern Surg Assoc 79:200–202
25. Phillips WL, Pallin S, Crostnopol P (1969) Diaphragmatic transplantation. Angiology 20:628–634
26. Macoviak JA, Stephenson LW, Spielman S, Greenspan A, Likoff M, St. John-Sutton M, Riechek N, Rashkind WJ, Edmunds LH (1980) Electrophysiological and mechanical characteristics of diaphragmatic autograft used to enlarge the right ventricle. Surg Forum 31:270–271
27. Macoviak JA, Stephenson LW, Spielman S, Greenspan A, Likoff M, St. John-Sutton M, Riechek N, Rashkind WJ, Edmunds LH (1981) Replacement of ventricular myocardium with diaphragmatic skeletal muscle: acute studies. J Thorac Cardiovasc Surg 81:519–527
28. Macoviak JA, Stephenson LW, Alavi A, Kelly AM, Edmunds LH (1981) Effects of electrical stimulation on diaphragmatic muscle used to enlarge the right ventricle. Surgery 90:271–277
29. Macovial JA, Stephenson LW, Kelly A, Likoff M, Reichek N, Edmunds LH (1981) Partial replacement of the right ventricle with a synchronously contracting diaphragmatic skeletal muscle autograft. Proceedings of II Meeting of the International Society for Artificial Organs 1981; 5 [Suppl 1]:550–555
30. Carpentier A, Chachques JC (1985) Myocardial substitute with a stimulated skeletal muscle: first successful clinical case. Lancet 1:1267
31. Magovern GJ, Park SB, Magovern GJ, Benckart DH, Tullis G, Rozar E, Kao R, Christlieb I (1986) Latissimus dorsi as a functioning synchronously paced muscle component in the repair of a left ventricular aneurysm. Ann Thorac Surg 41:116
32. Anderson WA, Andersen JS, Acker MA, Hammond RL, Chin AJ, Douglas PS, Salmons S, Stephenson LW (to be published) Skeletal muscle applied to the heart: a word of caution. Circulation
33. Kusserow BK, Clapp JF (1964) A small ventricle-type pump for prolonged perfusions: construction and initial studies including attempts to power a pump biologically with skeletal muscle. Trans Am Soc Artif Intern Organs 8:74–78
34. Vachon BR, Kunov H, Zingg W (1975) Mechanical properties of diaphragm muscles in dogs. Med Biol Eng 13:252–260
35. von Recum A, Stulc JP, Hamada O, Baba H, Kantrowitz A (1977) Long-term stimulation of a diaphragm muscle pouch. J Surg Res 23:422–427
36. Juffe A, Ricoy JR, Marquez J, Castillo-Olivares JL, Figuera D (1978) Cardialization: a new source of energy for circulatory assistance. Vasc Surg 12:10–17
37. Mommaerts WFHM (1982) Heart muscle. In: Fishman AP, Richards DW (eds) Circulation of the blood, man and ideas. American Phyiological Society, Bethesda, pp 127–198
38. Adams R, Schwartz A (1980) Comparative mechanisms for contraction of cardiac and skeletal muscle. Chest 78:123–139
39. Dewar ML, Drinkwater DC, Wittnich C, Chiu RCJ (1984) Synchronously stimulated skeletal muscle graft for myocardial repair. J Thorac Cardiovasc Surg 87:325–331

40. Chiu RCJ, Walsh GL, Dewar ML, De Simon JH, Khalafalla AS (1987) Implantable extra-aortic balloon assist powered by transformed fatigue-resistant skeletal muscle. J Thorac Cardiovasc Surg 94:694–701
41. Chachques J, Grandjean P, Vasseur B, Hero M, Perier P, Bourgeois I, Fardeau M, Carpentier A (1985) Electrophysiological conditioning of latissimus dorsi muscle flap for myocardial assistance. In: Nose Y, Kjellstrand C, Ivanovich P (eds) Progress in artificial organs. ISAO Press, Cleveland, pp 409–412
42. Mannion JD, Velchik M, Alavi A, Stephenson LW (1985) Blood flow in conditioned and unconditioned latissimus dorsi muscle (abstract). Second Vienna Muscle Symposium, 1985, p 28
43. Glenn W, Phelps M (1985) Diaphragm pacing by electrical stimulation of the phrenic nerve. Neurosurgery 17:974–984
44. Ciesielski TE, Fukuda Y, Glenn W, Gorfien J, Jeffery K, Hogan JF (1983) Response of the diaphragm muscle to electrical stimulation of the phrenic nerve. J Neurosurg 58:92–100
45. Kim JH, Manuelidis EE, Glenn W, Fukuda Y, Cole DS, Hogan JF (1983) Light- and electron-microscopic studies of phrenic nerves after long-term electrical stimulation. J Neurosurg 58:84–91
46. Buller JC, Eccles JC, Eccles RM (1960) Differentiation of fast and slow muscles in the cat hind limb. J Physiol (Lond) 150:399–416
47. Buller JC, Eccles JC, Eccles RM (1960) Interactions between motor neurons and muscles in respect of the characteristic speeds of their responses. J Phyiol (Lond) 150:417–439
48. Salmons S, Vrbova G (1969) The influence of activity on some contractile characteristics of mammalian fast and slow muscles. J Physiol (Lond) 210:535–549
49. Chi et al. (1986) Chronic stimulation of mammalian muscle: enzyme changes in individual fibers. Am J Physiol C633–C642
50. Macoviak JA, Stephenson LW, Armenti F, Kelly AM, Alavi A, Mackler T, Cox J, Palatianois GM, Edmunds LH (1982) Electrical conditioning of in situ skeletal muscle for replacement of myocardium. J Surg Res 32:429–439
51. Armenti FR, Bitto T, Macoviak JA, Kelly AM, Chase CT, Hoffman BK, Rubinstein NA, St. John-Sutton M, Edmunds LH, Stephenson LW (1984) Transformation of skeletal muscle for cardiac replacement. Surg Forum 35:258–260
52. Bitto T, Mannion J, Hammond R, Cox J, Yamashita J, Duckett SW, Salmons S, Stephenson LW (1985) Preparation of fatigue-resistant diaphragmatic muscle grafts for myocardial replacement. In: Nose Y, Kjellstrand C, Ivanovich P (eds) Progress in artificial organs. ISAO Press, Cleveland, pp 441–446
53. Mannion JD, Bitto T, Hammond R, Rubinstein N, Stephenson LW (1986) Histochemical fatigue characteristics of conditioned canine latissimus dorsi muscle. Circ Res 58:298–304
54. Mannion JD, Acker MA, Hammond RL, Stephenson LW, Khalafalla A, Henriksson J, Salmons S (in press) Chronic burst stimulation of canine latissimus dorsi muscle: a further step towards the use of skeletal muscle for cardiac augmentation. Proceedings, Padova muscle symposium, 1986
55. Acker MA, Mannion JD, Brown WE, Salmons S, Henriksson J, Bitto T, Gale DR, Hammond R, Stephenson LW (1987) Canine diaphragm muscle after one year of continuous electrical stimulation: its potential as a myocardial substitute. J Appl Physiol 62:1264–1270
56. Clark BJ, Acker MA, Subramanian H, McCully K, Hammond B, Salmons S, Chance B, Stephenson LW (1988) In vivo P-NMR spectroscopy of electrically conditioned skeletal muscle. Am J Physiol 254:C-258–266
57. Acker MA, Anderson WA, Hammond RL, Di Meo F, McCullum J, Staum M, Velchik M, Brown WE, Gale D, Salmons S, Stephenson LW (1987) Oxygen consumption of fatigue-resistant muscle. J Thorac Cardiovasc Surg 94:702–709
58. Stevens L, Brown J (1986) Can noncardiac muscle provide useful cardiac assistance? Am Surg 52:423–427
59. Neilson IR, Brister SJ, Khalafalla AS, Chiu RCJ (1985) Left ventricular assistance in dogs using a skeletal muscle-powered device for diastolic augmentation. J Heart Transplant 4:343–347

45. Design and Stimulation of Biological Cardiac Assist Systems

A. S. KHALAFALLA and A. M. MALEK

Introduction

The feasibility of enhancing cardiac output of a patient suffering from end-stage heart failure has recently been demonstrated without resorting to heart transplantation or using a mechanical artificial heart. Previous work [1, 2] has shown that autogenous skeletal muscle can be used as a power source to drive an extra-aortic balloon and increase cardiac output by up to 20%, thereby circumventing the delicate issues of immune rejection and high cost associated with transplantation and artificial devices.

An encouraging possibility exists, therefore, for augmenting a patient's cardiac output by harnessing his own muscle power to perform the required work. This subject could then lead a normal life after implantation of a small cardiomyostimulator, similar to the ordinary pacemaker, with no need for outside power sources or wires protruding from the subject's chest.

As an alternative to the apico-aortic balloon pump that can assist, or even replace a failing left ventricle, one can induce circulatory counterpulsations by an extra-aortic balloon pump; both are driven by muscle power. The latter concept can replace on a permanent basis the temporarily applied intra-aortic balloon pump that is driven pneumatically.

Optimization of Cardiac Assist Systems

An important new concept in this mode of cardiac assistance is that of adjusting the balloon or pump size and shape as well as the mass of muscle activating it to match the hemodynamic requirements of the subject's body and somatic type. Such impedance and compliance matchings would undoubtedly synchronize blood flow to body needs, thus averting the disturbing mismatches that often complicate artificial heart programs, usually through localized strokes and/or other organ failures.

In a preceding publication [3] we presented some classical (first-generation) calculations to optimize the balloon size, shape, and required valve and connecting tube radii. By "classical" we mean that the fluid is assumed to be Newtonian and that its flow is laminar. Fine-tuned, or second-generation computations will have to take into account the fact that blood is a non-Newtonian suspension of corpuscles in fluid plasma. Its viscosity increases sharply at low shear rate in contrast to the Newtonian plasma, whose viscosity is independent of shear rate. Also,

Assisted Circulation 3
F. Unger (Ed.)
© Springer-Verlag Berlin Heidelberg 1989

although blood flow in veins and most arteries is laminar, there is some incipient turbulence [4] in the ventricle and branching aorta, to which laminar flow is inapplicable.

Classical calculations [3] for a device capable of delivering a stroke volume of 70 ml at a systolic pressure of 120 mmHg (16 000 N/m^2) and ejection ratio of 0.5 gave two useful rules of thumb. These two rules are helpful in designing an artificial left ventricle, i.e., a cylindrical or ellipsoidal balloon to be inserted between the subject's left ventricle and descending aorta and sandwiched into a suitable mass of innervated muscle tissue:

$$m = 2 \times 10^{-4} P \tag{1}$$

where m is the muscular mass in grams and P is the balloon's ejection pressure (or systolic pressure) in dyne/cm^2.

The second rule relates the radius, r, of the tube connecting the balloon with the descending aorta to the balloon average radius, R, thus

$$r^6 P = 4 \times 10^3 R^2 \tag{2}$$

These two rules form the basis for optimizing the balloon and muscle dimensions in a cardiac assist system. For example, in order to achieve the human systolic pressure of 120 mmHg (1.6×10^5 dyne/cm^2 or 1.6×10^4 Pa) in a 140-ml balloon that delivers a stroke volume of 70 ml, the required muscular mass is about 32 g.

The average left ventricle weight in adults (25–30 years) is reported [5] by the Federation of American Societies for Experimental Biology as being 100 g (range 73–125 g). The cardiac muscle structure indicates that the inner surfaces [6] of both the atria and ventricles are lined with connective tissue, the endocardium, which also covers the valves. Over the outer surface of the heart lies another layer of connective tissue, the epicardium. The intermediate layer is the ventricular myocardium, which lies between the epicardium and the endocardium. This consists of a series of overlapping sheets of muscle bundles which arise from the fibrous base of the heart. The myocardium itself is therefore approximately one third of the ventricular volume or mass. With the average human ventricular weight of 100 g, the average weight of the cardiac muscle required to pump the left ventricular chamber is about 33 g. This is very close to our calculated muscle fiber mass requirement of 32 g as predicted from rule 1 for a muscle-wrapped artificial left ventricle.

Rule 2 guides in the design of the cardiac assist system by relating the radius, r, of the tube connecting the balloon to the aorta with the average balloon radius, R. Thus, for R for 1.5 cm, the radius, r, of the valve connecting the bladder to the descending aorta is estimated to be 0.53 cm. Increasing R to 2.0 cm will correspondingly increase r to 0.69 cm. In order to use the commercial aortic valve with an orifice at 1.6 cm ($r = 0.8$ cm), a balloon with an average radius R of 3.2 cm would be needed. This is also close to the average radius of 2.8 cm for a normal ventricle [6] in the working human heart. This can increase to 4.5 cm in the dilated ventricle.

It is somewhat surprising that classical first-generation calculations would give close agreements with the real system. Starting from a few simple mechanical and hydrodynamic principles [3], one can end up with configurations that simulate the actual left ventricular function, thus exemplifying the profounder's beauty which comes from the harmonius ordering of the parts, and illustrating that nature has already chosen the best designs.

It appears that partial cancellation of errors lies behind the relatively good agreement of the theory [3] and the actually observed results. Poiseuille's law for laminar flow of a Newtonian fluid in cylindrical tubes expresses the flow rate, f, as

$$f = \frac{\pi P r^4}{8 L \eta} \tag{3}$$

where P is the driving pressure, L is the tube length, r is the tube radius, and η is the fluid viscosity coefficient in poise. This can be written as

$$f = \frac{P}{(8 L \eta / \pi r^4)} = \frac{P}{R} \tag{4}$$

where R is the hydrodynamic resistance to flow. A plot of f against P/R should give a straight line of unit slope in the ideal case as shown in Fig. 1.

The two debatable approximations in the classical treatment are based on two assumptions:

1. Flow is laminar. It is known that this is not entirely true, especially for early blood pumping, where flow is somewhat turbulent.

2. Blood is Newtonian. This is not true; blood is a non-Newtonian fluid whose viscosity decreases as its flow rate increases. The plot of f against P/R would therefore give a curvilinear relationship that bends downward from the ideal as shown in curve B, Fig. 1. This is because with increasing flow, f, the resistance R decreases because of the decrease in η ($R = 8 L \eta / \pi r^4$) and therefore P/R increases more than expected from the ideal straight line. Likewise, increasing turbulence at constant P/R would yield flows that increase at faster rates than predicted by the ideal Poiseuille straight line. This is shown in curve A of Fig. 1, which bends upward from the ideal straight line. The partial cancellation of errors

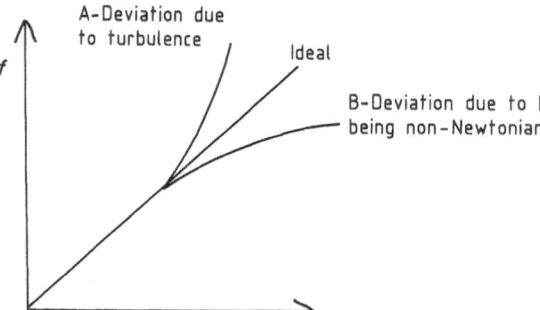

Fig. 1. Partial cancellation of errors due to neglect of turbulence and non-Newtonian flow characteristics gives apparent agreement with the ideal case

in curves A and B would result in the ideal case being a close representation of the actual system.

This analysis should by no means stop us from performing a second-generation mathematical analysis for the real system. This is the subject of following papers that will take into account the real features and actual hydrodynamic properties of blood flow.

The results of these calculations, especially when aided with computer modeling, would ultimately apply a CAD/CAM system leading to an exact size and shape fit of the cardiac assist device to the actual body needs.

The remainder of this paper will deal with the experimental determination of muscle power and stimulation modalities.

Nerve Versus Muscle Stimulation for Power Generation

We chose the latissimus dorsi muscle (LDM) to provide the driving power for the extra-aortic balloon pump (EABP) system because of this muscle's substantial mass and strength, as well as its nonessential nature in day-to-day activity.

The EABP can be used in various configurations. Some of these are shown in Fig. 2. The EABP can be placed in series with the descending aorta as shown in type A, in parallel as in type C, or in an adjacent configuration as in type B. In all three types of configuration, the muscle is wrapped around the bladder (dashed lines) in order to generate the required pressure upon contraction of its fibers. Each configuration has its advantages and drawbacks. Actually, fluid dynamics modeling and research will have to be conducted before a final bladder configuration is chosen. In all of the three types shown here, the blood is in direct contact with the inner wall of the bladder, thus raising the important issue of platelet and clot formation as well as thrombosis in regions of the bladder where the flow is stagnant.

This important area of research is currently advancing under the auspices of the American National Heart and Blood Institute of the NIH. The most advanced state-of-the-art material will be used to fabricate these balloons for actual human

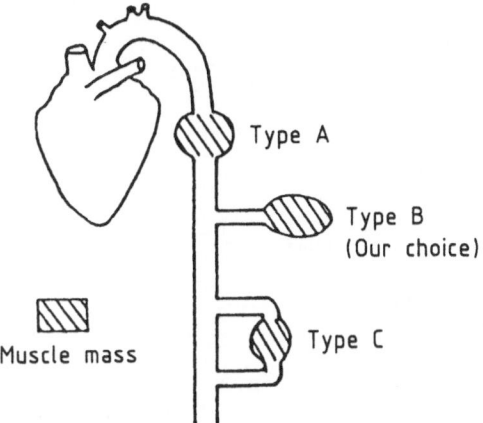

Fig. 2. Various extra-aortic balloon pump (EABP) cardiac assist configurations

usage. In this research, we used Biomer (made under an NIH grant) a material that showed sufficient compliance, biocompatibility and impermeability to blood for the manufacture of the bladders.

Methods and Materials

Since our goal was to obtain a quantitative measure of the power that can be generated by the LDM, and in order to avoid the trauma of placing the animal on a heart-lung machine and actually carrying the anastomosis of the bladder to the descending aorta of our experimental models, we decided to simply use the experimental setup shown in Fig. 3. The bladder is of type B shown in Fig. 2 and is connected via a stiff Teflon tube to a U-shaped glass tube filled with a 15% glycerol solution. The glycerol was added to reduce the oscillation of the fluid column following a contraction. We must keep in mind that this increase in viscosity probably resulted in frictional losses.

The pressure was measured inside the bladder and the volume alongside the glass column; the volume flow at this point is expected to be the same as that at the exit of the bladder because of the very low compliance in the Teflon and glass tubing.

Surgical Procedure

Five male mongrel dogs weighing 20–25 kg were anesthetized with sodium pentobarbital, kept on a ventilator, and intravenously injected with lactated Ringer's solution. These dogs had not undergone any muscle conditioning prior to the operation. An incision to the left of the thorax was made to expose the left LDM, which was then transected at its origin. Care was taken to maintain all blood vessels and nerve fibers intact. Once isolated, the LDM flap was then wrapped around the 150-ml Biomer bladder (1.5–2 turns).

In four experiments, the muscle was stimulated indirectly via the thoraco-dorsal nerve (TDN). This was identified, and a Medtronic Model 4080 nerve-cuff bi-

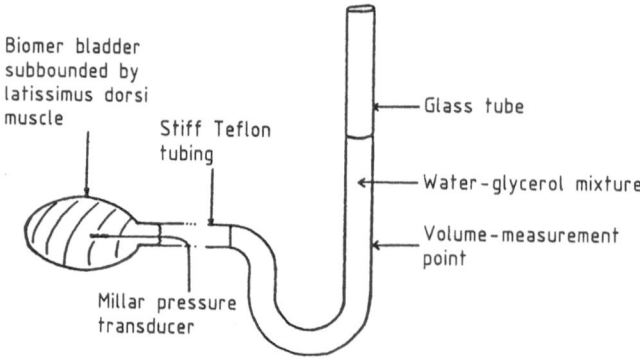

Fig. 3. Experimental setup

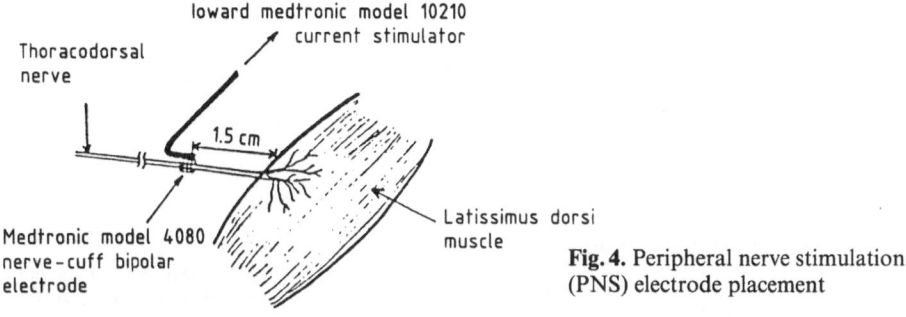

Fig. 4. Peripheral nerve stimulation (PNS) electrode placement

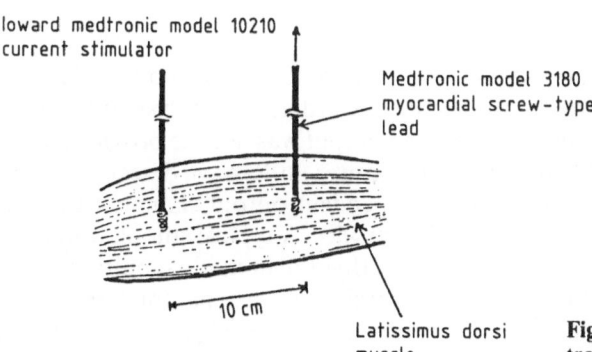

Fig. 5. Muscle stimulation (MS) electrode placement

polar electrode[1] was wrapped around it at a distance of 1.5 cm from the neuro-muscular junction point, as shown in Fig. 4.

In the fifth experiment, the LDM was stimulated directly, using a pair of Medtronic Model 3180 myocardial unipolar screw-type electrodes[1]. These were inserted, as shown in Fig. 5, into the mass of the LDM for a depth of 1 cm; the two electrodes were separated by a distance of 10 cm along an axis that would ensure that the electric field lines be parallel to the msucle fibers. We must keep in mind that the LDM was not curarized, and all nerve conduction pathways inside the muscle mass were therefore intact and active in this stimulation scheme. Thus, intramuscular stimulation included not only direct stimulation to muscle fibers, but also, and more importantly, indirect stimulation of the nerve network within the LDM.

It is well known that the force that a muscle fiber can generate is dependent on the length of the fiber at rest. This so-called length-tension relation, when extrapolated to a volume-pressure domain, gives Starling's law of the heart.

In order to maintain the muscle fibers distended in accordance with the skeletal muscle-fiber length-tension relation, we subjected the bladder in all experiments to a preload pressure of 30 mmHg by setting the height of the liquid column at 40 cm above the level of the bladder.

---

[1] Reference to trade names is given for identification purposes only and does not imply endorsement of the product.

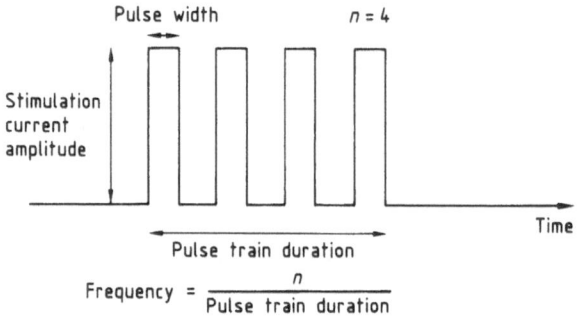

Fig. 6. Parameters of the current stimulation pulse train

Stimulation Apparatus

We chose to use a current-source stimulator for both the nerve and muscle stimulation experiments. A Medtronic Model 10210 Cardiac Assist System External Stimulator (CASES)[1] with inductively coupled output was used to provide a train of biphasic current pulses. The model 10210 features an R-wave detector to trigger the stimulation; it also provides four independent output channels, thus allowing the use of more than a single pair of electrodes. A typical stimulation wave is shown schematically in Fig. 6 (note, however, that the individual pulses, unlike the ones shown, are actually biphasic). The stimulation wave parameters such as pulse width, pulse frequency, and total duration of the pulse train are selectable. An adjustable delay that allows setting the time period between the time of cardiac R-wave detection and the onset of stimulation is also adjustable to allow for use of the EABP in a counterpulsation mode.

It is envisaged either that the muscle will be conditioned prior to installation of the cardiac assist device or that conditioning will start shortly after the installation. In the latter case it will be crucial to know the response characteristics of the muscle, which will be stronger, though more prone to fatigue than the conditioned muscle. Such knowledge will help us to avoid overdriving the system by generating high levels of power, which could be harmful to the lining of the aorta.

Since the bladder is not connected to the circulation, synchronization issues were not critical in this work. The dog's ECG was recorded for monitoring purposes but not connected to the stimulator's R-wave detector. Instead, we strived to obtain low muscle fatigue by stimulating the LDM every 7 s. This allowed for an approximate 10% drop in the peak pressure achieved by the muscle over a period of 5 h. Here we were more interested in the response characteristics of an untrained muscle than in its fatigue time course, which will be the subject of future studies.

Modeling of the Experimental Setup

The experimental setup shown in Fig. 3 does not exactly mimic the type of load that the muscle-bladder complex will be subjected to in the final system. It does,

---

[1] (See footnote on page 517).

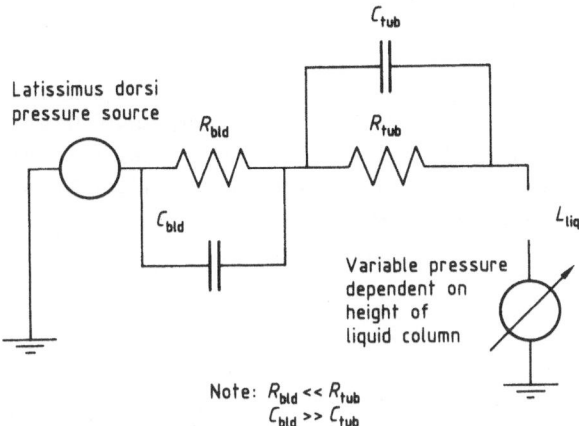

Fig. 7. Electrical equivalent circuit of the experimental setup. R, Resistance; C, compliance; L, inertness

however, provide a realistic impedance that can be used to measure the amount and type of work that the wrapped LDM can furnish. An electrical equivalent circuit of the experimental setup is shown in Fig. 7.

The left portion of the circuit deals with the bladder with its associated compliance and resistance, along with the LDM, which is represented as a voltage (i.e., pressure) source. The middle section is made up of the compliance and resistance of the Teflon and glass tubes. The inertness due to the mass of the liquid in this tube is shown on the left, as is a voltage (pressure) source. The latter is variable because the pressure faced by the bladder is proportional to the height of the top of the liquid column above the bladder. This characteristic is not realistic and could be avoided by adding a shunt from a certain level on the glass tube back to the Teflon tubing; this was not done here for the sake of simplicity.

By analyzing the pressure wave, one can better see the suitability of the proposed equivalent circuit. At the onset of muscle contraction, we observed a rapid rise in pressure which is measured at the midpoint of the circuit in Fig. 7, followed by a slower decrease. This happens once the inertness, L_{liq}, is overcome and the flow becomes nonzero. The inertness element encountered in this setup is usually not so substantial in cardiovascular fluid systems and is usually neglected. It is worthwhile to note that the compliance of the bladder, C_{bld}, is believed to be lower than that of the tubes, C_{tub}. The resistance of the bladder, R_{bld}, however, is lower than that of the tubes, R_{tub}. Furthermore, C_{bld}, is nonlinear; at low volumes it is substantially more compliant that at higher ones, where it becomes nearly impossible to stretch the bladder beyond its 150-ml volume. Assuming laminar flow (which is something that has to be verified), Poiseuille's equation yields a value of the resistance of the tubes. Furthermore, the addition of glycerol to the water served to increase the resistance and thus to damp the inherent oscillations present in this underdamped system.

Results

The threshold for both modes of stimulation – peripheral nerve stimulation (PNS) and muscle stimulation (MS) – were defined as the magnitude of the current that resulted in a pressure peak of around 5 mmHg. These threshold measurements were conducted at the following set of stimulation parameters deemed optimal on the basis of earlier research by Nielson et al. [1]:

Pulse width	230 µs
Pulse frequency	36 Hz
Train duration	190 ms
Number of pulses	7

The threshold values were found to be 220 µA for PNS and 2 mA for MS, using the electrodes described previously.

Our first efforts were concentrated on determining the effect of increasing stimulation current beyond the threshold and studying its effect on the characteristics of the muscle contraction. To do so, we fixed our stimulation parameters to be the optimal set described above and varied the amplitude of the current train pulse. The most basic characteristics of the contraction are the pressure peak and the pressure wave duration.

Peak Pressure

Figure 8 shows the dependence of the peak pressure on the log of current amplitude for both PNS and MS. One notices that in the case of nerve, it is possible to consistently reach lower and higher pressures than with muscle.

For PNS the maximum peak pressure reached was 175 mmHg as compared with 115 mmHg for MS. This points up the fact that MS does not activate as many muscle fibers simultaneously as PNS; that is, MS causes more localized muscle contraction than PNS, which seems to cause the muscle to contract as a unit. This is also due to the fact that PNS makes use of the nerve and thus the

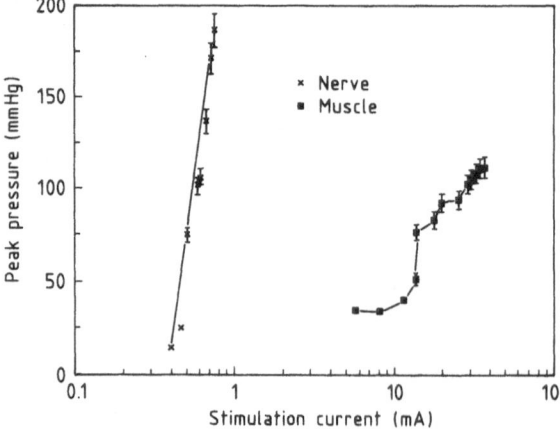

Fig. 8. Variation of peak pressure with stimulation current

conduction pathway already present in the muscle; it therefore relies on the various junctional delays and branchings of the natural muscle.

In contrast, MS uses a more irregular conduction, in part due to the unnatural location of the foci of excitation, chosen arbitrarily, and also due to the incomplete spread of the wave of excitation, even though the latter spreads partly via existing nerve pathways.

The most significant point is that to achieve the same level of pressure, MS requires a tenfold increase in current is compared with PNS. Furthermore, though PNS allows us to reach the maximum pressure at 880 µA (with a threshold of 220 µA), resulting in a range of 600 µA (300% of the threshold), MS requires 40 mA to reach the maximum (with a threshold of 2 mA) with a consequent range of 38 mA (1900% of the threshold). Thus, it appears more efficient, though more tricky, to modulate the peak pressure by PNS than by MS. From a qualitative standpoint, the dependence of peak pressure, and probably the number of recruited fibers, appears to be a logarithmic function of current, whereas no such obvious dependence can be coined for MS. It would seem that this dependence in the case of MS will depend on various individual factors such as the patient's anatomy and electrode placement, all of which are variable. All the above findings seem to point to PNS as the better mode of stimulation.

Pressure Duration

Pressure duration is a very important variable that has to be carefully considered in cardiac assistance because of the synchronization constraints imposed by counterpulsation. At a heart rate of 60 bpm, assuming that diastole requires about two thirds of the heart beat, then the duration should be shorter than 600 ms. At 120 bpm, that duration will have to be less than 300 ms. Since we were using a mock setup that does not truly reproduce the impedance of the circulation, the pressure durations obtained here are not expected to be the same as the ones in the actual cardiac assist system.

Regardless of the above note of caution, the results shown in Fig. 9 largely reflect the behavior of the muscle contraction. It is safe to assume that the rising

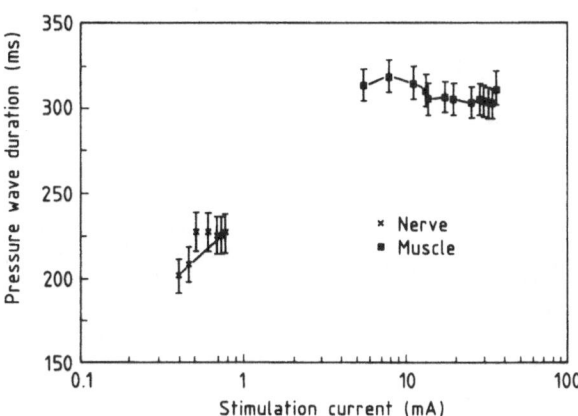

Fig. 9. Variation of pressure wave duration with stimulation current

part of the pressure wave is governed mainly not by the system's impedance, but more importantly by the characteristics and recruitment of the stimulation. The most striking feature is that the durations of MS lasted an average of 100 ms longer than the ones for PNS. This is important, and points to the slower conduction velocity of the muscle fibers as compared with the nerve. A more detailed frequency analysis might have separated the contributions of direct and indirect (via nerve) muscle fiber stimulation. Another feature worth mentioning is that duration increases somewhat with increased current amplitude in the case of PNS, whereas it does not show any significant dependence for MS. In both cases, the ranges of pressure duration were less than 25 ms (approximately 15% of total value), thus refuting current amplitude as a possible method for modulation of the duration of contraction.

Power Output of the LDM

Having measured both pressure inside and the volume displacement out of the bladder, it was possible to compute the power and energy using:

power = pressure × flow

work = power.dt = pressure × flow.dt

Figure 10 shows the dependence of average power achieved using both PNS and MS. One can observe that up to 1.8 W were achieved, a level that compares favorably with the recommended [7] value of 3 W for a totally implantable artificial heart. As expected, the ranges of currents needed to achieve the full range of power are the same, thus leading to a more easily controllable (though over a narrower range) power source under PNS than MS.

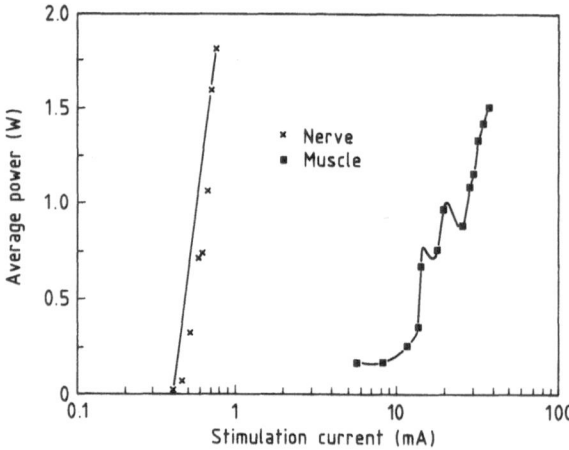

Fig. 10. Variation of output power with stimulation current

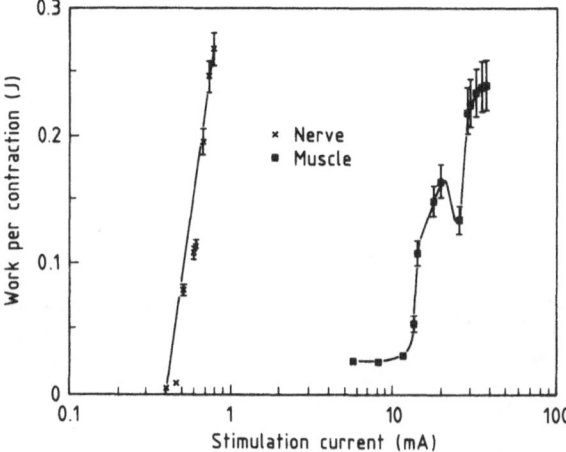

Fig. 11. Variation of muscular work with stimulation current

Work Performed by LDM

One can integrate the power output of the muscle over the period of positive pressures to obtain the amount of work supplied by the muscle in this type of setup. Figure 11 shows the results, which resemble those obtained for power. The interesting feature is that levels of work are comparable for both PNS and MS, even though the pressure peaks achieved under PNS were significantly higher than those under MS; this can be due to the somewhat higher flow and the longer duration of contraction of MS as compared with PNS.

Gain Factor

Since the method of stimulation finally chosen will have to permit a totally implantable system, it is critical to know how efficiently both PNS and MS achieve a certain level of output. Having measured the power output of the muscle, and knowing the power required to stimulate the nerve or muscle for every set of stimulation parameters, it is possible to calculate the gain factor, G. This is simply the ratio of work expended by the LDM to the electrical energy required to achieve that type of stimulation. The electrical energy was obtained by multiplying the current pulse train by the extrapolated voltage wave.

The value obtained is quite instructive, because it offers the answer to our need for a low-energy, totally implantable device. It is here that PNS appears most significantly the better choice. In fact, PNS appears to be ten times more efficient at high amplitudes of current. Another interesting feature, shown in Fig. 12, is the fact that with increased current amplitudes, the efficiency increases for PNS while it decreases on the average for MS. This means that increasing the CAS device's flow on demand would not have as detrimental an effect on battery life in PNS as it would in MS.

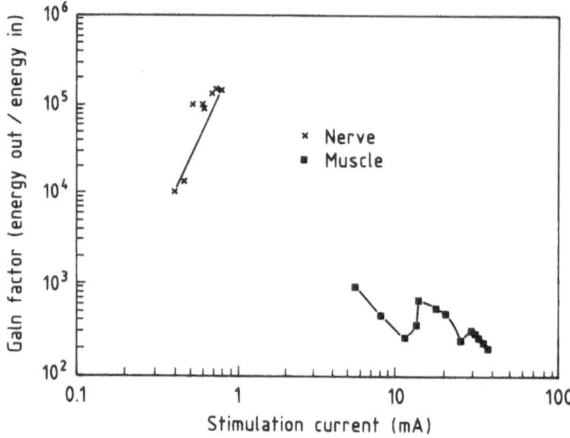

Fig. 12. Variation of muscular gain factor with stimulation current

Conclusion

Properly stretched and conditioned skeletal muscle can provide a viable option for energizing a cardiac assist system. This biomechanical approach to cardiac augmentation has obvious advantages over total biological transplantation on the one hand, and the total mechanical or artificial heart on the other hand. In this paper, the design and optimization of the muscle-wrapped balloon pump are discussed. Considerable skill is required to denervate, stretch, and orient the available muscular tissue to surround the balloon pump. Balloon design parameters and their optimization have been discussed. It appears that the system can be computer-optimized for the particular hemodynamic needs of each patient without much difficulty. A reasonable range of balloon sizes and orifice diameters should therefore be made available to the operating physician. A new experimental procedure for determining muscular power output has been developed. The procedure was adopted to articulate the advantages of nerve stimulation over direct muscle stimulation for performing the needed work in the cardiac assist device. The ultimate goal is, of course, to implant a muscle stimulator of the pacemaker type to power the cardiac assist device, thus providing the subject with an adequate quality of life.

References

1. Neilson IR, Brister SJ, Khalafalla AS, Chiu RS (1985) Left ventricular assist using a skeletal muscle-powered device for diastolic augmentation – a canine study. J Heart Transplant 4:343
2. Macoviak JA, Stephenson LW (1981) Replacement of ventricular myocardium with diaphragmatic skeletal muscle. J Thorac Cardiovasc Surg 18:519
3. Khalafalla AS (1986) Muscle mass and design requirements for cardiac assist systems. In: Chiu RC-J (ed) Biomechanical cardiac assist. Futura, p 151
4. Shepherd JT, Vanhoutte PM (1980) The human cardiovascular system – facts and concepts. Raven, New York, p 19
5. Altman PL, Dittmer DS (1968) Respiration and circulation. Federation of American Societies of Experimental Biology, Bethesda, MD, p 232
6. Katz AM (1977) Physiology of the heart. Raven, New York, pp 3, 222
7. Watson JT (1985) The present and future of cardiac assist devices. Artif Org 9:138

46. Dynamic Cardiomyoplasty to Improve Ventricular Function

J. C. Chachques, P. A. Grandjean, I. Bourgeois, and A. Carpentier

Introduction

Autologous electrostimulated latissimus dorsi muscle (LDM) may be used to assist myocardial contraction in order to prolong and improve the quality of life in patients with severe congestive heart failure refractory to adequate pharmacological support. This is not applied to patients in the last stage. Significant and consistent improvement of ventricular function and functional circulatory capacity have been demonstrated experimentally and clinically using the cardiomyoplasty procedure [1, 2].

Dynamic cardiomyoplasty involves the use of an electrically stimulated skeletal muscle wrapped around part of the heart to restore or augment myocardial contractility. In our approach, a latissimus dorsi muscle flap (LDMF) (Fig. 1) is transferred to the heart via a partial resection of the second rib and sutured around the ventricles. The muscle flap is stimulated in synchrony with heart contractions using a burst of impulses delivered by a Cardio-myostimulator implantable pulse generator via intramuscular original electrodes [3, 4].

We proposed three types of dynamic cardiomyoplasty:

1. Ventricular reinforcement, consisting of an electrostimulated LDMF wrapped around akinetic or hypokinetic ventricles (Fig. 2a).
2. Ventricular substitution after aneurysmal or tumoral resection, by means of a new biological cardiac wall composed of a patch of autologous pericardium as neoendocardium and the electrostimulated LDMF as myocardium (Fig. 2b).

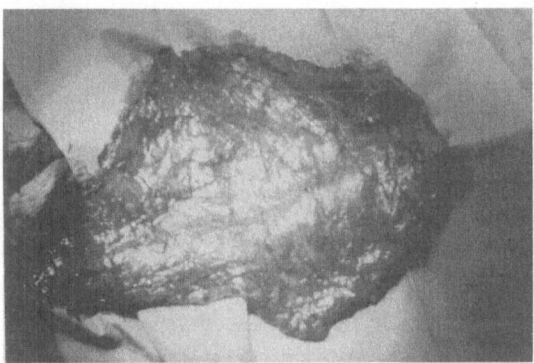

Fig. 1. Human latissimus dorsi muscle flap (LDMF)

Assisted Circulation 3
F. Unger (Ed.)
© Springer-Verlag Berlin Heidelberg 1989

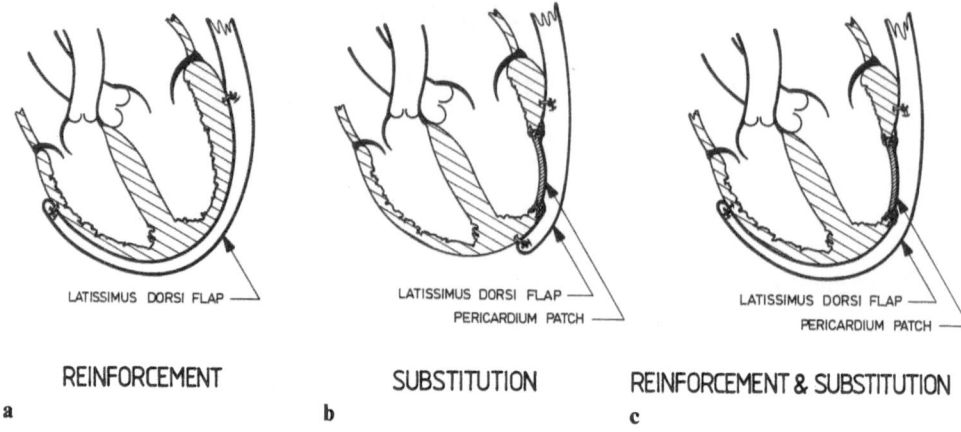

Fig. 2 a–c. Different approaches of dynamic cardiomyoplasty

3. Ventricular substitution and reinforcement of the remaining akinetic ventricular wall (combination of procedures 1 and 2; Fig. 2c).

The LDMF was chosen for cardiomyoplasty because the vascular supply,
principally via the axillary pedicle, ensures the muscle flap vitality, its functional
loss is minimal, its anatomy allows easy entrance into the thoracic cavity, and its
range intrathoracically can reach and cover ventricular walls. The volume occu-
pied by a LDMF is approximately 5%–10% of the hemithorax, and pulmonary
function should thus not be affected appreciably, if at all [5].

Historical Review

The surgical uses of skeletal muscle on the heart have been reported in the following chronologic sequence:

1933, Leriche and Fontaine: pectoralis muscle grafts in dogs for repair of in-
      farcted myocardial tissue [6].
1935, Beck: a new blood supply to the heart by pectoralis muscle pedicled grafts
      on the ventricles [7].
1959, Kantrowitz and McKinnon: experimental use of electrostimulated
      diaphragm wrapped around the heart and around the aorta [8].
1961, Petrovsky: surgical treatment of human cardiac aneurysms using diaphrag-
      matic pedicled grafts [9].
1964, Nakamura and Glenn: electrostimulated diaphragm flap to enlarge the
      right atrium and to assist ventricles [10].
1966, Termet et al.: pedicled LDM around dog hearts [11].
1974, Spotnitz et al.: rectus abdominis muscle pouch as a muscle-powered ar-
      tificial ventricle [12].
1980, Macoviak and Stephenson: replacement of right ventricular myocardium
      with acutely stimulated diaphragmatic muscle [13].

1980, Drinkwater and Chiu: myocardial repair and powered pouches using the stimulated rectus abdominis muscle [14].

1982, Chachques et al.: latissimus dorsi dynamic cardiomyoplasty [15, 16].

1983, Carpentier and Chachques: progressive and sequential muscle stimulation protocol simulating cardiac rhythm [17, 18].

1984, Chachques, Grandjean, and Carpentier: new design of intramuscular electrodes and principles of neuromuscular electrostimulation; basis of an implantable pulse-train generator (Cardio-myostimulator) [4, 17, 19].

1985, Carpentier and Chachques: dynamic cardiomyoplasty; first successful clinical case, electrostimulated LDMF wrapped around ventricles after resection of a cardiac tumor [2].

1986, Chachques and Carpentier: experimental left and right ventricle "full-tickness" dynamic cardiomyoplasty with pericardial neoendocardium; new sensing myocardial electrode [20, 21].

1986, Magovern et al.: clinical cardiomyoplasty for repair of a resected left ventricular ischemic aneurysm [22].

1987, Carpentier and Chachques: full-tickness dynamic cardiomyoplasty with pericardial neoendocardium: first successful clinical case, after extensive left ventricular aneurysm resection [23].

1987, Acker and Stephenson: skeletal muscle ventricles in circulation as a biomechanical diastolic counterpulsation system [24].

Functional Electro-Myostimulation

The growing interest in the use of skeletal muscle flaps in plastic and reconstructive surgery stimulated our interest to develop this new technique. It has only been in recent years that experimental functional electrostimulation of skeletal muscle has been possible, and interest in this tissue has increased accordingly. Chronic electrical activation of skeletal muscle is already used in various clinical situations, such as chronic generation of correcting forces to reduce developing skeletal deformities (e.g., scoliosis), muscle stimulation to restore functions lost as a result of trauma or disease, and diaphragmatic stimulation for respiratory support [25].

The natural process of neuromuscular activity can be considered as a machine which converts biochemical energy into mechanical work. The work output is produced against a load of mechanical resistance. The muscular contraction implies three distinct processes: (a) the generation of nerve impulses (action potentials) in muscle nerve(s), either naturally by the central nervous system or artificially by electrical stimulation; (b) the biochemical processes that produce energy for muscle contraction; and (c) the adaptation of the muscular structure to the new work output.

Skeletal muscles consist of two types of fibers. Type I, oxidative fatigue-resistant fibers, use aerobic metabolism and contract slowly. Type II, glycolytic fatigue-sensitive fibers, use anaerobic metabolism and contract rapidly. The composition of muscles is variable with respect to these fibers, the proportions de-

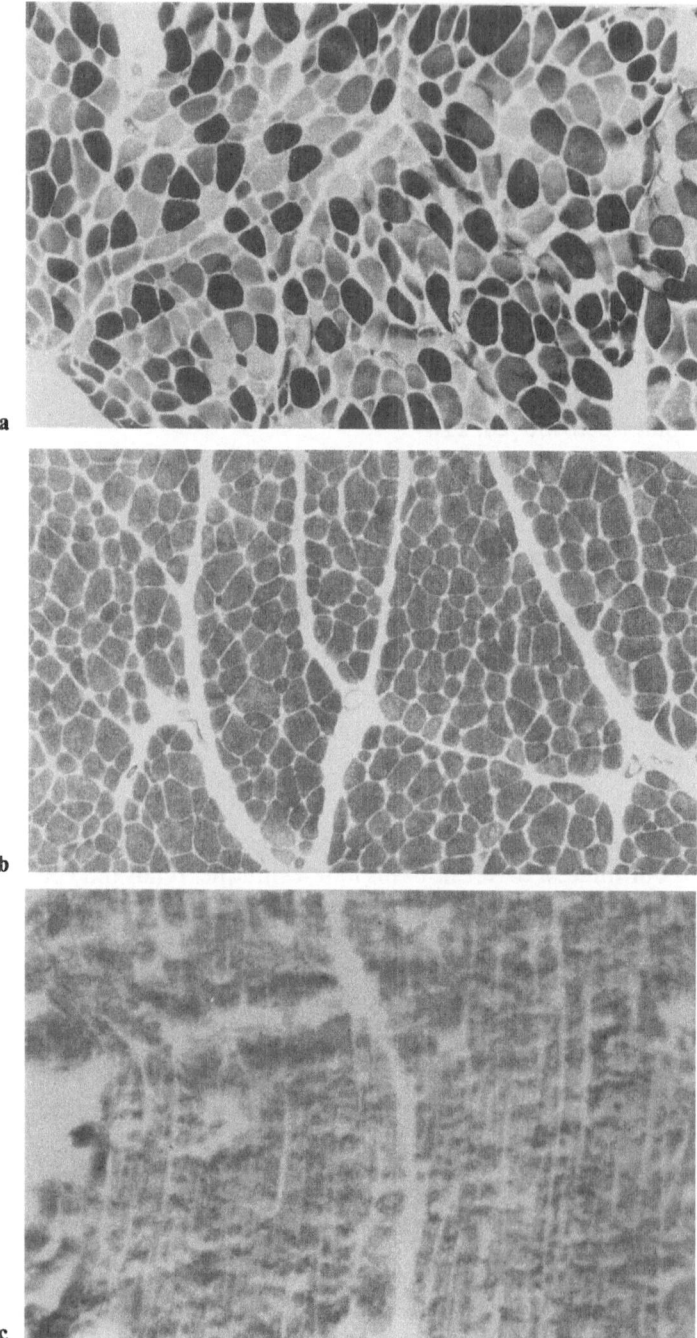

Fig. 3 a–c. Histochemical muscular studies. Cross-sections stained for ATPase (pH 9.4). **a** Non-stimulated control LDM. *Light-stained* fibers are classified as type I, oxidative fatigue-resistant fibers; *dark-stained* fibers as type II, glycolytic fatigue-sensitive fibers. **b** LDM stimulated by pulse trains for 6 months. Complete conversion to type I, oxidative fibers. **c** Myocardium stained for ATPase, showing similar histochemical characteristics to stimulated LDM

pending upon the specific function of the muscle and upon genetic factors. Furthermore, the particular metabolism of a particular fiber is not immutable but, rather, can adapt to demand, which is determined by the neuromotor input transmitted to the muscle motor units. Electrical myostimulation, when taking over from normal neuromotor input, must adequately mimic the same effects. Put practically, this fundamental principle means that it is necessary to provide the muscle with a repeatable and defined quantity of work [26, 27].

Physiological, histological, metabolic, and biochemical properties of skeletal muscle alter in response to chronic electrical stimulation. Histochemical and electrophysiological studies of conditioned LDMF show that muscle fatigue resistance can be greatly improved after training. The cardiomyoplastic postoperative muscle electrostimulation protocol provides a full fiber conversion from glycolytic to oxidative fatigue-resistant type, with similar histochemical characteristics to myocardium (Fig. 3). This adaptive response of skeletal muscle to working demands, such as those required for myocardial assistance, is the basic principle for a cardiac support function.

Cardiomyoplasty – Surgical Technique

Cardiomyoplasty can be performed using either the left or the right LDM. The choice depends on the localisation of the heart disease. With the patient in a lateral position, the cutaneous incision is performed at the level of the lateral border of the scapula (Fig. 4). The mean length of incision in adults was 33 ± 5 cm ($n =$

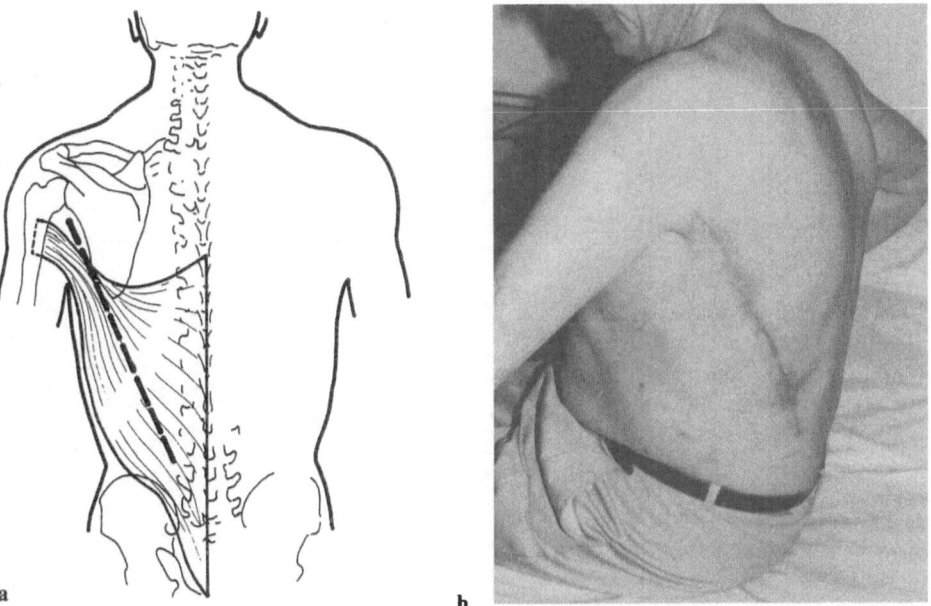

a   b

Fig. 4. a Cutaneous incision for LDM dissection. **b** Patient 2 months after dynamic cardiomyoplasty

12). For cardiomyoplasty using the left LDM, the muscle is dissected free from the iliac crest, vertebra, and rib insertions. Particular attention is necessary to identify the anterior muscle insertions, in continuity with the obliquens abdominis externus. Dissection of the LDM flap must be performed carefully, mainly with scissors. Electrocoagulation, if needed, is used with great care and with low intensity, especially over the muscle surface, to minimize damage to the vascularization. LDM flap hemostasis is completed when the collateral blood vessels arising from intercostal arteries are divided during dissection of the distal part of the flap. After the flap has been freed of its distal insertions, the neurovascular bundle (thoracodorsal pedicle) is identified and carefully preserved.

A 6-cm segment of the anterior arc of the second rib including periostium is then removed to allow transposition of the LDMF into the chest. Two intramuscular pacing electrodes (Medtronic SP 5528) are implanted into the proximal area of the LDMF for chronic neuromuscular stimulation. The cathode is placed in close proximity to the distribution of main nerve branches into the muscle to perform a neuromuscular stimulation. The anode is implanted transversally into the muscle, 6–8 cm distal from the cathode (Fig. 5). Electrophysiological tests

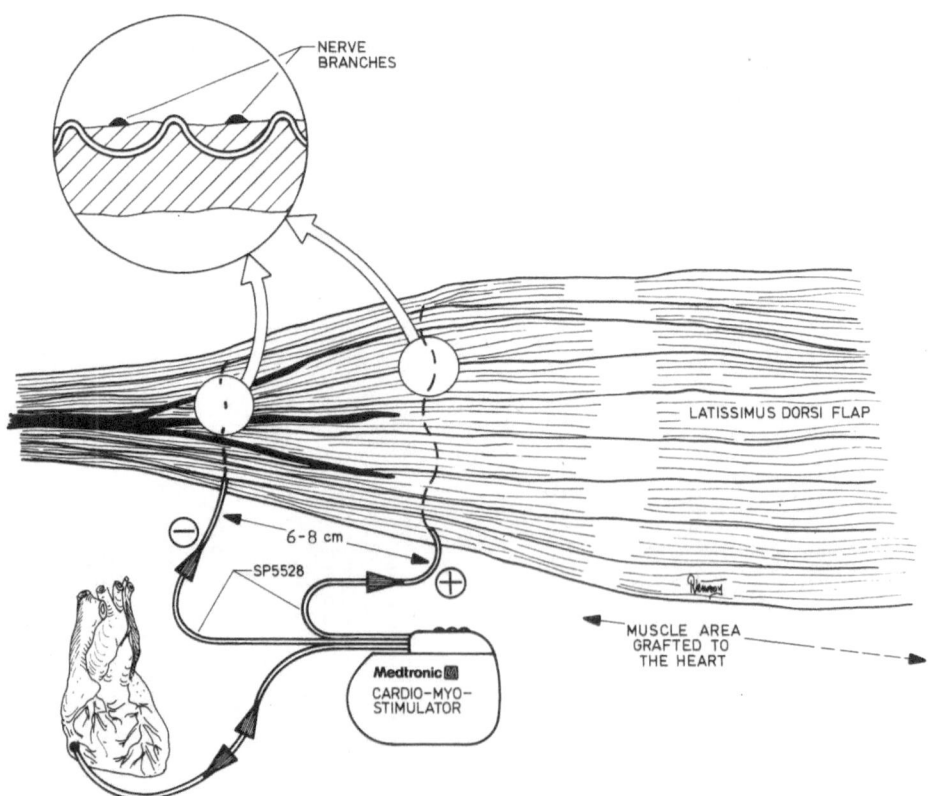

Fig. 5. Placement of electrodes into the LDMF. The cathodic lead located near the nerve branches results in neuromuscular stimulation

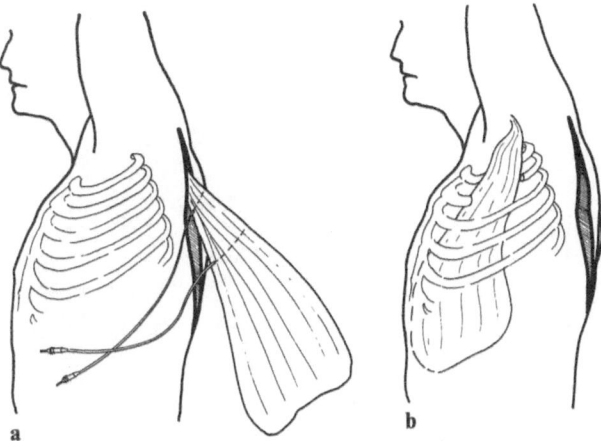

Fig. 6. a LDMF with stimulation leads. b LDMF transposed
into the left pleural cavity

(thereshold, impedance) are recorded. To perform these tests it is important to anesthetize patients without curare. Leads as well as the LDMF are transposed into the left pleural cavity (Fig. 6). A pleural drain is positioned, and the muscle is fixed with four interrupted sutures to the intercostal muscles at the level of the resection of the rib. This fixation is intented to avoid traction of the stimulated LDMF over its neurovascular pedicle and to close the pleural cavity. To avoid any motion of the left arm during electrostimulation, the latissimus dorsi humeral tendon is then severed at its most proximal part. Three subcutaneous aspiratory drains are implanted between the cutaneous flaps and the chest wall. The dissected cutaneous flaps are then fixed with interrupted absorbable sutures to the thoracic wall. The wound is then closed. This surgery lasts about 110–130 min.

In a second surgical step, the patient is placed in the supine position. The heart is exposed through a midline sternotomy and pericardiotomy. Access to the LDMF and leads is possible with a long longitudinal incision in the left mediastinal pleura.

Depending on cardiac lesions, two approaches can be considered: ventricular reinforcement and ventricular substitution.

Ventricular Reinforcement. To wrap ventricles with the LDMF, a cardiopulmonary bypass is generally not required. The internal layer (anterior fascia) of the LDM is in contact with the heart surface. Wrapping begins in the diaphragmatic ventricular wall (Fig. 7). The heart is lifted, and five to seven interrupted myocardial sutures (3/0 braided polyester) are placed beginning at the posterior atrioventricular junction, longitudinally in the intercoronary spaces, to the spinal border of the flap (Fig. 8).

After the muscle flap fixation behind the heart, two sensing intramyocardial leads (Medtronic SP 5548) are implanted into the diaphragmatic and the anterior right ventricular wall (Fig. 9). The amplitude of the R wave is measured, and the lead with best values is selected to be connected to the sensing chamber of the Cardio-myostimulator (Medtronic SP 1005). The muscle stimulator is triggered by the QRS complex. The other intramyocardial lead is capped and kept as a spare electrode. The wrapped one is then completed with sutures placed between the lat-

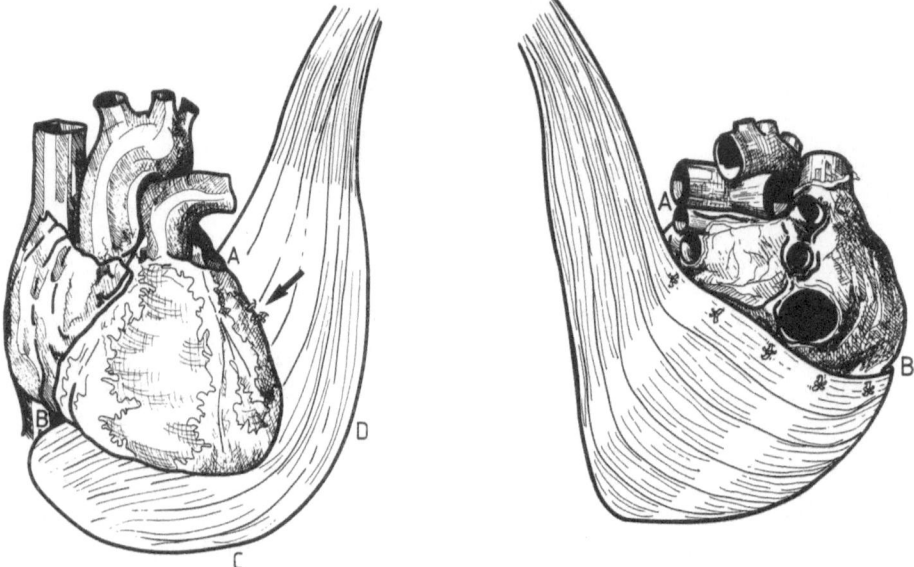

Fig. 7. Surgical technique of latissimus dorsi cardiomyoplasty. The LDMF in the thoracic cavity is positioned behind the heart

Fig. 8. The muscle is first fixed on the diaphragmatic ventricular wall in the proximity of the atrioventricular junction

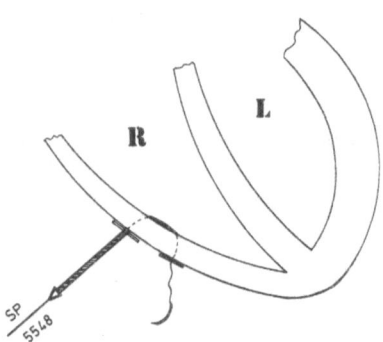

Fig. 9. Intramyocardial electrode used to detect the QRS signal, in contact with endo-, myo-, and epicardium

eral and anterior wall of the right and left ventricles and the LDMF (Fig. 10). A single complementary suture must be placed between the middle part of the LDMF and the lateral wall of the left ventricle to provoke the muscle adhesion to this area (Fig. 7, arrow).

If during fixation of the LDMF behind the heart a severe hemodynamic disfunction is verified, suture of the flap over the diaphragmatic ventricular wall can be suppressed.

In cases in which the dilatation of the heart does not allow total muscle wrapping because of insufficient LDM mass, it can be completed by a piece of autol-

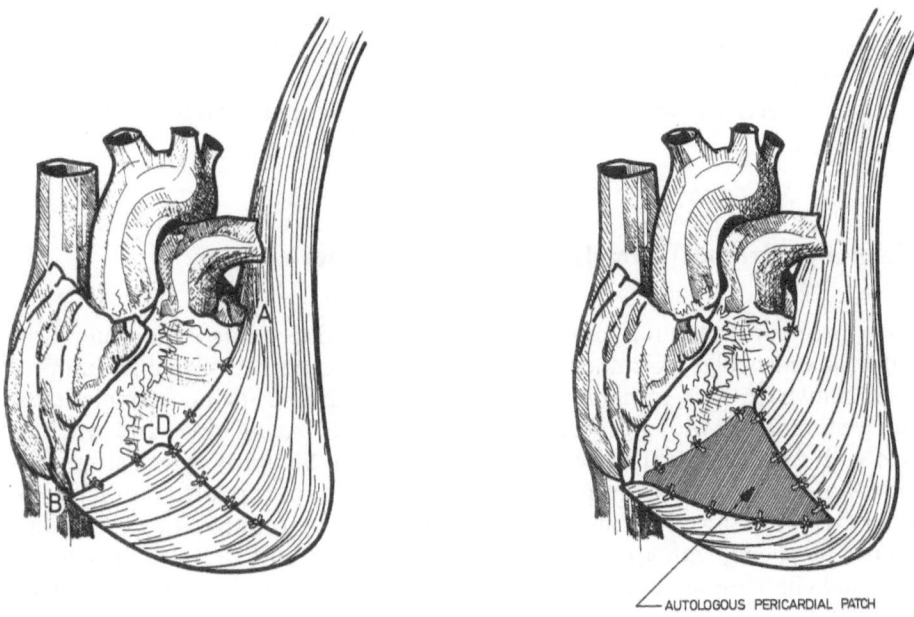

AUTOLOGOUS PERICARDIAL PATCH

Fig. 10. Muscle wrapped onto the anterior part of the heart and sutured to the myocardium

Fig. 11. Wrapping completed with autologous pericardium, to be used in cases with insufficient LDM mass

ogous pericardium. This pericardial patch must be implanted in continuity with the LDMF and placed in front of the right ventricle (Fig. 11).

A pocket for the Cardio-myostimulator is then fashioned beneath the right rectus abdominis muscle. Muscular and cardiac leads are tunnelled to the pocket and coupled with the stimulator. Drains of left pleural cavity and pericardial cavity are exteriorized at the left side of epigastrium, far from the electronic device. The pericardium is left open, and sternotomy is closed.

Ventricular Substitution. The LDM dissection in ventricular substitution is performed as in the case of ventricular reinforcement, above. The patient is placed on cardiopulmonary bypass and the ventricular pathology is treated (e.g., resection of an extensive left ventricular aneurysm or ventricular tumor). A piece of pericardium is resected to be used as neoendocardium. It is treated intraoperatively with glutaraldehyde (0.62%, 10 min minimum). This treatment is required to allow a sufficient degree of collagen cross-linking to insure pericardium stability. Pericardial shrinkage, thickening, fibrosis, and aneurysm development in high-pressure circulatory areas are some of the drawbacks of nontreated pericardium [28].

To obtain a new ventricular wall with antithrombogenic characteristics, the tanned pericardial patch (fixed to endo- and myocardium by a running 4/0 suture) is used to close the ventricular cavity as an interface between blood and the LDMF. It also avoids bleeding problems after the ventricular reconstruction and a latissimus dorsi interfascicular hematoma. The pericardial neoendocardium and the remaining left ventricular wall are then covered by the LDMF, fixed on to the ventricular surface with interrupted sutures (Fig. 2 b, c).

Sensing electrodes and the Cardio-myostimulator are implanted as described above.

Stimulation Protocol – Implantable Electronic Device

In our preclinical research, our attention has been directed to conditioning the LDM for ventricular assistance using an original postoperative stimulation protocol, similar to that of cardiac contraction [18, 29]. Until now, implantable muscle stimulators with a programmable burst as the pacing mode and synchronous with cardiac rhythm have not been available. Similarly, preexisting electrodes have not been able to produce a diffused and appropriate contraction of the LDM. We designed an implantable electronic device for providing cardiac assistance by pacing with appropriate contractions the LDM wrapped around the heart and enabling recruitment of all muscle fibers. The leads are provided with electrode surface areas which can be varied at the time of surgical implantation (Fig. 5). Despite the fact that our electrodes were placed inside the muscle body, stimulation was carried out mostly by nerve branch depolarization, as has been confirmed by complementary curare tests. The programmable pulse generator (Cardio-Myostimulator, Medtronic SP 1005) includes a heart monitor, a myostimulator, and a synchronization circuit processing the heart and muscle activities. If necessary, it can be used simultaneously as a heart and muscle stimulator [4, 19].

The protocol for the sequential and progressive stimulation of the skeletal muscle (Fig. 12), coordinated with the systolic-diastolic cycle, starts with single impulses, followed by bursts of impulses (minimum synchronization delay, 4 ms) (Fig. 13). For skeletal muscles, single-pulse stimulation results in single-twitch evoked force. Larger and longer muscular contraction elicited by multiple stimulation pulses (burst of impulses) spaced in time in such a way that temporal summation occurs. Its duration is physiologically adapted to ventricular systolic activity. In our muscle stimulation protocol (experimental and clinical) we use bursts of impulses composed of 210 μsec balanced cathodic pulses occurring at a frequency of 30 Hz. This stimulation rate (30 Hz) generates action potentials occurring at frequencies similar to the natural physiological nerve discharge. A duty cycle of chronic muscle electrostimulation with 25% of time "on" (185-ms burst duration) and 75% of time "off" (555 ms; synchronization ratio 1:1, 81 ppm) has been shown to produce repeated and sustained muscle work without significant fatigue and/or fiber degeneration [21, 30] (Fig. 14).

Furthermore, in our early clinical experience commercially available epicardial leads were found to be inadequate for detecting the R wave signal due to myocardial diseases resulting in nonhomogeneous cellular signal transduction. Intramyocardial lead (Medtronic SP 5548) with structure similar to our intramuscular lead has been found to be more adequate in our experimental and clini-

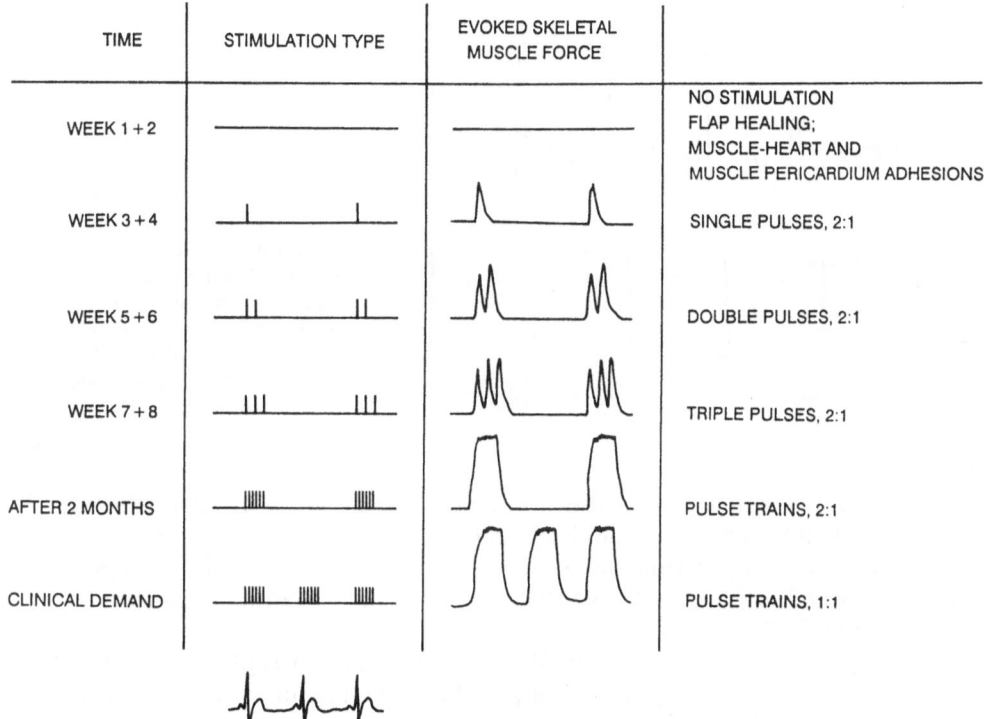

TIME	STIMULATION TYPE	EVOKED SKELETAL MUSCLE FORCE	
WEEK 1 + 2			NO STIMULATION FLAP HEALING; MUSCLE-HEART AND MUSCLE PERICARDIUM ADHESIONS
WEEK 3 + 4			SINGLE PULSES, 2:1
WEEK 5 + 6			DOUBLE PULSES, 2:1
WEEK 7 + 8			TRIPLE PULSES, 2:1
AFTER 2 MONTHS			PULSE TRAINS, 2:1
CLINICAL DEMAND			PULSE TRAINS, 1:1

Fig. 12. Postoperative skeletal muscle stimulation protocol

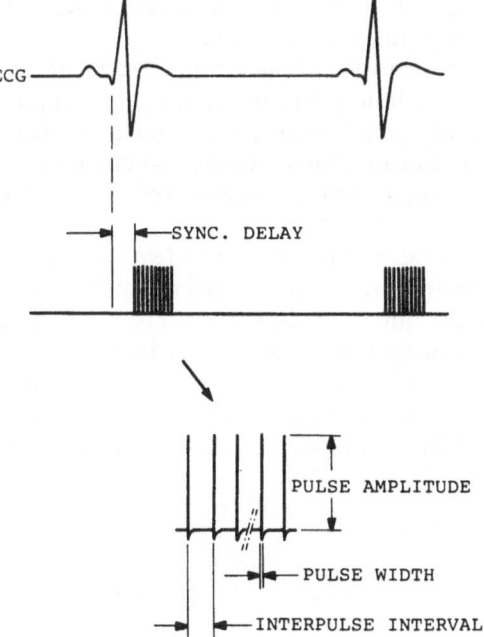

ECG

SYNC. DELAY

PULSE AMPLITUDE

PULSE WIDTH

INTERPULSE INTERVAL

Fig. 13. Output burst synchronized on the ventricle and its characteristics

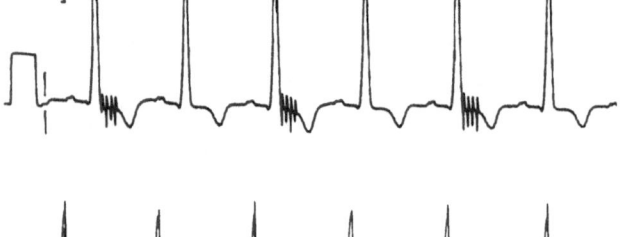

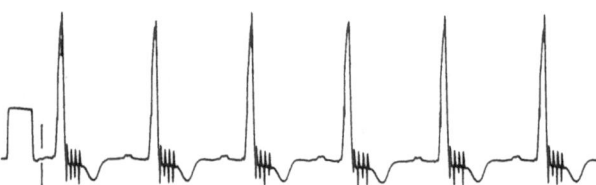

Fig. 14. ECG recorded during the Cardio-myostimulator activity (burst 30 Hz, 6 pulses, synchronization delay 4 ms, heart/muscle contraction ratio 2:1 and 1:1). The first two spikes are superimposed to R wave

cal experience to synchronize muscle stimulation with cardiac rhythm (Fig. 14). Its contact with the epi-, myo-, and endocardium is very useful for proper detection in hearts with myocardial diseases. No mechanical or electrochemical problems were found in long-term investigations using these platinum-iridium alloy electrodes (SP 5528, SP 5548) [19].

In our postoperative LDMF stimulation protocol, electrostimulation starts 2 weeks after cardiomyoplasty. This protocol (Fig. 12) takes into account the delay of gradual conversion of fast-twitch glycolytic muscular fibers into slow-twitch oxidative, fatigue-resistant fibers as well as the healing time required by the muscle after cardiomyoplasty to recover collateral blood circulation and to adhere to the heart. The adhesion between the external surface of the LDMF and the pericardium is also important because it avoids upper traction of the heart during muscle stimulation and its hemodynamic consequences.

Histological studies showed that after cardiomyoplasty the skeletal muscle structure was retained. The muscle-myocardium relationship has shown a good adaptability. The present investigation has demonstrated that electrostimulated skeletal muscles can survive for a long time in an ectopic situation when the vascular and nerve supply are carefully preserved, and when a progressive electrostimulation protocol is used [3].

After cardiomyoplasty the LDMF was shown to maintain adequate contractile force and to increase its fatigue resistance by gradual conversion of glycolytic fatigue-sensitive to oxidative fatigue-resistant muscular fibers (100%). Histochemical and biochemical studies of chronically stimulated muscles showed the total transformation of muscle fast myosin into slow myosin with similar characteristics to myocardium (Fig. 3). Electron microscopy showed preserved myofibrillar cytoarchitecture and an increase in the mitochondrial density in the cell [1].

Conclusions

We undertook this study to examine the potential advantages of using electrically stimulated autologous striated muscle to reconstruct the heart and to augment its function. In particular, we were interested in developing a biomechanical system for functional cardiac augmentation. Our approach has been to investigate the substitution or the reinforcement of the ventricular wall by a contractile tissue that possesses the potential for growth and differentiation, while maintaining the kinetic characteristics of the entire cardiac muscle.

We have considered the possibility of increasing the cardiac output of the patient's own failing heart by substituting skeletal muscle for myocardial tissue, and we have attempted to train that muscle to operate in the same way as a ventricular wall. In preclinical research and later in patients we demonstrated the surgical feasibility of cardiomyoplasty, the long-term histological and histochemical adaptability, and the adequate electrophysiological properties of the stimulated LDMF transferred to a heterotopic position over the heart. In several clinical cases we were able to carry out cardiomyoplasty without cardiopulmonary bypass, facilitated by the close proximity of the LDM to the heart, the length of its neurovascular bundle, and the ability of the muscle mass itself to stretch without problem. The flap provides a large mass of contractile tissue and can be moulded around the heart.

The LDMF was not electrically stimulated during the first 2 weeks after surgery. This was then followed by progressive stimulation. There is a great danger of flap ischemia due to vascular thrombosis and postoperative lymphedema caused by surgical muscle trauma during the days following surgery. We consider that these 2 weeks are very important because this is a very critical period for redevelopment of collateral vascular circulation.

The cardiomyoplasty procedure is intented for use in patients with chronic low cardiac output refractory to pharmacological support, due to myocardial deficiences of ischemic, neoplastic, dysplastic, infectious, or congenital origins, before the end-stage period when the only possibility is the heart transplantation or mechanical assist device. The experimental work has allowed us to progress to the first clinical application of the technique in the human (January 1985) [2]. At present our successful clinical experience (patients discharged from the hospital with improved ventricular function) involves twelve patients with severe preoperative cardiac disfunction (class III and IV, New York Heart Association) [23]. This early experience (follow up, 3–50 months) demonstrates that dynamic cardiomyoplasty was effective in patients after the electrical muscle stimulation has been instituted. Postoperative technetium heart scan (Fig. 15), ultrasonic echocardiography (Fig. 16), and hemodynamic studies show the improvement of ventricular function and no tendency of the LDMF to compress or constrict the heart. All these patients are now in functional class I or II. Electromyograms were performed postoperatively using the extrathoracic segment of the LDMF. Results showed a preserved motor neuron and a physiologic involuntary contraction of muscle mass [1].

In our opinion, one of the most suitable indications for this technique is the ischemic cardiomyopathy. In these cases, the cardiomyoplasty procedure can be

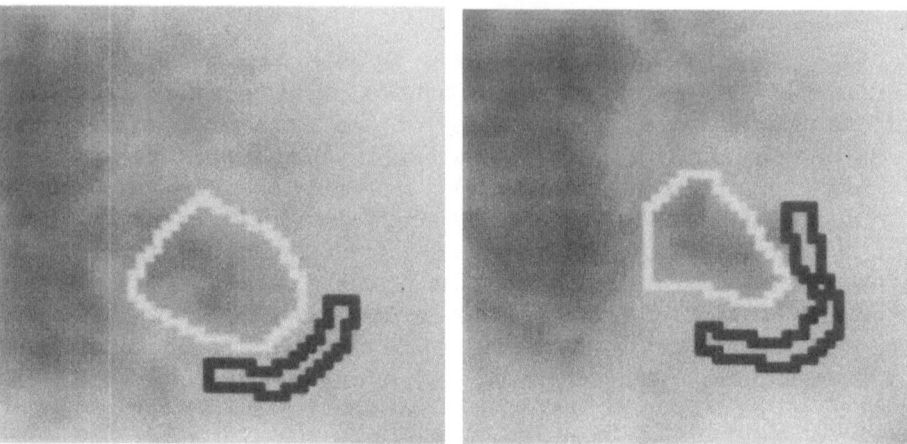

Fig. 15. ^{99m}Tc heart scan following cardiomyoplasty. *White line* represents systole. *Left*, without LDMF stimulation; *right*, with synchronous skeletal muscle stimulation. In this clinical case, stimulation improves ejection fraction by 23%

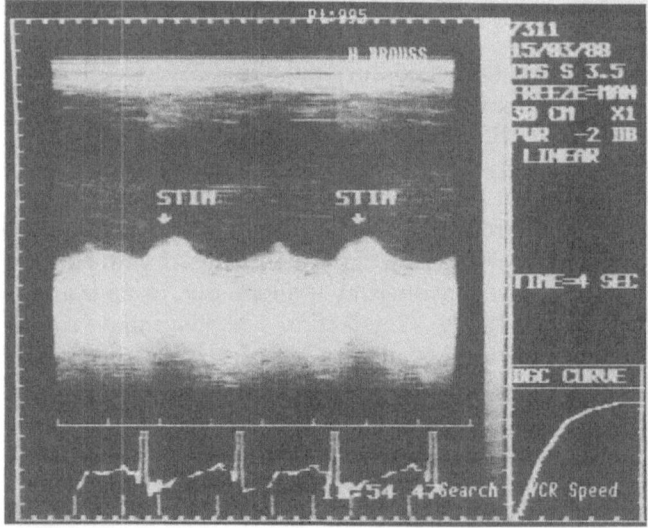

Fig. 16. Echocardiographic study of left ventricular wall after human cardiomyoplasty (reinforcement approach). Heart/LDMF stimulation ratio 2:1. Evidence of increase of wall motion during muscle electrostimulation (*STIM*)

considered after coronary surgery has failed to bring further improvement or in cases in which a direct revascularization of coronary arteries was not possible owing the lesions of the coronary system and the myocardium, principally in extensive left ventricular aneurysms with decrease in contractility of the remaining ventricular wall [22, 23, 31]. When selecting patients during the course of evolution of the disease, one must consider the remaining ventricular function, since the postoperative regimen does not allow the patient to benefit fully from the cardiomyoplasty in the first few weeks after surgery [32].

Cardiomyoplasty also has a considerable potential in the treatment of myocardial failure due to parasitic diseases, such as Chagas' disease (South American trypanosomiasis). There are about 3.5 million people, aged between 30 and 50 years, with some degree of the myocarditis of Chagas' disease in Latin America. The myocardial lesions comprise degenerative muscular necrobiosis, followed by intense interstitial fibrosis and aneurysm development, for which at present there is not treatment [33].

Furthermore, we think that cardiomyoplasty could be indicated whenever cardiac transplantation is contraindicated. Finally, the dilated cardiomyopathy [31] without significant valvular insufficiency or major arrythmia problems before the end-stage period could benefit from this type of biomechanical cardiac assistance. Our current understanding of this procedure is that dynamic cardiomyoplasty acts in two ways: (a) more vigorous systolic contraction and (b) limitation of heart dilatation. We think that dynamic cardiomyoplasty offers a new horizon and hope for the treatment of profound refractory chronic myocardial failure.

Acknowledgments. The authors wish to acknowledge the collaboration of the following persons: M. Fardeau MD, K. Schwartz PhD, B. Swynghedauw MD, S. Mihaileanu MD, P. Perier MD, F. Fontaliran MD, A. Sebille MD, N. Languillat MD, M. Levy MD, M. Hassler MS, N. Goussef, C. Gaiche, B. Martinet, H. Rebai, K. Smits, L. Herpers, B. Terpstra, J. de Jonge, P. Van Venroy, R. Pidet, S. McCann, and F. Fort.

References

1. Chachques JC, Grandjean PA, Schwartz K, Mihaileanu S, Fardeau M, Swynghedauw B, Fontaliran F, Romero N, Wisnewsky C, Perier P, Chauvaud S, Bourgeois I, Carpentier A (1988) Effect of latissimus dorsi dynamic cardiomyoplasty on ventricular function. Circulation 78 (Suppl 3):203–216
2. Carpentier A, Chachques JC (1985) Myocardial substitution with a stimulated skeletal muscle: first successful clinical case. Lancet I:1267
3. Chachques JC, Mitz V, Hero M, Arhan P, Gallix P, Fontaliran F, Vilain R (1985) Experimental cardioplasty using the latissimus dorsi muscle flap. J Cardiovasc Surg (Torino) 26:457–462
4. Chachques JC, Grandjean PA, Carpentier A (1986) Dynamic cardiomyoplasty: experimental cardiac wall replacement with a stimulated skeletal muscle. In: Chiu RCJ (ed) Biomechanical cardiac assist. Futura, New York, pp 59–84
5. Shesol BF, Clarke JS (1980) Intrathoracic application of the latissimus dorsi musculocutaneous flap. Plast Reconstr Surg 66:842–845
6. Leriche R, Fontaine R (1933) Essai expérimental de traitement de certains infarctus du myocarde et de l'anévrisme du coeur par une greffe de muscle strié. Bull Soc Nat Chir 59:229–232
7. Beck CS (1935) A new blood supply to the heart by operation. Surg Gynecol Obstet 61:407–410
8. Kantrowitz A, McKinnon WMP (1959) The experimental use of the diaphragm as an auxiliary myocardium. Surg Forum 9:266–268
9. Petrovsky BV (1966) Surgical treatment of cardiac aneurysms. J Cardiovasc Surg (Torino) 7:87–91

10. Nakamura K, Glenn WWL (1964) Graft of the diaphragm as a functioning substitute for the myocardium. J Surg Res 4:435–439
11. Termet H, Chalencon JL, Estour E, Gaillard P, Favre JP (1966) Transplantation sur le myocarde d'un muscle strié excité par pacemaker. Ann Chir Thorac Cardiovasc 5:568–571
12. Spotnitz HM, Merker C, Malm JR (1974) Applied physiology of the canine rectus abdominis. Trans Am Soc Artif Intern Organs 20:747–755
13. Macoviak J, Stephenson LW, Spielman S et al. (1980) Electrophysiological and mechanical characteristics of diaphragmatic autograft used to enlarge right ventricle. Surg Forum 31:270–271
14. Drinkwater DC, Chiu RCJ, Modry D, Wittnich C, Brown PR (1980) Cardiac assist and myocardial repair with synchronously stimulated skeletal muscle. Surg Forum 31:271–274
15. Chachques JC, Mitz V, Hero M, Arhan P (1982) Evolution expérimentale du muscle grand dorsal pédiculé, transposé dans le thorax du chien. Proceedings of the 27th congress of the Société Francaise de Chirurgie Plastique et Reconstructive, Paris, 1982, p 7
16. Chachques JC, Mitz V, Hero M, Arhan P, Gallix P, Fontaliran F, Jach S (1984) Transfert d'un muscle innervé sur le coeur. In: Magalon G, Mitz V (eds) Les lambeaux pédiculés musculaires et musculo-cutanés. Masson, Paris, pp 5–6
17. Chachques JC, Chauvaud S, Carpentier A (1983) Development of a non-tiring stimulation of the latissimus dorsi flap as a myocardial substitute. Proceedings of the first Vienna international workshop on functional electrostimulation. Vienna, 1983, p 114
18. Carpentier A, Chachques JC, Grandjean PA, Perier P, Mitz V, Bourgeois I (1985) Transformation d'un muscle squelettique par stimulation séquentielle progressive en vue de son utilisation comme substitut myocardique. C R Acad Sci 301:581–586
19. Grandjean PA, Herpers L, Smits K, Bourgeois I, Chachques JC, Carpentier A (1986) Implantable electronics and leads for muscular cardiac assistance. In: Chiu RCJ (ed) Biomechanical cardiac assist. Futura, New York, pp 103–114
20. Chachques JC, Grandjean PA, Vasseur B, Perier P, Mitz V, Bourgeois I, Carpentier A (1986) Cardiomyoplasty: a new approach to cardiac assistance. Eur Surg Res 18:89–90
21. Chachques JC, Grandjean PA, Tommasi JJ, Perier P, Chauvaud S, Bourgeois I, Carpentier A (1987) Dynamic cardiomyoplasty: a new approach to assist chronic myocardial failure. Life Support Syst 4:323–327
22. Magovern GJ, Heckler FR, Park SB, Christlieb IY, Magovern GJ, Kao RL, Benckart DH, Tullis G, Rozar E, Liebler GA, Burkholder JA, Maher TD (1987) Paced latissimus dorsi used for dynamic cardiomyoplasty of left ventricular aneurysms. Ann Thorac Surg 44:379–388
23. Carpentier A, Chachques JC, Grandjean P, Perier P, Chauvaud S, Mihaileanu S (in press) Dynamic cardiomyoplasty: early clinical experience and preliminary conclusions. J Thorac Cardiovasc Surg
24. Acker MA, Anderson WA, Hammond RL, Chin AJ, Buchanan JW, Morse CC, Kelly AM, Stephenson LW (1987) Skeletal muscle ventricles in circulation. J Thorac Cardiovasc Surg 94:163–174
25. Glenn WWL, Phelps ML (1985) Diaphragm pacing by electrical stimulation of the phrenic nerve. Neurosurgery 17:974–984
26. Salmons S, Henriksson J (1981) The adaptative response of skeletal muscle to increased use. Muscle Nerve 4:94–105
27. Pette D, Vrbovà G (1985) Neural control of phenotypic expression in mammalian muscle fibers. Muscle Nerve 8:676–689
28. Chachques JC, Vasseur B, Perier P, Balansa J, Chauvaud S, Carpentier A (1988) A rapid method to stabilize biological materials for cardiovascular surgery. Ann NY Acad Sci 529:184–186
29. Chachques JC, Grandjean PA, Vasseur B, Hero M, Perier P, Bourgeois I, Fardeau M, Carpentier A (1986) Electrophysiological conditioning of latissimus dorsi muscle flap for myocardial assistance. In: Nosé Y, Kjellstrand C, Ivanovich P (eds) Progress in artificial organs. ISAO Press, Cleveland, pp 409–412
30. Chachques JC, Grandjean PA, Vasseur B, Hero M, Perier P, Bourgeois I, Carpentier A (1987) Preclinical research and first successful clinical myocardial substitution with a stimulated skeletal muscle. Ann NY Acad Sci 494:445–448

31. Franciosa JA, Wilen M, Ziesche S, Cohn JN (1983) Survival in men with severe chronic left ventricular failure due to either coronary heart disease or idiopathic dilated cardiomyopathy. Am J Cardiol 51:831–836
32. Carpentier A, Chachques JC (1987) Latissimus dorsi cardiomyoplasty to increase cardiac output. In: Rabago G, Cooley DA (eds) Heart valve replacement and future trends in cardiac surgery. Futura, New York, pp 473–486
33. Castagnino HE, Jorg ME, Thompson AC (1982) Ventricular aneurysms in chronic Chagas' cardiopathy. J Cardiovasc Surg (Torino) 23:28–33

47. Drive and Management of Circulation Support Systems [1]

H. Thoma and H. Schima

Introduction

After three decades of intensive research, circulation support systems have attained considerable importance in clinical work. Today, intra-aortic balloon pumping (IABP) is acknowledged in clinical use. The development and construction of ventricular assist devices (VAD) and the total artificial heart (TAH) have further progressed. Because of their inherent limitations, up to now these devices are not intended for permanent use. However, impressive results have been achieved in bridging patients to transplantation. In recent years, over a hundred implantations have been performed for bridging purposes, and a reasonably high percentage of these procedures have been successful.

This clinical practice has brought up a number of new aspects in the adjustment and monitoring of these cardiac prostheses. Nevertheless, the application of these systems is very expensive and quite complex, and they need careful driving management and cautious intensive care to be successful. Many problems of design and application of controls and drives, as well as of safety and clinical management, arise on close inspection and demand an optimal solution. Reliable detection of signals and parameters used for control is another difficult task. Even the adjustments for IABP differ in various publications. International requirements and standardization seem to be necessary.

In addition, each pump, if not fully automated, should be monitored and controlled continuously while in use. Expensive fail-safe systems sometimes seem useless, because these systems are usually switched off or reset without a check.

Moreover, extensive problems are caused by the persistent and growing psychic strain on patients connected to mechanical circulation aids. This article covers not only the problems of mechanical aid systems, but also the practical problems of their application.

The Intra-aortic Balloon Pump (IABP)

The IABP permits increase of circulatory pressure during diastole and decrease of circulatory pressure during systole of the heart. This method is an application

[1] Sponsored by the Ludwig Boltzmann Gesellschaft and the Fonds zur Förderung der wissenschaftlichen Forschung.

of the counterpulsation principle. Unfortunately, the optimal adjustment of balloon pulsation is incorrectly described in many publications and in manufacturers' operating manuals. It is agreed that pump action should be initiated immediately after the aortic valve has closed, but there are differing statements regarding control of the balloon deflation point. Since the gas volume which displaces the balloon is usually smaller than the ejection volume of the heart, the positive supporting effect is possible only during the end diastole or directly in the systole. It is correct that the end-diastolic pressure decrease shortens the isometric tension time of the ventricle.

But there are some disadvantages:

1. End-diastolic deflation leads to a reversal of coronary flow.
2. It is not possible to reduce the work done by the heart, since the volume is displaced during the beginning of the systole and is not available at the systolic maximum.
3. With this method the mean aortic pressure normally decreases or is equal to nonaugmentation.

We are of the opinion that it is usually better to decrease the systolic peak by balloon deflation.

The advantages are:

1. Optimal decompression to reduce the work done by the heart
2. Optimal coronary flow during the entire diastole
3. Increase in the mean aortic pressure.

Figure 1 illustrates the two timing methods. The optimal control of IABP should be discussed in connection with the patient's disease. Should priority be given to aortic pressure, coronary function, or reduction of the work done by the heart, or is it better to decrease the systolic peak? Patients with limp muscle, for instance, those suffering from cardiomyopathy or ventricular aneurysm, are probably better supported by an end-diastolic pressure decrease if their aortic pressure is high enough.

The incorrect rule for balloon-pump timing probably derives from animal experiments. For purposes of comparison, these experiments use balloon catheters with great volume. If the displacement volume of the balloon is greater than the

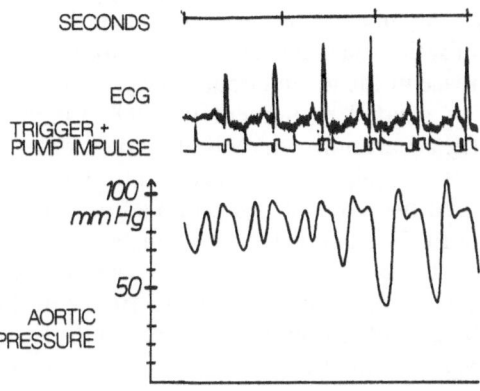

Fig. 1. Clinical application of the IABP. The augmentation can be used either for reduction of the systolic peak or to reduce end-diastolic pressure

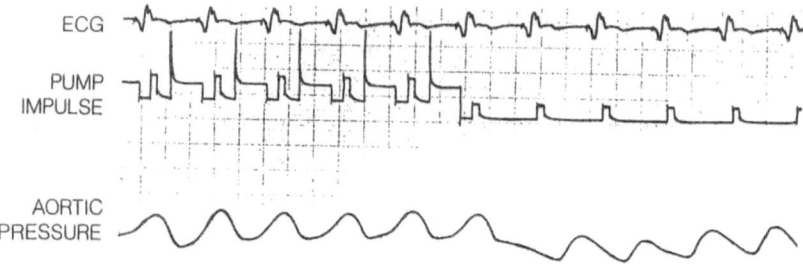

ECG

PUMP
IMPULSE

AORTIC
PRESSURE

Fig. 2. Clinical application of the IABP. "Total counterpulsation" takes place owing to volume loss. Systolic wave disappears completely and mean arterial pressure rises considerably

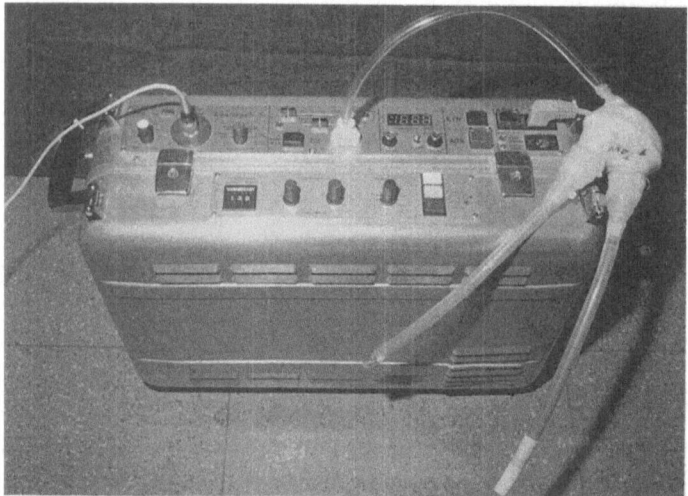

Fig. 3. Portable suitcase unit to drive the IABP and assist pumps, specially developed for easy clinical application

ejection volume of the heart, a systolic pressure loss is obtained, despite the fact that the pump is adjusted for end-diastolic decrease. But in clinical applications this is the exception to the rule (Fig. 2). Only in extreme cases and when the ejection volume is low may total counterpulsation be achieved. In this case the balloon pulsation causes considerable increase in the mean circulatory pressure.

We began developing drives and associated equipment in 1968. Figure 3 shows a portable driving unit of the fifth generation, which is able to drive both intra-aortic balloons and assist pumps. The equipment is mainly automatic and easy to handle, with only two switches and two controls for pump adjustment.

For triggering, the amplitude of the ECG is stabilized at a constant voltage and the actual trigger threshold is computed on the basis of the preceding heart action. The trigger range comprises R-peak amplitudes from 0.1 to 10 mV of the input signal. The information "low voltage" and "ripple interference" in the ECG is processed electronically. "Low voltage" means that the input voltage of the

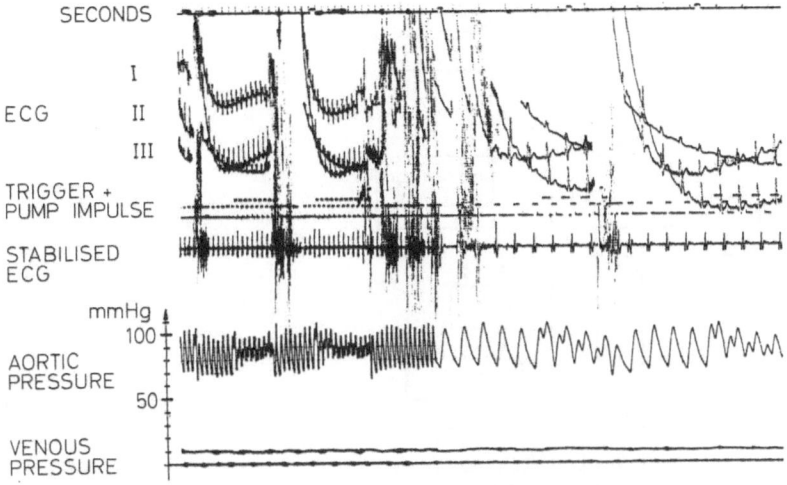

Fig. 4. Application of the IABP during surgery. Pulsation is interrupted if artifacts appear in the ECG; it switches back when the influences have ceased

ECG is below 0.1 mV, and the ripple danger signal is an alarm for 50% AC interference in the ECG. This indicates poor positioning of the electrodes.

Recognizing the initiation of the heart beat is one of the great problems, for which an optimal solution has yet to be found. The reason is that patients treated with IABP have atypical ECG waveforms. Another point is that the cardiac heart rhythm and ECG characteristics of these patients change frequently.

The previous RR distance serves as a basis for computing the pump impulse. Only QRS complexes that are hemodynamically effective are used. For individual adaptation for each patient, the pump timing and pump duration are adjusted by means of two sliding potentiometers before the pump action is switched on. If arrhythmic beats occur, the deviation of the momentary cycle duration from the integrated cycle duration signals alarm. In case of tachycardia the apparatus also sets off an alarm and stops. When interferences ("ripple," "arrhythmic") cease, the pump will start to work again automatically. Therefore, it is not necessary to operate the unit manually during electrocauterization in surgery (Fig. 4). With the help of modern microprocessor technology complex algorithms can be calculated using only a few components.

Automatic Mode

Immediate initiation of counterpulsation after closure of the valve and maximum decrease of the systolic peak or end-diastolic depression can be automated (we developed such an automatic system in 1972). Figure 5 shows the principal layout; the literature contains a detailed description.

The ECG is picked up by means of two channels, one of which may be wireless; the optimal R peak, selected by logical decisions, drives the following automatic trigger. The trigger output pulse serves as the clock input of the digital store

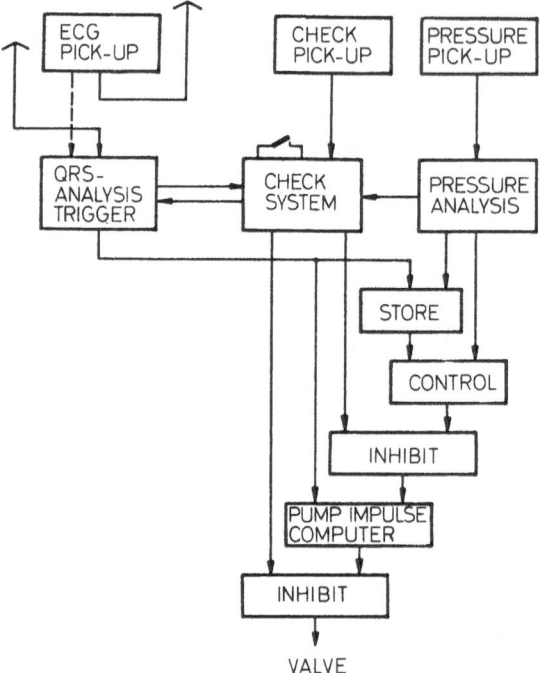

Fig. 5. Basic block diagram of the automatic control system (Counter-pulse IV) for IABP

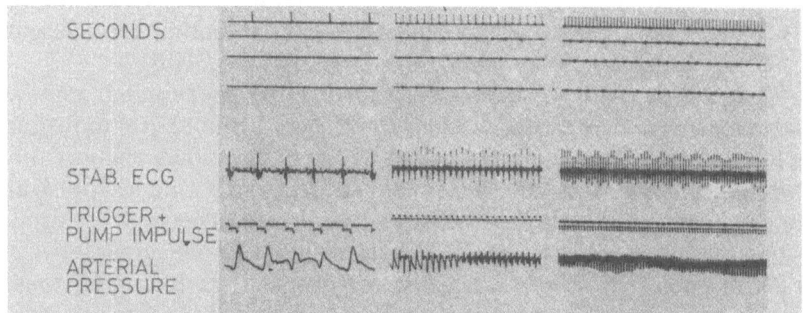

Fig. 6. Clinical application of Counterpulse IV. At the beginning (*left*) the unit compares values measured during pulsation and when it is switched off. In the *middle*, the unit switches over to continuous mode. *Right*: In automatic operation control deviations of the arterial pressure can be seen

and as the input of the pump pulse computer. From the pressure signal, important parameters such as systolic peak and valve closing are analyzed and stored.

The values necessary for the control are the one stored from the measuring cycles and the actual values during pulsation. The control influences control timing, primarily computed by means of a loop, which is closed by the balloon action. Following logical decisions the particular phases of the control are timed, starting at the primary setting when the valve is switched on. The check system monitors the balloon movement, balloon gas flow, rhythm and frequency of heart action, amplitude and pulse width of the R peak, hum noise in the ECG, pattern of pressure curves, synchronization of ECG, and pressure; it opens the loop if the limits are exceeded and cuts off pulsation if necessary. A control without automatic monitoring and automatic cut-off does not qualify for clinical application.

Figure 6 shows three phases during a clinical application of the device. In the first part of the figure, the adjustment for optimal pump start is made immediately after the pump is switched on. The drive stops after two pump cycles, having completed two measuring cycles. The system optimizes itself within 60 s; from then on it is not necessary to stop the pump to obtain reference values. Note the control deviations in the circulatory pressure and the respiratory variation of the ECG amplitude.

Safety

The application of pneumatically driven cardiac-assist devices (CAD) is inherently dangerous. Each leak in the pump membrane releases air into the circulatory system. Opinions differ: According to the so-called Helsinki Agreement, the insertion of air-filled catheters into cardiovascular systems is strictly prohibited. The American Society for Internal Artificial Organs (ASAIO) and the Association for the Advancement of Medical Instrumentation (AAMI) have established a committee which stipulates definite regulations for using IABP. These regulations are relatively strict. The regulations require that if any leakage occurs in the balloon, the maximum gas volume emerging into the circulation system should be limited to 1 balloon volume (30 ml). This value is only theoretical, because pressurized gas is present in the drive and in the supply lines, and the effective volume is accordingly much greater than the 30 ml maximum.

Fortunately, we have not had such an accident yet. It has been proved in animal experiments that a small gas volume in the coronary system irreversibly impairs the animal's heart. The question of which kind of gas is more dangerous for the circulation system seems secondary. The actual infiltration of gas into the coronaries is the hazard of balloon rupture. Even more fatal is a leak in the bypass ventricle pump, because the bypass ventricle needs about five times the balloon volume. This leads us to conclude that both intra-aortic balloon pumps and ventricular-assist device drives should have a leakage detection to switch off the device immediately in the case of membrane rupture.

With the total artificial heart the situation is different: In case of membrane rupture, especially of the left ventricle, the patient would die because of the loss of circulation; fortunately, however, this has never occurred in clinical use to date. Therefore, most of the TAHs have hitherto been driven by so-called open systems (described below) with no possibility of detecting a leakage.

The mechanics and safety features of a drive system for clinical use (see Fig. 3) are described below. The safety drive consists of a cylinder in which gas is displaced by a piston. This piston is the armature of a solenoid (Fig. 7). It divides the cylinder into two areas: a small-volume/high-pressure area between piston and electromagnet and behind this a low-pressure area. The cylinder is sealed and

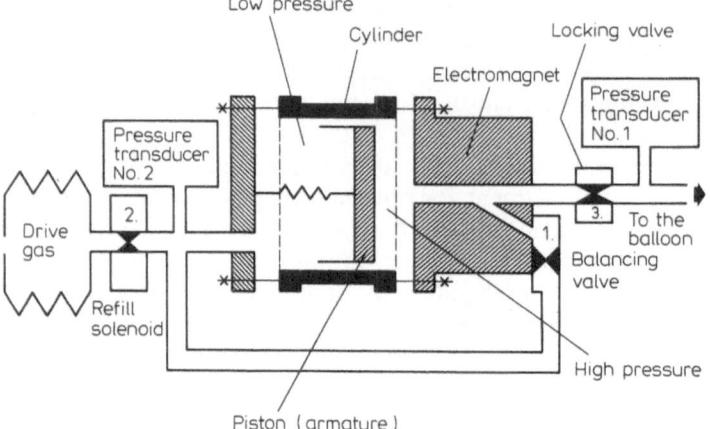

Fig. 7. Layout of the safety piston drive

can be opened only by solenoid valves. All types of gas can be pumped by means of a flexible gas tank.

This very simple mechanical unit is controlled by complex logic by means of a microprocessor. High and low pressure are sensed, together with the position of the piston. The movement of the piston is controlled by a closed loop to guarantee full action using a minimum of electrical energy. The piston is returned by three return springs. The device offers twofold safety:

1. High leakage can be detected by measuring high pressure beat to beat; in this case the pump is switched off automatically.
2. Small amounts of leakage can be detected by monitoring the trend of gas pressure (i.e., the volume of gas in the low-pressure system).

An important feature of this drive unit is the so-called locking valve (Fig. 7, no. 3). This valve is closed immediately after the pump is filled. Thus, neither a piston lock nor a holding current in the electromagnet is necessary. This feature, together with a low displacement of about 10 mm, makes possible a very fast rise and response time. Using helium as the drive gas, full action of the balloon is possible up to 200 cycles/min.

The recording shown in Fig. 8 was made in a mock test. The balloon was positioned in a closed chamber in which a circulation pressure of 90 mmHg was simulated. Balloon action (inflation) can be detected by measuring the chamber pressure signal (top recording in Fig. 8). The high-pressure signal (middle recording) indicated an initial high-pressure impulse, which is necessary for a quick gas exchange. Plateau pressure is about two thirds of the peak value and is necessary to hold the balloon in an active position. At the end of the active cycle the locking valve mentioned above is opened. The high pressure drops with a response time of only 20 ms. Due to the sealed system, the low pressure demonstrated in the bottom recording is negative during the high-pressure period. The bottom recording indicates the electrical pump impulse of the control unit. With helium as the drive gas a maximum frequency of 280/min is reached.

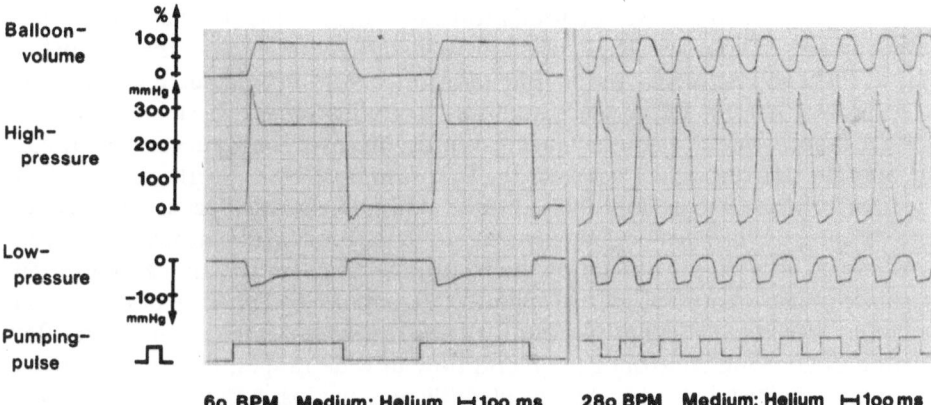

60 BPM Medium: Helium ⊢⊣100 ms   280 BPM Medium: Helium ⊢⊣100 ms

Fig. 8. Recording of the safety solenoid drive function

We use a defined leak system to avoid high friction and to ensure the long-term reliability of the piston cylinder. During the compression phase gas escapes between the cylinder wall and the piston. During the idle period the gas returns via the balancing valve (no. 1 in Fig. 7) to the low-pressure part of the cylinder or vice versa.

Due to this balancing effect, the leak rate of the piston is unimportant. The efficiency of this drive unit is relatively high because the solenoid has to be switched on for only 30–40 ms. A power consumption of 40 W is quite low, compared with other drives.

The drive unit is automatically adjusted by means of light barriers which control the position of the piston, a procedure which has proved to be very reliable. The electronics guarantee continuous monitoring and analysis of the pump pressure and check the drive status. A refill period is initiated automatically in the event of a drop in low pressure by means of refill solenoid no. 2. Refill time as an indication for a small amount of leakage in the gas line or the balloon catheter is controlled by the leakage test logic. High pressure is adjusted by piston displacement using an electric servomotor. This system has been used clinically during the past 6 years.

Drive of Ventricular Assist Devices

If the intra-aortic balloon pump is not sufficient for stabilizing the patient's circulatory system, the application of an assist device or a total artificial heart may become necessary. During recent years pneumatically driven assist devices have been used with increased frequency in two clinical applications: On the one hand, they are used to support patients after acute myocardial failure until their own heart recovers. On the other hand, they are used to support the patient's circulation until a donor heart is available – this procedure is called "bridging."

Compared with the use of a total artificial heart, this method has both advantages and disadvantages: The application of assist devices is easier than the orthotopic TAH implantation and can be performed without a heart-lung machine. The natural heart is left in place and is a – certainly limited – backup in case of device failure. Nevertheless, achieving a sufficient cardiac output can be difficult. If only the left ventricle is assisted, the flow is limited by the performance of the patient's right ventricle, and this ventricle might deteriorate because of the additional charge. Furthermore, the necessity of up to four (in biventricular assist applications) transcutaneous inflow and outflow cannulas remains an enormous problem, first because of the risk of infection and second because of driving difficulties. Whereas an orthotopic total artificial heart has short inflow and outflow cannulas allowing control of the blood flow in wide ranges, the transcutaneous cannulas of assist devices cause considerable pressure loss because of their length, the small inner diameter required, and the pulsating flow characteristics. Thus, the blood flow is limited to 4, at the most 6 l/min maximum, which might be too low in some situations.

Inflow characteristics also depend on the kind of cannulation used. When bridging to transplantation is intended and it is not necessary to spare the original heart, the ventricle itself can be cannulated through its apex to support the filling of the pump. In contrast, atrial cannulation, which induces minor injury to the heart muscle, might easily result in inflow obstruction. From the mechanical point of view, both drives for the total artificial heart (if they provide a sufficiently high vacuum) and balloon pumps (if they can manage the stroke volume required) can be used to drive assist devices.

However, assist devices require particular controls supporting the specific algorithms of assist pumping, which can be classified into three modes:

First, the pump can be driven at a fixed frequency as a total artificial heart (see below) usually completely ejecting and partially filling.

Second, the heart rate and also the systolic time interval can be altered depending on the filling and ejection speed: The ventricle is switched after detection of complete systole and complete diastole (similar to the "optimal timing control" of the TAH; see below, which leads to a minimum frequency. Because of the decreased pulsatility and accordingly reduced friction losses in the inflow and outflow cannulas, this mode is very useful to attain maximum cardiac output.

With a slight modification, this mode can be applied to synchronize the assist device with the heart frequency without evaluation of the ECG: If the detection of complete filling is used for starting systole, but the systolic time interval is fixed, the moment of complete filling, and in this way the start of ejection, correlates with the peak of inflow pressure caused by the heart.

Third, pumping activity can be synchronized with the ECG. In this mode the timing of filling and ejection can be adjusted to optimize the preload and afterload of the natural heart. This may be especially important if the recovery of the patient's own heart is aimed at.

Because of the limitation of the pump frequency it may be necessary to trigger the pump on every second or third heartbeat only; however, this can lead to irritations of the heart rhythm. Heart frequency and ejection volume have to be observed so that a switch to the fixed-rate mode can be made if a regular ECG is

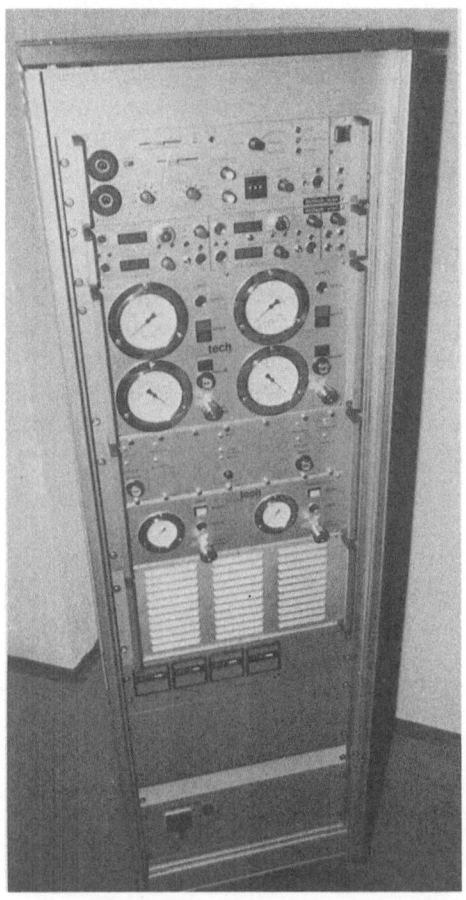

Fig. 9. Unit for general use in animal experiments

not available. (For this reason conventional IABPs cannot be used for driving assist devices: They switch off in the case of an irregular ECG!)

Figure 9 shows a typical drive unit for general experimental use. This unit was developed for widespread use with assist systems, IABP and TAH. It consists of two separated drivers, backup power and pressure supply, and an ECG-synchronization unit suitable for IABP and assist devices. For the latter, this unit has a window discriminator to preselect synchronous drive frequencies. If tachyarrhythmia or bradycardia occurs or the ECG detection fails, the automatic control unit will switch to a fixed frequency.

Drive and Control of the Total Artificial Heart

Drivers for the Pneumatically Driven TAH

Pneumatically driven total artificial hearts (TAH) are used in a number of hospitals to bridge patients to transplantation. Although these prostheses are not intended for permanent use because of the inconvenience and risks involved, some patients develop contraindications against transplantation and thus need chronic support over some months or even for the rest of their lives. The requirements for drivers used during implantations and in the early postoperative period are different from those for chronic patients:

During operation and in the early postoperative period it must be possible to change all or most of the drive parameters easily. Extensive monitoring and facilities for data collection are required.

The system should be as silent as possible and offer comfortable handling, but size and weight need not be minimized, because the patient is generally immobile and kept in a special transplantation unit to minimize the risk of infection. In case of emergency nursing staff will be available to take action immediately.

Nevertheless, when the patient becomes mobile or can even leave the hospital with an artificial heart, it is essential to have small portable drivers available that work completely automatically and can react even to severe system breakdown. Figures 10–12 show a TAH driver that was especially designed for clinical application.

In normal use the device is connected to the hospital power and pressure supply. If one or both of these lines are disconnected, batteries and a compressor

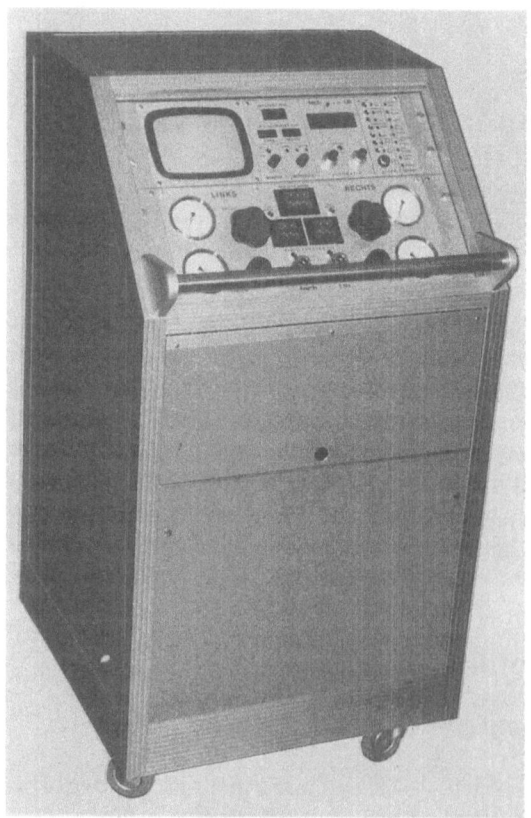

Fig. 10. Driving system for clinical use of TAH

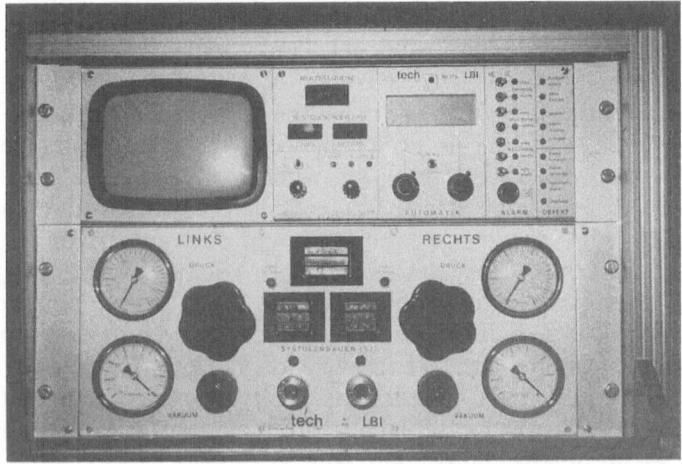

Fig. 11. Control panel of the driving system shown in Fig. 10

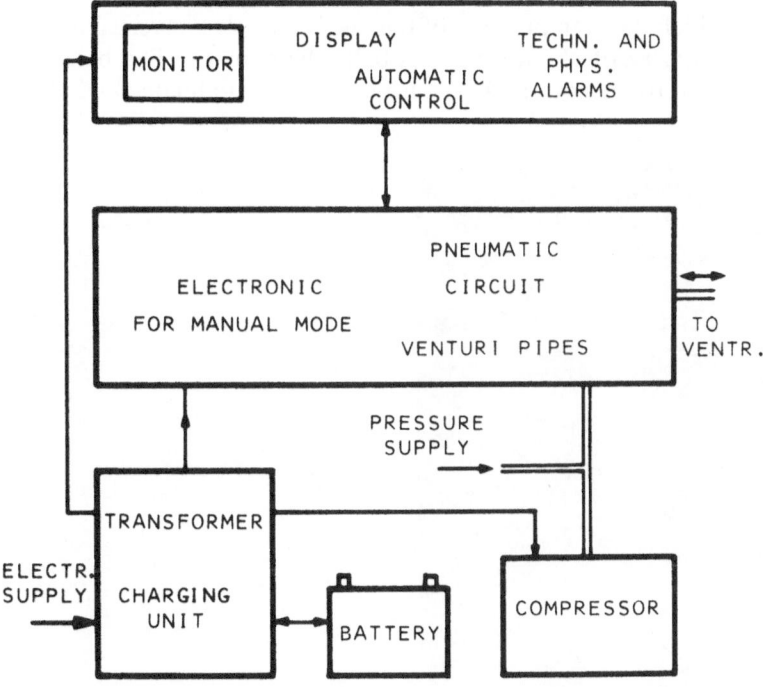

Fig. 12. Block diagram of the driving system shown in Fig. 10

automatically take over the energy support. The functional units, and especially the electric current supply, are divided into various stages with different priorities, so that a minimum operating mode will be provided even if major parts of the system fail. Nevertheless, an emergency driver has to be placed standby in the event of catastrophic breakdowns.

Driving pressure, vacuum, and – in manual mode – heart rate and systolic time intervals can be adjusted on the lower control panel. The system is an "open system": Systolic pressure is built up in a storage chamber by a regulatory valve out of the pressure supply, and a three-way valve switches the ventricle from this storage chamber to the outlet. A throttle is placed between the systolic storage chamber and the three-way valve to restrain dp/dt, which is important to minimize the water hammer caused by the valves. Magnetic safety valves with high hysteresis are positioned in the pneumatic circuit to avoid overpressure on the ventricle in case of severe failure of the regulatory elements. Vacuum, if necessary, is generated by specially designed venturi pipes, which are small, have minimum pneumatic resistance, and need only little primary flow. Because no motors are required in normal mode, the system has an extremely low noise performance.

The upper control panel contains a monitor for observing gas pressure and gas flow in the drive lines, displays of the actual heart rate, systolic time intervals and alarm conditions, an automatic control unit, which can work in two modes, and an alarm unit with a number of physiological and technical alarms (see section "Surveillance").

To permit the patient some mobility within the care unit, a small driver has been designed in which the high pressure of the line is directly converted into the driving pressure by the use of a high-frequency ball valve (Fig. 13). This ball valve, working at a constant frequency of 400 Hz, is pulse-width modulated and allows

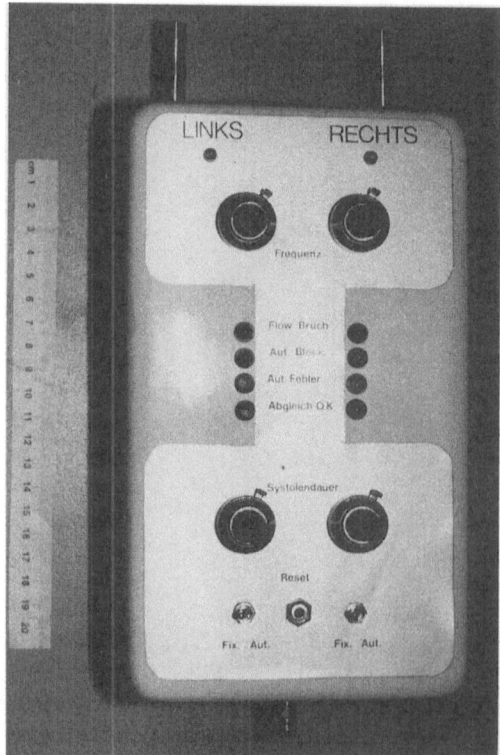

Fig. 13. Miniaturized driver with direct pressure conversion by means of high-frequency ball valves

the generation of various pressure patterns, thus minimizing dp/dt. Control of timing and pressure is effected by a miniaturized automatic control unit based on a microprocessor 8051.

The system is connected to the power supply by a long "umbilical line" and the TAH recipient has to carry only a case $23 \times 14 \times 9$ cm in size and weighing 1.9 kg. At the moment it is under experimental testing.

Automatic Control of the Total Artificial Heart

Many theoretical and experimental studies on the control of total artificial heart replacement have been carried out during the past two decades. However, in recent years clinical application has pointed out some new aspects which are obviously related to the severe preoperative condition of TAH recipients.

In general, control strategies should provide normal hemodynamic pressure and flow values and at the same time guarantee gentle treatment of the blood and the device itself. In the pneumatically driven device four parameters can usually be adjusted for each pump: frequency, duration of the systole, systolic driving pressure, and diastolic vacuum. The cardiac output required can be obtained by a number of different adjustments of these four parameters; e.g., a very high driving pressure can eject the whole ventricle even in a very short systolic time. Careful setting is necessary to minimize the number and speed of valve movements and thus the traumatic effects on the blood, and at the same time to provide sufficient washout to avoid thromboembolism.

The pump can be driven in different modes: In the complete-ejection/partial-filling mode the device ejects completely during systole and is filled incompletely during diastole, thus providing an adaptation to the filling pressure similar to the Frank-Starling mechanism. This mode, which can be operated without any automatic unit, leads to a heart frequency higher than necessary. The timing can be optimized by observing the membrane movement and switching over between diastole and systole exactly after complete filling and complete ejection. Figure 14 shows the "optimal control": The gas flow applied to the ventricle is measured continuously by a thermistor flow probe (which is cooled by the moving gas and therefore cannot distinguish the flow direction). When the ventricle is filled or emptied completely, the gas flow approaches zero, and this information can be used to switch the valve (Fig. 14a). Therefore, "optimal control" is defined as the highest frequency which just enables complete filling and ejection at given hemodynamic and driving pressures.

A further improvement is acquired by skipping the very last time period of ejection, in which the membrane is overstretched and nearly no pumping effect is obtained (Fig. 14b): The control circuit monitors the gas volume during systole by linearizing and integrating the flow signal. It switches over to diastole after approximately 90% of ejection. This "stroke volume control" leads to a further increase of available cardiac output by avoiding time delays due to membrane still-stand. Furthermore, it provides smoother valve movements in the switchover from systole to diastole.

The control of timing is only a first step to automatic control. In a second step automatic adjustment of drive pressure or vacuum according to the recipient's ar-

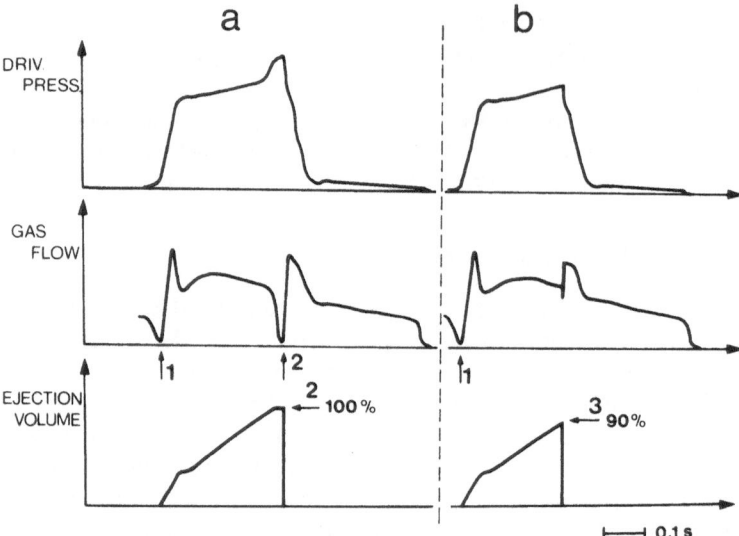

Fig. 14a, b. Gas-pressure and gas-flow patterns in optimal control of timing: *1*, detection of end-diastolic position: gas flow stops; *2*, detection of end-systolic position: gas flow stops; *3*, beat volume limited to 90% of complete ejection volume; *a*, switchover caused by flow zero at the end of diastole and systole; *b*, volume control: switchover takes place before the ejection is completed

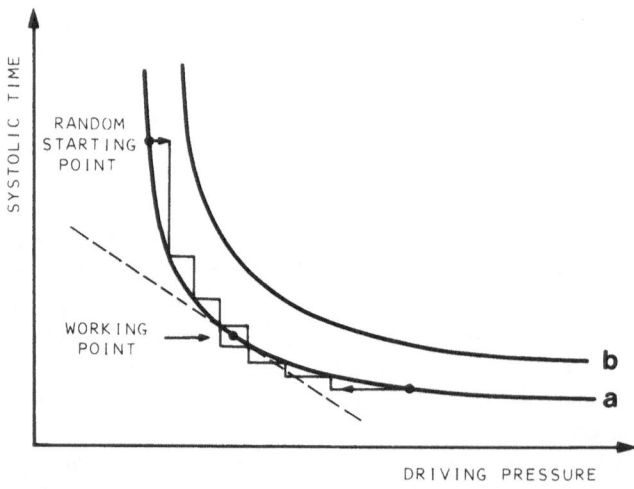

Fig. 15. Economic control of driving pressure by observation of the relation of driving pressure and ejection time

terial and filling pressures is necessary. One method developed by our group is based on the hyperbolic connection between driving pressure and systolic time and is called "economic control" (Fig. 15): Increases of peripheral vascular resistance at a constant driving pressure would prolong the systolic duration and therefore decrease the heart rate and the cardiac output. On the other hand, decreasing peripheral resistance requires a lower driving pressure for effective and gentle pumping. The optimal working point is defined as a constant average Tsys/Pdriv at the vertex of the hyperbola. If the circulatory resistance changes, the hyperbola of working points will shift. The driving pressure is adjusted automatically in small steps to achieve the predefined Tsys/Pdriv. Adjustment of Tsys/Pdriv depends on the cardiac output required. The same principle could be used to adapt the vacuum according to the filling time.

In addition to these control strategies for the driving of the single pump, the definition of the necessary cardiac output as well as a coordination of the interaction between the left and right ventricles is necessary. Most of these algorithms are based on inflow pressure values (which are an indicator of venous return) or pressure changes in the aorta. In animal experiments we usually use the left ventricle to specify cardiac output. The right ventricle is adjusted to keep the left atrial pressure within a proper range.

Monitoring of other physiological parameters, such as action of the sinus node, blood temperature, oxygen utilization, or lactate level, is normally not done in animal experiments, first because the pressure levels seem to represent the demands of the recipient to a very high extent, second because of the hypersensitivity of some of these signals, and third because of the difficulties in reliable online analysis.

These complex functions of pattern recognition, monitoring, and automatic control are appropriately implemented on microprocessors. We designed an automatic control unit based on a single-chip controller 8051. This unit monitors gas pressures and flows for both ventricles, carries out the necessary calculations for automatic adjustment of digital and analogous valves, and transmits registration data to a computer terminal. Certainly, the use of microprocessors in such vital systems requires special safety precautions (see below).

TAH Control in the Early Postoperative Stage

Control strategies for the TAH have generally been based on experience with healthy animals under stable hemodynamic conditions and with working autoregulation of the vascular bed. Human candidates for TAH implantation, however, typically suffer from severe cardiac insufficiency and correlated organ impairments when the cardiac prosthesis is finally implanted. In all patients we observed very low peripheral resistance in the early postoperative stage, sometimes followed by periods of eminent vasoconstriction. Infusions and blood transfusions to normalize the liquid balance influence the venous pressure levels. Moreover, we observed, on the one hand, instabilities of the vascular resistance immediately after implantation and, on the other hand, hyperstability in a case of sepsis. Figure 16 shows a strip chart of a patient, done 12 h postoperatively, who developed rhythmical changes of the vascular resistance with a cycle time period of approximately 15 min and extreme highs of up to 2000 dyn/s/cm^5 and extreme lows down to 500 dyn/s/cm^5. This phenomenon occurred in a phase of very deep unconsciousness and disappeared completely when the patient recovered. Figure 17 shows the pressure values of a septic patient; when the cardiac output

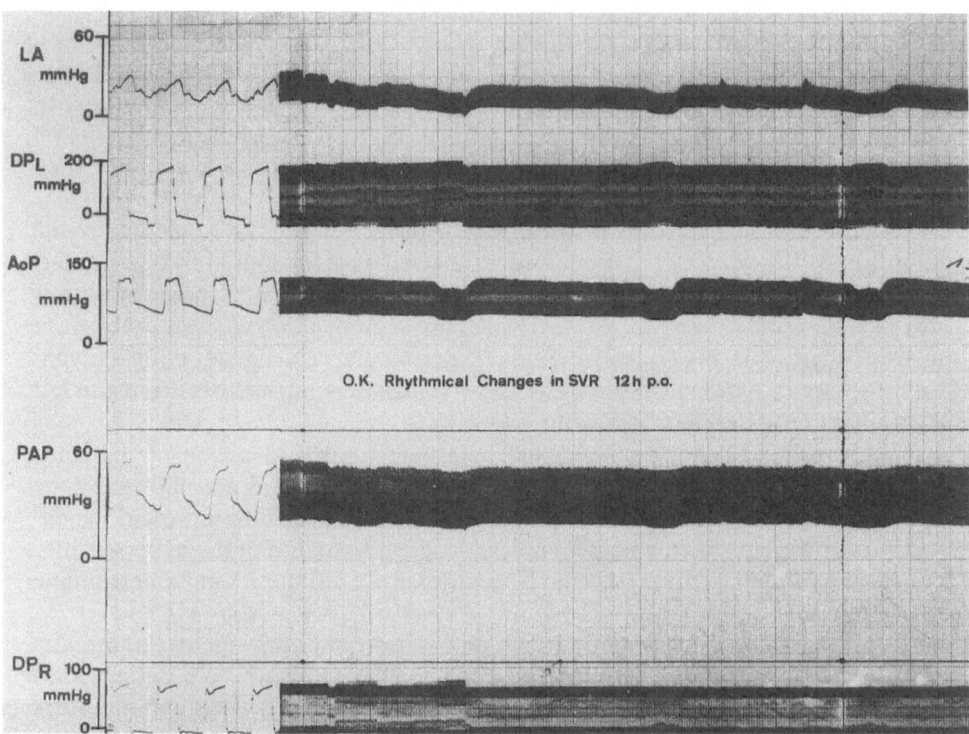

Fig. 16. Rhythmic changes of vascular resistance in the early postoperative phase of a TAH patient (see text for details)

was altered within 25%, the monitored pressure values stayed completely stable.

Because of these observations we lost our confidence in regulating the cardiac output depending on pressure values alone. We chose the O_2X ratio (which is the difference between arterial and venous oxygen content divided by the arterial O_2 content) to evaluate the necessary flow.

Intending to keep the O_2X ratio within a range of 20%–25% we obtained cardiac indices between 3.3 and 4.4 $l/m^2/min$ (CO 6–8 l/min) in noninfected patients, which is higher than COs reported by other groups. As much as 10.5 l/min were necessary to obtain an O_2X ratio of 32% in the septic patient. This strategy led to stable driving management and brought about rapid hemodynamic stabilization and general improvement of the patient's condition. Undoubtedly, many more studies have to be done in this field, in which the evaluation of the superior methods is certainly difficult. The choice of the optimal method depends on the specific situation of each patient and might change with his or her state of health.

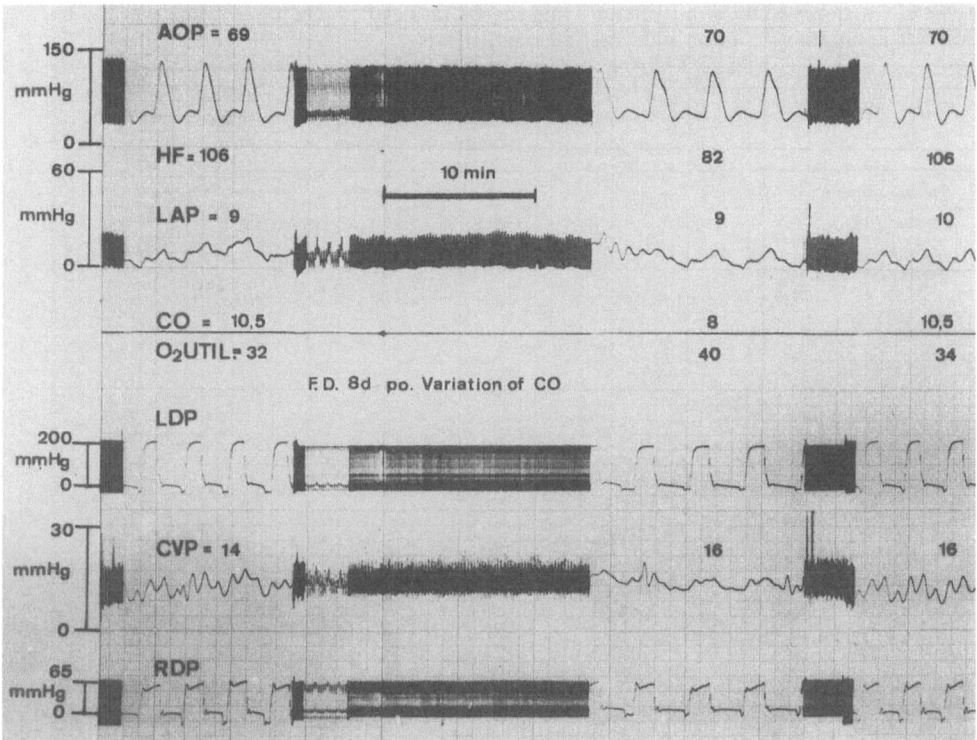

Fig. 17. Recording of an arbitrary reduction of CO causing no pressure changes but only a variation of O_2X ratio (see text for details)

Surveillance and Reliability

Measuring systems and surveillance are two of the main elements of artificial heart development. There is no doubt that a defect of these components can induce a vital crisis for the patient, similar to pump failure. The reliability of measuring systems is indispensable, especially when they are used for automatic control.

Of course, the availability of parameters depends on the specific conditions of the application. Many parameters can be monitored in the intensive-care unit, where the staff is used to sophisticated apparatus. In chronic animal experiments there are far fewer facilities, and on an outpatient basis no complicated evaluations could be done.

Furthermore, some of these methods include inherent risks, such as of infections when catheters are used, so that only a limited number of parameters are available and beneficial. Redundancy of parameters may be useful to limit detection errors, but the staff members may get confused if they have too many data to observe. Table 1 lists the parameters monitored by nine different research groups.

Table 1. Crossover study of nine centers working on artificial circulation. Parameters used in different applications; number indicates frequency of use

	In vitro test	Animal experi- ment	Human appli- cation	Temporary appli- cation	Chronic appli- cation
1. Device parameter					
Rate right	4	6	4	3	4
left	4	6	4	3	5
Stroke volume right	4	6	4	2	4
left	4	6	3	2	4
Others (% systole)	1	–	–	–	–
2. Hemodynamic					
Pressure arterial	3	4	2	3	2
venous	3	4	2	3	1
arterial right	3	5	3	3	3
arterial left	3	6	3	3	3
volume	2	2	2	2	2
others (PCP)	–	–	1	1	–
3. Device surveillance					
Parameters energy	2	5	4	3	4
drive	1	4	2	2	2
pressure	4	8	6	4	7
volume	2	6	4	2	5
vacuum	3	5	4	3	5
leakage	1	3	2	2	4
4. Medical surveillance					
Breathing parameters	–	3	3	2	2
Temperature	1	5	4	2	2
Blood gases	2	6	6	5	3
Hematology	2	5	5	4	3
Coagulation test	1	5	5	5	4
Blood chemistry	1	4	5	4	3
Urine analysis	–	3	4	2	1
Fluid balance	–	5	5	4	1
5. Patient observation					
Continuous	–	2	3	1	–
Discontinous	2	3	3	4	4
6. All-over all-alarm system	1	3	5	4	4
7. Backup	–	3	5	4	4

We are monitoring the following parameters to guarantee proper adjustment of the total artificial heart:

Technical: power and pressure supplies, temperature, valve function
Hemodynamics: heart frequency, % systole left and right, driving pressures and vacua, aortic pressure, central venous pressure, left atrial pressure, cardiac output and output balance
Other parameters (absolute minimum): arterial and venous oxygen content, coagulation parameters, hemolysis

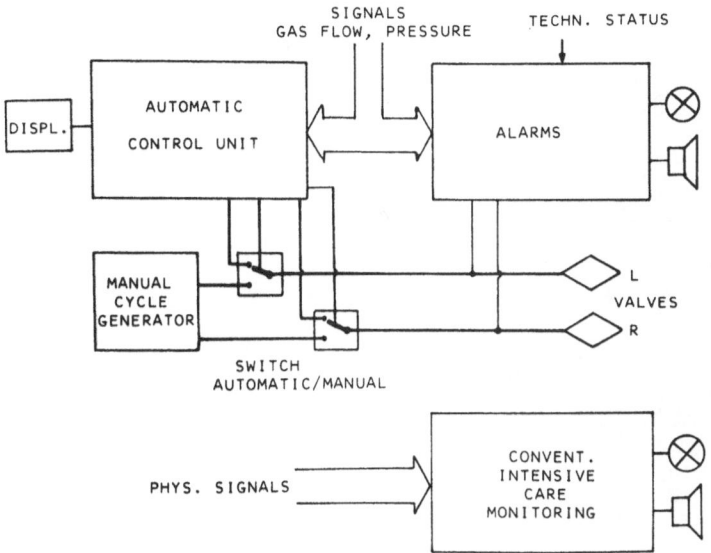

Fig. 18. Control and monitoring components in TAH application

Most of the parameters calculated within the driver are processed by micro-controllers, as with the driver shown in Fig. 10. However, microprocessors are not fail-safe, so many different security precautions have been established to guarantee proper observation of the patient (Fig. 18):

– Continuous monitoring of driving parameters is done by the automatic control unit itself. Systolic and diastolic time intervals, systolic and diastolic pressures, and the cardiac output must be within certain limits; left and right cardiac output must correspond. If the controller observes atypical conditions which it cannot manage by changing control parameters within a few seconds, it sends optical error messages and acoustic alarms and switches over to a backup timing unit, which is designed with conventional logic and is connected to a separate power supply.

– The performance of the control unit is observed by a hardware watchdog, which requires action of the microprocessor at defined intervals of approximately 10 ms. In the case of other intervals it switches over to the backup and resets the controller.

– A completely separate alarm unit calculates the alarm conditions in parallel to the controller. In addition, it observes technical parameters of the driver such as power and pressure supplies, battery voltage, and temperature. It has both optical and acoustic alarm, some of which can be blocked by the nursing staff in the case of atypical but not dangerous conditions.

– At least in the early postoperative stage, instrumentation with blood-pressure catheters using conventional intensive-care equipment is done, which also gives an alarm in the case of atypical blood pressure.

These precautions guarantee that minor failure conditions are handled by the system itself. However, in the case of severe breakdowns, e.g., of the three-way

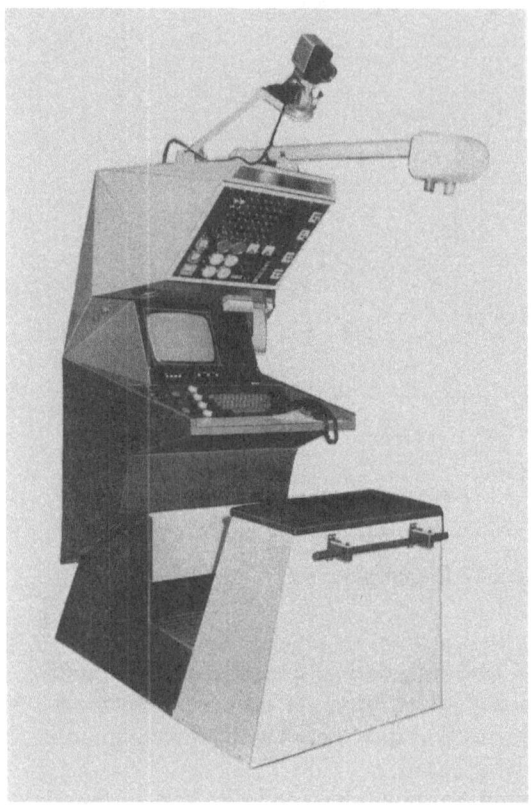

Fig. 19. Driving system for total artificial hearts with complete protection against first failure

valve, immediate action on the part of the staff – switching to the backup driver – is necessary. Basically, it is possible to develop drivers which are completely protected against first failure. Figure 19 shows a driving unit which is completely redundant in power and pressure supply as well as in the main system components. In case of technical failure it switches over automatically to the backup system. However, the definition of switching conditions is critical, and unnecessary switching can occur under unusual driving conditions. Furthermore, these drivers – if really redundant – tend to be enormous. Therefore, this safety standard is not used in intensive care but would be a necessity if the patient is unattended.

Nonpneumatic Drive Systems

Although pneumatic drive systems are widely employed nowadays, they are limited to temporary use because of their inconveniences. Numerous attempts have been made to achieve nonpneumatic driving systems for membrane pumps: spring mechanism in Stanford, ball-screw drive in Hershey, electrohydraulic drives in Utah and Cleveland.

Changing the concept of the pulsatile membrane pump, Biomedicus and Medtronic Inc. developed centrifugal pumps for external use. There are some advantages to such rotary pumps: they need no valves and no plastic membranes. If they are used in the nonpulsatile mode, pressure losses in inflow and outflow cannulas are far lower than in pulsatile devices, which is important in extracorporeal applications. Driving can be done with comparably simple motors.

Nevertheless, these devices present a number of different problems that must be considered: Little information exists about the nonpulsatile effects on the body. Efficient sealing of the rotor shaft is necessary, the rotors have to spin at a comparatively high speed, and in case of pump failure the device becomes an additional load for the ventricle it was intended to assist. However, these questions may be solved if more efforts are made in this field.

The general problem of centrifugal pumps is that they are at a development status comparable to that of membrane pumps at the very beginning of this new technology. It is therefore not fair to compare the results with the high standard of pneumatically driven membrane pumps today. The first step that must be taken is to reach a really high standard in this field in order to make the next step possible: an exact evaluation of nonpulsatile circulatory effects on the organism.

Figure 20 shows a centrifugal pump with a vaneless rotor and a brushless electric motor that was developed in our laboratory. This pump has a diameter of 80 mm and a height of 40 mm and delivers 6 l/min against a pressure of 150 mmHg when rotating at 4000 rpm. It can be fully implanted and was tested first in animal experiments over 2 days without severe thrombogenicity: Plasma-free hemoglobin could be kept below 20 mg%.

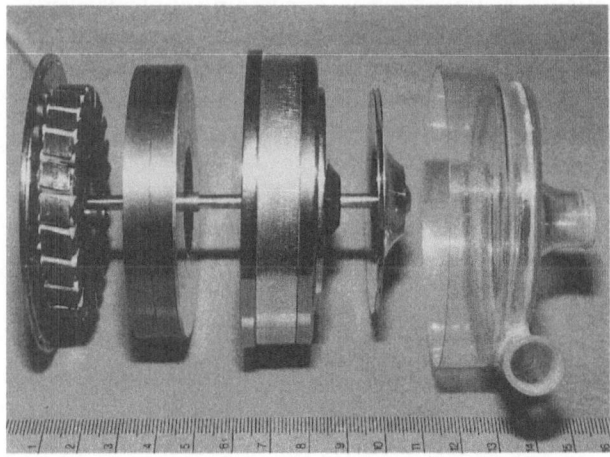

Fig. 20. Implantable centrifugal pump with integrated brushless motor, exploded view

Management

Critique

There is no doubt that the past several decades have seen a great deal of progress in the fields of assisted circulation and total heart replacement. Today, IABP treatment is performed worldwide in about 30 000 patients a year (industry calculations). Left heart assist, biventricular bypass, and TAH replacement are performed by an increasing number of groups. These first successful implantations have encouraged patients, industry, and research groups. Nevertheless, this step forward has affected only a small group of patients, which is certainly limited by the number of grafts available for transplantation.

So far there are no standards for the clinical application of bypass pumps in either the medical or the engineering field. With regard to the blood pump, there is no alternative today to the conventional membrane pump, and problems such as calcification and pannus formation have yet to be solved. At the moment there is nearly a stillstand in the field of chronic TAH replacement because of the poor biocompatibility and bioresistance of these membrane pumps. The long-term durability of plastic materials therefore seems to be limited to 1–2 years inside the body.

Another point of criticism concerns the complexity and costs of the treatment and the devices. For a routine long-term application of mechanical circulation pumps it would be necessary to reduce the costs of today's technology. But such a simplification is still impossible. On the contrary, current devices and instrumentation do not even approximately suit the necessary requirements for safety, reliability, and ease of operation. Practice shows that even the technology of the IABP is not satisfactory, despite the fact that it has been in constant clinical use since 1967 in thousands of patients. Many problems concerning controls, drives, safety, and especially clinical organization must be solved.

Clinical application of assist devices results in management problems, justifying the statement that these methods have advantages for the patient only if they are routinely applied. Sporadic applications tend to show many symptoms of a clinical experiment.

The effect of applying mechanical circulation must be clearly estimated. It is known that the effect of the IABP is quite minimal. Therefore, all precautions must be taken to ensure the optimal effect. This makes continuous monitoring of pump timing and other drive parameters necessary. Small deviations from the optimum could destroy the effect of the IABP, making it completely useless. Management expense in the hospital should not be underestimated.

This applies not only to possible medical complication checks, but also to the monitoring of the entire system.

Usually, the staff does not continuously monitor the devices during clinical application. Theoretical explanations of the so-called safety drive sound good, especially in those publications advertising material of manufacturers or sponsored by them. In practice, however, these features are often impractical. What is the use of the best alarm circuit announcing a leak in the membrane, if one of the staff presses the reset button almost automatically? Interrogation of groups doing routine balloon pulsation has revealed that no group does extensive leakage monitoring of IABP; instead, the ominous reset button is pressed. Why do we develop and construct complicated safety drives if no check of the balloon's airtightness is made following the alarm?

Moreover, the IABP and, far more, the implantation of assist devices and total artificial hearts cause a great psychological strain on the patient. Because the relatives and also the intensive-care staff are not used to the application of this new and in some ways frightening technology, they often avoid talking with the patient about his anxiety. Therefore, psychohygienic precautions must be taken.

Practice

It is desirable to apply all methods of mechanical circulation support routinely. This, of course, depends on the number and frequency of operations. Patients should be treated centrally if possible, according to agreements between hospitals. Requirements increase with the complexity of the method: While a breakdown of a balloon pump can be somehow backed up by the natural heart, a failure of a total artificial heart could be immediately lethal. Mercifully, up to now no TAH patient has died because of technical failure.

All staff members involved – physicians, nurses, and engineers – must undergo training to become acquainted with the new method. This training, which must be performed frequently in addition to the regular work, can be bothersome: most of the important things to know are necessary only in case of emergency, and fortunately, emergency situations occur very seldom (to date not one patient has died due to device failure!). But in the case of alarm, correct emergency actions have to be initiated within seconds.

Systems should be operated and checked by trainer personnel, experienced in the application of such devices (for instance, from animal experiments). This applies to checking and eliminating leaks and kinked pneumatic tubes, loose or disconnected electrodes, and additional ground loops on the patient.

The necessary team has to be on duty 24 h a day, weekends included. It must be guaranteed that the unit is completely checked after one operation and prepared for the next by the ward technician. A technician assisting during operations is advantageous. Use of blood pumps allows no interruption. Consequently, each care unit must at least have two drivers. If the device depends on external power or gas supplies, its functions must be guaranteed in case one or both supplies fail. At least one unit should be reserved for the patient's transportation to or from the operating room or to the angiography room or other areas. Transportation should be a routine procedure. If during bridging the transplantation procedure is delayed, the patient usually arrives at a suitable state of health. Then a miniaturized driver is indispensable to provide for his mobilization. Unfortunately, many industrial devices are becoming more complicated, heavier, and difficult to transport.

Another problem is synchronization with the patient's heart. These patients usually have highly pathological ECGs, making the correct derivation difficult to find. We therefore use twin isolation amps exclusively. Two ECG amps are connected so that only three electrodes, placed in a triangle, have to be fixed on the patient's body. The amplitude of positive and negative signals of both derivations is displayed by light modulation of LEDs. The operator then selects one or more derivations by means of four push-button triggers. The utilization of isolation amps protected against electrocoagulation is a must!

Another problem is the machinery and array of equipment in the intensive-care ward. Aggregates are growing increasingly larger. The patient's isolation caused by the wall of machinery is certainly a negative aspect of intensive-care wards. Unfortunately, miniaturization of devices is not yet a quality criterion. Relocation of aggregates to the periphery would be a possibility.

The utilization of measuring devices during mechanical support of the circulation is an important issue: Is it better to use the parts available in the stock of the intensive-care unit, or should they be a part of the drive aggregate? In the first case the ward staff know the instrumentation better and the inventory of the care unit need not be enlarged, in the second, a better adaptation to the specific requirements of the driver is possible.

Finally, recording methods should be used for later analysis and check. A trend analysis is of great importance, especially during utilization of VAD or TAH.

Psychohygienic Intervention

Any unbiased observer of activities on an intensive-care ward will immediately realize that intensive care imposes a great psychological strain on the patients. This is especially valid for the cardiac patients, who are usually not at all prepared for the intensive-care field.

Except for extreme situations, arising in conjunction with the cardiac patient's disease and recovery, the patient has to contend with additional facts such as strain reactions due to noxiousness. Of course, such reactions occur only if the patient is at least partially conscious and brain activity is not blocked. The patient must be aware of his or her situation and face it critically. Reactions due to extreme strain on the mentally stable human being can best be described as "shock reactions." Abnormal strain reactions such as emotional weakness, semi-consciousness, or depression appear when patients are disordered in their identity.

Other restrictions are due to ward rules and are the result of the perfect organization in an intensive-care ward. These include therapeutic, attending, and management precautions, of which the following are obvious examples:

1. Dictation of the day's schedule; the patient cannot influence it
2. Noise and activity around him the whole day and even all night
3. Insufficient possibilities for individual and productive activity
4. Restriction of trivial needs, e.g., eating and drinking
5. Restricted movement for therapeutic reasons
6. Insufficient information

If, in addition, 20 interested observers are admiring the "wonder of mechanical circulation support," and this extraordinary progress is explained over and over by a "guide," it is no wonder that the patient suffers.

Considering the time consumed by psychic care, the following possibilities are given:

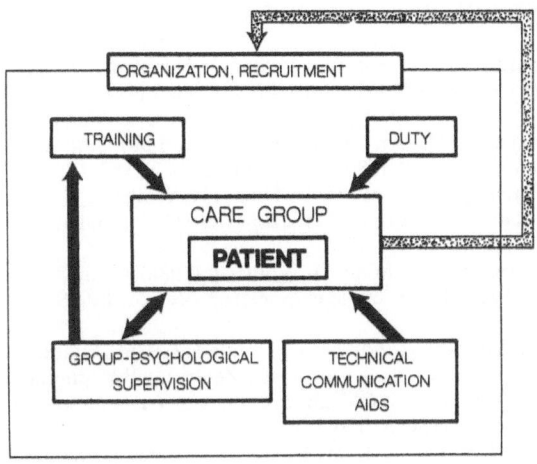

Fig. 21. Management of psychohygienic intervention

1. Radical increase of visiting time for relatives and friends; a suitable visitor (the spouse, if possible) can do wonders, especially for the cardiac patient.
2. Integration of psychological care and supervision intervals by the attending personnel, during the shift.
3. Integration of a special care group (social care duty). Persons who are interested in such service and will do it with pleasure and at no cost are invited to the organization. The only requirement is that these persons like personal contact. In the project run by the author, the special care group was trained in seminars (Fig. 21). Duties should be directed by the ward personnel. The social care group should attend group-dynamic sessions once a week, because great psychic strain is exerted on the care personnel, as well. These sessions could improve the training of novices. Such a group can reconstitute itself by means of public relations or advertising campaigns. Technical aids are necessary.
4. Development and purchase of technical communication aids, such as radio, tape recorder, TV, telephone, and video telephone.

All these modifications of communication – e.g., increasing visiting time, integration of conversation intervals during the shift of attending personnel, institution of a special social care group – add a bit of "human confusion" to the perfect organization of an intensive-care ward, but psychosomatic and social rules seem to justify them.

References

1. Affeld K (ed) (1986) Nonpulsatile blood pumps. ESAO workshop 1985. Hermann Föttiger Institut der TU Berlin
2. Horcher E (1980) Regulation und Kontrolle des künstlichen Herzens. Hydrodynamische, tierexperimentelle and pharmakologische Studien. Fakultas, Vienna
3. Imachi K, Fujimasa I, Nakajima M, Miyamoyo A, Takido N, Inou N, Tsukagoshi S, Abuchi K, Motomura K, Kouno A, Ono T, Atsumi K (1984) Evaluation of the metabolic state

in a total artificial heart circulatory system. In: Progress in artificial organs – 1983. ISAO Press, Cleveland, pp 252–265

4. Mays JB, Hastings L, Williams MA, Barker LE, De Vries WC (1986) Drive system management of emergency conditions in three permanent total artificial heart patients. Trans Am Soc Artif Intern Organs 32:221–225
5. Olsen DB, Riebman JB, Paulis R, Durrant G, Nielsen S (1987) Registry and tabulations of orthotopic total artificial hearts in humans. Trans Am Soc Artif Int Organs 33:182–189
6. Schima H, Huber H, Prodinger A, Schmallegger H, Spitaler F, Thoma H, Wolner E (1985) Driving the artificial heart with constant air pressure or constant flow. ESAO, Annual Meeting, Athens, 1985
7. Schima H, Losert U, Prodinger A, Rokitansky A, Thoma H, Wolner E (1986) A miniaturized automatic control unit for the TAH based on a single-chip microprocessor. Life Supp Syst 4 [Suppl 2]:S23–25
8. Schima H, Schauflinger U, Losert U, Rokitansky A, Spitaler F, Thoma H (1986) Hämodynamische and experimentelle Untersuchungen an einer flügellosen Zentrifugalblutpumpe. In: Medizin-Technik und Medizinische Informatik 86. Oldenbourg, Vienna, Wien, pp 61–64 (Schriftenreihe der österreichischen Computer Gesellschaft 34)
9. Schima H, Trubel W, Coraim F, Huber L, Müller MR, Redl G, Losert U, Thoma H, Wolner E (to be published) Control of the total artificial heart: new aspects in human versus animal experiments. Artif Organs
10. Snyder AJ, Imachi K, Hennig E (1986) Control. In: Buecherl, Moeller (eds) Proceedings, second world symposium on a artificial heart analysis. Vieweg, Braunschweig, pp 165–210 (Advances in system analysis)
11. Takatani S, Tanaka T, Nakatani T, Takano H, Akutsu T, Kohno H, Nudeshima H, Takahashi A (1985) Development of hemoglobin oxygen optical sensors for automatic control of artificial heart output. Trans Am Soc Artif Intern Organs 31:45–49
12. Thoma H, Deutsch M, Fasching W, Wolner E, Navratil J, Polzer K (1969) Controlling the intra-aortic balloon pump. Proceedings, international symposium devices for heart transplantation and heart substitution. Prague, p 113
13. Thoma H (1973) Automatic control of circulation pumps synchronized to the heart. Z Biomed Tech 18:3
14. Thoma H, Deutsch M, Fasching W, Haider W, Horcher E, Stellwag F, Losert U, Mohl W, Oster H, Schedl R, Unger F, Weisskirchner R, Wolner E, Polzer K, Navratil J (1976) In vivo testing of a closed loop driving unit for artificial hearts. ESAO Proc 3:360–377
15. Thoma H, Losert U, Schwanda G, Stöhr H, Wolner E (1984) Development of implantable centrifugal pumps. In: Progress in artificial organs – 1983. ISAO Press, Cleveland, pp 152–157
16. Thoma H, Losert U, Prodinger A, Schima H, Wolner E (1985) Control and drive of blood pumps: design, application and results. Proceedings of the 7th annual conference of the IEEE engineering in medicine and biology society, Chicago, 1985, pp 809–814
17. Thoma H, Heimes HP, Baer P (1986) Measuring systems and surveillance. In: Buecherl, Moeller (eds) Proceedings, second world symposium on artificial heart analysis. Vieweg, Braunschweig, pp 165–210 (Advances in system analysis)
18. Thoma H, Losert U, Prodinger A, Schima H, Stöhr H, Wolner E (1986) First animal experiments with a fully implanted control and drive unit for the total artificial heart. In: Progress in artificial organs – 1985. ISAO Press, Cleveland, pp 393–399
19. Thoma H (1986) Some aspects of medical ethic from the perspective of bioengineering. Theor Med 7:305–317
20. Trubel W, Losert U, Schima H, Roktiansky A, Spiss CK, Coraim F, Laszkowics A, Wolner E (1987) Total artificial heart bridging: a temporary support for deteriorating HTX candidates. Thorac Cardiovasc Surg 277
21. Wolner E, Thoma H, Deutsch M, Enenkel W, Fasching W, Leodolter S, Navratil J (1971) Application of the intra-aortic balloon pump during experimental cardiac infarction. J Exp Surg Res 4:2
22. Yozu R, Shimomitsu T, Jacobs G, Watanabe T, Morimoto T, Stacy G, Nose Y (1985) Use of the anaerobic threshold for evaluating various total artificial heart control algorithms in calves. Artif Organs 9:279–287

48. Transcutaneous Energy Transmission for Assisted Circulation

Y. Mitamura, A. Hirano, E. Okamoto, and T. Mikami

Introduction

Pneumatic total artificial hearts and cardiac assist systems have been successfully applied clinically. However, this method involves the permanent piercing of the chest wall by energy-carrying lines. Both for psychological reasons and from the viewpoint of minimizing the danger of infection, there are objections to compromising the integrity of the tissue barrier.

The next generation of artificial hearts and permanent cardiac assist systems will be actuated electrically rather than by compressed gases. Electrical actuation permits the design of systems free of tubes and wires passing through the skin. Electric systems promise dramatic improvements in the quality of life of pump-dependent patients.

Electric artificial hearts and heart assist systems require significant power levels which cannot be met by implanted battery systems. Although power requirements of artificial hearts depend on the efficiency of artificial hearts and on conditions of exercise, the current power requirement is 22 W.

Although there are a variety of possible methods for transporting energy into the body, schemes involving electromagnetic coupling are currently receiving the most attention. Coupling types fall essentially into two broad categories: (a) audio-frequency transmission by means of closed or nearly closed magnetic systems, in which the coils are wound around a magnetic material to achieve coupling [1–3], and (b) radio-frequency transmission by means of pancake air core coils in which magnetic material is not required [4–10].

Air core transformers have some potential disadvantages, such as large size, bulkiness, and less coupling between the external and internal coils. To solve these problems a new transformer was formed from a pair of concave and convex ferrite cores. The transcutaneous energy transmission system includes output voltage regulation and an implanted rechargeable backup battery. These functions keep the power supply to a load constant even in cases of dislocation of coils, drop of primary battery voltage, etc. It is the purpose of this study to demonstrate the feasibility of this transcutaneous energy transmission system for delivering the required power of 22 W.

Assisted Circulation 3
F. Unger (Ed.)
© Springer-Verlag Berlin Heidelberg 1989

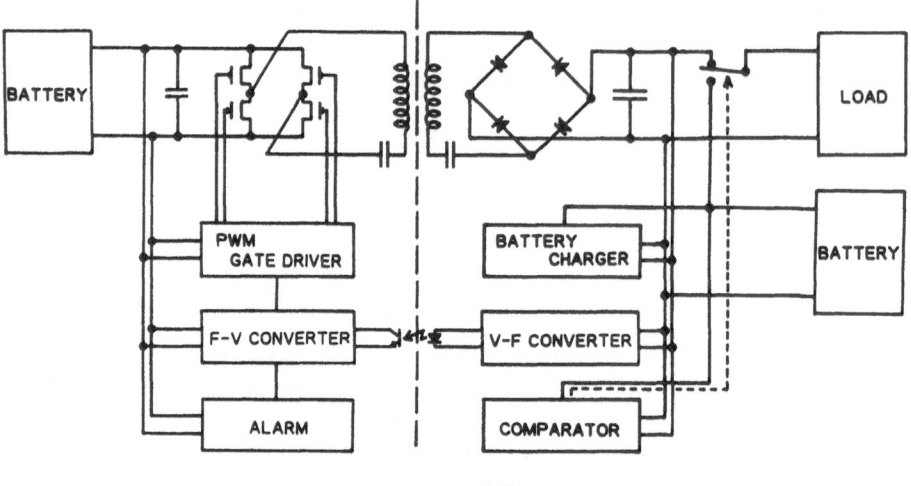

SKIN ➡ THE INTERIOR OF THE BODY

Fig. 1. Transcutaneous energy transmission system

Materials

The transcutaneous energy transmission system that has been developed for use with electric artificial hearts comprises a transcutaneous transformer, a power oscillator, an output power-conditioning system, a rechargeable backup battery, and an alarm system (Fig. 1).

Transcutaneous Transformer

Three types of transcutaneous transformer have been developed: those with a concave/convex core, a pot core, and an air core (Fig. 2). The concave/convex core transformer is formed from two ferrite cores (TDK, specific permeability of 3300). A problem which has been observed in other devices of this type is that the external part moves with respect to the implanted part, resulting in reduced coupling and higher loss. To minimize this possibility, the external device is concave at the base, and the upper surface of the internal device is convex. The internal device causes a bulge in skin. This mound serves to locate a primary core the inner diameter of which approximates the perimeter of the mound. This prevents lateral motion of the primary core. The implanted secondary device of the transformer is a ferrite core measuring 5.6 cm in diameter at the base, 4.0 cm in diameter at the upper surface, 1.3 cm in height and weighing 96 g. The windings have 20 turns of Litz wire (diameter, 012/45) (0.12 mm in diameter/45 wires twisted).[1] The superficial primary coil contains 15 turns of the same wire wound inside a concave ferrite core with a diameter of 6.2 cm at the base, a diameter of 4.4 cm at the top surface, and a weight of 97 g.

---

[1] Each wire has a diameter of 0.12 mm. Forty five wires were twisted to make a Litz wire.

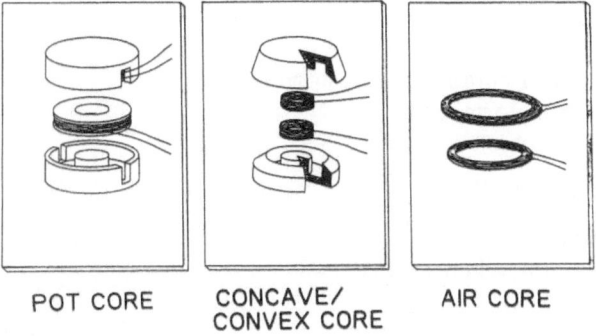

POT CORE   CONCAVE/   AIR CORE
           CONVEX CORE

Fig. 2. Three types of transcutaneous transformer: those with pot core, concave/convex core, and air core

Each half of the pot core transformer is a ferrite core (TDK, P36/22, specific permeability of 2794), 3.6 cm in diameter, and 1.1 cm thick. The windings have 25 turns of Litz wire. The weight of each unit is 30 g.

The secondary coil of the air core transformer contains 25 turns of Litz wire wound in a tight spiral with an inner diameter of 5.0 cm and a weight of 20 g. The superficial primary coil contains 20 turns of the same wire wound in a tight spiral with an inner diameter of 7.0 cm and a weight of 25 g.

Theoretical Considerations

In the transcutaneous energy transmission system, both the primary and secondary coils are series-tuned at the operating frequency using capacitors (Fig. 1). To ascertain the conditions for minimizing losses in the coils, we shall first consider the equivalent circuit of Fig. 3. Solving the loop and node equations for operation at the resonant frequency:

$$V_1 = R_1 I_1 + jwMI_2 \tag{1}$$

$$V_2 = jwMI_1 + R_2 I_2 \tag{2}$$

$$V_2 = -R_L I_2 \tag{3}$$

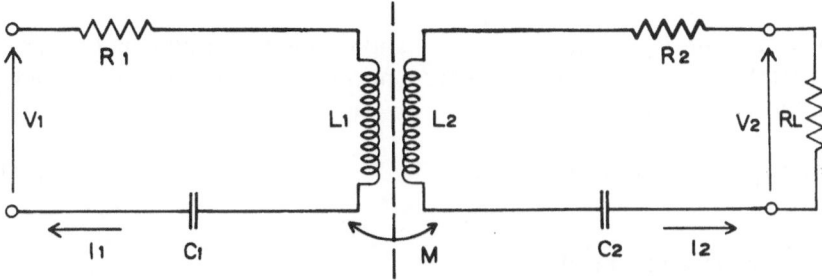

Fig. 3. Equivalent circuit of transcutaneous transformer

where

M = the mutual inductance of the two coils
V_1 = the voltage applied to the transcutaneous transformer
V_2 = the output voltage of the transformer
I_1 = the current supplied by the source
I_2 = the current in the load
R_1 = the loss in the primary coil
R_2 = the loss in the secondary coil
From Eqs. 2 and 3, the primary coil current is

$$I_1 = -(R_L + R_2)\, I_2/jwM. \tag{4}$$

The power loss is given by

$$P_{loss} = (R_1|I_1|^2 + R_2|I_2|^2)/2. \tag{5}$$

Equations 4 and 5 yield

$$P_{loss} = (R_1(R_L + R_2)^2/(w^2 M^2) + R_2)|I_2|^2/2. \tag{6}$$

The received load power is given by

$$P_{load} = (R_L|I_2|^2)/2 \tag{7}$$

Equations 6 and 7 yield

$$P_{loss} = P_{load}/R_L(R_1(R_L + R_2)^2/w^2 M^2 + R_2). \tag{8}$$

At this point, it is convenient to introduce a set of dimensionless quantities to eliminate R_1 and R_2. These parameters are defined by

$$D_1 = R_1/wL_1;\ D_2 = R_2/wL_2. \tag{9}$$

Using Eq. 9, Eq. 8 becomes

$$P_{loss} = P_{load}/R_L(D_1(R_L + wL_2 D_2)^2/wk^2 L_2 + wL_2 D_2) \tag{10}$$

where k is the coefficient of coupling $(M = k\sqrt{L_1 L_2})$.

By differentiating P_{loss} with respect to L_2 and setting the result equal to zero, one finds that the load condition for minimum power loss under the power supply of P_{load} to the load R_L is

$$L_2 = R_L/(w\sqrt{D_2^2 + D_2 k^2/D_1}) = N_2^2 L_{2S} \tag{11}$$

where
N_2 = turns of the secondary coil
L_{2S} = self inductance for $N_2^2 = 1$.

When the resistance R_1 is small enough, Eq. 1 can be approximated by

$$|V_1| = wM|I_2| = wN_1N_2M_S|I_2| \tag{12}$$

where
N_1 = turns of the primary coil
N_2 = turns of the secondary coil
M_S = mutual inductance for $N_1 = N_2 = 1$
Equation 7 gives the unique current $|I_2|$ which provides the load R_L with the power of P_{load}. Therefore, for a given V_1, Eq. 12 becomes

$$wN_1N_2M_S = |V_1/I_2| = \text{const.} \tag{13}$$

Equations 11 and 13 yield the optimum number of turns which provides the load with the given power.

Power System and Output Voltage Regulation

The power MOS-FETs (Hitachi, 2SJ122 and 2SK428) convert the power drawn from an external 18-V DC source into a 10- to 100-kHz square wave to excite the transformer primary coil. The loaded transformer presents a low impedance to the power FET at the fundamental frequency of the square wave and relatively high impedance at the frequencies of the higher harmonics. The result is that the primary current waveform approximates the sine wave. The implanted portion of the system contains the secondary coil and series capacitor (polypropylene capacitor), followed by full-wave rectifier (Schottky barrier diodes, Toshiba 5FWJ2S41) and filter.

The output power-conditioning circuitry is responsible for holding its output voltage constant as the external battery voltage falls, as coupling between the coils varies, and as the load current changes. This circuit is a variation on the switching regulator. The output voltage is converted into its proportional pulse frequency by a V–F converter (National Semiconductor, LM566). The information on pulse frequency is transcutaneously transmitted by a photocoupler (Sharp, GL513F and PT550F). The pulse frequency is proportionally changed into voltage by an F–V converter (National Semiconductor, LM2917). This voltage is compared with the nominal value for the ouput voltage, and according to the error signal, the duty cycle of the primary pulse is varied by switching a regulator control circuit (Motorola MC-3420).

Rechargeable Backup Battery and Alarm System

A sealed rechargeable lead storage battery (Matsushita, LCT-812 0.8 Ah, 12 V DC) measuring $61 \times 25 \times 95$ mm and weighing 320 g was connected in parallel to the load through a relay. A constant voltage was applied from the DC-DC regulator (Maxim, MAX 630) to the battery terminals sufficient to maintain an ap-

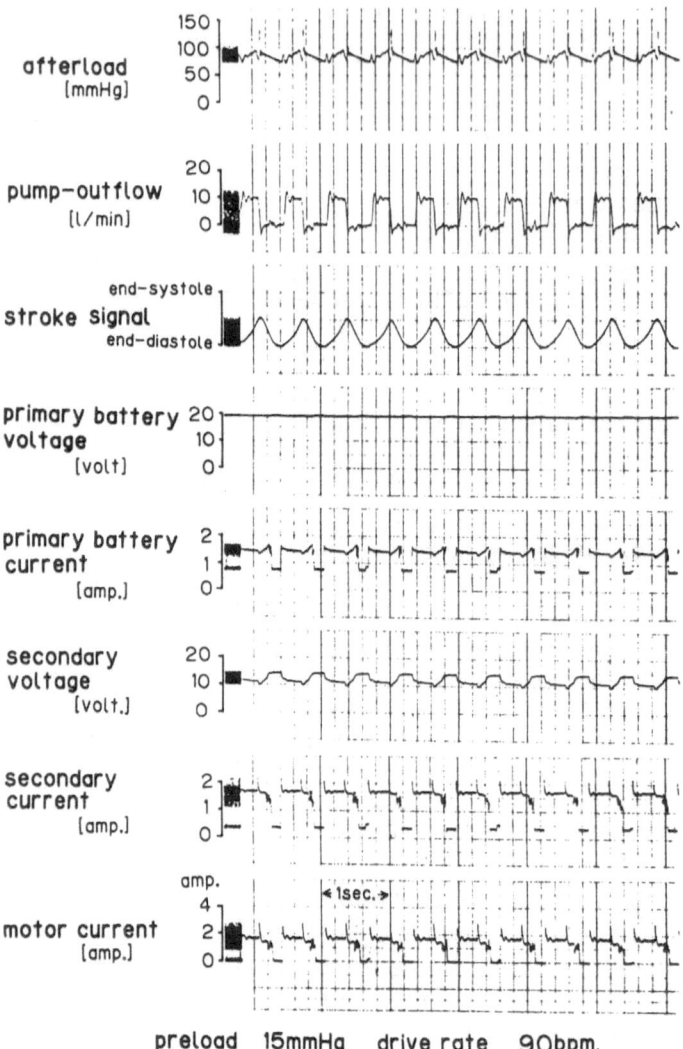

Fig. 4. Fluid dynamics of the motor-driven artificial heart powered by the transcutaneous energy transmission system

proximately constant storage of charge. If transcutaneous energy transmission is interrupted due to dislocation of transformers, the comparator drives the relay, and electric energy is supplied from the backup battery for at least 10 min. If the voltage to the load becomes normal, the comparator switches the relay, and the backup battery is disconnected from the load and recharged.

The alarm system always monitors the transmitted infrared signal. If the amplitude decreases below a threshold level due to dislocation of transformers, or if pulse frequency drops below a threshold level due to the decrease of output voltage, the alarm system gives a warning signal.

Experimental Studies

Efficiency of the energy transmission system was measured when a current of 20 W was transmitted at a core separation of 5 mm. Overall efficiency was 69% in the air core transformer, 75% in the concave/convex core transformer, and 78% in the pot core transformer at 50 kHz.

Output voltage control for the changes in tissue gap and radial misalignment was tested in the pot core transformer [11]. The output voltage was kept almost constant for the changes in tissue gaps of 3–8 mm. Output voltage was also maintained almost constant for the changes in radial displacement of 0–10 mm.

Feasibility of the transcutaneous energy transmission system was tested by using a motor-driven artificial pump. The motor-driven assist pump was developed in our laboratory [12, 13]. The artificial pump consists of a high-speed DC brushless motor driving a ball screw, and its mating blood pump. The basic drive system consists of a ball screw and plastic magnet. The screw is connected to a plate, to which the plastic magnet is firmly fixed. As the ball screw is rotated in one direction, the plastic magnet moves forward, pushing an iron pusher plate (emptying phase). As the ball screw reverses, the pusher plate and plastic magnet move together backward. When pump filling is poor, and the pusher plate moves backward more slowly than the plastic magnet, the pusher plate is pulled back by the magnetic force of the plastic magnet (active filling). However, if pressure lower than -25 mmHg is applied to the blood pump, the plastic magnet is automatically detached from the pusher plate, and excess negative pressure is not applied to the pump. The blood pump has been specifically designed for use with the motor drive. The blood-contacting surface of the pump housing is coated with segmented polyurethane. The smooth blood-contacting diaphragm within the pump cases is also fabricated of segmented polyurethane. The motor housing is machined from stainless steel. The maximum stroke volume of the pump is 89 ml and the stroke of the pusher plate is 12 mm. The motor driven pump is connected to a mechanical mock loop.

Pump outflow, arterial pressure, pusher plate displatement, motor current, and secondary voltage were monitored when the pump was driven at a rate of 90 bpm, under a preload of 15 mmHg, and against an afterload of 95 mmHg (Fig. 4). Electric energy was transmitted at a core separation of 5 mm. At the beginning of the emptying phase, a large pulse current flowed to the motor. During the following emptying phase, a motor current of 1.8 A flowed, and the secondary voltage of the transformer decreased from 14 to 11 V. During the filling phase, a motor current of 1.3 A flowed, and the secondary voltage returned to the preset level of 14 V. During the later period of the filling phase, the motor was at a standstill, and a current of 0.7 A flowed through the control circuit from the primary battery.

Figure 5 demonstrates that the motor was driven by the backup battery when energy transmission through the transformer was interrupted. When energy transmission was interrupted, the secondary voltage suddenly dropped to zero. The drop in secondary voltage was sensed by the comparator, and 1 s later the backup battery was connected to the motor by the relay. Almost the same stroke volume of the artificial pump was maintained by the backup battery.

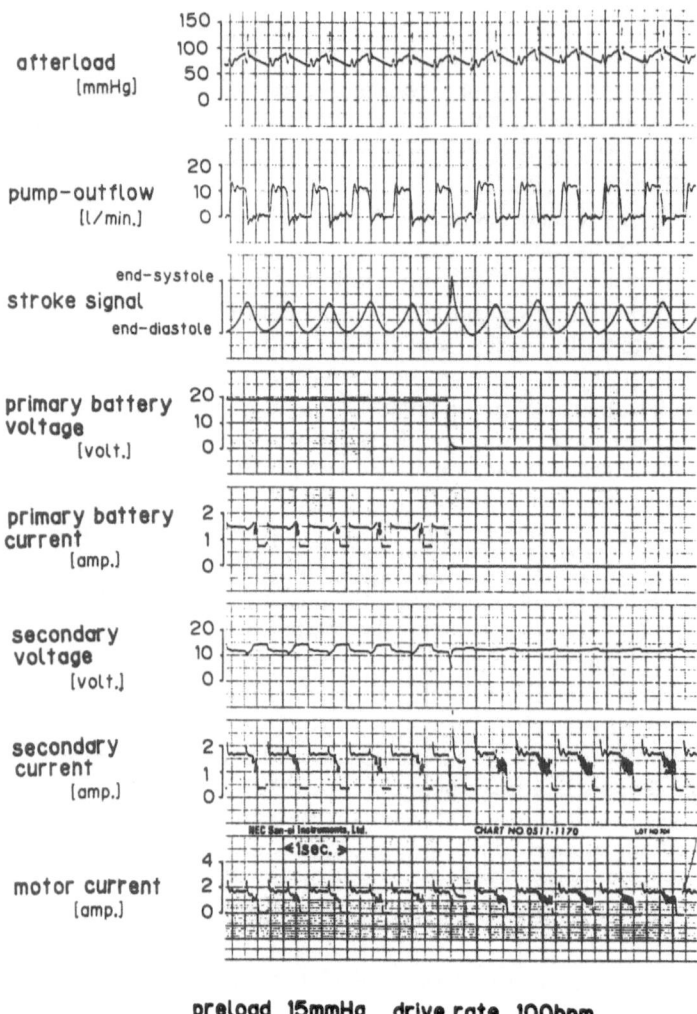

afterload [mmHg]

pump-outflow [l/min.]

stroke signal
end-systole
end-diastole

primary battery voltage [volt.]

primary battery current [amp.]

secondary voltage [volt.]

secondary current [amp.]

motor current [amp.]

preload 15mmHg   drive rate 100bpm

Fig. 5. Continuous pumping of the motor-driven artificial heart by the backup battery during interruption of transcutaneous energy transmission

Temperature rise was tested in a chronic experiment by implanting the device in a dog and measuring with implanted thermisters. The dog was anesthetized and the secondary core inserted just beneath the skin of the back. The coil was fixed in position by means of several sutures around the coil. The leads from this core were tunneled beneath the skin and removed at a remote location. After the dog recovered from the surgical procedure, a core similar to that inserted was placed on the surface of the back in such a position as to be coaxial with the core inside the animal. The leads from the coil within the body were connected to a resistance load (incandescent lamp). Three thermisters were used: one on the outside of the internal core, one in the tissue, and one on the outside of the external core. Temperature monitored as the power delivered to the lamp load was varied from 10 to 30 W. The temperature rise in the tissue was less than 1 °C when 30 W was transmitted.

Discussion

Various types of transcutaneous energy transmission systems have been developed to power implanted electric artificial hearts [1–10]. However, several problems remain to be solved: increase of transmission efficiency, allowable temperature rise, easy fitting, regulation output voltage, and safety.

High energy transmission efficiency is essential for a battery-powered biomedical system because it prolongs the life of the external battery and minimizes the possibility of burns due to high temperature. High transmission efficiency was realized in our system by employing the optimum number of windings and by using MOS-FETs and Schottky barrier diodes with low on-resistance. Total efficiency of 75%–78% in our systems is reasonably high compared with other reported values; total efficiency was 65%–80% for nominal loads of 12–24 W [7] and 53% –67% for 10 W supply [8].

Temperature rise in the tissue when 30 W was transmitted was within 1 °C. This temperature rise may not produce harmful effects on the skin. Heat diffusion in the pot core and heat removal by blood flow probably limited the temperature rise. Similar temperature rises have been reported by other researchers; maximum tissue temperature of 39.7 °C was observed at the transmission of 1 kW power [6], and temperature rises were less than 1 °C in the surface of the implanted coils [7].

In a number of applications it is important to keep the received power within narrow limits despite coupling variations. Several effective means were included in our study to achieve this goal. To minimize the possibility of lateral motion of the coils, the concave/convex core type of transformer was developed. Since the internal device causes a bulge in skin, the projections on the external portions can engage the internal portion and prevent lateral motion. Although several approaches have been developed to prevent lateral motion of cores, these have employed an additional device such as a shallow cup [2] or annular permanent ferrite magnets [3]. The output voltage control circuit is another effective method for maintaining constant received power despite some degree of coupling variations. In this study the information on the voltage to an implanted motor was transcutaneously transmitted by infrared pulses. Optical transmission has advantages over conventional radio-frequency transmission. The optical signal is not interfered with by radio-frequency signals induced by the transcutaneous energy transmission system and motor. In this study the duty cycle of the primary pulse was varied to maintain constant secondary voltage. Sherman reported that 6 W was dissipated when power to the output stage was switched off by short-circuiting the output of the tuned secondary transformer to keep motor voltage constant, while the losses were reduced from 6 to 0.75 W when the primary voltage was reduced by a factor of 10 [7]. Energy loss due to output voltage regulation is less when primary voltage is regulated rather than when secondary voltage is regulated.

The concept of using an implanted rechargeable cell as a backup battery in the case of complete power interruption is attractive and essential for continuous power supply. However, the chemical and physical requirements for the components of secondary cells are much more restrictive than those needed for primaries. Therefore, the list of viable candidates is very narrow. In fact, to date only two rechargeable systems, nickel oxide/cadmium cells and mercuric oxide/zinc cells, have been successfully implanted in human patients. In this study a recently developed, hermetically sealed lead storage battery was utilized. This has several advantages. The volumetric energy density is as high as 0.066 Wh/cm^3, whereas the energy density of the nickel oxide/cadmium cell is 0.056 Wh/cm^3 [11]. The rate of self-discharge is 0.36%/per day at a temperature of 40 °C. This compares to values of -0.3%/per day at body temperature with the nickel oxide/cadmium cell. The sealed lead storage battery can be recharged repeatedly after full discharge. A capacity of 90%–100% can be restored after recharge. Provision of telemetry of battery voltage would allow continuous battery status assessment to avoid an overcharge.

In vitro testing of the developed transcutaneous energy transmission system used with the motor-driven artificial heart demonstrates that it is feasible for operating the motor-driven pump (Fig. 4). Figure 5 demonstrates that continuous pumping of the artificial heart is assured by the implanted lead storage battery even when transcutaneous energy transmission is interrupted.

From the above results it can be concluded that this constitutes a potential transcutaneous energy transmission system for implanted electric artificial hearts.

References

1. Andren CF, Fadall MA, Gott VL, Topaz SR (1968) The skin tunnel transformer: a new system that permits both high efficiency transfer of power and telemetry of data through the intact skin. IEEE Trans Biomed Eng 15:278–280
2. Myers GH, Reed GE, Thumin A, Fascher S, Cortes L (1968) A transcutaneous power transformer. Trans Am Soc Artif Intern Organs 14:210–214
3. Sutton GW, Rivera LM, Kirby PT (1981) A miniaturized device for electrical energy transmission through intact skin: concepts and results of initial tests. Artif Organs 5 [Suppl]:437–440
4. Schuder JC, Stephenson HE, Townsend JF (1961) High-level electromagnetic energy transfer through a closed chest wall. IRE Int Conv Record 9:119–126
5. Fuller JW (1968) Apparatus for efficient power transfer through a tissue barrier. IEEE Trans Biomed Eng 15:63–65
6. Schuder JC, Gold JH, Stephenson HE (1971) An inductively coupled RF system for the transmission of 1 kW of power through the skin. IEEE Trans Biomed Eng 18:265–273
7. Sherman CW, Clay WC, Dasse KA, Daly BDT (1985) A transcutaneous energy transmission system for high-power prosthetics. Proc IEEE 7th Annu Conf Eng Med Biol Soc, The Institute of Electrical and Electronics Engineers, Inc. New York, The IEEE Engineering in Medicine and Biology Society, pp 804–808
8. Koshiji K, Utsunomiya T, Takatani S, Takano H, Nakatani T, Kinoshita M, Noda H, Fukuda S, Akutsu T (1987) Analysis of efficiency and experimental consideration of energy transmission system to drive total implanted artificial hearts. Jpn J Artif Organs 16:167–170

9. Abe Y, Fujumasa I, Imachi K, Nakajima M, Chinzei T, Maeda K, Orime Y, Asano M, Hata H, Hosaka S, Kouno A, Ono T, Atsumi K (1987) Development of transcutaneous energy transmission system for totally implanted artificial hearts: effect of coreless coils. Jpn J Artif Organs 16:212–215

10. Portner P, Oyer P, Jassawalla J, Chen H, Miller P, LaForge D, Green G, Shumway N (1984) A totally implantable ventricular assist device for end-stage heart disease. In: Unger F (ed) Assisted circulation 2. Springer, Berlin Heidelberg New York Tokyo, pp 115–141

11. Mitamura Y, Hirano A, Okamoto E, Mikami T (1988) Development of trancutaneous energy transmission system. In: Akutsu T (ed) Artificial heart 2. Springer, Berlin Heidelberg New York Tokyo, pp 265–271

12. Mitamura Y, Okamoto E, Mikami T (1986) Motor-driven artificial pump. In: Akutsu T (ed) Artificial heart 1. Springer, Berlin Heidelberg New York Tokyo, pp 71–75

13. Mitamura Y, Okamoto E, Hirano A, Mikami T (1987) Development of motor driven assist pump systems. Joye Leinberger (ed) Proc 9th Conf IEEE Engineering in Medicine and Biology Society, The Institute of Electrical and Electronics Engineers, Inc., New York, pp 184–185

14. Holleck GL (1986) Rechargeable electrochemical cells as implanted power sources. In: Owen BB (ed) Batteries for implantable biomedical devices. Plenum, New York, pp 275–284

49. Endothelialization
of Artificial Heart Materials

R. Fasol and P. Zilla

Since the beginning of artificial heart research and the first clinical applications of total artificial hearts (TAH), thromboembolism has represented the major limiting factor for successful long-term clinical trials [1]. One of the main reasons for this undesired complication is the contact-induced platelet activation by artificial surfaces of cardiac prostheses [2, 3]. This thrombocyte activation is not affected by anticoagulation therapy. In addition, the value of antiaggregatory treatment of artificial heart patients is limited, and only recently we were able to demonstrate that antiaggregatory treatment does not fully inhibit blood platelet activation [4].

Following disappointing attempts to find an ideal nonthrombogenic material that would prevent platelet, plasma protein, and red cell adhesion to artificial surfaces, attention has turned to create the de novo formation of a so-called pseudoneointima (PNI) [5–7]. Since it was discovered that the vessel wall's antithrombotic properties depend on a lining of living endothelial cells, which actively synthesize antithrombotic agents such as prostacyclin and heparin-like substances, the focus began to shift toward creating viable endothelial linings on biomaterials as early as 1968 [8]. At a time when most research groups were still involved in PNI studies. Adachi et al. [9] reported the cultivation of bovine microvascular endothelial cells (EC) on silastic material in 1971, and Mansfield et al. [10] tried autologous lining of artificial surfaces with cultured endothelial cells in calves in 1975. However, in artificial heart research this idea was taken up only long after its initiation [11–13]; the concept was successfully adapted to peripheral vascular surgery in 1978, when Herring introduced endothelial cell seeding for use in Dacron velour vascular grafts [14]. To date, many research groups have performed seeding studies, including ones with small-diameter polytetrafluorethylene (PTFE) grafts. However, first clinical trials showed that seeding does not lead to complete endothelialization until the 14th week after implantation [15]. To offer endothelial cells a suitable substratum for adherence and spreading, the prosthetic surface of artificial implants must be either preclotted or precoated with protein substances. However, blood preclotting procedures for vascular grafts differ markedly from precoating procedures for nonporous materials suitable for TAH constructions.

Since a cell loss of up to 96% is found in the first 24 h after implantation of endothelial cell-seeded grafts [16], the technique of seeding endothelial cells does not seem feasible for endothelialization of artificial heart ventricles, and this emphasizes the necessity of alternative solutions like the confluent endothelialization of a synthetic surface prior to implantation. For this purpose, two approaches

Assisted Circulation 3
F. Unger (Ed.)
© Springer-Verlag Berlin Heidelberg 1989

seem to be promising: microvessels as an EC source for immediate high-density "sodding" [17–19], or culture techniques in combination with a two-staged procedure [20–24]. When microvascular endothelial cells are used the possible uncertainties of cell culture outside the operating room can be avoided – as can a significant time delay required for cell culture – since large quantities of cells can be rapidly isolated from adipose tissue [17]. However, it remains to be proven whether or not the immature cytoskeleton of freshly "sodded" cells is ready to withstand shear forces after implantation. In venous endothelial cells, parallel stress fibers – the most prominent feature of the cytoskeleton of human arterial endothelial cells in situ – were already shown to be inducible by shear forces. Moreover, the formation of the "dense peripheral band" of microfilament bundles, which is thought to be the site of strong cell adhesion [25], seems to require a cultivation period of 8–12 days [26]. Taking this delay into consideration, a two-step in vitro cultivation of endothelial cells on artificial surfaces prior to implantation seems to be the most promising approach to providing, in vitro, a confluent and shear stress-resistant endothelial lining for artificial hearts at the time of implantation.

Harvest and Growth Characteristics of Endothelial Cells

The first step in any attempt to endothelialize artificial surfaces is the procedure of harvesting endothelial cells. The first approaches were the enzymatical harvest method using veins everted on a steel rod [27] and the mechanical "scrapping" technique [28]. The steel rod technique was hampered by contamination with fibroblasts and smooth muscle cells, but the introduction of a vein-cannulation technique by Sharefkin solved this problem [29]. Nevertheless, vein harvesting by the surgeon is the first important step, significantly influencing the further endothelialization process.

Importance of Vein Handling for Subsequent Culture of Endothelial Cells

If a vein segment is surgically harvested, the technique used is of crucial importance for the subsequent harvest and culture of endothelial cells. The cytotoxic effects of surgical glove powder particles on human vascular endothelial cells have been described [30], as have the detrimental effects of not employing the "no-touch technique" [31]. To evaluate the importance of a careful, no-touching vein harvest, we compared the endothelial cell harvest efficiency and the culture behavior of spahenous vein segments harvested either carefully, with the "no-touch technique," or in the normal, routine way.

No-touch technique: The mean number of cells harvested was $44\,000/cm^2$ vein. In 45 primary cultures the cells from only two vein segments failed to grow. After 10 days of cultivation [population doubling number (PDN) 3.4; population doubling time (PDT) 1.2] the mean number of EC was $64\,000/cm^2$.

Touch technique: The mean number of cells harvested was $18\,000/cm^2$ vein. In 40 primary cultures the cells from 16 vein segments failed to grow. After 10 days of cultivation (PDN: 2.8; PDT: 1.4) the mean number of EC was $31\,000/cm^2$.

Our data show that the surgical handling of veins is of utmost importance if a subsequent attempt to endothelialize artificial surfaces is to be successful. Avoidance of the cytotoxic effects of surgical glove powder particles, as well as of rough surgical handling during vein harvesting, is a prerequisite for subsequent endothelial cell culture.

Growth Characteristics of Patient's Endothelial Cells

In an attempt to gain more information concerning the growth characteristics of endothelial cells of a potential group of patients for TAH implantation, we studied the reproductive capacity of saphenous vein endothelial cells from smoking and nonsmoking coronary bypass patients by a replicate microwell technique using human fibronectin for precoating.

Previous reports have indicated that smoking has a detrimental effect on the efficiency of autologous endothelial seeding (AES) in vascular surgery [32]. One reason for these discouraging results may be that cigarette smoking impairs endothelial cell prostacyclin production [33, 34]. Such impaired endothelial cells – deprived of the most potent antiaggregatory substance at their apical surface – may represent an even more thrombogenic substratum than a nonendothelialized surface. Moreover, endothelial cell injuries such as swelling, blebbing, and opening of cell junctions [34, 35] – the result of cigarette smoking – may subsequently cause reduced reproductive capacity of the endothelium. A lower reproductive capacity of EC in smokers, however, would result in incomplete EC coverage of artificial surfaces at a time when the group of nonsmokers had already produced a closed EC monolayer.

Applying an enzymatic harvest method, vein remnants of 21 smoking and 18 nonsmoking coronary bypass patients were incubated with collagenase (CLS II) for either 15 or 7 min. The different collagenase exposure times were applied to detect possible negative influences of the protease digestion on EC growth behavior. In smokers, the harvest efficiency of EC for the two respective periods of collagenase exposure was 41% ($P<0.02$) and 30% ($P<0.2$) lower than in nonsmokers. Moreover, the PDN between viable cell yield (VCY) and day 10 in cells exposed to 15 or 7 min of collagenase was 4.5 ± 0.5 and 4.3 ± 1.3 in nonsmokers but only 2.4 ± 2.1 and 1.8 ± 1.3 in smokers. Thirteen of 18 cultures from vein donors who smoked showed an absence of logarithmic proliferation, while the few exponentially proliferating cultures from the remaining smokers displayed a PDT-log of 30 ± 9 h during the logarithmic growth, which was similar to the 32 ± 7 h obtained in nonsmokers.

The much lower PDN and lack of exponential growth in the majority of cultures, in addition to a distinctly reduced harvest efficiency, provide in vitro evidence for the possible failure of clinically applied endothelialization trials [32] in smokers.

Since our in vitro conditions were characterized by growth-promoting circumstances, the actual in vivo situation might even be worse. Our results indicate that growth characteristics of endothelial cells of smokers – a possible group of patients for TAH implantation – could alter the successful outcome of trials of autogenic endothelialization of artificial heart ventricles.

Characteristics of Biomaterials (Porous, Nonporous)

Considering that artificial hearts consist of (a) a nonporous surface of the ventricle and the driving membrane and (b) a porous surface of the atrial part, we evaluated the growth behavior of endothelial cells on various artificial heart materials.

Since the final purpose of an endothelialized artificial surface is long-term implantation into the bloodstream, it must be excluded that growth characteristics do not change after monolayer growth has been achieved. For this reason, we evaluated the primary attachment rate of endothelial cells seeded onto differently precoated materials, investigated surface characteristics of different porous and nonporous biomaterials which can potentially be used for artificial heart construction, and compared different precoating procedures to ensure optimal cultivation conditions for endothelial cells. Finally, we investigated the shear-stress resistance of these endothelialized surfaces.

Porous Materials

Primary Attachment of Endothelial Cells
Since the efficiency of endothelialization of artificial surfaces is related to initial cell adherence and spreading on the underlying substratum, we examined these parameters in order to determine the most suitable precoating procedure for artificial surfaces. Using our specially designed microprocessor-controlled rotation device, we seeded 30 000 EC/cm^2 of precoated PTFE graft. The different surface precoatings investigated were:

- The glycoproteins fibronectin and laminin
- Type-I and type-IV collagen
- Epsilon-amino capronic acid (EACA)-inhibited fibrin glue.

Immediately and 4 h after the 60-min seeding procedure we determined the percentage of adherent cells and the cell area using an image-analyzing system for morphometric measurement of scanning electron micrographs.

The results of this study (Fig. 1 a, b) revealed a significantly higher initial adherence of endothelial cells seeded onto surfaces precoated with collagen type I/ IV, post-treated with fibronectin (HFN). Considering the cell surface area as a parameter for ideal spreading and adherence of endothelial cells, our study showed a significantly higher cell area of endothelial cells on fibrin glue-precoated surfaces than on others. Therefore, fibronectin-coated collagen I/IV and EACA-inhibited fibrin glue offer the best underlying substrata with regard to primary cell adherence and cell spreading.

To verify these results of our initial study and to investigate the shear-stress resistance of such endothelialized surfaces, we exposed in vitro endothelialized porous surfaces to pyhsiological shear stress in subsequent experiments.

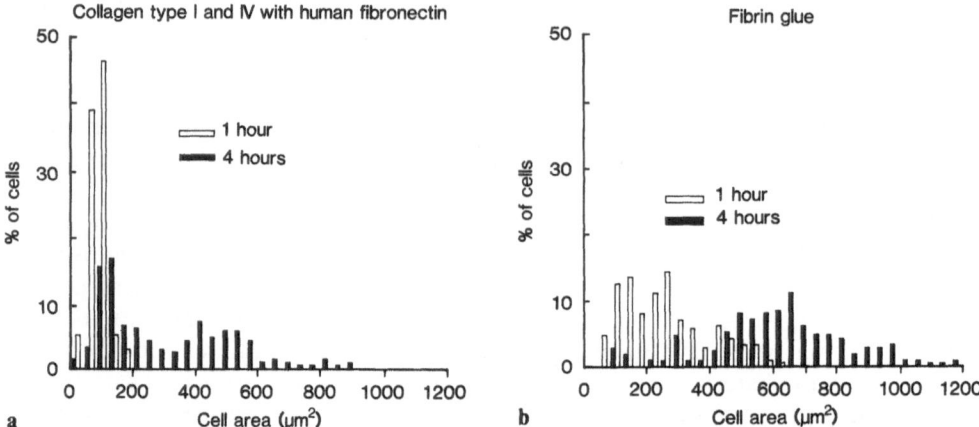

Fig. 1 a, b. Primary attachment of endothelial cells on differently precoated surfaces 1 and 4 h after seeding. Morphometric analysis revealed a significantly higher initial adherence on collagen- and HFN-precoated surfaces (**a**), but a better spreading and adherence on fibrin glue-precoated surfaces after 4 h (**b**)

In Vitro Endothelialization and Shear-Stress Exposure
of Porous Materials

In vitro growth of endothelial cells on artificial surfaces was shown to be dependent on surface precoating with either fibronectin, collagen, or fibrin [12, 20–22, 24, 36, 37]. In previous trials with in vitro endothelialization of vascular prostheses, however, high seeding densities of up to 5×10^5 EC/cm^2 [20, 22, 24] were necessary to achieve confluent monolayers.

In order to improve this unsatisfying seeding efficiency we had used a pH- and temperature-controlled rotation device [15, 21, 38]. This technique made a low inoculum of 2×10^5 EC/cm^2 graft possible and produced an instant confluent monolayer [21, 23].

In contrast to the well-reproduced growth evidence of EC on synthetic surfaces [12, 13, 20, 24, 37], data on the shear-stress resistance of such in vitro endothelialized artificial surfaces are scare [21, 22, 25]. Using nonpulsatile flow conditions, Sentissi et al. [22] found only a moderate detachment rate after a 1-h short-term perfusion of bovine endothelial cells on collagen-coated PTFE grafts. Similar experiments of our own group with cryopreserved human saphenous vein EC on fibronectin-coated PTFE grafts resulted in a major cell loss after 16 h of shear-stress exposure [21]. Taking these results, as well as those of our spreading and primary-attachment study, as indicative of the necessity for a surface which provides not only fibronectin but also a sufficient attachment area for seeded EC, we decided to use a precoating substratum that contained fibronectin and filled the PTFE interspaces.

Since EACA-inhibited fibrin glue is an easily accessible and obvious substratum, and since it had proven to result in the best spreading and adherence behavior of endothelial cells, we found it opportune to try it as the underlying material for in vitro endothelialization. However, in regard to the finding that hemoglobin from lysed erythrocytes is capable of inhibiting EC attachment [39] and that betathromboglobulin – one of the major release products of aggregating platelets – was shown to inhibit the prostacyclin production of EC [40], we avoided whole-blood preclotting and used cell-free fibrin of a clinically approved fibrin glue [38].

To evaluate the shear-stress resistance of cultivated EC on this fibrin substratum, we applied a previously described mock circulation [41], which enabled us to simulate the physiological pulsatile flow and the shear forces of the superficial femoral artery (Fig. 2a–c). According to our previous results [21], a short-term

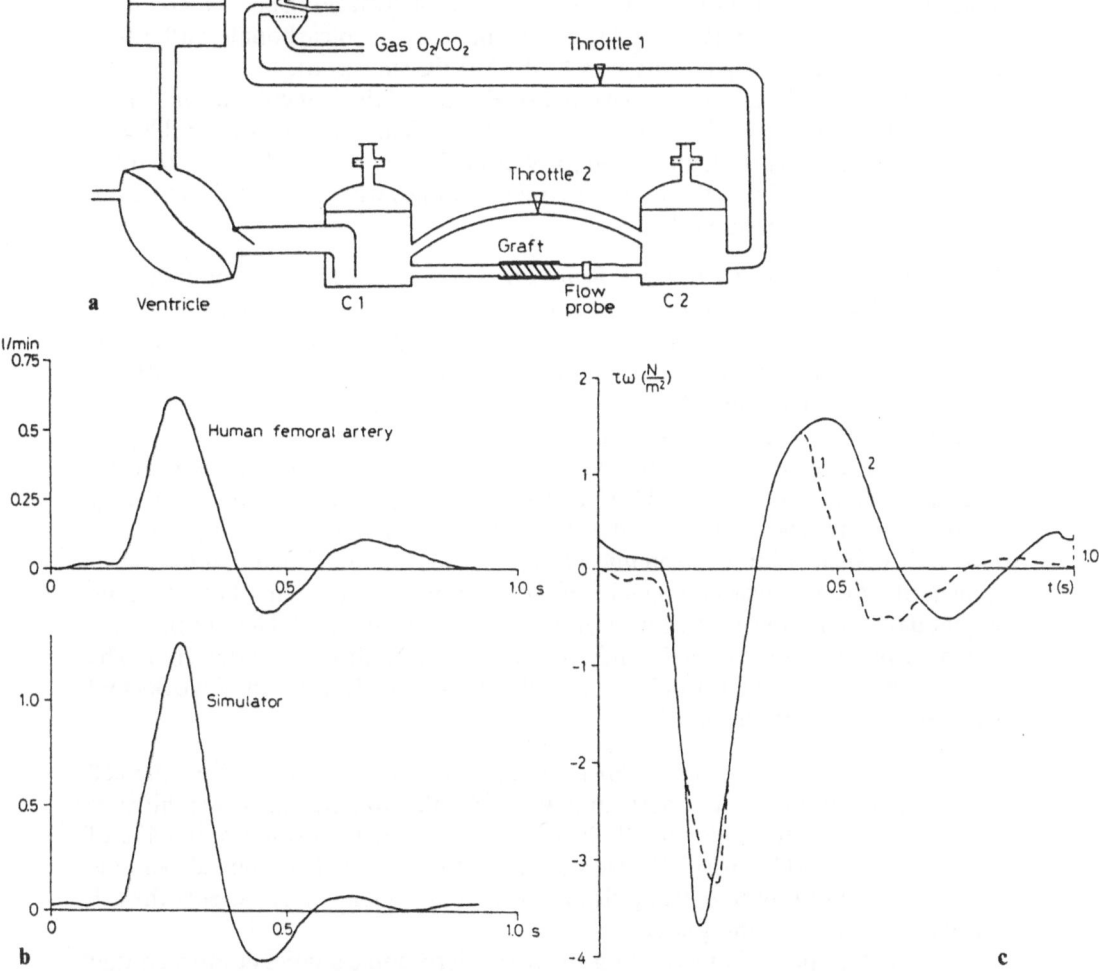

Fig. 2 a–c. a Mock circulation, using a ventricle of an artificial heart to simulate the damped oscillating-wave pattern by a hydraulic resonant circuit. **b** Flow pattern in the common femoral artery and flow pattern obtained in the simulator. **c** *1*, Shear stress calculated for physiological volume-rate flow in the common femoral artery; *2*, Shear stress calculated for a volume-rate flow in the circulatory device simulating the shear stress in the superficial femoral artery. (From Schima et al. [41])

perfusion of 1 h – as applied by others [22, 36] – seemed to be too short to predict the extent of shear force-induced cell loss. For this reason we perfused our in vitro endothelialized grafts for a long-term period of 48 h.

Endothelialization of Porous PTFE Material. Adult human saphenous vein endothelial cells (AHSVEC) were harvested and cultivated from vein remnants $(1.7 \pm 1.2 \text{ cm}^2)$, normally discarded after coronary bypass surgery, according to a previously published technique [23].

In all our experiments expanded PTFE graft material (Gore-Tex) was used: this was preclotted with a dilution of a clinically approved fibrin glue (Immuno). The preclotting procedure was as previously described [38]. To guarantee an even distribution of EC, a rotation device with adjustable rotation speed, a constant temperature of 37 °C, and a 5% CO_2 atmosphere for the bicarbonate buffer was used [21, 38]. The seeding density was 12.0×10^4 EC/cm^2 graft.

To evaluate the shear-stress resistance of EC after 9 days of cultivation, a pulsatile mock circulation using a ventricle of an artificial heart was assembled as previously described [41]. Cultivation for 9 days allowed endothelial cells to form the "dense peripheral band" of microfilament bundles which is thought to be the site of strong cell adhesion [26].

Endothelialized Surfaces Prior to Shear-Stress Exposure. The control counts of the final cell suspension showed an actual seeding density of $10.8 \pm 0.7 \times 10^4$ for AHSVEC. After 3 h of rotation, 43% of the AHSVEC ($4.6 \pm 1.2 \times 10^4$) were adherent to the graft surface. Saphenous vein endothelial cells showed a significant increase in cell density of 42% between seeding and cultivation day 9. Thus, the preperfusion cell density was $6.6 \pm 1.5 \times 10^4$ $AHSVEC/cm^2$.

Scanning electron microscopic (SEM) studies showed a confluent endothelial monolayer right after seeding. Until cultivation day 9 an increase in cell density together with a higher degree of interdigitation of marginal overlapping could be observed. Transmission electron microscopy (TEM) demonstrated that the development of marginal overlapping had already begun, but the extent of overlapping was moderate and no specific intercellular contacts were found. Neither basal attachment plaques nor luminal condensations of microfibrils were detected. The TEM appearance of the fibrin layer varied between fine fibrillar meshworks and dense amorphous structures.

Endothelialized Surfaces During Shear-Stress Exposure. For AHSVEC the cell loss during the initial 24 h of perfusion was 23%; this was statistically significant $(P < 0.05)$. During the following 24 h the trend persisted, showing only 64% of the preperfusion EC density. Thus, $4.3 \pm 1.2 \times 10^4$ AHSVEC remained per cm^2 graft after 48 h of physiological pulsatile perfusion, which still represents the cell density of a confluent monolayer.

After 24 h of perfusion, scanning electron microscopic studies confirmed that the cell layer still entirely covered the surface. Only a few single detached ECs were detected, that had lost their contact to the underlying matrix and adhered with only spider-like intercellular bridges to the neighboring cells. TEM showed a decrease in the extent of marginal overlapping and only luminal condensations of microfibrils.

Following 48 h of shear-stress exposure, SEM showed a grossly cell covered surface with a distinctly lower cell density and an even higher degree of single-cell detachment within the EC layer. Wherever cell detachment disclosed the underlying matrix, the fibrin layer was found to be well preserved, covering the PTFE structure completely. TEM revealed that intercellular contacts were further reduced, to an extent where cell margins were only rarely overlapping. Junctional complexes were not found at all. Covering larger areas, cells were distinctly flattened. However, the detection of nutritional changes in the medium – due to a changing pattern of lipoproteins – on top of the myelin figures found with TEM, suggests that the moderate cell loss after 48 h is due mainly to metabolic disturbances, related to the mock circulation. Assuming ideal nutritional conditions in vivo, this moderate cell loss might be considered negligible.

In summary, we showed that microprocessor-controlled low-density seeding produces instant EC monolayers on fibrin glue-precoated PTFE surfaces. The addition of fibrinolytic inhibitors to the fibrin glue and an extended cultivation period of 9 days resulted in a moderate 23% cell loss after 24 h of physiological pulsatile shear-stress exposure and in a well-preserved underlying fibrin layer. At this stage in vivo experiments seem to be reasonable to obtain further proof of the value of this technique.

Nonporous Materials

Surface Characteristics

To evaluate the possibility of providing an endothelial lining for artificial hearts in vitro we investigated the surface characteristics of various nonporous polyurethane and silicone-rubber materials. For each material the angle at the margin of a spreading droplet of distilled water was measured to determine the surface tension and thus the degree of hydrophobia (Table 1).

In a preliminary study the influence of precoating on the proliferation rate and mitotic activity of endothelial cells was investigated, following initial seeding of 10000 endothelial cells and cultivation for 7 days on fibronectin (HFN)- or glycosaminoglycane (GAG)-precoated surfaces compared with uncoated control surfaces. The advantage of fibronectin coating turned out to be more significant after 7 days ($P < 0.05$) of cultivation than after 2 or 3 days (Fig. 3).

[^{3}H]thymidine uptake was measured in order to compare the effect of the various precoating procedures on the mitotic rate of endothelial cells. A 3-h pulse of

Table 1. Hydrophobia of nonporous materials (spreading angle)

Polyurethane	1 s/30 s	Silicone rubber	1 s/30 s
Biomer	88°/ 82°	Medical adhesive	107°/104°
Cardiomat 610	70°/ 68°	3145 RTV	106°/103°
Lycra	87°/ 80°	Elasotosil E43	108°/106°
Mitrathane	72°/ 65°	PVC Tygon	88°/ 85°
Pelethane	75°/ 72°		
Cardiothane 51	104°/103°	Teflon PTFE	104°

Cell count (x 10⁶)

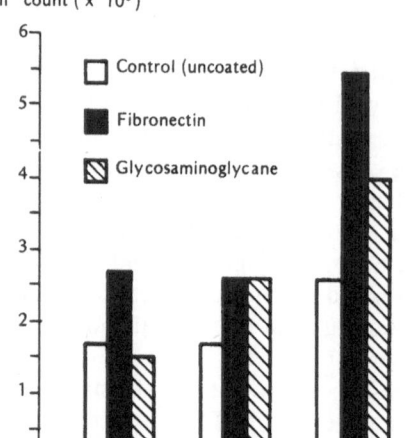

Fig. 3. Influence of precoating procedures on the proliferation rate of human endothelial cells. The advantage of fibronectin precoating turned out to be significant in this short-term experiment

Table 2. Influence of precoating on ^{3}H thymidine uptake

Fibronectin	Glycosaminoglycane	Uncoated control
10216 ± 182 cpm	8382 ± 182 cpm	6862 ± 182 cpm

1 µCi/20 000 cells 16 h later yielded $10\,216 \pm 182$ cpm with endothelial cells growing on fibronectin-coated surfaces. In contrast, only 83282 ± 182 cpm were counted after GAG cultivation and 6862 ± 182 cpm in the control cultures ($P < 0.05$; Table 2).

In Vitro Endothelialization of Nonporous Materials
For further experiments, glass coverslips 12 mm in diameter were coated with the biomaterials most commonly used for artificial heart construction [12]. Endothelial cells were obtained from human umbilical veins by the method of Jaffe [42] and cultivated according to a previously published procedure [13]. Culture surfaces were coated with fibronectin to improve growth and adhesion of endothelial cells, according to our previous studies, which had proved the advantage of fibronectin precoating [12]. Three types of growth behavior were found as a result of this preliminary study: endothelial cell monolayer growth, cell islands with sharply defined margins, and single cell growth, which sometimes even displayed signs of cytotoxicity.

Comparing fibronectin-coated biomaterials, we found that cell growth seemed to be strikingly dependent on hydrophobia. Monolayer growth could be achieved only on hydrophobic materials showing more than a 103 ° spreading angle. On the hydrophilic surfaces (less than 85 ° spreading angle), either isolated cell islands with low cell spreading or cells with cytotoxic vacuolization which had not spread were found.

In a subsequent study – to evaluate the possibility of providing endothelialized artificial heart surfaces – we cultivated adult human endothelial cells on two polyurethane and two silicone-rubber surfaces over a period of 11 days [13]. We investigated the resulting cell proliferation and morphology by means of light- and scanning electron microscopy. On the silicone-rubber surfaces, seeding of 200 000 human saphenous vein endothelial cells per cm^2 produced an ideal cobblestone monolayer within a single day. In contrast, the polyurethane surfaces displayed an uneven, patchy distribution of endothelial cells. Scanning electron microscopy revealed microvilli and marginal overlapping in both groups. After the first day, the cell count on the polyurethane surfaces increased, whereas the cell count on the silicone-rubber surfaces decreased. Morphological investigations revealed that the ideally shaped cells initially found on the silicone rubbers had begun to overspread and subsequently became detached, leaving denuded spheroid areas. Moreover, cultivation for 11 days on the polyurethane surfaces resulted in an unevenness of cell distribution that even exceeded that seen on day 1. Thus, despite the fact that materials with a high surface tension (such as silicone rubbers) seem to be ideal for initial cell spreading, subsequent cultivation results in cell detachment. On materials with a lower surface tension (such as polyurethanes), the less-differentiated monolayers do at least proliferate, although their morphology remains unsatisfactory (Fig. 4).

In an further attempt to determine the "ideal" precoating procedure, most suitable for artificial heart endothelialization, we investigated three different hydrophobic silicone rubbers (Medical Adhesive Silicone Type A Silastic:; Elastosil E 43; 3145 RTV) and three different hydrophilic polyurethanes (Biomer; Enka; Pellethane).

For this experiment 9-mm glass coverslips were coated with these three silicone rubbers and three polyurethanes and all investigated materials were individually precoated with:

Group 1: 3.3 µg/ml human fibronectin (HFN) for 1 h
Group 2: fibroblast-derived extracellular matrix, by seeding murine fibroblasts (FB) L-929 onto the synthetics at a density of 1.5×10^4/cm^2 and lysing the fibroblasts with hypo-osmolaric buffer after having achieved confluence
Group 3: 3.3 µg/ml HFN (1 h), preceded by the seeding of 1.5×10^4/cm^2 L-929 FB onto the synthetic surfaces. On cultivation day 6 the monolayer was preserved with 2% glutaraldehyde; this was followed by a thorough rinsing procedure and additional incubation with 3.3 µg/ml HFN for 1 h.

After seeding of 2.5×10^4/cm^2 second-passage human umbilical vein endothelial cells, the surface morphology was investigated by SEM and TEM, and the cell kinetics was investigated using the crystal violet technique. Parallel series were examined on days 1, 5, 9, and 13.

The results of this experiment are shown in Figs. 5 and 6. Morphological analysis of the results showed for group 1, that up to day 5 endothelial cells reached confluence on both groups of materials precoated with HFN. However, a far better developed cobblestone relief was seen on silicone rubbers, the endothelial cells

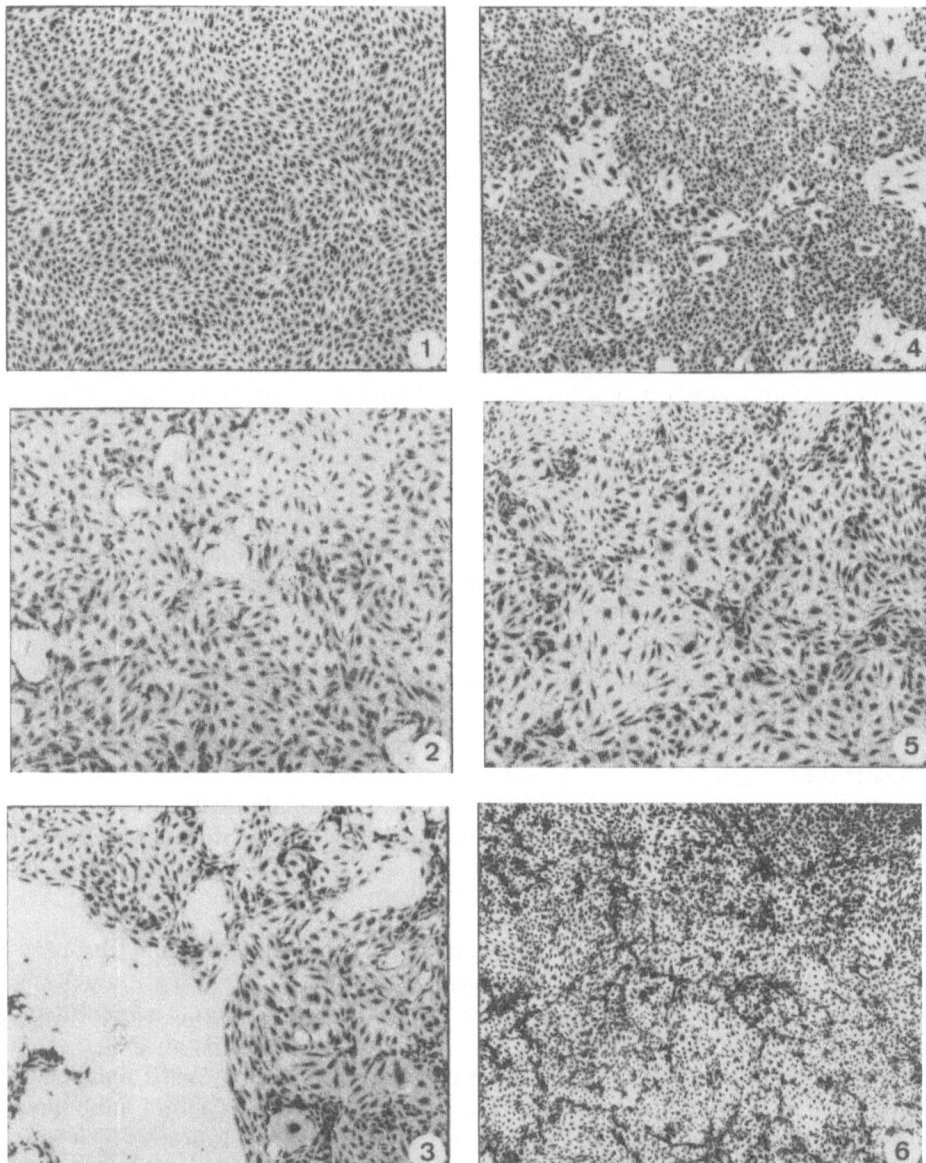

Fig. 4. Human saphenous vein endothelial cells on the silicone rubber Elastosil E43 (*1–3*) and the polyurethane Pellethane (*4–6*). On day 1 after seeding, the Elastosil E43 surface showed an ideal cell morphology (*1*), whereas the Pellethane surface showed numerous giant cells unevenly distributed throughout the monolayer (*4*). On day 5, the endothelial cells on both surfaces revealed overspreading (*2*, *5*), but typical denuded areas on the silicone rubber were already visible (*2*). On day 11, large areas of Elastosil E43 appeared denuded; the remaining cells were overspread and sometimes giant cells were seen (*3*). The cell count on the Pellethane surface had increased remarkably, but the cell distribution was uneven and patchy (*6*). (From Fasol et al. [13]) ×90

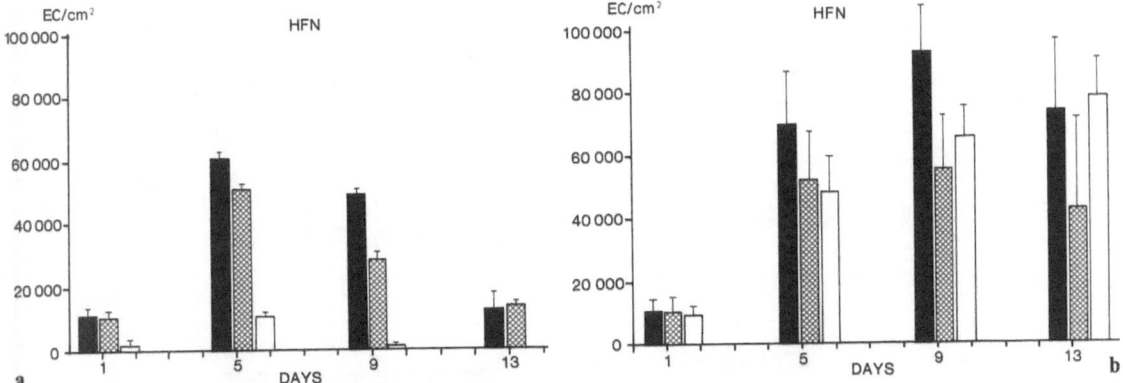

Fig. 5 a, b. Results of experiments to evaluate the "ideal" precoating procedure for endothelial cells cultivated on fibronectin-precoated silicone rubbers (**a**): ■ Medical Adhesive Silicone Type A Silastic, ▨ 3145 RTV, ☐ Elastosil E 43; and fibronectin precoated polyurethanes (**b**): ■ Biomer, ▨ Enka, ☐ Pellethane. Up to day 5, endothelial cells reached confluence on both groups of materials precoated with HFN. Between cultivation days 5 and 13, cell numbers increased on polyurethanes from 1×10^4 to $8 \times 10^4/cm^2$ (**b**), but decreased on silicone rubbers from 8×10^4 to $1 \times 10^4/cm^2$ (**a**) due to the detachment of large spheroid areas of cells

growing on polyurethanes being uneven and patchy. Between cultivation days 5 and 13, cell numbers increased on polyurethanes from 1×10^4 to $8 \times 10^4/cm^2$ (Fig. 5 b), but decreased on silicone rubbers to $1 \times 10^4/cm^2$ (Fig. 5 a) due to the detachment of large spheroid areas.

In group 2, growth behavior on fibroblast-derived extracellular matrix was similar in the polyurethane group to that of group 1 up to day 13, but no growth at all was found on silicone rubbers (Fig. 6 a, b). Prelining with glutaraldehyde-preserved fibroblasts (group 3) resulted not only in the highest cell density $(9–10 \times 10^4 EC/cm^2)$ and the best-differentiated cobblestone morphology over the whole period of investigation on all endothelialized polyurethane materials (Fig. 6 d), but also in the highest cell density $(8 \times 10^4\text{-}EC/cm^2)$ with no subsequent cell detachment on two of the three silicone rubbers (Fig. 6 c).

Summarizing the results of our experiments, we showed that endothelial cells cultivated on fibronectin-precoated nonporous materials with a high surface tension detached after a few days, although the initial morphology and proliferation capacity seemed to be promising.

The results of our subsequent studies demonstrated that glutaraldehyde-preserved and additionally fibronectin-precoated fibroblasts enabled us to cultivate well-differentiated endothelial cell monolayers on both hydrophobic and hydrophilic synthetic materials (Fig. 7 a, b).

Since the final purpose of an endothelialized artificial surface is long-term implantation into the blood stream, the possibility must be excluded that endothelial cells detach after being exposed to physiological flows after implantation.

We therefore endothelialized synthetic tubes made of the previously investigated artificial heart materials and investigated the flow- and shear-stress resistance of such endothelialized surfaces in pilot experiments. To evaluate the flow-

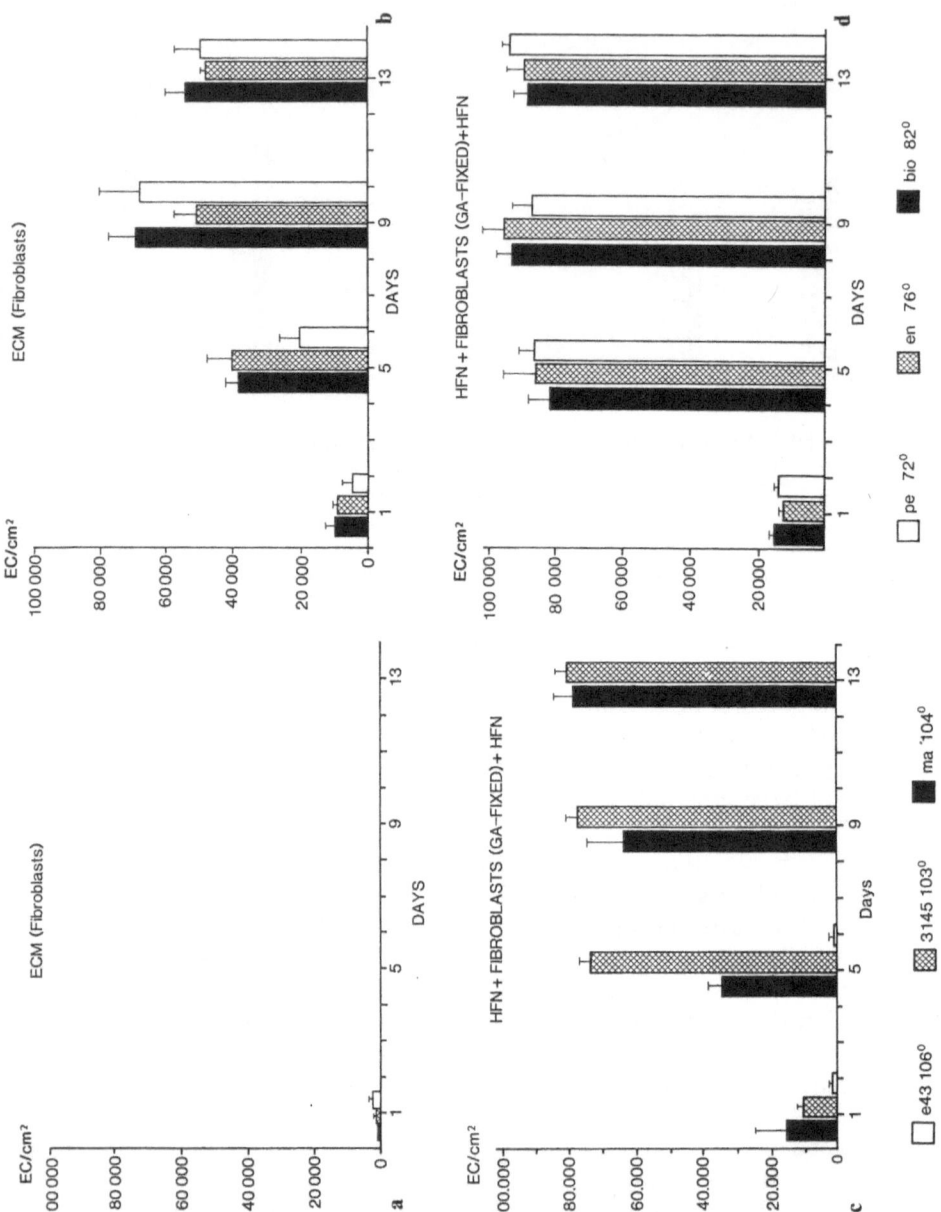

Fig. 6 a–d. Experiments to evaluate the "ideal" precoating procedure for endothelial cells cultivated on fibroblast-derived extracellular matrix (ECM)-precoated artificial heart materials: hydrophobic silicone rubbers (**a**), hydrophilic polyurethanes (**b**). Surfaces prelined with glutaraldehyde-preserved fibroblasts and additional HFN precoating: silicone rubbers (**c**), polyurethanes (**d**). Up to day 13, growth behavior on fibroblast-derived extracellular matrix was similar in the polyurethane group (**b**) to that on HFN-precoated polyurethane surfaces (Fig. 5 b), but as a striking difference, no growth at all was found on silicone rubbers (**a**). Prelining with glutaraldehyde (*GA*)-preserved fibroblasts and additional HFN precoating resulted not only in the highest cell density and the best-differentiated cobblestone morphology over the whole period of investigation on all polyurethane materials (**d**), but also in the highest cell density with no subsequent cell detachment in two of the three silicone rubbers (**c**)

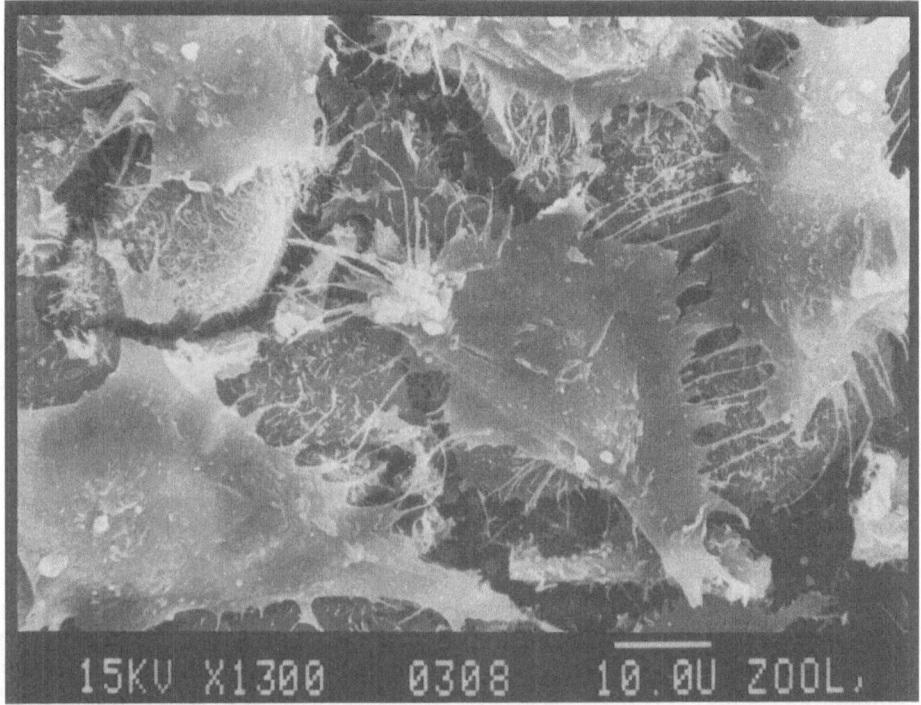

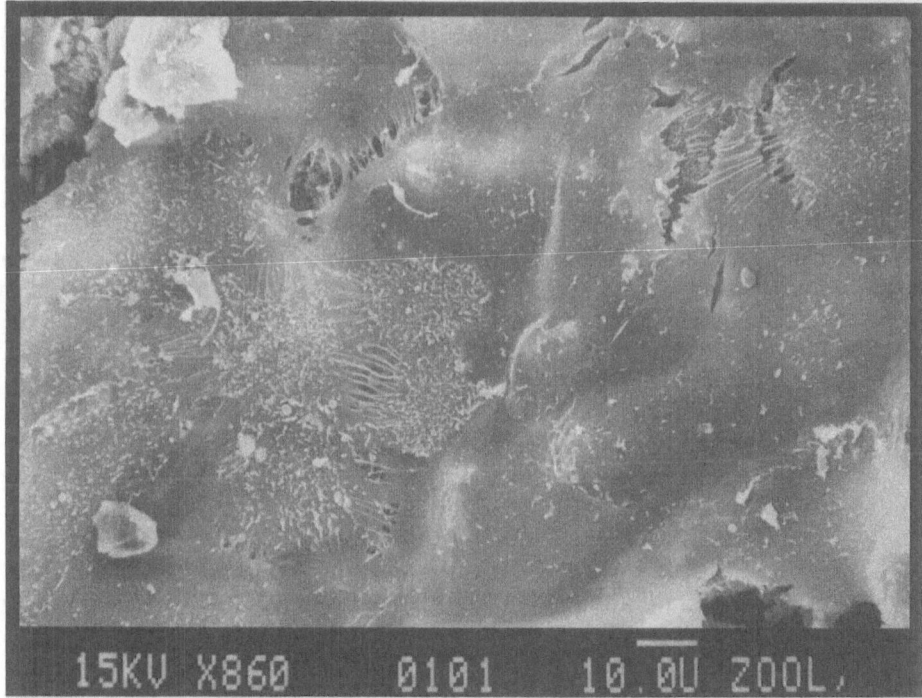

Fig. 7. a Scanning-electron micrograph showing the spreading of endothelial cells 1 day after seeding on the polyurethane Pellethane, prelined with GA-preserved fibroblasts and additional HFN precoating. × 1300. **b** Scanning-electron micrograph showing the confluent endothelial cell monolayer on the polyurethane Pellethane after 13 days of cultivation. The underlying fibroblasts are exposed in some areas due to shrinkage artifacts caused by fixation and drying. × 860

and shear-stress resistance we employed our mock circulation unit (Fig. 2a), which allowed us to simulate a physiological, pulsatile flow and shear forces similar to those of a superficial femoral artery [41] (Fig. 2b, c). This pilot experiment showed significant cell detachment in the first 2 h of shear-stress exposure. The cell count per cm^2 dropped from 120000 EC/cm^2 to 90000 EC/cm^2. In the following period the rate of cell detachment was not significant. Scanning-electron microscopy demonstrated that even after 48 h the surfaces of the investigated materials were confluently covered by an endothelial cell monolayer.

These results are quite promising compared with those of previous experiments with endothelial cell-seeded vascular grafts, where a cell detachment rate of more than 90% was found in the initial period after exposure to the bloodstream [16].

Conclusion

In order to develop an antithrombogenic surface for artificial heart prostheses, we evaluated the growth behavior of endothelial cells on various materials. Why endothelial cells? The classical view of endothelium is that of a passive, blood-compatible lining, forming a selective barrier between blood and tissue. Early studies indicated a functional role for endothelium in the control of hemostasis; Todd et al. demonstrated that living endothelial cells could lyse a fibrin clot [43]. Endothelium is now known to be an important modulator of many aspects of vascular homeostasis, including blood coagulation, blood platelet aggregation, leukocyte emigration, and vascular tone: heparin sulfate was known to exist on endothelial surfaces in 1976, and prostacyclin was also discovered [44]. In 1980 the plasminogen activator function was described [45], and in 1983 thrombin binding and inhibition [46], thromboxane A2 synthesis [47], the antithrombin-3-function [48], and the binding of clotting factor Xa [49]. In 1984 thrombospondin was discovered, as well as the protein-C function [50], thrombomodulin activity [51], the plasminogen-activator inhibitory functions [52], the platelet-activating factor [53], nexin production [49], and the binding of coagulation factors IX and IXa to endothelial cells [54].

Endothelium has been shown to possess unrealized metabolic properties that may play vital roles in the control of hemostasis and thrombosis, and – in the context of synthetic surfaces lined with endothelial cells – the ability of the resulting monolayer to function appropriately, particularly with regard to hemocompatibility, is paramount.

Based on clinical experience showing that autologous tissue is the best arterial substitute [55, 56] and that an intact endothelium is a most important element in such substitutes, the idea of lining synthetic materials with these same cells seemed attractive. But it is yet not known whether endothelial cells growing on a synthetic material continue to express their desirable "normal" function, as do endothelial cells that line the normal blood vessels in vivo. Endothelial cells growing on artificial surfaces lack the underlying basement membrane, extracellular matrix, as well as underlying smooth muscle cells. Since many of the important functions of endothelial cells take place on its abluminal surface, it has yet to be demonstrated that endothelial cells in the absence of such elements function in the normal way. It is also not known whether endothelial cells perceive the prosthetic material as an injurious or inflammatory stimulus and express undesired functions [57].

There is a growing awareness of the importance of intensive investigative efforts in an attempt to overcome the problems of the high failure rate of cardiovascular implants. Future research must therefore be directed at the many complex interactions between endothelial cells, the constituents of the blood, the prosthetic surface, the technique for harvesting and culturing endothelial cells, and the relationship between all of these elements. Nevertheless, recent advances in research and results of experiments to date provide reason for cautions optimism.

We have demonstrated that polyurethane, the standard biomaterial for artificial heart construction, can be lined with well-differentiated endothelial cell monolayers if glutaraldehyde-preserved fibroblasts are the underlying substratum. In addition, these endothelialized surfaces showed a confluent endothelial lining even after 48 h of pyhsiological shear-stress exposure.

Our experiments lead us to believe that if a shear-stress-resistant endothelial lining can be achieved under the turbulent flow conditions of an artificial heart ventricle, as well as on the moving driving membrane of an artificial heart, long-term implantation of total artificial hearts could regain its earlier attractiveness in modern cardiac surgery.

References

1. Levinson MM, Smith RG, Cork RC, Emery RW, Icenogle TB, Ott RA, Burns GL, Copeland JG (1986) Thromboembolic complications of the Jarvik-7 total artificial heart: a case report. Artif Organs 10:236
2. Mueller MM, Wohlfahrt A, Nowak H, Lee A, Trubel W, Buxbaum P, Zilla P, Fasol R (1988) Observations of human thrombocytes during TAH replacement: effects of ASA on thromboembolism risk. Artif Organs (in press)
3. Fasol R, Zilla P, Fischlein T, Deutsch M (1988) Surface morphology of circulating platelets: a suggested parameter for the monitoring of endothelial cell-seeded grafts. J Cardiovasc Surg (in press)
4. Zilla P, Groscurth P, Varga G, Fischlein T, Fasol R (1987) PGI^2 and PGE^1 induce morphological alterations in human platelets similar to those observed in the initial phase of activation. Exp Haematol 15:741
5. Trono R, Hibbs CW, Fuqua JM, Edmonds CH, Holub DA, Brewer AM, Igo SR, Norman JC (1978) Quantitative methods for testing pseudoneointima developing on textured blood-interfacing surfaces within left ventricular assist devices (LVADS). Trans Am Soc Artif Intern Organs 24:352
6. Trono R, Holub DA, McGee MG, Fuhrmann TM, Hibbs CW, Fuqua JM, Edmonds CH, Sturm JT, Bossat MI, Milan JD, Norman JC (1979) Human pseudoneointimal (PNI) accretion kinetics during abdominal left ventricular assist device (ALVAD) utilization in man: a replication sequence. Trans Am Soc Artif Intern Organs 25:311
7. Harasaki H, Kambic H, Whalen R, Murray J, Snow J, Murabayashi S, Hillegass D, Ozawa K, Kiraly R, Nose Y (1980) Comparative study of flocked versus biolized surfaces for long-term assist pumps. Trans Am Soc Artif Intern Organs 26:470

8. Mansfield PB, Wechezak AR (1968) Tissue-cultured cells as an endothlial lining of prosthetic materials. In: Norman JC (ed) Organ perfusion and preservation. Appleton-Century-
   Crofts, New York, p 189
9. Adachi M, Suzuki M, Kennedy JH (1971) Neointimas cultured in vitro for circulatory assist
   devices. I. Comparison of cultured cells derived from autologous tissues of various organs.
   J Surg Res 11:483
10. Mansfield PB, Wechezak AR, Sauvage LR (!975) Preventing thrombus on artificial vascular
    surfaces: true endothelial cell linings. Trans Am Soc Artif Intern Organs 21:264
11. Nichols WK, Gospodarowisz D, Kessler TR, Olsen DB (1981) Increased adherence of
    vascular endothelial cells to Biomer precoated with extracellular matrix. Trans Am Soc Artif
    Intern Organs 27:208
12. Fasol R, Zilla P, Groscurth P, Wolner E, Moser R (1985) Experimental in vitro cultivation
    of human endothelial cells on artificial surfaces. Trans Am Soc Artif Intern Organs 31:276
13. Fasol R, Zilla P, Deutsch M, Fischlein T, Kadletz M, Griesmacher A, Mueller MM (1987)
    Endothelialization of artificial surfaces: does surface tension determine in vitro growth of
    human saphenous vein endothelial cells? J Tex Heart Inst 14:119
14. Herring MB, Gardner AL, Glover J (1978) A single-staged technique for seeding vascular
    grafts with autologous endothelium. Surgery 84:498
15. Zilla P, Fasol R, Deutsch M, Fischlein T, Minar E, Hammerle A, Krupicka O, Kadletz M
    (1987) Endothelial cell seeding of PTFE vascular grafts in humans: a preliminary report. J
    Vasc Surg 6:535
16. Rosenman JE, Kempczinski RF, Pearce WH, Roedersheimer LR, Berlatzky Y, Ramanlan-
    jaona G (1985) Kinetics of endothelial cell seeding. J Vasc Surg 2:778
17. Jarrell BE, Williams SK, Stokes G, Hubbard FA, Carabasi RA, Koolpe E, Greener D, Pratt
    K, Moritz MJ, Radomski J, Speicher L (1986) Use of freshly isolated capillary endothelial
    cells for the immediate establishment of a monolayer on a vascular graft at surgery. Surgery
    100:392
18. Pearce WH, Rutherford RB, Whitehill TA, Rosales C, Bell CP, Patt A (1987) Successful en-
    dothelial seeding with omentally derived microvascular endothelial cells. J Vasc Surg 5:203
19. Radomski JS, Jarrell BE, Williams SK, Koolpe EA, Greener DA, Carabasi RA (1987) Initial
    adherence of human capillary endothelial cells to Dacron. J Surg Res 42:133
20. Foxall TL, Auger KR, Callow AD, Libby P (1986) Adult human endothelial cell coverage
    of small-caliber Dacron and poly-tetrafluorethylene vascular prostheses in vitro. J Surg REs
    41:158
21. Kadletz M, Moser R, Preiss P, Deutsch M, Zilla P, Fasol R (1987) In vitro lining of fibro-
    nectin-coated PTFE grafts with cryopreserved saphenous vein endothelial cells. Thorac Car-
    diovasc Surg 35:143
22. Sentissi JM, Ramberg K, O'Donnell TF, Connolly RJ, Callow AD (1986) The effect of flow
    on vascular endothelial cells grown in tissue culture on polytetrafluorethylene grafts. Surgery
    99:337
23. Zilla P, Fasol R, Kadletz M, Preiss P, Groscurth P, Schima H, Tsangaris S, Moser R, Herold
    CH, Griesmacher A, Mostbeck G, Deutsch M, Wolner E (1987) In vitro lining of PTFE
    grafts with human saphenous vein endothelial cells: physiological shear stress exposure. In:
    Zilla P, Fasol R, Deutsch M (eds) Endothelialization of vascular grafts. Karger, Basel,
    p 195
24. Anderson JS, Price TM, Hanson SR, Harker LA (1987) In vitro endothelialization of small-
    caliber vascular grafts. Surgery 101:577
25. Gottlieb AI, Spector W, Wong MKK, Lacey C (1984) In vitro reendothelialization: micro-
    filament bundle reorganization in migrating porcine endothelial cells. Arteriosclerosis 4:91
26. Schnittler HJ, Franke RP, Fuhrmann R, Petermeyer M, Jung F, Mittermayer CH,
    Drenckhahn D (1987) Influence of various substrates on the actin filament system of cul-
    tured human vascular endothelial cells exposed to fluid shear stress. In: Zilla P, Fasol R,
    Deutsch M (eds) Endothelialization of vascular grafts. Karger, Basel, p 183
27. Herring M, Dilley R, Jersild RA, Boxer L, Gardner A, Blover J (1979) Seeding arterial pros-
    theses with vascular endothelium. The nature of lining. Ann Surg 190:84
28. Ryan US, Mortara M, Whitacer C (1980) Methods for microcarrier culture of bovine pul-
    monary artery endothelial cells avoiding the use of enzymes. Tissue Cell 12:619

29. Watkins MT, Sharefkin JB, Zajtchuk R, Maciag TM, D'More PA, Ryan UAS, van Wart H, Rich NM (1984) Adult human saphenous vein endothelial cells. Assessment of their reproductive capacity for use in endothelial cell seeding of vascular prostheses. J Surg Res 36:588

30. Sharefkin JB, Fairchild KD, Albus RA, Cruess DF, Rich NM (1986) The cytotoxic effects of surgical glove powder particles on adult human vascular endothelial cell cultures: implications for clinical use of tissue-culture techniques. J Surg Res 41:463

31. LoGefro FW, Haudenschild C, Quist WC (1984) A clinical technique for prevention of spasm and preservation of endothelium in saphenous vein grafts. Arch Surg 119:1212

32. Harring MB, Gardner A, Glover J (1984) Seeding human arterial prostheses with mechanically derived endothelium: the detrimental effect of smoking. J Vasc Surg 1:279

33. Reinders JH, Brinkman HJM, van Mourik JA, de Groot PH (1986) Cigarette smoke impairs endothelial cell prostacyclin production. Arteriosclerosis 6:15

34. Pittilio RM, Mackie IJ, Rowles PM, Machin SJ, Woolf N (1982) Effects of cigarette smoking on the ultra-structure of rat thoracic aorta and its ability to produce prostacyclin. Thromb Haemost 48:173

35. Asmussen I, Kjelsen K (1975) Intima ultrastructure of human umbilical arteries: observations of arteries from newborn children of smoking and non-smoking mothers. Circ Res 36:579

36. Kessler KA, Herring MB, Arnold MP, Glover JL, Hee-Myung P, Helmus MN, Bendick PJ (1986) Enhanced strength of endothelial attachment on polyester elastomer and polytetrafluorethylene graft surfaces with fibronectin substrate. J Vasc Surg 3:58

37. Williams SK, Jarrell BE, Friend L, Radomski JS, Carabasi A, Koolpe E, Mueller S, Thornton SC, Marinucci T, Levine E (1985) Adult human endothelial cell compatibility with prosthetic graft material. J Surg Res 38:618

38. Fasol R, Zilla P, Deutsch M, Fischlein T, Minar E, Hammerle A, Wolner E (1987) Endothelial cell seeding: experience and first clinical results. In: Zilla P, Fasol R, Deutsch M (eds) Endothelialization of vascular grafts. Karger, Basel, p 233

39. Klebe RJ, Bentley KL, Schoen RC (1981) Adhesive substrates for fibronectin. J Cell Physiol 109:481

40. Hope W, Martin TJ, Chesterman CN, Morgan FJ (1979) Nature 282:210

41. Schima H, Tsangaris S, Zilla P, Fasol R, Kadletz M (1987) Simulation of pulsatile wall shear stress in peripheral arteries by means of a mock circulation. In: Zilla P, Fasol R, Deutsch M (eds) Endothelialization of vascular grafts. Karger, Basel, p 189

42. Jaffe EA (1980) Culture of human endothelial cells. Transplant Proc 12 [Suppl] 1:49

43. Todd AG (1959) The historical localisation of fibrinogen activator. J Pathol Bacteriol 78:281

44. Moncada S, Gryglewski R, Bunting S, Vane JR (1976) An enzyme isolated from arteries transforms prostaglandin endoperoxides to an unstable substance that inhibits platelet aggregation. Nature 263:663

45. Laug WE (1980) Secretion of different plasminogen activators and anchorage-independent growth of bovine endothelial cells. Biol Vasc Endothelial Cell, Cold Spring Harbor, NY, p 21

46. Dryjski M, Olsson P, Swedenborg J (1983) The vascular endothelium as an inhibitor of thrombin. Thromb Res 5:67

47. Eldor A, Vlodavsky I, Hy-Am E, Atzmon R, Weksler B et al. (1983) Cultured endothelial cells increase their capacity to synthesize prostacyclin following the formation of a contact-inhibited cell monolayer. J Cell Physiol 114:179

48. Bauer P, Machovich R, Aranyi P, Buki K, Csonka E, Horvath I (1983) Mechanism of thrombin binding to endothelial cells. Blood 61:368

49. Jaffe EA (1985) Physiologic functions of normal endothelial cells. Ann NY Acad Sci 454:279

50. Boffa MC, Bourin MC, Dmoszyska A, Machovich R (1984) Bovine protein C cofactor actively separated from other thrombomodulin effects. Circulation 70(II):53

51. Johnson AE, Esmon NL, Esmon CT (1984) The active site of thrombin is altered by association with thrombomodulin. Circulation 70(II):61

52. van Hinsberg V, Bertina R, van Wijngaarden A, Elmeis J (1984) Production of plasminogen activator by cultured human endothelial cells: effect of activated protein C. 3rd Int Symp Biology Vasc Endothelial Cell. MIT, Cambridge, p 1
53. Prescott SM, Zimmermann GA, McIntyre TM (1984) Human endothelial cells in culture produce a platelet-activating factor when stimulated with thrombin. Proc Natl Acad Sci USA 81:3534
54. Nawroth PP, Stern DM (1985) A pathway of coagulation on endothelial cells. J Cell Biochem 28:253
55. Szilagyi DE, McDonald RT, SMith RF et al. (1957) Biologic fate of human arterial homografts. Arch Surg 75:506
56. Wylie EM (1965) Vascular replacement with arterial autografts. Surgery 57:14
57. Libby P, Birinyi LK (1987) The dynamic nature of vascular endothelial functions. In: Zilla P, Fasol R, Deutsch M (eds) Endothelialization of vascular grafts. Karger, Basel, p 80

Part VII
Horizons

50. Horizons –
How Has Assisted Circulation Developed
and Where Is It Headed?

F. UNGER

Beginning with the first volume, distinguished experts in the field have commented on the present status of assisted circulation, where it stands and where it is going. In 1979, ten experts gave their opinions. Dr. Bücherl, from Berlin, stated that, in view of the great number of cardiac patients and the shortage of donors, the development of an artificial heart was desired, for temporary use. Dr. Cooley, from Houston, who performed the first bridge in 1969, said that at many cardiac centers countless opportunities for gaining much-needed human experience were being wasted while philosophers and critics pondered the social implications. Dr. De Bakey, also from Houston, who performed the first clinical LVAD operation in 1962, felt that a temporary application could be expedient.

Dr. Frommer, of Washington, D.C., had a very critical outlook, but he felt that the first clinical trials were justified by the fact that the prognosis for patients with a 95%–100% chance of mortality could improve significantly within 48 h.

Dr. Moulopoulos, from Athens, who designed the first IABP, was sure that it would have temporary application. Dr. Nosé, from Cleveland, was convinced that a safe implantable total artificial heart would be available by 1985. Dr. Polzer, from Vienna, felt that the temporary application of LVADs would produce clinical results that led to development of a TAH. Dr. Senning, from Zurich, was of the opinion that mechanical circulatory assistance belonged to the future. Dr. Watson, from Washington, D.C., was convinced that the first clinical trials would be the basis of future development.

In 1984, in the second volume, Dr. Björk, from Stockholm, stated that he could imagine temporary support, but he was very skeptical about permanent implantation. Dr. Cortesini, from Rome, was optimistic that the TAH would be available in the near future. Dr. Frommer from Washington, D.C., stated that research must be continued in a manner that justified public confidence in both the direction and the methods. Dr. Nosé now predicted that a permanently implantable artificial heart would be ready by 1990. In 1988, however, at the ESAO meeting in Prague, he stated that the totally implantable artificial heart was unrealistic, but that the permanent LVAD was a reasonable target. Dr. Pierce from Hershey, Pennsylvania, gave a very critical analysis and found that real progress takes place in small steps.

Dr. Polzer, who died in 1985, was very excited about the first clinical attempts and found that the measurable progress justified continuous support for research. Dr. Watson, from Washington, D.C., was convinced that the late 1980s would see permanent replacement in selected patients.

Assisted Circulation 3
F. Unger (Ed.)
© Springer-Verlag Berlin Heidelberg 1989

In this third volume we have the statements of six most distinguished experts. Dr. Björk foresees a permanent TAH in the not too distant future. Dr. Cortesini hopes that mechanical devices will soon replace the pneumatically driven devices, and thinks that in 3 years the first clinical applications could be made in selected cases. Drs. Emoto, Fujimoto, and Nosé, from Cleveland, expect to see an increasing number of pneumatically activated devices for temporary use. Drs. Morea and De Paulis, from Turin, think that the energy source and driving and control systems can be improved, while the biomaterials remain the greatest challenge. Dr. Pierce, from Hershey, imagines that in 1990 electrical assist pumps will be in clinical use. Finally, Dr. Watson, from Washington, D.C., feels that, in view of the great progress that has been made, it is necessary to initiate the clinical evaluation of electrically powered implantable ventricular assist devices.

It is fascinating to watch how the exciting field of assisted circulation evolves. I have been personally involved in this area of research since 1972. Anticipation was especially high in 1975, after the first clinical attempts in Houston made by Norman. I recall the first European implantation in 1977, by Navratil in Vienna, where the E-LVAD was implanted postoperatively in a cardiac patient. The patient was weaned off and the pump explanted. We felt that a real breakthrough with this method could be expected soon. Feelings were the same in 1986, with my first clinical bridge in Europe using the Ellipsoid heart. There has certainly been some amount of frustration; measured against the progress with the IABP, the clinical establishment of TAH and assist devices was expected earlier. This reflects on the industry, which has taken a wait-and-see attitude.

The clinical results for the 513 patients overall, with a survival rate of 25%, should be evaluated critically. Most of the patients had a survival prognosis of only 0%–5%, and so the results should serve as a stimulus for new investigations. The basic feasibility of temporary devices has been clearly demonstrated. It is now necessary to better identify the patients who are candidates, especially for bridging, and the devices themselves must be refined, particularly in terms of pump design.

The totally implantable artificial heart will certainly be realized in the distant future, but clinical investigations must continue, in a manner worthy of public confidence and support.

51. The Total Artificial Heart 1987

V. O. Björk

It has now been proven that the total artificial heart saves lives and is reliable for a short period of time (some weeks or months) in patients with acute irreversible rejection or severe myocarditis, and in those with end-stage cardiac failure when more time is needed to find an optimal donor heart.

Prolonged use of the presently available total artificial hearts seems to involve an unphysiological and fixed high cardiac output and to cause problems in handling the balance between anticoagulation and bleeding and later infection via the drive tubes. The quality of life, once complications have begun, is not acceptable.

However, considering the results already achieved, and in view of the intensive ongoing research to improve the surfaces and thereby anticoagulation-related bleeding, to improve the physiological regulation of cardiac output, and to place the electrical driving power source under the skin, significant improvements of function, leading toward much longer-term use, can be expected in the not-too-distant future.

Assisted Circulation 3
F. Unger (Ed.)
© Springer-Verlag Berlin Heidelberg 1989

52. Horizons in Heart Substitution

R. Cortesini and P. Berloco

Cardiac transplantation is an established therapeutic modality for selected patients with end-stage heart disease. Approximately 25 000 patients could benefit from heart transplantation each year, while only about 1500 acceptable heart donors could be procured from the present donor pool. Better education of the medical communities and increasing public information could enlarge the current pool of donors. The death of a patient who is waiting for a heart donor is a repetitively frustrating experience and emphasizes the need for developing a cardiac support or replacement pump. In fact, the development of temporary or permanent mechanical cardiac support devices for adults and xenotransplantation for pediatric patients represent the future alternatives for cardiac replacement in patients with end-stage heart disease [1].

During the past decade, advances have been made in the clinical application of cardiac transplantation. Survival rates have improved dramatically. Proper selection criteria, improved treatment of infections, cardiac biopsy, and the use of cyclosporin have contributed to current survival rates (80%–85% 1-year survival). Improvement in immunosuppressive techniques and monitoring for rejection may lead to even better statistics [2]. At the present time, the indications for heart transplantation are not clear in all cases, but survival and quality of life after transplantation are well documented [3].

Potential candidates for transplantation are all patients with end-stage heart disease and limited life expectancy for whom no other form of therapy is available. Contraindications to heart transplantation have evolved as the immunosuppressive protocols have changed [4]. It is clear that heart transplantation has developed from an experimental procedure with minimally acceptable results to a true therapeutic option. With the technique firmly established and immunosuppression relatively standardized, heart transplantation centers are expanding almost exponentially. In 1982 and 1986 respectively, 103 and over 1400 heart transplants were performed, attesting to the growing acceptance of heart transplantation as an effective therapeutic modality. We believe that every available heart donor should be utilized to allow end-stage cardiac patients the chance of life [5]. Research should continue in an effort to prolong the period that an allograft may be safely preserved outside the body, so that some of the current logistic problems can be alleviated and the availability and utilization of heart donors increased. Meanwhile, xenografts may provide one approach to resolving organ-procurement problems for clinical transplantation, and the monoventricular or biventricular assist devices, placed intra- or extracorporeally and providing an ad-

Assisted Circulation 3
F. Unger (Ed.)
© Springer-Verlag Berlin Heidelberg 1989

equate blood flow, are the best way to support the life of a dying patient until a heart transplantation can be performed [6, 7].

At present, some questions need to be addressed formally: Which of the available support devices should be used? What indications are reasonable for implantation or transplantation? Among the techniques used, only one method of temporary left ventricular assistance – intra-aortic balloon pumping – has gained wide clinical acceptance [8]. About 50 000 patients a year are now treated by intra-aortic balloon pumping. Although this technique is still used to treat patients in cardiogenic shock, the main indications for its use are inability to discontinue cardiopulmonary bypass after open-heart surgery and unstable angina. Pneumatically powered assist pumps are now in clinical trials in patients with profound that reversible heart failure after open-heart surgery or in patients with cardiogenic shock. As with other forms of therapy, these devices have specific indications. The appropriate pump for a particular patient is the simplest unit that will provide the circulatory support required. The temporary (severed days to a week) ventricular assist pump is the only unit that has been shown to be lifesaving in clinical application: survival rates as high as 50% in a heretofore lethal condition have been encouraging [9, 10]. Excluding total heart replacement, permanently implanted left ventricular assist devices (LVAD) have fared less well. The wonder, however, is not that progress has been slow, but that a remarkable number of difficult problems have been solved. The need for a permanent LVAD for irreversible failure is obvious. After two decades of support by the National Heart, Lung and Blood Institute devices branch, a cluster of totally implantable left ventricular assist systems are now being readied for clinical trial. Today, the major application for these devices is likely to be as a bridge to cardiac transplantation [11].

In the initial group of five patients who received permanent artificial hearts between 1982 and 1985 the average survival was approximately 9 months; all were very complex medical cases requiring an extraordinary amount of follow-up care and chronic hospitalization. Only one patient was rehabilitated to sufficient strength to experience a modest degree of mobility using the portable artificial heart drive system and to leave the hospital frequently. Experience with permanent clinical application of the TAH has shown that long-term life support is possible. These patients experienced many medical complications, related in part to their pre-existing disease, in part to the lack of experience with management while on the artificial heart, and in part to some inherent features of the devices themselves. Significant improvements in the quality of life of permanent TAH patients are expected through better medical management based on the experience to date, including the experience with many "bridge-to-transplant patients." From January 1985 to March 1987, 61 patients were treated with the TAH as a bridge to transplantation (51 with the Jarvik-7) and 49 patients have undergone successful transplantation [12, 13]. This has been possible in part through improvements in the TAH and drive system and in part due to a better understanding of the postoperative care of TAH patients. During the usual period of 1–2 weeks on the artificial heart the condition of most of the patients improved dramatically, including correction of pulmonary edema, marked improvement in lung function, reversal of renal insufficiency, diuresis with resolution of peripheral edema, and improvement of nutritional status. Several surgeons have noted that patients whose condition is dramatically improved by the artificial heart prior to transplantation may be better candidates for a transplant and may do better for that reason.

The utilization of the TAH as a temporary support prior to cardiac transplantation is growing rapidly and, although this application is in its early phases, it is clear that a high percentage of patients can be saved [7]. At present, it appears that interim placement of the TAH provides three primary therapeutic advantages. First, the TAH reproduces normal circulatory hemodynamics and thus preserves life in patients with inadequate cardiac output and perfusion when medical therapy has failed. Second, a period of stable physiologic support on the TAH allows organ dysfunction caused by end-stage heart failure to resolve. This improves the likelihood of successful transplantation when a suitable donor is finally located. Third, patients who may have reversible acute organ failure such as hepatic or renal insufficiency, and thus are not candidates for primary transplantation, can improve markedly following removal of the diseased heart and TAH support of the circulation.

In the near future the pneumatically assisted devices will be replaced by electromechanically driven units that are more reliable and flexible. Regarding the permanent and totally implantable artificial heart, we believe that this will be an electromechanical device powered by an external battery with the energy transferred across the skin by electromagnetic induction. An implanted intracorporeal battery will make the patient autonomous, thus giving him or her a reasonable quality of life.

These devices are now in experimental testing, and many improvements will be made in the present models. We believe that in the next 3 years many problems will be solved, allowing clinical application in selected cases.

References

1. Sadeghi AM, Robbins RC, Smith CR, Kurlansky RA, Michler RE, Rechntsma F, Rose EA (1987) Cardiac xenograft survival in baboon treated with cyclosporin in combination with conventional immunosuppression. Transplant Proc 19(1):1149
2. Solis E, Kaye MP (1986) The registry of the International Society for Heart Transplantation: third official report – June 1986. J Heart Transplant 5:2
3. Pennock JK, Oyer PE, Reitz BA, Jamieson SW, Bieber CP, Wallwork J, Stinson EB, Shumway NE (1982) Cardiac transplantation in perspective for the future: survival, complications, rehabilitation and cost. J Thorac Cardiovasc Surg 83:168
4. Copeland JG, Emery RW, Levinson MM, Cenogle TB, Cavrier M, Ott RA, Copeland JA, Nicholson SM (1987) Transplantation of the heart: selection of patients for cardiac transplantation. Circulation 75(I):2–9
5. Evans RW, Manninen DL, Garrison LP Jr, Mainer AM (1986) Donor availability as the primary determinant of the future of heart transplantation. JAMA 255:1892
6. Cortesini R, Cucchiara G (1979) Total artificial heart replacement with consecutive heart transplantation. In: Unger F (ed) Assisted circulation 1. Springer, Berlin Heidelberg New York, p 388
7. Jojce LD, Johnson KE, Pierce RNW, De Vries WC, Semb BKH, Copeland JG, Griffith BP, Cooley DA, Frazier OH, Cabrol C, Keon WJ, Unger F, Bucherl ES, Wolner E (1986) Summary of the world experience with clinical use of total artificial hearts as heart support devices. J Heart Transplant 5:229–235
8. Kantrowitz A (1987) Introduction of left ventricular assistance. Trans Am Soc Artif Intern Organs 33:39–48

9. Kolff J, Deeb GM (1985) Artificial heart and left ventricular assist devices. Symposium on the latest advances in cardiac surgery. Surg Clin North Am 65:3
10. Pae WE (1987) Temporary ventricular support: current indications and results. Trans Am Soc Artif Intern Organs 33:4
11. Griffith BP, Hardesty RL, Kormos RL, Trento A, Borovetz HS, Thompson ME, Bahnson HT (1987) Temporary use of the Jarvik-7 total artificial heart before transplantation. N Engl J Med 316:130
12. Pierce WS, Pae WE (1987) Clinical registry of mechanical ventricular assist pumps and artificial hearts. Hershey Medical Center Combined Registry of ASAIO, Hershey, Penn
13. Olsen DB, Riebman JB, De Paulis R, Durrant G, Nielsen SD (1987) Registry and tabulations of orthotopic total artificial heart in man. Trans Am Soc Artif Intern Organs (in press)

53. Horizons in Assisted Circulation

H. Emoto, L. K. Fujimoto, and Y. Nosé

Research on the artificial heart was initiated about 30 years ago, many types of circulatory assist devices intended for different clinical applications have been developed and introduced. Although enthusiastically pursued by many investigators, the ultimate goal, a totally implantable permanent artificial heart, still requires many years of research. This mechanical system has a great potential not only to extend the life expectancy of the patient but also to provide an acceptable quality of life. When compared with heart transplantation it presents several advantage in terms of off-the-shelf availability and application for a large number of end-stage heart disease patients.

Somewhat less complex than the ultimate total artificial heart are the totally implantable ventricular assist systems intended for end-stage chronic ventricular failure patients. These permanent assist systems are currently at the level of device readiness testing; first clinical trials are expected within the next few years.

Figure 1 shows a permanent electric left ventricular assist system (E3C LVAS) developed by Nimbus Inc. and the Cleveland Clinic Foundation. The titanium blood pump and the variable-volume device (VVD) are implanted in the left chest cavity, the energy converter in a resected rib space, and the internal battery and the secondary transformer of the transcutaneous energy transmission system in the subcutaneous tissue. Uniquely, the entire internal surface of the blood pump is coated with cross-linked gelatin to result in a seamless, smooth hydrophilic surface. Gelatin is composed of denatured collagen molecules and large volumes of water. After contacting blood, this water is gradually replaced by the recipient's plasma proteins. Therefore, this type of gel surface contributes to the excellent blood compatibility associated with biolized surfaces [1]. Biolized surfaces, in conjunction with the use of bioprosthetic valves, have eliminated the need for anticoagulant drugs in blood pump recipients. The diaphragm is easily formed by a compression-mold technique from polyolefin rubber (Hexsyn), a material with an outstanding flex live.

The VVD consists of a center layer of butyl rubber covered with polyester velour fabric. The highly impermeable rubber minimizes the problem of gas diffusion and the texturized surface in contact with the lung assures minimal tissue encapsulation. The electrohydraulic energy converter consists of a high-speed, continuously running motor driving a hydraulic gear pump. The motor speed varies according to the heart rate, thus assuring minimal energy demand and optimal synchronization with the natural heart. The performance features of the energy converter integrated with the biolized blood pump and the VVD were demonstrated during animal tests for periods of up to 196 days [2].

Assisted Circulation 3
F. Unger (Ed.)
© Springer-Verlag Berlin Heidelberg 1989

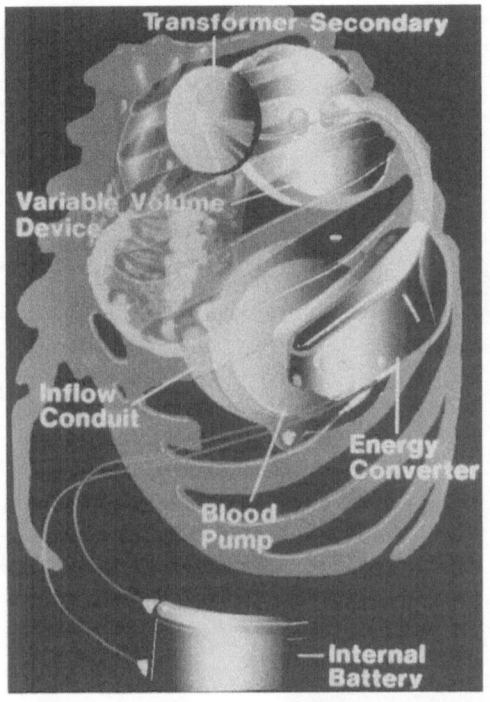

Fig. 1. Nimbus, Inc./Cleveland Clinic Foundation E3C electrohydraulic ventricular assist system

Modern technology has been adapted and data accumulated over the last several years on totally implantable electrically driven ventricular assist systems intended for chronic use. It is conceivable that a completely implantable system for total heart replacement (CITAH) with high reliability, optimal physiological performance, acceptable biocompatibility, minimal noise or vibration, and optimal anatomical compatibility for a large number of patients will be available for the first clinical trials before the end of this century. Figure 2 shows the anatomical placement of an electrohydraulic CITAH designed by the Cleveland Clinic Foundation and Nimbus, Inc., based on the technology gained in the development of the E3C system. Except for small design changes to the energy converter to physiologically match the output of the right and left pump and changes in the external configuration of the blood pump/energy converter unit to match anatomical constraints, the overall design concept of the complete system, including materials, is the same as that of the LVAS.

The ideal system in terms of prolonged tether-free operation would use implantable radioisotopes as a power source. Currently, the use of such a power source is not considered sociologically practical. In the United States this concept was abandoned in 1973. The thermal systems now under development are considered the most promising tether-free systems [3, 4]. Different from the electric systems, whose internal battery provides only 30–40 min of complete tether-free operation, the thermal systems store thermal energy within the body in a molten salt storage unit sufficient to power the assist system for 8–10 h, thus providing more freedom and consequently an enhanced quality of life for the recipient (Fig. 3).

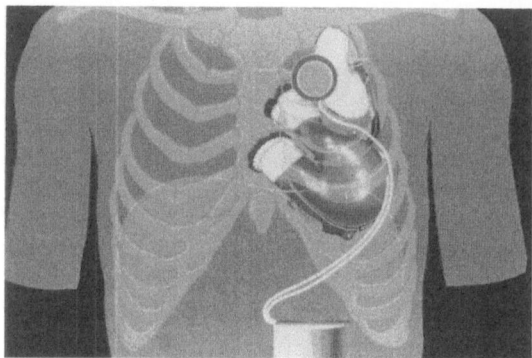

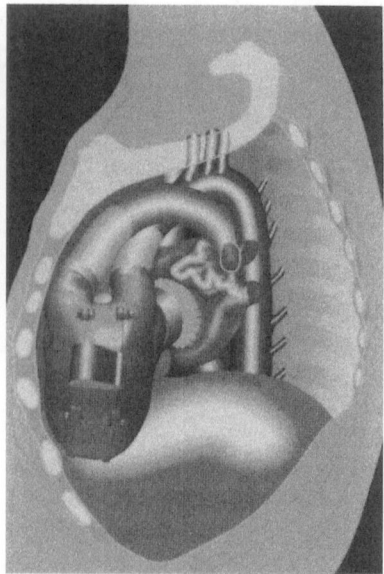

Fig. 2. Nimbus, Inc./Cleveland Clinic completely implantable system for a total heart replacement (CITAH)

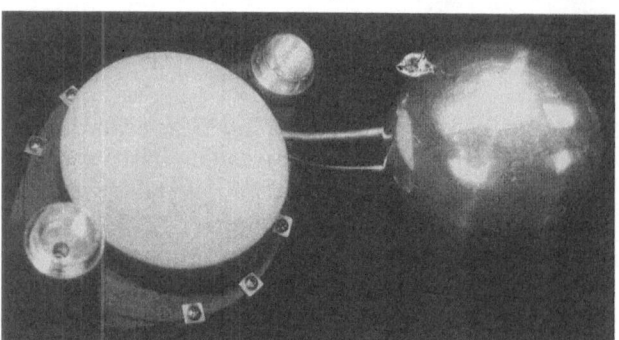

Fig. 3. Electrothermohydraulic ventricular assist system under development by the University of Washington, Cleveland Clinic, and Whalen Biomedical Inc. The thermal storage module is shown on the right

The left ventricular assist thermopneumatic and thermohydraulic systems are currently in the developmental stage. Within a few years the preclinical testing of these systems is expected to begin.

Centrifugal pumps have received increasing attention from many investigators during the past few years. Conceptually different from the conventional pulsatile device, the centrifugal pump generates nonpulsatile flow and offers many desirable features for long-term implantability, such as its reduced size and the absence of valves or the VVD. However, continued research and development are still necessary for the centrifugal pump to become a reliable implantable device for long-term circulatory support. One of the major areas of investigation is related to the problem of blood deposition at the shaft-seal interface of these devices. The issue of pulsatile or nonpulsatile flow is still debatable. Experimental data demonstrate that the organism can adapt to nonpulsatile flow, provided that adequate pump output is maintained [5].

Finally, for the next several years the clinical use of pneumatic-actuated devices for temporary use, either as ventricular assist devices or total artificial hearts, is expected to increase. Their usefulness as a bridge to heart transplantation has been demonstrated at many centers, and important information has been gained from these clinical trials. The continuous tether to an external drive system and the risk of thromboembolism and infection at the skin entrance points of the driving tube constitute major restrictions for long-term application. However, the shortage of donor hearts, in addition to the progressive accumulation of clinical experience with better patient management, optimization of the devices, and confidence, may result in more and more patients remaining as chronic recipients. This may be inevitable for the next few years at least, until implantable systems become a more attractive alternative to heart transplantation.

References

1. Emoto H, Murabayashi S, Kambic HE, Zimmerman M, Goldcamp J, Horiuchi T, Harasaki H, Nosé Y (1987) Plasma protein and gelatin surface interactions: kinetics of protein adsorption. Trans Am Soc Artif Intern Organs 33:606
2. Moise J, Butler K, Payne J, Wampler R, Smith W, Fujimoto L, Kiraly R, Harasaki H, Nosé Y (1985) Experimental evaluation of complete electrically powered ventricular assist system. Trans Am Soc Artif Intern Organs 31:202
3. Sugita Y, Navarro RR, White M, Whalen R, Kiraly R, Harasaki H, Nosé Y (1986) In vivo evaluation of a permanently implantable thermal ventricular assist system. Trans Am Soc Artif Intern Organs 32:242
4. Blubaugh AL, Butler KC, Schneider JA, Moise JC, Fujimoto LK, Kiraly RJ, Smith WA, Nosé Y (1984) Thermally and electrically powered left ventricular assist. In: Progress in artificial organs – 1983. ISAO Press, Cleveland, p 91
5. Yada I, Golding LR, Harasaki H, Jacobs G, Koike S, Yozu R, Sato N, Fujimoto LK, Snow J, Olsen E, Murabayashi S, Venkatesen VS, Kiraly R, Nosé Y (1983) Physiopathological studies of nonpulsatile blood flow in chronic models. Trans Am Soc Artif Intern Organs 29:392

54. The Future of the Artificial Heart

M. Morea and R. De Paulis

The Italian language has two words to identify future events: "predizione" and "previsione". Their meanings are very different; the former means "guess," the latter "forecast," i.e., based on the available information about uncertain events. To forecast without having information is therefore close to guessing. In the particular case of the total artificial heart (TAH) and, to some extent, of the ventricular assist device (VAD), it is important to determine the probability of outcomes. This is achieved through personal experience, and allows one to weigh the utility (payoff). Forecasting then becomes a decision-making tool for future choices.

The reliability of the TAH and the VAD is determined by the their efficiency, durability, and lack of complications. Nowadays, we think it is difficult to forecast the future of the TAH as a permanent substitute for traditional cardiac surgery or the heart transplant. On the other hand, we can forecast the reliability of the TAH and VAD *components*: the drive system, the control system, the biocompatibility, etc. In this short comment, based on our daily experience with prosthetic valves, we will therefore dwell only briefly upon the expected reliability of artificial heart valves.

Based upon more than 20 years of clinical experience, the reliability of mechanical and biological valve prostheses is correlated to their failure rate. The failure rate depends on the type of valve, its position, and the duration of implantation, and its derivative (i.e., hazard function) may be constant or not constant: decreasing, increasing, J-shaped. Most of the complications are directly related to the prosthesis: disk fracture, thrombosis, aging process, calcification; some are caused indirectly by the prosthesis itself: thromboembolism, hemorrhage, infection. Embolism, thrombosis, and hemorrhage are typical for any kind of prosthesis. However, they cannot be considered solely related to the prosthesis but are also related to the patient's pathophysiological status: atrial thrombosis, systemic infection, incorrect anticoagulation regimen. The hazard function of these complications is constant over time and, in the particular case of hemorrhage, as long as the anticoagulation therapy is continued.

What is the incidence of these complications after valvular surgery and how might we extrapolate these complications to the use of the TAH or VAD? We are aware of a rate varying from 0% for the incidence of thrombosis of a bioprosthetic aortic valve to 5.25% patient/year for all the negative events related to the mechanical valve in the mitral position [1] (see Table 1).

An incidence of 5.25%/patient/year means a probability that 50% of the patients will develop a major complication over a 10-year follow-up period. Ten years is the minimum survival that can be offered to a patient undergoing valve

Assisted Circulation 3
F. Unger (Ed.)
© Springer-Verlag Berlin Heidelberg 1989

Table 1. Major complications of prosthetic heart valves

Valve type	Aortic		Mitral		Mitro-aortic	
	Nonfatal	All	Nonfatal	All	Nonfatal	All
Mechanical		(y=)		(y=)		(y=)
Embolism	1.66		2.35		2.27	
Thrombosis	0.12		0.38		0.2	
Hemorrhage	1.7		1.84		1.0	
		3.6		5.25		4.15
Biological						
Embolism	1.07		1.51		1.98	
Thrombosis	0		0.03		0.06	
Hemorrhage	0.21		0.62		0.65	
		1.4		2.5		3.12

y, Mean incidence of all fatal and nonfatal events (embolism, thrombosis, hemorrhage)/ 100 patients/year.

replacement but, as in the case of mitral valve replacement with a mechanical prosthesis, with the probability that one patient in two will develop a major complication.

When we transfer these data to the TAH, even without considering problems related to the pumping chamber, we have to deal with the presence of four prosthetic valves and an obvious increase in the above-mentioned incidence of complications. In effect, as reported by others [2, 3], patients with three prosthetic valves had a higher incidence of systemic thromboembolism than did those with two left-sided prostheses. Therefore, in order to decrease the incidence of thromboembolism we should use four bioprostheses. However, since their durability is not longer than 10 years, the possibility of replacing them without replacing the artificial heart is desirable or, as an alternative, we should consider a valveless device. Finally, although remarkable progress in biocompatibility has been made in the past year with the use of smooth polyurethane, it is still our belief that biologically derived tissue should be used to cover the inside of the blood chamber. In this way, problems related to anticoagulation therapy will also be avoided.

In conclusion, we think that problems related to the energy source and to transmission, driving, and control systems can be solved in the coming years, while biocompatibility will remain the greatest challenge, along with the threatening incidence of infection in the presence of large areas of foreign material.

References

1. Edmunds LH (1987) Thrombotic and bleeding complications of prosthetic heart valves. Ann Thorac Surg 44:430
2. Gersh BJ, Schaff HV, Vatterott PJ (1985) Results of triple valve replacement in 91 patients: perioperative mortality and long-term follow-up. Circulation 72:130
3. Macmanus Q, Grunkemeier G, Starr A (1978) Late results of triple valve replacement. J Thorac Cardiovasc Surg 74:20

55. Horizons in Assisted Circulation

W. S. Pierce

A decade ago, artificial heart development and cardiac transplantation were viewed as competing forms of therapy. We now recognize the complementary nature of these two areas. Also recognized is the scarcity of donor hearts, indicating a need for a mechanical counterpart.

As a variety of assist devices and artificial hearts are put into clinical use, the benefits, problem areas for improvement, and future potential become apparent.

Assist Pump Use Following Cardiac Operations

Only within the past decade has there been realization of the potential for the damaged heart to regain functional capacity in a time frame measured in days. Fortunately, we now have techniques to sustain the patient during this time while the healing process takes place, using paracorporeal assist pumping. This form of therapy applied to the patient with post-cardiotomy cardiogenic shock results in a 30%–40% survival rate. Clinical studies to date suggest the importance of applying assist pumping only with appropriate indications, limiting the time of cardiopulmonary bypass, and employing biventricular support in a larger percentage of patients than had earlier been predicted. Accordingly, results will improve, just as the early results associated with intra-aortic balloon use have improved. The development of techniques to apply ventricular assist pumping without requiring surgery stimulate our thought processes, but an effective, practical system remains elusive.

Bridge to Transplantation

Spectacular results have been achieved in supporting the circulation in cardiac transplant candidates with profound circulatory failure using paracorporeal assist pumps and artificial hearts. In the past, such patients died because no donor heart was available. Now a survival rate of 62% has been achieved (in 219 patients) where transplantation followed mechanical pump use. Not clear, however, is the optimal technique for support. The patient with isolated left ventricular failure, from either cardiomyopathy or myocardial infarction, would appear to be optimally supported by a left ventricular assist pump. Insertion is readily accom-

Assisted Circulation 3
F. Unger (Ed.)
© Springer-Verlag Berlin Heidelberg 1989

plished using left ventricular apex and aortic cannulae. With this technique, the cardiac structures are only minimally disturbed and all vascular suture lines associated with the circulatory support are excised at the time of transplantation. Clearly, the patient with clinical evidence of biventricular failure should have mechanical support of both the pulmonary and systemic circulation. This can be and has been accomplished using two paracorporeal pumps or, if chest size is ample, employing an intrathoracic artificial heart. Adequate comparison of the results of these two techniques is not available, but it serves as a focus of discussion and exchange of ideas at international meetings. Moreover, use of the intrathoracic artificial heart in this application has allowed important statements to be made regarding the usefulness of the pneumatic artificial heart as a permanent form of circulatory support. Evident shortcomings relate to risk of infection at the drive-line sites and to the bulk of the pneumatic power unit and associated safety devices.

Permanent Circulatory Support

There is every indication that the ideal permanent circulatory support device that will take us into the next century will be electrically powered, with energy transmission via inductive coupling and data transmission via telemetric techniques. A major landmark in this field was reached in 1987 with the first implantable blood pump, powered by the inductive coupling techniques. The electric assist pump is far simpler than the artificial heart and will come into clinical use before 1990. Reliability will continue to improve, just as the reliability of implanted cardiac pacemakers has improved as intense focus has been directed at critical components. The important lessons learned with the electric assist device will be easily transported to the more complex electric total heart. Importantly, effective electronic control techniques are already available.

The field of research associated with ventricular assist pumps and artificial hearts continues to serve as a challenge to a variety of disciplines in engineering and medicine. The spectacular achievement now on the horizon will serve as ample reward for the efforts currently being expended.

56. Horizons in Assisted Circulation III

J. T. Watson

In 1985, the Working Group on Mechanical Circulatory Support of the National Heart, Lung, and Blood Institute (NHLBI) reconfirmed that cardiac transplantation, or a potential mechanical analog, continues to be the most effective procedure for treating end-stage heart disease. Furthermore, no new technologies were envisaged by the Working Group for the next 5–15 years that might make the artificial heart obsolete. However, much more research and development must be carried out before we can expect safe and effective mechanical support devices for long-term therapeutic applications.

Although death from heart disease has declined steadily for the past 20 years, the incidence and prevalence of congestive heart failure continue to increase. While this represents only a fraction of patients with heart disease, and while estimates vary, many authorities agree that in the future a significant portion of these patients will benefit from some form of a safe, effective, and reliable mechanical assist or replacement device for the failing heart. Certainly, prevention remains our hope for controlling heart disease, and this may eventually be achieved. For the present, however, mechanical circulatory support offers promise for the rehabilitation of some patients with end-stage disease and is improving our understanding of heart and vascular disease.

Clinical results with cardiac transplantation are outstanding and provide a standard for quality of life and longevity that must be approached by other therapies. Registry tabulation of temporary mechanical ventricular assist and artificial hearts suggests an increasing clinical experience for their use as bridges to heart transplantation and in post-cardiotomy cardiogenic shock. During 1988 it is expected that assist and replacement devices will be used in 150–200 patients worldwide for bridging or cardiogenic shock. On the one hand, results demonstrate that the devices are safe, with few instances of technical dysfunction, and, on the other hand, that they are effective, as a major fraction of the bridges to cardiac transplant are fully successful and nearly half of the shock patients benefit from treatment.

Enthusiasm for these early results is tempered by several clinical complications: hemorrhage, renal failure, respiratory failure, thrombosis, embolism, and infection. Beyond 100 days with an implant, patients universally experience the complication constellation of infection, embolism, and stroke. For all patients the management of the balance between adequate clot retardation and potential hemorrhage remains partially undefined. In summary, temporary use of mechanical circulatory support provides a favorable benefit/risk ratio for a few indicated pa-

Assisted Circulation 3
F. Unger (Ed.)
© Springer-Verlag Berlin Heidelberg 1989

tients. Continued clinical experience should lead to better patient management and fewer clinical complications.

On the horizon, we expect the continued use of pneumatically activated temporary mechanical support devices for laboratory research and clinical application, as noted above. Current commercially available devices are expensive and clumsy to use. There is a need for devices designed for 3–6 months of use and costing a small fraction of what present models cost. These devices should build on past experience, incorporating improved flow patterns, physiological rate of pressure changes, appropriate valves, and improved materials.

As noted earlier, long-term implantable ventricular assist and replacement devices are needed for patients with end-stage heart disease. The NHLBI has focused its resources on the development of safe, effective, and reliable implantable, electrically powered ventricular assist systems (VASs) capable of 2 years of uninterrupted service. Toward this objective the NHLBI is currently coordinating the formal testing of these systems in its Device Readiness Program.

Four versions of a VAS fabricated to standards equaling or exceeding the FDA Good Manufacturing Procedures are undergoing reliability tests on laboratory mock loops. Each VAS being tested includes a blood pump integrated with an electrical energy converter, a miniature control system, variable volume mechanism (if required), and implantable batteries. Twelve devices are being tested against a guideline of 80% reliability at a confidence level of 65%, i.e., no more than one system failure over the 2 years of testing. Failure is defined as a reduction of device cardiac output below 4 l/min for 1 min owing to an irreversible process or component dysfunction. It is envisioned that a majority of problems with the VAS will result in patient symptoms of low cardiac output rather than in a sudden complete loss of function.

Animal performance studies will also ensure that during 25 animal months the VAS provides physiological support and responds to both acute and chronic biological requirements and environmental conditions. Eighteen medical grade systems are required to complete the laboratory and animal studies for VAS validation testing prior to clinical use, which will be complete in about 2 years.

The NHLBI is planning to initiate the clinical evaluation of electrically powered, implantable ventricular assist systems in the late 1980s. Studies will be undertaken in 50–100 carefully selected patients who meet all the criteria for heart transplantations except institutional age criteria. Patients will be adequately studied and characterized, assessed for their overall suitability for the VAS, and adequately informed. Long-term device implantations will not be performed on an emergency basis or in patients with cardiogenic shock.

Three additional devices are on the horizon to further foster and broaden the scientific foundation for assisted circulation. The first is a biologically activated cardiac assistance which offers a unique approach to the support of end-stage heart disease patients in a less obtrusive manner than is currently envisioned for mechanical systems. The demonstration that skeletal muscle, after appropriate electrical stimulation, acquires many of the biochemical, morphological, and physiological characteristics of myocardial tissue is remarkable. Animal results have provided evidence of muscle fatigue resistance for over a year at a beat rate of 120 under no-load conditions. Also, reports have been published on a few weeks of fatigue-resistant skeletal muscle function under moderate-load conditions. Prospects are promising that the next 5–10 years will see the demonstration of a biologically activated energy converter capable of assuming the full pressure and volume work of the right ventricle and possibly the left ventricle.

Since the inception of the NHLBI Artificial Heart Program in 1964, research support has been for a spectrum of devices to eventually treat the many manifestations of end-stage heart disease. Beginning in 1987, the Institute initiated research and development of an electrically powered, implantable artificial heart designed for 5 years of operation. The typical implantable, tether-free system will be capable of supporting the circulation with a continuous left-sided output of 8 l/min, pumping into a mean systemic arterial pressure of 110 mmHg and a mean pulmonary pressure of 25 mmHg. As a result of the past 10 years of research, it is anticipated that this new generation of high-technology devices will be more versatile and will be further reduced in weight and volume.

While available biomaterials are adequate for current research, development, and clinical evaluation of mechanical device implants, future studies should emphasize the known clinical problems of implanted cardiovascular devices. Toward these objectives the NHLBI is now promoting a new scientific opportunity for conducting interdisciplinary basic and applied research into the mechanisms of vascular healing. Biological mediators, rheological factors, physical properties, and the chemical composition of grafts will be assessed. These investigations and others should provide new information that may reduce the thromboembolic and infection complications of most long-term implanted grafts or cardiovascular devices.

Clinical reports on temporary circulatory support continue to provide evidence suggesting that safe, effective, and reliable mechanical circulatory assist and replacement devices will provide clinical benefit. Clinical experience has been gained in a few hundred patients with reversible ventricular dysfunction and in a small number of patiens with irreversible ventricular dysfunction. Long-term VAS readiness testing is underway. Quality control and quality assurance are being introduced in the animal testing laboratory and into device fabrication and characterization. We can expect to see continued, orderly progress toward cardiac assist and replacement devices that may provide a means for reducing death and disability from heart disease and also unlock new information about the disease process itself that will aid in its eventual prevention.

Subject Index